American Heart Association®

Learn and Live SM

AF722651

2005 American Heart Association Guidelines for Cardiopulmonary Resuscitation and Emergency Cardiovascular Care

Supplement to *Circulation* • Volume 112 • Issue 24 • December 13, 2005

This special supplement to *Circulation* is freely available at http://www.circulationaha.org

Suggested Citation Format

Authors citing this publication may use this form of reference as an example:

2005 American Heart Association Guidelines for Cardiopulmonary Resuscitation and Emergency Cardiovascular Care, Part 4: Adult Basic Life Support. *Circulation*. 2005;112(suppl IV):IV-19–IV-34.

ISBN 0-87493-459-1

Supplement to

Circulation

JOURNAL OF THE AMERICAN HEART ASSOCIATION

Volume 112 ■ Number 24
December 13, 2005

Editorials

CIRCULATION (ISSN 0009-7322) is published weekly except combined the first two weeks in January and the last two weeks in December by Lippincott Williams & Wilkins at 16522 Hunters Green Parkway, Hagerstown, MD 21740. Business offices are located at 530 Walnut Street, Philadelphia, PA 19106-3621. Production offices are located at 351 West Camden Street, Baltimore, MD 21201-2436. Individuals may subscribe for their personal use at the following rates: $216 for members of an American Heart Association scientific council and $303 for nonmembers; international: $371 for members of an American Heart Association scientific council and $519 for nonmembers. Periodicals postage paid at Hagerstown, MD, and additional mailing offices. POSTMASTER: Send address changes to CIRCULATION, American Heart Association, Lippincott Williams & Wilkins, 16522 Hunters Green Parkway, Hagerstown, MD 21740.

2005 American Heart Association Guidelines for Cardiopulmonary Resuscitation and Emergency Cardiovascular Care

Editors

Mary Fran Hazinski, RN, MSN, *Senior Science Editor*
Leon Chameides, MD, *Pediatric, Neonatal, and First Aid Editor*
Bob Elling, EMT-P, MPA, *BLS and Stroke Editor*
Robin Hemphill, MD, MPH, *ACLS and ACS Editor*

Acknowledgments

The editors and science volunteers gratefully acknowledge the extraordinary efforts of F.G. Stoddard, PhD, AHA ECC Editor-in-Chief; and others of the AHA staff, including Tanya Semenko, Kara Robinson, Gabrielle Hayes, and David Barnes. In particular, we wish to acknowledge the wisdom and dedication of the ECC Director of Product Development from 1996 through 2005, Mary Ann McNeely, PhD.

Part 1: Introduction

This publication presents the 2005 American Heart Association (AHA) guidelines for cardiopulmonary resuscitation (CPR) and emergency cardiovascular care (ECC). The guidelines are based on the evidence evaluation from the 2005 International Consensus Conference on Cardiopulmonary Resuscitation and Emergency Cardiovascular Care Science With Treatment Recommendations, hosted by the American Heart Association in Dallas, Texas, January 23–30, 2005.[1] These guidelines supersede the *Guidelines 2000 for Cardiopulmonary Resuscitation and Emergency Cardiovascular Care*.[2]

As with all versions of the ECC guidelines published since 1974,[2–6] the *2005 AHA Guidelines for CPR and ECC* contain recommendations designed to improve survival from sudden cardiac arrest and acute life-threatening cardiopulmonary problems. These guidelines, however, differ from previous versions in several ways. First, they are based on the most extensive evidence review of CPR yet published.[1] Second, these guidelines were developed under a new structured and transparent process for ongoing disclosure and management of potential conflicts of interest. Third, the guidelines have been streamlined to reduce the amount of information that rescuers need to learn and remember and to clarify the most important skills that rescuers need to perform.

Evidence Evaluation Process

The evidence evaluation process that was the basis for these guidelines was accomplished in collaboration with the International Liaison Committee on Resuscitation (ILCOR),[1] an international consortium of representatives from many of the world's resuscitation councils. ILCOR was formed to systematically review resuscitation science and develop an evidence-based consensus to guide resuscitation practice worldwide. The evidence evaluation process for these guidelines was built on the international efforts that produced the *ECC Guidelines 2000*.[2]

To begin the process, ILCOR representatives established 6 task forces: basic life support, advanced life support, acute coronary syndromes, pediatric life support, neonatal life support, and an interdisciplinary task force to address overlapping topics such as education. The AHA established 2 additional task forces—on stroke and first aid. The 8 task forces identified topics requiring evidence evaluation. They formulated hypotheses on these topics, and the task forces appointed international experts as worksheet authors for each hypothesis.

The worksheet authors were asked to (1) search for and critically evaluate evidence on the hypothesis, (2) summarize the evidence review, and (3) draft treatment recommendations. They then completed worksheets that provided the format for a structured literature review (Table 1). The worksheet authors identified key research studies, recorded the levels of evidence (Table 2) of the studies, and drafted recommendations. When possible, two worksheet authors, one from the United States and one from outside the United States, were recruited to complete independent reviews of each topic. This process is described in detail in the *2005 International Consensus on Cardiopulmonary Resuscitation and Emergency Cardiovascular Care Science With Treatment Recommendations*[1] and the accompanying editorial.[7]

A total of 281 worksheet authors completed 403 worksheets on 276 topics. To obtain feedback from the resuscitation science community, in December 2004 the worksheets and worksheet author conflict of interest disclosures were posted on the Internet at *http://www.C2005.org*. Journal advertisements and emails invited comment from healthcare professionals and the resuscitation community. The comments were then referred to the task forces and worksheet authors for consideration. Worksheets are available through *http://www.C2005.org*.

Expert reviews began in 2002, and individual topics were presented and discussed at 6 international meetings, culminating in the 2005 Consensus Conference. The evidence was presented, discussed, and debated, with task forces and resuscitation councils meeting daily to draft summaries. The consensus statements on the science of resuscitation developed at the conference were incorporated into the *ILCOR 2005 CPR Consensus*, published simultaneously in *Circulation* and *Resuscitation* in November 2005.[1]

Guidelines and Treatment Recommendations

During the evidence evaluation process the ILCOR task forces weighed the evidence and developed consensus statements on the interpretation of the scientific findings. If the task forces agreed on common treatment recommendations, the recommendations were included with the science statements in the *ILCOR 2005 CPR Consensus*.[1] The consensus document was designed to serve as the science foundation for the guidelines to be published by many ILCOR member councils in 2005–2006.

Classes of Recommendation

Following the 2005 Consensus Conference, AHA ECC experts adapted the ILCOR scientific statements and expanded the treatment recommendations to construct these new guidelines. In developing these guidelines, the ECC experts used a recommendation classification system that is consistent with that used by the American Heart Association–American College of Cardiology collaboration on evidence-based guidelines.

The classes of recommendation used in this document are listed in Table 3. These classes represent the integration of the

(*Circulation.* **2005;112:IV-1-IV-5.**)

This special supplement to *Circulation* is freely available at http://www.circulationaha.org

DOI: 10.1161/CIRCULATIONAHA.105.166550

TABLE 1. Steps in Evidence Integration

Integrate all evidence following these steps:

1. Perform literature review and record search terms and databases searched.
2. Select studies relevant to hypothesis.
3. Determine level of evidence based on methodology (see Table 2).
4. Perform critical appraisal *(poor to excellent)*.
5. Integrate evidence into a science summary and possible treatment recommendation.

Experts must develop consensus based on scientific evidence. Steps used include:

Evidence evaluation and worksheet preparation by experts, plus

2005 Consensus Conference presentations and discussions

ILCOR Task Force discussions and development of 2005 International Consensus on CPR and ECC Science With Treatment Recommendations publication[1]

Review and discussions by AHA ECC Committee and Subcommittees with development of specific recommendations and algorithms with classes of recommendations

Final editorial review and approval by AHA ECC Committee and Subcommittees

Blinded peer review

Review and approval by AHA Science Advisory and Coordinating Committee

Publication

weight of scientific evidence with contextual factors such as expert assessment of the magnitude of benefit, usefulness, or efficacy; cost; educational and training challenges; and difficulties in implementation. For Class I recommendations, high-level prospective studies support the action or therapy, and the risk substantially outweighs the potential for harm. For Class IIa recommendations, the weight of evidence supports the action or therapy, and the therapy is considered acceptable and useful.

Ideally all CPR and ECC recommendations should be based on large prospective randomized controlled clinical trials that find substantial treatment effects on long-term survival and carry a Class I or Class IIa label. In reality few clinical resuscitation trials have sufficient power to demonstrate an effect on intact survival to hospital discharge. As a result the experts were often confronted with the need to make recommendations on the basis of results from human trials that reported only intermediate outcomes, nonrandomized or retrospective observational studies, animal models, or extrapolations. Recommendations were generally labeled Class IIb when the evidence documented only short-term benefits from the therapy (eg, amiodarone for pulseless ventricular fibrillation cardiac arrest) or when positive results were documented with lower levels of evidence.

Class IIb recommendations fall into 2 categories: (1) optional and (2) recommended by the experts despite the absence of high-level supporting evidence. Optional interventions are identified by terms such as "can be considered" or "may be useful." Interventions that the experts believe should be carried out are identified with terms such as "we recommend."

TABLE 2. Levels of Evidence

Evidence	Definition
Level 1	Randomized clinical trials or meta-analyses of multiple clinical trials with substantial treatment effects
Level 2	Randomized clinical trials with smaller or less significant treatment effects
Level 3	Prospective, controlled, nonrandomized cohort studies
Level 4	Historic, nonrandomized cohort or case-control studies
Level 5	Case series; patients compiled in serial fashion, control group lacking
Level 6	Animal studies or mechanical model studies
Level 7	Extrapolations from existing data collected for other purposes, theoretical analyses
Level 8	Rational conjecture (common sense); common practices accepted before evidence-based guidelines

Algorithms

The 12 AHA CPR and ECC algorithms contained in these guidelines highlight essential assessments and interventions recommended to treat cardiac arrest or a life-threatening condition. These algorithms have been developed using a template with specific box shapes and colors. Memorizing the box colors and shapes is not recommended, nor is it necessary for use of the algorithms. But in response to requests from the AHA training network and from clinicians, we briefly describe the template used.

Box shape distinguishes action boxes from assessment boxes. Boxes with square corners represent interventions or therapies (ie, actions); rose-colored boxes with round corners represent assessment steps that typically create a decision point in care.

TABLE 3. Applying Classification of Recommendations and Level of Evidence

Class I	Class IIa	Class IIb	Class III
Benefit>>>Risk	Benefit>>Risk	Benefit≥Risk	Risk≥Benefit
Procedure/treatment or diagnostic test/assessment should be performed/administered.	It is reasonable to perform procedure/administer treatment or perform diagnostic test/ assessment.	Procedure/treatment or diagnostic test/assessment may be considered.	Procedure/treatment or diagnostic test/assessment should not be performed/administered. It is not helpful and may be harmful.

Class Indeterminate.

- Research just getting started
- Continuing area of research
- No recommendations until further research (eg, cannot recommend for or against)

Colors of the boxes distinguish types of actions. As noted above, the rose boxes indicate assessment steps. In general, treatments that involve electrical therapy or drugs are placed in blue boxes, and simple action steps are placed in tan boxes. In order to emphasize the fundamental importance of good basic CPR in all ECC algorithms, action steps involving support of airway, breathing, and circulation are placed in green boxes. In addition, all advanced cardiovascular life support (ACLS) and pediatric advanced life support (PALS) algorithms contain a green "reminder" box to assist the clinician in recalling helpful information, including fundamentals of CPR. The algorithm box color-coding is not absolute because some boxes contain combinations of several types of actions.

Three algorithms have unique features. In the basic life support (BLS) healthcare provider adult and pediatric algorithms, the actions that are completed by only healthcare providers are bordered with a dotted line. In the ACLS Tachycardia Algorithm, several boxes are printed with screening (the text contained in screened boxes appears lighter than regular text). These screened boxes include actions that are intended to be accomplished in the in-hospital setting or with expert consultation readily available. Information in non-screened boxes is intended to apply to the out-of-hospital or the in-hospital setting. In the ACLS Tachycardia Algorithm, to create visual separation between actions for wide-complex versus narrow-complex tachycardia, boxes containing therapy for wide-complex tachycardia are shadowed with yellow, and boxes with treatment for narrow-complex tachycardia are shadowed with blue.

Management of Conflict of Interest

The world's leading experts in resuscitation science have established their expertise by undertaking and publishing research and related scholarly work. Some investigators' activities are supported by industry, thereby creating the potential for conflicts of interest.[8,9] Grants and other support for scientific research, speaker fees, and honoraria can also create potential financial conflicts of interest. Nonfinancial conflicts of interest include in-kind support, intellectual collaboration or intellectual investment in personal ideas, and long-term research agendas in which investigators have invested a substantial amount of time.

To protect the objectivity and credibility of the evidence evaluation and consensus development process, the AHA ECC Conflict of Interest (COI) policy was revised before the 2005 Consensus Conference to ensure full disclosure and comprehensive management of potential conflicts. A process was developed for managing potential conflicts of interest during the evidence evaluation process and the 2005 Consensus Conference. Each speaker's COI statement was projected on a dedicated screen during every presentation, question, and discussion period. The COI policy is described in detail in an editorial in this supplement[10] and the corresponding editorial in the *ILCOR 2005 CPR Consensus*.[11] Potential conflicts of interest disclosed by the editors and science volunteers of this document are listed in this supplement (page B4). Potential conflicts of interest disclosed by members of the ECC Committee and subcommittees who wrote and reviewed this document are listed online as a COI supplement (available through *http://www.C2005.org*). Worksheet authors' potential conflicts of interest are included on each worksheet, which can be accessed through *http://www.C2005.org*.

New Developments

The most significant changes in these guidelines were made to simplify CPR instruction and increase the number of chest compressions delivered per minute and reduce interruptions in chest compressions during CPR. Following are some of the most significant new recommendations in these guidelines:

- Elimination of lay rescuer assessment of signs of circulation before beginning chest compressions: the lay rescuer will be taught to begin chest compressions immediately after delivering 2 rescue breaths to the unresponsive victim who is not breathing (Parts 4 and 11).
- Simplification of instructions for rescue breaths: all breaths (whether delivered mouth-to-mouth, mouth-to-mask, bag-mask, or bag-to–advanced airway) should be given over 1 second with sufficient volume to achieve visible chest rise (Parts 4 and 11).
- Elimination of lay rescuer training in rescue breathing without chest compressions (Parts 4 and 11).
- Recommendation of a single (universal) compression-to-ventilation ratio of 30:2 for single rescuers of victims of all ages (except newborn infants). This recommendation is designed to simplify teaching and provide longer periods of uninterrupted chest compressions (Parts 4 and 11).
- Modification of the definition of "pediatric victim" to preadolescent (prepubescent) victim for application of pediatric BLS guidelines for healthcare providers (Parts 3 and 11), but no change to lay rescuer application of child CPR guidelines (1 to 8 years).
- Increased emphasis on the importance of chest compressions: rescuers will be taught to "push hard, push fast" (at a rate of 100 compressions per minute), allow complete chest recoil, and minimize interruptions in chest compressions (Parts 3, 4, and 11).
- Recommendation that Emergency Medical Services (EMS) providers may consider provision of about 5 cycles (or about 2 minutes) of CPR before defibrillation for unwitnessed arrest, particularly when the interval from the call to the EMS dispatcher to response at the scene is more than 4 to 5 minutes (Part 5).
- Recommendation for provision of about 5 cycles (or about 2 minutes) of CPR between rhythm checks during treatment of pulseless arrest (Parts 5, 7.2, and 12). Rescuers should not check the rhythm or a pulse immediately after shock delivery—they should immediately resume CPR, beginning with chest compressions, and should check the rhythm after 5 cycles (or about 2 minutes) of CPR.
- Recommendation that all rescue efforts, including insertion of an advanced airway (eg, endotracheal tube, esophageal-tracheal combitube [Combitube], or laryngeal mask airway [LMA]), administration of medications, and reassessment of the patient be performed in a way that minimizes

interruption of chest compressions. Recommendations for pulse checks are limited during the treatment of pulseless arrest (Parts 4, 5, 7.2, 11, and 12).

- Recommendation of only 1 shock followed immediately by CPR (beginning with chest compressions) instead of 3 stacked shocks for treatment of ventricular fibrillation/pulseless ventricular tachycardia: this change is based on the high first-shock success rate of new defibrillators and the knowledge that if the first shock fails, intervening chest compressions may improve oxygen and substrate delivery to the myocardium, making the subsequent shock more likely to result in defibrillation (Parts 5, 7.2, and 12).
- Increased emphasis on the importance of ventilation and de-emphasis on the importance of using high concentrations of oxygen for resuscitation of the newly born infant (Part 13).
- Reaffirmation that intravenous administration of fibrinolytics (tPA) to patients with acute ischemic stroke who meet the NINDS eligibility criteria can improve outcome. The tPA should be administered by physicians in the setting of a clearly defined protocol, a knowledgeable team, and institutional commitment to stroke care (Part 9).
- New first aid recommendations (Part 14).

For further information about these and other new developments in these guidelines, see the editorial "The Major Changes in the 2005 AHA Guidelines for Cardiopulmonary Resuscitation and Emergency Cardiovascular Care"[12] in this supplement and the guidelines sections noted.

The recommendations in the *2005 AHA Guidelines for CPR and ECC* confirm the safety and effectiveness of many approaches, acknowledge that other approaches may not be optimal, and recommend new treatments that have undergone evidence evaluation. *These new recommendations do not imply that care involving the use of earlier guidelines is unsafe.* In addition, it is important to note that these guidelines will not apply to all rescuers and all victims in all situations. The leader of a resuscitation attempt may need to adapt application of the guidelines to unique circumstances.

Future Directions

The most important determinant of survival from sudden cardiac arrest is the presence of a trained rescuer who is ready, willing, able, and equipped to act. Although hypothermia has recently been shown to improve survival to hospital discharge for selected victims of VF SCA,[13] most advanced life support techniques have failed to improve outcome from SCA[14] or have only been shown to improve short-term survival (eg, to hospital admission).[15,16] Any improvements resulting from advanced life support therapies are less substantial than the increases in survival rate reported from successful deployment of lay rescuer CPR and automated external defibrillation programs in the community.[17–21]

Thus, our greatest challenge continues to be the improvement of lay rescuer education. We must increase access to CPR education, increase effectiveness and efficiency of instruction, improve skills retention, and reduce barriers to action for basic and advanced life support providers.[22] Resuscitation programs must establish processes for continuous quality improvement to reduce time to CPR and shock delivery and to improve the quality of CPR provided.[23,24]

The AHA and collaborating organizations will use these guidelines as the basis for developing comprehensive training materials. Once the training materials are available, the most important step will be to get them into the hands of rescuers who will learn, remember, and perform CPR and ECC skills.

References

1. International Liaison Committee on Resuscitation. 2005 International Consensus on Cardiopulmonary Resuscitation and Emergency Cardiovascular Care Science With Treatment Recommendations. *Circulation.* 2005;112:III-1–III-136.
2. American Heart Association in collaboration with International Liaison Committee on Resuscitation. Guidelines 2000 for Cardiopulmonary Resuscitation and Emergency Cardiovascular Care. *Circulation.* 2000; 102(suppl):I1–I384.
3. Standards for cardiopulmonary resuscitation (CPR) and emergency cardiac care (ECC). 3. Advanced life support. *JAMA.* 1974;227:(suppl): 852–860.
4. Standards and guidelines for cardiopulmonary resuscitation (CPR) and emergency cardiac care (ECC). *JAMA.* 1980;244:453–509.
5. Standards and guidelines for Cardiopulmonary Resuscitation (CPR) and Emergency Cardiac Care (ECC). National Academy of Sciences—National Research Council [published correction appears in *JAMA.* 1986; 256:1727]. *JAMA.* 1986;255:2905–2989.
6. Guidelines for cardiopulmonary resuscitation (CPR) and emergency cardiac care (ECC). *JAMA.* 1992;286:2135–2302.
7. Zaritsky A, Morley P. The evidence evaluation process for the 2005 international consensus on cardiopulmonary resuscitation and emergency cardiovascular care science with treatment recommendations. *Circulation.* 2005;112:III-128–III-130.
8. Davidoff F, DeAngelis CD, Drazen JM, Hoey J, Hojgaard L, Horton R, Kotzin S, Nicholls MG, Nylenna M, Overbeke AJ, Sox HC, Van Der Weyden MB, Wilkes MS. Sponsorship, authorship, and accountability. *Lancet.* 2001;358:854–856.
9. Choudhry NK, Stelfox HT, Detsky AS. Relationships between authors of clinical practice guidelines and the pharmaceutical industry. *JAMA.* 2002; 287:612–617.
10. Billi JE, Eigel B, Montgomery WH, Nadkarni V, Hazinski MF. Management of conflict of interest issues in the American Heart Association emergency cardiovascular care committee activities 2000–2005. *Circulation.* 2005;112:IV-204–IV-205.
11. Billi JE, Zideman D, Eigel B, Nolan J, Montgomery WH, Nadkarni V, from the International Liaison Committee on Resuscitation (ILCOR) and American Heart Association (AHA). Conflict of interest management before, during, and after the 2005 international consensus conference on cardiopulmonary resuscitation and emergency cardiovascular care science with treatment recommendations. *Circulation.* 2005;112:III-131–III-132.
12. Hazinski MF, Nadkarni VM, Hickey RW, O'Connor R, Becker LW, Zaritsy A. The major changes in the 2005 AHA guidelines for cardiopulmonary resuscitation and emergency cardiovascular care. *Circulation.* 2005;112:IV-206–IV-211.
13. Hypothermia After Cardiac Arrest Study Group. Mild therapeutic hypothermia to improve the neurologic outcome after cardiac arrest. *N Engl J Med.* 2002;346:549–556.
14. Stiell IG, Wells GA, Field B, Spaite DW, Nesbitt LP, De Maio VJ, Nichol G, Cousineau D, Blackburn J, Munkley D, Luinstra-Toohey L, Campeau T, Dagnone E, Lyver M. Advanced cardiac life support in out-of-hospital cardiac arrest. *N Engl J Med.* 2004;351:647–656.
15. Dorian P, Cass D, Schwartz B, Cooper R, Gelaznikas R, Barr A. Amiodarone as compared with lidocaine for shock-resistant ventricular fibrillation. *N Engl J Med.* 2002;346:884–890.
16. Kudenchuk PJ, Cobb LA, Copass MK, Cummins RO, Doherty AM, Fahrenbruch CE, Hallstrom AP, Murray WA, Olsufka M, Walsh T. Amiodarone for resuscitation after out-of-hospital cardiac arrest due to ventricular fibrillation. *N Engl J Med.* 1999;341:871–878.
17. Holmberg M, Holmberg S, Herlitz J. Effect of bystander cardiopulmonary resuscitation in out-of-hospital cardiac arrest patients in Sweden. *Resuscitation.* 2000;47:59–70.
18. Caffrey SL, Willoughby PJ, Pepe PE, Becker LB. Public use of automated external defibrillators. *N Engl J Med.* 2002;347:1242–1247.

19. The Public Access Defibrillation Trial Investigators. Public-access defibrillation and survival after out-of-hospital cardiac arrest. *N Engl J Med.* 2004;351:637–646.
20. White RD, Bunch TJ, Hankins DG. Evolution of a community-wide early defibrillation programme experience over 13 years using police/fire personnel and paramedics as responders. *Resuscitation.* 2005;65:279–283.
21. Valenzuela TD, Bjerke HS, Clark LL, et al. Rapid defibrillation by nontraditional responders: the Casino Project. *Acad Emerg Med.* 1998;5: 414–415.
22. Chamberlain DA, Hazinski MF. Education in resuscitation: an ILCOR symposium: Utstein Abbey: Stavanger, Norway: June 22–24, 2001. *Circulation.* 2003;108:2575–2594.
23. Jacobs I, Nadkarni V, Bahr J, Berg RA, Billi JE, Bossaert L, Cassan P, Coovadia A, D'Este K, Finn J, Halperin H, Handley A, Herlitz J, Hickey R, Idris A, Kloeck W, Larkin GL, Mancini ME, Mason P, Mears G, Monsieurs K, Montgomery W, Morley P, Nichol G, Nolan J, Okada K, Perlman J, Shuster M, Steen PA, Sterz F, Tibballs J, Timerman S, Truitt T, Zideman D. Cardiac arrest and cardiopulmonary resuscitation outcome reports: update and simplification of the Utstein templates for resuscitation registries. A statement for healthcare professionals from a task force of the international liaison committee on resuscitation (American Heart Association, European Resuscitation Council, Australian Resuscitation Council, New Zealand Resuscitation Council, Heart and Stroke Foundation of Canada, InterAmerican Heart Foundation, Resuscitation Council of Southern Africa). *Resuscitation.* 2004;63:233–249.
24. Peberdy MA, Kaye W, Ornato JP, Larkin GL, Nadkarni V, Mancini ME, Berg RA, Nichol G, Lane-Trultt T. Cardiopulmonary resuscitation of adults in the hospital: a report of 14720 cardiac arrests from the National Registry of Cardiopulmonary Resuscitation. *Resuscitation.* 2003;58: 297–308.

Part 2: Ethical Issues

The goals of emergency cardiovascular care are to preserve life, restore health, relieve suffering, limit disability, and reverse clinical death. CPR decisions are often made in seconds by rescuers who may not know the patient or know if an advance directive exists. As a result, administration of CPR may sometimes conflict with a patient's desires or best interests.[1] This section provides guidelines to healthcare providers for making the difficult decision to provide or withhold emergency cardiovascular care.

Ethical Principles

Ethical and cultural norms must be considered when beginning and ending a resuscitation attempt. Although physicians must play a role in resuscitation decision making, they should be guided by scientifically proven data and patient preferences.

Principle of Patient Autonomy

Patient autonomy is generally respected both ethically and legally. It assumes that a patient can understand what an intervention involves and consent to or refuse it. Adult patients are presumed to have decision-making capability unless they are incapacitated or declared incompetent by a court of law. Truly informed decisions require that patients receive and understand accurate information about their condition and prognosis, the nature of the proposed intervention, alternatives, and risks and benefits. The patient must be able to deliberate and choose among alternatives and be able to relate the decision to a stable framework of values. When decision-making capacity is temporarily impaired by factors such as concurrent illness, medications, or depression, treatment of these conditions may restore capacity. When patient preferences are uncertain, emergency conditions should be treated until those preferences can be clarified.

Advance Directives, Living Wills, and Patient Self-Determination

An advance directive is any expression of a person's thoughts, wishes, or preferences for his or her end-of-life care. Advance directives can be based on conversations, written directives, living wills, or durable powers of attorney for health care. The legal validity of various forms of advance directives varies from jurisdiction to jurisdiction. Courts consider written advance directives to be more trustworthy than recollections of conversations.

A "living will" is a patient's written direction to physicians about medical care the patient would approve if he or she becomes terminally ill and is unable to make decisions. A living will constitutes clear evidence of the patient's wishes, and in most areas it can be legally enforced.

Living wills and advance directives should be reconsidered periodically because the desires of patients and their medical condition may change over time. The Patient Self-Determination Act of 1991 requires healthcare institutions and managed-care organizations to inquire whether patients have advance directives. Healthcare institutions are required to facilitate the completion of advance directives if patients desire them.

Surrogate Decision Makers

When a patient has lost the capacity to make medical decisions, a close relative or friend can become a surrogate decision maker for the patient. Most states have laws that designate the legal surrogate decision maker (guardian) for an incompetent patient who has not designated a decision maker through a durable power of attorney for health care. The law recognizes the following order of priority for guardianship in the absence of a previously designated decision maker: (1) spouse, (2) adult child, (3) parent, (4) any relative, (5) person nominated by the person caring for the incapacitated patient, (6) specialized care professional as defined by law. Surrogates should base their decisions on the patient's previously expressed preferences if known; otherwise, surrogates should make decisions on the basis of the patient's best interest.

Children should be involved in decision making at a level appropriate for their maturity and should be asked to consent to healthcare decisions when able. Although persons <18 years of age rarely possess the legal authority to consent to their own health care except under specific legally defined situations (ie, emancipated minors and for specific health conditions such as sexually transmitted diseases and pregnancy), the dissent of an older child should be taken seriously. If parents and an older child are in conflict about a treatment plan, every effort should be made to resolve the conflict. The use of force is rarely appropriate in the delivery of medical care to adolescents.

Principle of Futility

If the purpose of a medical treatment cannot be achieved, the treatment is considered futile. The key determinants of medical futility are length and quality of life. An intervention that cannot establish any increase in length or quality of life is futile.

Patients or families may ask physicians to provide care that is inappropriate. Physicians, however, are not obliged to provide such care when there is scientific and social consensus that the treatment is ineffective.[2] An example is CPR for patients with signs of irreversible death. In addition, healthcare providers are not obliged to provide CPR if no benefit from CPR and advanced cardiovascular life support (ACLS) can be expected (ie, CPR would not restore effective circulation). Beyond these clinical circumstances and in the absence of advance directives or living wills, resuscitation should be offered to all patients.

(*Circulation*. 2005;112:IV-6-IV-11.)

This special supplement to *Circulation* is freely available at http://www.circulationaha.org

DOI: 10.1161/CIRCULATIONAHA.105.166551

A careful evaluation of the patient's prognosis for both length and quality of life will determine whether CPR is appropriate. CPR is inappropriate when survival is not expected. In conditions for which the chance of survival is borderline, the morbidity rate is relatively high, and the burden to the patient is high, the patient's desires or (when the patient's desires are unknown) the legally authorized surrogate decision maker's preferences about initiation of resuscitation should be supported. Noninitiation of resuscitation and discontinuation of life-sustaining treatment during or after resuscitation are ethically equivalent, and in situations in which the prognosis is uncertain, a trial of treatment should be considered while further information is gathered to help determine the likelihood of survival and expected clinical course.

Withholding and Withdrawing CPR

Criteria for Not Starting CPR

Scientific evaluation shows that few criteria can accurately predict the futility of CPR (see Part 7.5: "Postresuscitation Support"). In light of this uncertainty, all patients in cardiac arrest should receive resuscitation unless

- The patient has a valid Do Not Attempt Resuscitation (DNAR) order
- The patient has signs of irreversible death (eg, rigor mortis, decapitation, decomposition, or dependent lividity)
- No physiological benefit can be expected because vital functions have deteriorated despite maximal therapy (eg, progressive septic or cardiogenic shock)

Withholding resuscitation attempts in the delivery room is appropriate for newborn infants when gestation, birth weight, or congenital anomalies are associated with almost certain early death and when unacceptably high morbidity is likely among the rare survivors. Two examples from the published literature include extreme prematurity (gestational age <23 weeks or birth weight <400 g) and anencephaly.

Terminating Resuscitative Efforts

The decision to terminate resuscitative efforts rests with the treating physician in the hospital and is based on consideration of many factors, including time to CPR, time to defibrillation, comorbid disease, prearrest state, and initial arrest rhythm. None of these factors alone or in combination is clearly predictive of outcome.

Witnessed collapse, bystander CPR, and a short time interval from collapse to arrival of professionals improve the chances of a successful resuscitation.

In many reports of pediatric resuscitation outcomes, survival falls as the duration of resuscitative efforts increases.[3] In many reports of resuscitation outcome, the patient's chance of being discharged from the hospital alive and neurologically intact diminishes as the duration of the resuscitation attempt increases.[4–7] The responsible clinician should stop the resuscitation attempt if there is a high degree of certainty that the patient will not respond to further ACLS.

For the newborn infant, discontinuation of resuscitation can be justified after 10 minutes without signs of life despite continuous and adequate resuscitative efforts. The prognosis for survival or survival without disability has been shown to be extremely poor when there is a lack of response to intensive resuscitative efforts of >10 minutes' duration.[8–11]

In the past, children who underwent prolonged resuscitation and absence of return of spontaneous circulation (ROSC) after 2 doses of epinephrine were considered unlikely to survive,[12] but intact survival after unusually prolonged in-hospital resuscitation has been documented.[13–15] Prolonged efforts should be made for infants and children with recurring or refractory VF or VT, drug toxicity, or a primary hypothermic insult.

In the absence of mitigating factors, prolonged resuscitative efforts are unlikely to be successful.[16] If ROSC of any duration occurs, however, it may be appropriate to consider extending the resuscitative effort. Other issues, such as drug overdose and severe prearrest hypothermia (eg, submersion in icy water), should be considered when determining whether to extend resuscitative efforts.

DNAR Orders

Unlike other medical interventions, CPR is initiated without a physician's order, based on implied consent for emergency treatment. A physician's order is necessary to withhold CPR. Physicians must initiate a discussion about the use of CPR with all adults admitted for medical and surgical care or with their surrogates. Terminally ill patients may fear abandonment and pain more than death, so physicians should also reassure the patient and family that pain control and other aspects of medical care will continue even if resuscitation is withheld.

The attending physician should write the DNAR order in the patient's chart with a note explaining the rationale for the DNAR order and any other specific limitations of care. The limitation-of-treatment order should contain guidelines for specific emergency interventions that may arise (eg, use of pressor agents, blood products, or antibiotics). The scope of a DNAR order should be specific about which interventions are to be withheld. A DNAR order does not automatically preclude interventions such as administration of parenteral fluids, nutrition, oxygen, analgesia, sedation, antiarrhythmics, or vasopressors unless these are included in the order. Some patients may choose to accept defibrillation and chest compressions but not intubation and mechanical ventilation.

Oral DNAR orders are not acceptable. If the attending physician is not physically present, nursing staff may accept a DNAR order by telephone with the understanding that the physician will sign the order promptly. DNAR orders should be reviewed periodically, particularly if the patient's condition changes.

The attending physician should clarify both the DNAR order and plans for future care with nurses, consultants, house staff, and the patient or surrogate and offer an opportunity for discussion and resolution of conflicts. Basic nursing and comfort care (ie, oral hygiene, skin care, patient positioning, and measures to relieve pain and symptoms) must always be continued. DNAR orders carry no implications about other forms of treatment, and other aspects of the treatment plan should be documented separately and communicated to staff.

DNAR orders should be reviewed before surgery by the anesthesiologist, attending surgeon, and patient or surrogate to determine their applicability in the operating suite and postoperative recovery room.

Initiation of CPR in Patients With DNAR Orders

Studies about DNAR orders suggest that healthcare providers who respond to those in cardiac or respiratory arrest who do not exhibit signs of irreversible death (listed below) should promptly provide resuscitative measures to the best of their ability unless or until they receive legally valid instructions (interpretable advance directives, DNAR orders, or valid surrogate directives) not to intervene. Out-of-hospital DNAR orders apply to the patient with no signs of life.[17,18]

Withdrawal of Life Support

Withdrawal of life support is an emotionally complex decision for family and staff. Withholding and withdrawing life support are ethically similar. A decision to withdraw life support is justifiable when a patient is determined to be dead, if the physician and patient or surrogate agree that treatment goals cannot be met, or if the burden to the patient of continued treatment would exceed any benefits.

Some patients do not regain consciousness after cardiac arrest and ROSC. In most cases the prognosis for adults who remain deeply comatose (Glasgow Coma Scale Score <5) after cardiac arrest can be predicted with accuracy after 2 to 3 days.[19] Specific physical findings or laboratory tests may be helpful to assist with this process. A meta-analysis of 33 studies of outcome of anoxic-ischemic coma documented that the following 3 factors were associated with poor outcome:

- Absence of pupillary response to light on the third day
- Absence of motor response to pain by the third day
- Bilateral absence of cortical response to median nerve somatosensory-evoked potentials when used in normothermic patients who were comatose for at least 72 hours after a hypoxic-ischemic insult (see Part 7.5: "Postresuscitation Support")[20]

A recent meta-analysis of 11 studies involving 1914 patients[21] documented 5 clinical signs that were found to strongly predict death or poor neurologic outcome, with 4 of the 5 predictors detectable at 24 to 72 hours after resuscitation:

- Absent corneal reflex at 24 hours
- Absent pupillary response at 24 hours
- Absent withdrawal response to pain at 24 hours
- No motor response at 24 hours
- No motor response at 72 hours

Withdrawal of life support is ethically permissible under these circumstances.

Patients in the end stage of an incurable disease, whether responsive or unresponsive, should have care that ensures their comfort and dignity. Care is provided to minimize suffering associated with pain, dyspnea, delirium, convulsions, and other terminal complications. For such patients it is ethically acceptable to gradually increase the dosage of narcotics and sedatives to relieve pain and other symptoms, even to levels that might concomitantly shorten the patient's life.

Issues Related to Out-of-Hospital Resuscitation

Withholding CPR Versus Withdrawing CPR

BLS training urges the first-arriving lay responder at a cardiac arrest to begin CPR. Healthcare providers are expected to provide BLS and ACLS as part of their duty to respond. There are a few exceptions to this rule:

- A person lies dead, with obvious clinical signs of irreversible death (eg, rigor mortis, dependent lividity, decapitation, or decomposition).
- Attempts to perform CPR would place the rescuer at risk of physical injury.
- The patient/surrogate has indicated with an advance directive (DNAR order) that resuscitation is not desired.

Neither lay rescuers nor professionals should make a judgment about the present or future quality of life of a cardiac arrest victim on the basis of current or anticipated neurologic status. Such snap judgments are often inaccurate. Quality of life should never be used as a criterion to withhold CPR, because conditions such as irreversible brain damage or brain death cannot be reliably assessed or predicted.[22–37]

Out-of-hospital DNAR protocols must be clear to all involved (eg, physicians, patients, family members, loved ones, and out-of-hospital healthcare providers). Advance directives can take many forms (eg, written bedside orders from physicians, wallet identification cards, identification bracelets, and other mechanisms approved by the local emergency medical services [EMS] authority).

The ideal EMS DNAR form should be portable if the patient is transferred, and in addition to including out-of-hospital DNAR orders, the form should provide direction to EMS about whether to initiate or continue life-sustaining interventions in the patient who is not pulseless and apneic.

Advance Directives in the Out-of-Hospital Setting

A significant number of patients for whom 911 is called because of cardiac arrest are also chronically ill, have a terminal illness, or have a written advance directive (DNAR order). States and other jurisdictions have varying laws about out-of-hospital DNAR orders and advance directives.[38] In some cases in which a DNAR order exists, especially where there are differing opinions among family members, it may be difficult to determine whether resuscitation should be initiated. EMS professionals should initiate CPR and ACLS if there is reason to believe that

- There is reasonable doubt about the validity of a DNAR order or advance directive
- The patient may have changed his or her mind
- The best interests of the patient are in question

Sometimes within a few minutes of the start of a resuscitation attempt, relatives or other medical personnel will arrive and confirm that the patient had clearly expressed a wish that resuscitation not be attempted. CPR or other life support measures may be discontinued with the approval of medical direction when further information becomes available.

In situations in which the EMS professional cannot obtain clear information about the patient's wishes, resuscitative measures should be initiated.

Family members may be concerned that EMS personnel will not follow advance directives written in the hospital if an out-of-hospital arrest occurs. This should be dealt with by asking the physician to write an out-of-hospital DNAR order on the appropriate form used in the jurisdiction where the patient would be potentially attended by EMS. The DNAR order should be available and provided to EMS responders as soon as they arrive on the scene of an emergency involving the patient. In situations in which a DNAR order is not provided to EMS personnel, resuscitative efforts should be attempted. The key to preventing such dilemmas rests with the patient's regular physician who has been providing prearrest care.

Terminating a Resuscitation in a BLS Out-of-Hospital System

Rescuers who start BLS should continue until one of the following occurs:

- Restoration of effective, spontaneous circulation and ventilation.
- Care is transferred to a more senior-level emergency medical professional who may determine that the patient is unresponsive to the resuscitation attempt.
- Reliable criteria indicating irreversible death are present.
- The rescuer is unable to continue because of exhaustion or the presence of dangerous environmental hazards or because continuation of resuscitative efforts places other lives in jeopardy.
- A valid DNAR order is presented to rescuers.

Defibrillators are required standard equipment on ambulances in most states, so the absence of a "shockable" rhythm on the defibrillator after an adequate trial of CPR can be the key criterion for withdrawing BLS in the absence of timely arrival of ACLS. State or local EMS authorities must develop protocols for initiation and withdrawal of BLS in areas where ACLS is not rapidly available or may be significantly delayed. Local circumstances, resources, and risk to rescuers should be considered.

Transport of Patients in Cardiac Arrest

If an EMS system does not allow nonphysicians to pronounce death and stop resuscitative efforts, personnel may be forced to transport to the hospital a deceased victim of cardiac arrest who proved to be refractory to proper BLS/ACLS care. Such an action is unethical.

This situation creates the following dilemma: if carefully executed BLS and ACLS treatment protocols fail in the out-of-hospital setting, then how could the same treatment succeed in the emergency department? A number of studies have consistently observed that $<1\%$ of patients transported with continuing CPR survive to hospital discharge.

Delayed or token efforts, a so-called "slow-code" (knowingly providing ineffective resuscitation), that appear to provide CPR and ACLS are *inappropriate*. This practice compromises the ethical integrity of healthcare providers and undermines the physician-patient/nurse-patient relationship.

Many EMS systems authorize the termination of a resuscitation attempt in the out-of-hospital setting. Protocols for pronouncement of death and appropriate transport of the body by non-EMS vehicles should be established. EMS personnel must be trained to focus on dealing sensitively with family and friends.

Providing Emotional Support to the Family

Despite our best efforts, most resuscitations fail. Notifying family members of the death of a loved one is an important aspect of a resuscitation attempt that should be done compassionately, with care taken to accommodate the cultural and religious beliefs and practices of the family.[39,40]

Family members have often been excluded from being present during the attempted resuscitation of a child or other relative. Surveys have suggested that healthcare providers hold a range of opinions about the presence of family members at resuscitation attempts.[41–51] Several commentaries have noted the potential for family members to become disruptive or interfere with resuscitation procedures, the possibility of family member syncope, and the possibility of increased exposure to legal liability.

However, several surveys administered before observation of resuscitative efforts showed that the majority of family members wished to be present during a resuscitation attempt.[45–49] Family members with no medical background have reported that being at a loved one's side and saying goodbye during the final moments of life was comforting.[45,46,50] Family members also have reported that it helped them adjust to the death of their loved one,[50,51] and most indicated they would do so again.[50] Several retrospective reports note positive reactions from family members,[41–43] many of whom said that they felt a sense of having helped their loved one and of easing their own grieving.[44] Most parents surveyed wanted to be given the option to decide whether they would want to be present at the resuscitation of their child.[43,52]

Thus, in the absence of data documenting harm and in light of data suggesting that it may be helpful, offering select family members the opportunity to be present during a resuscitation seems reasonable and desirable (assuming that the patient, if an adult, has not raised a prior objection. Parents and other family members seldom ask if they can be present unless encouraged to do so by healthcare providers. Resuscitation team members should be sensitive to the presence of family members during resuscitative efforts, assigning a team member to the family to answer questions, clarify information, and otherwise offer comfort.[49]

Ethics of Organ and Tissue Donation

The ECC community supports efforts to respond to the need for organ and tissue donations. Medical directors of EMS agencies should discuss the following issues with the organ procurement program in their region:

- Need for tissue from donors pronounced dead in the field

- How permission for organ and tissue donations will be obtained from the patient's relatives
- How clearly defined guidelines for organ and tissue procurement will be available to all healthcare providers both in the hospital and out of the hospital
- Possible differences between applicable laws and societal values in procedures for organ procurement

Research and Training Issues

The use of newly dead patients for training raises important ethical and legal issues. The consent of family members is both ideal and respectful of the newly dead but not always possible or practical at the time of cardiac arrest. Research advocates argue that presuming consent in these situations serves a "greater good" that will benefit the living. Others claim that consent is unnecessary because the body is "non persona" and without autonomy or interests. These arguments, however, do not consider the potential for harm to surviving family members who may oppose using a recently deceased loved one for the purpose of training or research. This view also ignores significant cultural differences in the acceptance or nonacceptance of the use of cadavers.

Clinical research in patients with cardiorespiratory arrest is challenging. In general, research involving human subjects requires the consent of the subject or, in some cases, a legally authorized surrogate. This has proved to be a challenge for research involving patients in cardiac arrest because research interventions must frequently be implemented at a time when obtaining consent may be impossible. After much public discussion and in recognition of the value of this type of human research, the government, through the Food and Drug Administration and the National Institutes of Health, adopted regulations that allow an exception for the need to obtain informed consent in certain limited circumstances. Stringent preresearch directives require that researchers consult with experts plus representative laypersons who might be study patients and to make full public disclosure of the details of the study methodology. Investigators must engage in candid public discussion of the need for resuscitation research, acknowledge the lack of an evidence-based foundation for many current practices, and describe the many potential benefits of the research.

In 1996 Congress passed the Health Insurance Portability and Accountability Act, commonly referred to as HIPAA. As its name suggests, one of the primary goals of the HIPAA legislation was to ensure the availability and continuity of health insurance coverage, but it has been amended over the past few years to include provisions that protect the privacy of patients' health information and their medical records. For details see *http://www.hhs.gov/ocr/hipaa/finalreg.html*. Healthcare providers involved in training and research must be careful to protect patient privacy and the confidentiality of patient data.

References

1. Bossaert L. European Resuscitation Council Guidelines for Resuscitation. In: *The Ethics of Resuscitation in Clinical Practice*. Amsterdam, Netherlands: Elsevier; 1998:206–217.
2. Marco CA, Schears RM. Societal opinions regarding CPR. *Am J Emerg Med.* 2002;20:207–211.
3. Barzilay Z, Somekh M, Sagy M, Boichis H. Pediatric cardiopulmonary resuscitation outcome. *J Med.* 1998;19:229–241.
4. Ronco R, King W, Donley DK, Tilden SJ. Outcome and cost at a children's hospital following resuscitation for out-of-hospital cardiopulmonary arrest. *Arch Pediatr Adolesc Med.* 1995;149:210–214.
5. Schindler MB, Bohn D, Cox PN, McCrindle BW, Jarvis A, Edmonds J, Barker G. Outcome of out-of-hospital cardiac or respiratory arrest in children. *N Engl J Med.* 1996;335:1473–1479.
6. Torphy DE, Minter MG, Thompson BM. Cardiorespiratory arrest and resuscitation of children. *Am J Dis Child.* 1984;138:1099–1102.
7. O'Rourke PP. Outcome of children who are apneic and pulseless in the emergency room. *Crit Care Med.* 1986;14:466–468.
8. Davis DJ. How aggressive should delivery room cardiopulmonary resuscitation be for extremely low birth weight neonates? *Pediatrics.* 1993;92:447–450.
9. Jain L, Ferre C, Vidyasagar D, Nath S, Sheftel D. Cardiopulmonary resuscitation of apparently stillborn infants: survival and long-term outcome. *J Pediatr.* 1991;118:778–782.
10. Yeo CL, Tudehope DI. Outcome of resuscitated apparently stillborn infants: a ten year review. *J Paediatr Child Health.* 1994;30:129–133.
11. Casalaz DM, Marlow N, Speidel BD. Outcome of resuscitation following unexpected apparent stillbirth. *Arch Dis Child Fetal Neonatal Ed.* 1998;78:F112–F115.
12. Young KD, Seidel JS. Pediatric cardiopulmonary resuscitation: a collective review. *Ann Emerg Med.* 1999;33:195–205.
13. Reis AG, Nadkarni V, Perondi MB, Grisi S, Berg RA. A prospective investigation into the epidemiology of in-hospital pediatric cardiopulmonary resuscitation using the international Utstein reporting style. *Pediatrics.* 2002;109:200–209.
14. Lopez-Herce J, Garcia C, Rodriguez-Nunez A, Dominguez P, Carrillo A, Calvo C, Delgado MA. Long-term outcome of paediatric cardiorespiratory arrest in Spain. *Resuscitation.* 2005;64:79–85.
15. Parra DA, Totapally BR, Zahn E, Jacobs J, Aldousany A, Burke RP, Chang AC. Outcome of cardiopulmonary resuscitation in a pediatric cardiac intensive care unit. *Crit Care Med.* 2000;28:3296–3300.
16. Peberdy MA, Kaye W, Ornato JP, Larkin GL, Nadkarni V, Mancini ME, Berg RA, Nichol G, Lane-Trultt T. Cardiopulmonary resuscitation of adults in the hospital: a report of 14720 cardiac arrests from the National Registry of Cardiopulmonary Resuscitation. *Resuscitation.* 2003;58:297–308.
17. Naess AC, Steen E, Steen PA. Ethics in treatment decisions during out-of-hospital resuscitation. *Resuscitation.* 1997;33:245–256.
18. Partridge RA, Virk A, Sayah A, Antosia R. Field experience with prehospital advance directives. *Ann Emerg Med.* 1998;32:589–593.
19. Attia J, Cook DJ. Prognosis in anoxic and traumatic coma. *Crit Care Clin.* 1998;14:497–511.
20. Zandbergen EG, de Haan RJ, Stoutenbeek CP, Koelman JH, Hijdra A. Systematic review of early prediction of poor outcome in anoxic-ischaemic coma. *Lancet.* 1998;352:1808–1812.
21. Booth CM, Boone RH, Tomlinson G, Detsky AS. Is this patient dead, vegetative, or severely neurologically impaired? Assessing outcome for comatose survivors of cardiac arrest. *JAMA.* 2004;291:870–879.
22. Al-Mobeireek AF. Physicians' attitudes towards 'do-not-resuscitate' orders for the elderly: a survey in Saudi Arabia. *Arch Gerontol Geriatr.* 2000;30:151–160.
23. Becker LJ, Yeargin K, Rea TD, Owens M, Eisenberg MS. Resuscitation of residents with do not resuscitate orders in long-term care facilities. *Prehosp Emerg Care.* 2003;7:303–306.
24. Braun K, Onaka A, Horiuchi B. Advance directive completion rates and end-of-life preferences in Hawaii. *J Am Geriatr Soc.* 2002;49:1708–1713.
25. Danis MSL, Garrett JM, Smith JL, Hielema F, Pickard CG, Egner DM, Patrick DL. A prospective study of advance directives for life-sustaining care. *N Engl J Med.* 1991;324:882–888.
26. Dull SM, Graves JR, Larsen MP, Cummins RO. Expected death and unwanted resuscitation in the prehospital setting. *Ann Emerg Med.* 1994;23:997–1002.
27. Dunn PM, Schmidt TA, Carley MM, Donius M, Weinstein MA, Dull VT. A method to communicate patient preferences about medically indicated life-sustaining treatment in the out-of-hospital setting. *J Am Geriatr Soc.* 1996;44:785–791.
28. Ghusn HF, Teasdale TA, Jordan D. Continuity of do-not resuscitate orders between hospital and nursing home settings. *J Am Geriatr Soc.* 1997;45:465–469.

29. Guru V, Verbeek PR, Morrison LJ. Response of paramedics to terminally ill patients with cardiac arrest: an ethical dilemma. *CMAJ*. 1999;161: 1251–1254.
30. Hickman SE, Tolle SW, Brummel-Smith K, Carley MM. Use of the Physician Orders for Life-Sustaining Treatment Program in Oregon nursing facilities: beyond resuscitation status. *J Am Geriatr Soc*. 2004; 52:1424–1429.
31. Iserson KV, Stocking C. Standards and limits: emergency physicians' attitude toward prehospital resuscitation. *Am J Emerg Med*. 1993;11: 592–594.
32. Lahn M, Friedman B, Bijur P, Haughey M, Gallagher EJ. Advance directives in skilled nursing facility residents transferred to emergency departments. *Acad Emerg Med*. 2001;8:1158–1162.
33. Lee MA, Brummel-Smith K, Meyer J, Drew N, London MR. Physician orders for life-sustaining treatment (POLST): outcomes in a PACE program. Program of All-Inclusive Care for the Elderly. *J Am Geriatr Soc*. 2000;48:1219–1225.
34. Llovera IMF, Ryan JG, Ward MF, Sama A. Are emergency department patients thinking about advance directives? *Acad Emerg Med*. 1997;4: 976–980.
35. Marco CA, Schears RM. Prehospital resuscitation practices: a survey of prehospital providers. *J Emerg Med*. 2003;24:101–106.
36. Hanson LC, Rodgman E. The use of living wills at the end of life: a national study. *Arch Intern Med*. 1996;156:1018–1022.
37. Hayashi M, Hasui C, Kitamura F, Murakami M, Takeuchi M, Katoh H, Kitamura T. Respecting autonomy in difficult medical settings: a questionnaire study in Japan. *Ethics Behav*. 2000;10:51–63.
38. Tolle SW, Tilden VP, Nelson CA, Dunn PM. A prospective study of the efficacy of the physician order form for life-sustaining treatment. *J Am Geriatr Soc*. 1998;46:1097–1102.
39. Iserson KV. Notifying survivors about sudden, unexpected deaths. *West J Med*. 2000;173:261–265.
40. Bereavement. In: *Resuscitation Council UK Advanced Life Support Course Manual*; 1998.
41. Meyers TA, Eichhorn DJ, Guzzetta CE. Do families want to be present during CPR? A retrospective survey. *J Emerg Nurs*. 1998;24:400–405.
42. Robinson SM, Mackenzie-Ross S, Campbell Hewson GL, Egleston CV, Prevost AT. Psychological effect of witnessed resuscitation on bereaved relatives [comment]. *Lancet*. 1998;352:614–617.
43. Boie ET, Moore GP, Brummett C, Nelson DR. Do parents want to be present during invasive procedures performed on their children in the emergency department? A survey of 400 parents. *Ann Emerg Med*. 1999;34:70–74.
44. Adams S, Whitlock M, Higgs R, Bloomfield P, Baskett PJ. Should relatives be allowed to watch resuscitation? *BMJ*. 1994;308:1687–1692.
45. Boyd R. Witnessed resuscitation by relatives. *Resuscitation*. 2000;43: 171–176.
46. Hampe SO. Needs of the grieving spouse in a hospital setting. *Nurs Res*. 1975;24:113–120.
47. Offord RJ. Should relatives of patients with cardiac arrest be invited to be present during cardiopulmonary resuscitation? *Intensive Crit Care Nurs*. 1998;14:288–293.
48. Shaner K, Eckle N. Implementing a program to support the option of family presence during resuscitation. *The Association for the Care of Children's Health (ACCH) Advocate*. 1997;3:3–7.
49. Eichhorn DJ, Meyers TA, Mitchell TG, Guzzetta CE. Opening the doors: family presence during resuscitation. *J Cardiovasc Nurs*. 1996;10:59–70.
50. Doyle CJ, Post H, Burney RE, Maino J, Keefe M, Rhee KJ. Family participation during resuscitation: an option. *Ann Emerg Med*. 1987;16: 673–675.
51. Barratt F, Wallis DN. Relatives in the resuscitation room: their point of view. *J Accid Emerg Med*. 1998;15:109–111.
52. Beckman AW, Sloan BK, Moore GP, Cordell WH, Brizendine EJ, Boie ET, Knoop KJ, Goldman MJ, Geninatti MR. Should parents be present during emergency department procedures on children, and who should make that decision? A survey of emergency physician and nurse attitudes. *Acad Emerg Med*. 2002;9:154–158.

Part 3: Overview of CPR

We have always known that CPR is not a single skill but a series of assessments and interventions. More recently we have become aware that cardiac arrest is not a single problem and that the steps of CPR may need to vary depending on the type or etiology of the cardiac arrest. At the 2005 Consensus Conference researchers debated all aspects of detection and treatment of cardiac arrest. Yet the last summation returned to the beginning question: how do we get more bystanders and healthcare providers to learn CPR and perform it well?

Epidemiology

Sudden cardiac arrest (SCA) is a leading cause of death in the United States and Canada.[1–3] Although estimates of the annual number of deaths due to out-of-hospital SCA vary widely,[1,2,4,5] data from the Centers for Disease Control and Prevention estimates that in the United States approximately 330 000 people die annually in the out-of-hospital and emergency department settings from coronary heart disease. About 250 000 of these deaths occur in the out-of-hospital setting.[1,6] The annual incidence of SCA in North America is ≈0.55 per 1000 population.[3,4]

Cardiac Arrest and the Chain of Survival

Most victims of SCA demonstrate ventricular fibrillation (VF) at some point in their arrest.[3–5] Several phases of VF have been described,[7] and resuscitation is most successful if defibrillation is performed in about the first 5 minutes after collapse. Because the interval between call to the emergency medical services (EMS) system and arrival of EMS personnel at the victim's side is typically longer than 5 minutes,[8] achieving high survival rates depends on a public trained in CPR and on well-organized public access defibrillation programs.[9,10] The best results of lay rescuer CPR and automated external defibrillation programs have occurred in controlled environments, with trained, motivated personnel, a planned and practiced response, and short response times. Examples of such environments are airports,[9] airlines,[11] casinos,[12] and hospitals (see Part 4: "Adult Basic Life Support"). Significant improvement in survival from out-of-hospital VF SCA also has been reported in well-organized police CPR and AED rescuer programs.[13]

CPR is important both before and after shock delivery. When performed immediately after collapse from VF SCA, CPR can double or triple the victim's chance of survival.[14–17] CPR should be provided until an automated external defibrillator (AED) or manual defibrillator is available. After about 5 minutes of VF with no treatment, outcome may be better if shock delivery (attempted defibrillation) is preceded by a period of CPR with effective chest compressions that deliver some blood to the coronary arteries and brain.[18,19] CPR is also important immediately after shock delivery; most victims demonstrate asystole or pulseless electrical activity (PEA) for several minutes after defibrillation. CPR can convert these rhythms to a perfusing rhythm.[20–22]

Not all adult deaths are due to SCA and VF. An unknown number have an asphyxial mechanism, as in drowning or drug overdose. Asphyxia is also the mechanism of cardiac arrest in most children, although about 5% to 15% have VF.[23–25] Studies in animals have shown that the best results for resuscitation from asphyxial arrest are obtained by a combination of chest compressions and ventilations, although chest compressions alone are better than doing nothing.[26,27]

Differences in CPR Recommendations by Age of Victim and Rescuer

Simplification

The authors of the *2005 AHA Guidelines for CPR and ECC* simplified the BLS sequences, particularly for lay rescuers, to minimize differences in the steps and techniques of CPR used for infant, child, and adult victims. For the first time, *a universal compression-ventilation ratio (30:2) is recommended for all single rescuers of infant, child, and adult victims (excluding newborns).*

Some skills (eg, rescue breathing without chest compressions) will no longer be taught to lay rescuers. The goal of these changes is to make CPR easier for all rescuers to learn, remember, and perform.

Differences in CPR for Lay Rescuers and Healthcare Providers

Differences between lay rescuer and healthcare provider CPR skills include the following:

- *Lay rescuers* should immediately begin cycles of chest compressions and ventilations after delivering 2 rescue breaths for an unresponsive victim. Lay rescuers are not taught to assess for pulse or signs of circulation for an unresponsive victim.
- *Lay rescuers* will not be taught to provide rescue breathing without chest compressions.
- The lone *healthcare provider* should alter the sequence of rescue response based on the most likely etiology of the victim's problem.
  - *For sudden*, collapse in victims of all ages, the lone healthcare provider should telephone the emergency response number and get an AED (when readily available) and then return to the victim to begin CPR and use the AED.
  - For unresponsive victims of all ages with likely *asphyxial* arrest (eg, drowning) the lone healthcare provider should deliver about 5 cycles (about 2 minutes) of CPR before leaving the victim to telephone the emergency response number and get the AED. The rescuer should

(*Circulation*. 2005;112:IV-12-IV-18.)

This special supplement to *Circulation* is freely available at http://www.circulationaha.org

DOI: 10.1161/CIRCULATIONAHA.105.166552

then return to the victim, begin the steps of CPR, and use the AED.

- After delivery of 2 rescue breaths, *healthcare providers* should attempt to feel a pulse in the unresponsive, non-breathing victim for no more than 10 seconds. If the provider does not definitely feel a pulse within 10 seconds, the provider should begin cycles of chest compressions and ventilations.
- *Healthcare providers* will be taught to deliver rescue breaths without chest compressions for the victim with respiratory arrest and a perfusing rhythm (ie, pulses). Rescue breaths without chest compressions should be delivered at a rate of about 10 to 12 breaths per minute for the adult and a rate of about 12 to 20 breaths per minute for the infant and child.
- *Healthcare providers* should deliver cycles of compressions and ventilations during CPR when there is no advanced airway (eg, endotracheal tube, laryngeal mask airway [LMA], or esophageal-tracheal combitube [Combitube]) in place. Once an advanced airway is in place for infant, child, or adult victims, 2 rescuers no longer deliver "cycles" of compressions interrupted with pauses for ventilation. Instead, the compressing rescuer should deliver 100 compressions per minute continuously, without pauses for ventilation. The rescuer delivering the ventilations should give 8 to 10 breaths per minute and should be careful to avoid delivering an excessive number of ventilations. The 2 rescuers should change compressor and ventilator roles approximately every 2 minutes to prevent compressor fatigue and deterioration in quality and rate of chest compressions. When multiple rescuers are present, they should rotate the compressor role about every 2 minutes. The switch should be accomplished as quickly as possible (ideally in less than 5 seconds) to minimize interruptions in chest compressions.

Age Delineation

Differences in the etiology of cardiac arrest between child and adult victims necessitate some differences in the recommended resuscitation sequence for infant and child victims compared with the sequence used for adult victims. Because there is no single anatomic or physiologic characteristic that distinguishes a "child" victim from an "adult" victim and no scientific evidence that identifies a precise age to initiate adult rather than child CPR techniques, the ECC scientists made a consensus decision for age delineation that is based largely on practical criteria and ease of teaching.

In these 2005 guidelines the recommendations for newborn CPR apply to newborns in the first hours after birth until the newborn leaves the hospital. Infant CPR guidelines apply to victims less than approximately 1 year of age.

Child CPR guidelines for the *lay rescuer* apply to children about 1 to 8 years of age, and adult guidelines for the lay rescuer apply to victims about 8 years of age and older. To simplify learning for lay rescuers retraining in CPR and AED apropos the 2005 guidelines, the same age divisions for children are used in the 2005 guidelines as in the *ECC Guidelines 2000.*[28]

Child CPR guidelines for *healthcare providers* apply to victims from about 1 year of age to the onset of adolescence or puberty (about 12 to 14 years of age) as defined by the presence of secondary sex characteristics. Hospitals (particularly children's hospitals) or pediatric intensive care units may choose to extend the use of Pediatric Advanced Life Support (PALS) guidelines to pediatric patients of all ages (generally up to about 16 to 18 years of age) rather than use onset of puberty for the application of ACLS versus PALS guidelines.

Use of AED and Defibrillation for the Child

When treating a child *found* in cardiac arrest in the out-of-hospital setting, *lay rescuers and healthcare providers* should provide about 5 cycles (about 2 minutes) of CPR before attaching an AED. This recommendation is consistent with the recommendation published in 2003.[29] As noted above, most cardiac arrests in children are not caused by ventricular arrhythmias. Immediate attachment and operation of an AED (with hands-off time required for rhythm analysis) will delay or interrupt provision of rescue breathing and chest compressions for victims who are most likely to benefit from them.

If a healthcare provider *witnesses* a *sudden* collapse of a child, the healthcare provider should use an AED as soon as it is available.

There is no recommendation for or against the use of AEDs for infants (<1 year of age).

Rescuers should use a pediatric dose-attenuating system, when available, for children 1 to 8 years of age. These pediatric systems are designed to deliver a reduced shock dose that is appropriate for victims up to about 8 years of age (about 25 kg [55 pounds] in weight or about 127 cm [50 inches] in length). A conventional AED (without pediatric attenuator system) should be used for children about 8 years of age and older (larger than about 25 kg [55 pounds] in weight or about 127 cm [50 inches] in length) and for adults. A pediatric attenuating system should *not* be used for victims 8 years of age and older because the energy dose (ie, shock) delivered through the pediatric system is likely to be inadequate for an older child, adolescent, or adult.

For in-hospital resuscitation, rescuers should begin CPR immediately and use an AED or manual defibrillator as soon as it is available. If a manual defibrillator is used, a defibrillation dose of 2 J/kg is recommended for the first shock and a dose of 4 J/kg for the second and subsequent shocks.

Sequence

If more than one person is present at the scene of a cardiac arrest, several actions can occur simultaneously. One or more trained rescuers should remain with the victim to begin the steps of CPR while another bystander phones the emergency response system and retrieves an AED (if available). If a lone rescuer is present, then the sequences of actions described below are recommended. These sequences are described in more detail in Part 4: "Adult Basic Life Support," Part 5: "Electrical Therapies," and Part 11: "Pediatric Basic Life Support."

For the unresponsive adult, the *lay rescuer* sequence of action is as follows:

- The lone rescuer should telephone the emergency response system and retrieve an AED (if available). The rescuer should then return to the victim to begin CPR and use the AED when appropriate.
- The lay rescuer should open the airway and check for normal breathing. If no normal breathing is detected, the rescuer should give 2 rescue breaths.
- Immediately after delivery of the rescue breaths, the rescuer should begin cycles of 30 chest compressions and 2 ventilations and use an AED as soon as it is available.

For the unresponsive infant or child, the *lay rescuer* sequence for action is as follows:

- The rescuer will open the airway and check for breathing; if no breathing is detected, the rescuer should give 2 breaths that make the chest rise.
- The rescuer should provide 5 cycles (a cycle is 30 compressions and 2 breaths) of CPR (about 2 minutes) before leaving the pediatric victim to phone 911 and get an AED for the child if available. The reasons for immediate provision of CPR are that asphyxial arrest (including primary respiratory arrest) is more common than sudden cardiac arrest in children, and the child is more likely to respond to, or benefit from, the initial CPR.

In general, the rescue sequence performed by the *healthcare provider* is similar to that recommended for the lay rescuer, with the following differences:

- If the lone healthcare provider witnesses the *sudden* collapse of a victim of any age, after verifying that the victim is unresponsive the provider should first phone 911 and get an AED if available, then begin CPR and use the AED as appropriate. *Sudden* collapse is more likely to be caused by an arrhythmia that may require shock delivery.
- If the lone healthcare provider is rescuing an unresponsive victim with a likely *asphyxial* cause of arrest (eg, drowning), the rescuer should provide 5 cycles (about 2 minutes) of CPR (30 compressions and 2 ventilations) before leaving the victim to phone the emergency response number.
- As noted above, the healthcare provider will perform some skills and steps that are not taught to the lay rescuer.

Checking Breathing and Rescue Breaths

Checking Breathing

When lay rescuers check breathing in the unresponsive adult victim, they should look for *normal* breathing. This should help the lay rescuer distinguish between the victim who is breathing (and does not require CPR) and the victim with agonal gasps (who is likely in cardiac arrest and needs CPR). Lay rescuers who check breathing in the infant or child should look for the presence or absence of breathing. Infants and children often demonstrate breathing patterns that are not normal but are adequate.

The healthcare provider should assess for adequate breathing in the adult. Some patients will demonstrate inadequate breathing that requires delivery of assisted ventilation. Assessment of ventilation in the infant and child is taught in the PALS Course.

Rescue Breaths

Each rescue breath should be delivered in 1 second and should produce visible chest rise. Other new recommendations for rescue breaths are these:

- Healthcare providers should take particular care to provide *effective* breaths in infants and children because asphyxial arrest is more common than sudden cardiac arrest in infants and children. To ensure that a rescue breath is effective, it may be necessary to reopen the airway and reattempt ventilation. The rescuer may need to try a couple of times to deliver 2 effective breaths for the infant and child.
- When rescue breaths are provided without chest compressions to the victim with a pulse, the healthcare provider should deliver 12 to 20 breaths per minute for an infant or child and 10 to 12 breaths per minute for an adult.
- As noted above, once an advanced airway is in place (eg, endotracheal tube, Combitube, LMA) during 2-rescuer CPR, the compressor should provide 100 compressions per minute without pausing for ventilation, and the rescuer delivering breaths should deliver 8 to 10 breaths per minute.

Chest Compressions

Both lay rescuers and healthcare providers should deliver chest compressions that depress the chest of the infant and child by one third to one half the depth of the chest. Rescuers should *push hard, push fast* (rate of 100 compressions per minute), allow complete chest recoil between compressions, and minimize interruptions in compressions for all victims.

Because children and rescuers can vary widely in size, rescuers are no longer instructed to use a single hand for chest compression of all children. Instead the rescuer is instructed to use 1 hand or 2 hands (as in the adult) as needed to compress the child's chest to one third to one half its depth.

Lay rescuers should use a 30:2 compression-ventilation ratio for all (infant, child, and adult) victims. *Healthcare providers* should use a 30:2 compression-ventilation ratio for all 1-rescuer and all adult CPR and should use a 15:2 compression-ventilation ratio for infant and child 2-rescuer CPR.

For the Infant

Recommendations for lay rescuer and healthcare provider chest compressions for infants (up to 1 year of age) include the following:

- Lay rescuers and healthcare providers should compress the infant chest just below the nipple line (on lower half of sternum).
- Lay rescuers will use 2 fingers to compress the infant chest with a compression-ventilation ratio of 30:2.
- The lone healthcare provider should use 2 fingers to compress the infant chest.
- When 2 healthcare providers are performing CPR, the compression-ventilation ratio should be 15:2 until an advanced airway is in place. The healthcare provider who is compressing the chest should, when feasible, use the 2-thumb–encircling hands technique.

For the Child

Recommendations for lay rescuer and healthcare provider compressions for child victims (about 1 to 8 years of age) include the following:

Summary of BLS ABCD Maneuvers for Infants, Children, and Adults (Newborn Information Not Included)

Maneuver	Adult Lay rescuer: ≥8 years HCP: Adolescent and older	Child Lay rescuers: 1 to 8 years HCP: 1 year to adolescent	Infant Under 1 year of age
Airway	Head tilt–chin lift (HCP: suspected trauma, use jaw thrust)		
Breathing Initial	2 breaths at 1 second/breath	2 effective breaths at 1 second/breath	
HCP: Rescue breathing without chest compressions	10 to 12 breaths/min (approximate)	12 to 20 breaths/min (approximate)	
HCP: Rescue breaths for CPR with advanced airway	8 to 10 breaths/min (approximately)		
Foreign-body airway obstruction	Abdominal thrusts		Back slaps and chest thrusts
Circulation HCP: Pulse check (≤10 sec)	Carotid		Brachial or femoral
Compression landmarks	Lower half of sternum, between nipples		Just below nipple line (lower half of sternum)
Compression method Push hard and fast Allow complete recoil	Heel of one hand, other hand on top	Heel of one hand or as for adults	2 or 3 fingers HCP (2 rescuers): 2 thumb–encircling hands
Compression depth	1½ to 2 inches	Approximately one third to one half the depth of the chest	
Compression rate	Approximately 100/min		
Compression-ventilation ratio	30:2 (one or two rescuers)	30:2 (single rescuer) HCP: 15:2 (2 rescuers)	
Defibrillation AED	Use adult pads Do not use child pads	Use AED after 5 cycles of CPR (out of hospital). Use pediatric system for child 1 to 8 years if available **HCP: For sudden collapse (out of hospital) or in-hospital arrest use AED as soon as available.**	No recommendation for infants <1 year of age

Note: Maneuvers used by only Healthcare Providers are indicated by "HCP."

- Lay rescuers should use a 30:2 compression-ventilation ratio for CPR for all victims.
- Rescuers should compress over the lower half of the sternum, at the nipple line (as for adults).
- Lay rescuers should use 1 or 2 hands, as needed, to compress the child's chest to one third to one half the depth of the chest.
- Lay rescuers and lone healthcare providers should use a compression-ventilation ratio of 30:2.
- Healthcare providers (and all rescuers who complete the healthcare provider course, such as lifeguards) performing 2-rescuer CPR should use a 15:2 compression-ventilation ratio until an advanced airway is in place.

For the Adult

Recommendations for lay rescuer and healthcare provider chest compressions for adult victims (about 8 years of age and older) include the following:

- The rescuer should compress in the center of the chest at the nipple line.
- The rescuer should compress the chest approximately 1½ to 2 inches, using the heel of both hands.

Comparison of CPR skills used for adult, child, and infant victims are highlighted in the Table.

CPR for Newborns

Recommendations for the *newborn* are different from recommendations for infants. Because most providers who care for newborns do not provide care to infants, children, and adults, the educational imperative for universal or more uniform recommendations is less compelling. There are no major changes from the *ECC Guidelines 2000* recommendations for CPR in newborns[28]:

- The rescue breathing rate for the newborn infant with pulses is approximately 40 to 60 breaths per minute.
- When providing compressions for newborn infants, the rescuer should compress to one third the depth of the chest.
- For resuscitation of the newborn infant (with or without an advanced airway in place), providers should deliver 90 compressions and 30 ventilations (about 120 events) per minute.
- Rescuers should try to avoid giving simultaneous compressions and ventilations.

Important Lessons About CPR

What have we learned about CPR? To be successful, CPR must be started as soon as a victim collapses, and we must therefore rely on a trained and willing public to initiate CPR and call for professional help and an AED. We have learned that when these steps happen in a timely manner, CPR makes a difference.[30–32] Sadly we have also learned that bystander CPR is performed in about only a third of witnessed arrests or fewer[31,32] and that when CPR is performed, even by professionals, it is often not done well. Excessive ventilation is provided during CPR for victims with advanced airways, with a resulting decrease in cardiac output[33]; compressions are interrupted too frequently,[34–37] with a resulting drop in coronary perfusion pressure and worse outcomes[38–40]; and chest compressions are often too slow and too shallow.

These guidelines have addressed issues of CPR quality by stressing good CPR—"push hard, push fast, allow full chest recoil after each compression, and minimize interruptions in chest compressions," —and by simplifying recommendations to make it easer for lay rescuers and healthcare providers alike to learn, remember, and perform these critical skills. To minimize interruptions, other changes have been made in recommendations regarding CPR and debrillation (see Part 5: Electric Therapies).

Why are bystanders reluctant to perform CPR? We don't have enough data to answer this important question definitively, but a number of possible reasons have been suggested:

- Some claim that CPR has been made too complicated with too many steps that tax the memory. In these guidelines we have tried to simplify the steps whenever the science allows it. For example, the compression-ventilation ratio for lay rescuers is now the same for infants, children, and adults, and the same technique can be used for chest compressions for children and adults.
- Some feel that our training methods are inadequate, and skills retention has been shown to decline fairly rapidly after training.[41] The American Heart Association has established an ECC education subcommittee to find better and more efficient educational methods. We must also try to apply the lessons of self-efficacy from the field of psychology to understand why people with the same knowledge apply it so differently in emergencies.
- Others point out that the public is afraid of transmitted diseases and is reluctant to perform mouth-to-mouth resuscitation.[42–45] The guidelines emphasize that the data shows that transmission of infection is very low.[46] The guidelines encourage anyone who is still concerned about infection to use a barrier device to give ventilations, although simple barrier devices (ie, face shields) may not reduce the risk of bacterial transmission.[47] The guidelines also encourage those who would rather not give mouth-to-mouth ventilations to call for help and start chest compressions only.

About 10% of newborns require some of the steps of CPR to make a successful transition from uterine to extrauterine life. The Neonatal Resuscitation Program (NRP), which is based on these guidelines, has trained more than 1.75 million providers worldwide. The NRP is used throughout the United States and Canada and in many other countries. The educational challenges for resuscitation of the newborn are quite different from those applying to education of rescuers for response to SCA: because most births in the United States occur in hospitals, resuscitations are performed by healthcare personnel.

Quality Improvement

Processes for continuous quality improvement are essential for the success of out-of-hospital and in-hospital resuscitation programs. For out-of-hospital resuscitation programs the Utstein Registries provide templates to facilitate outcome monitoring.[48–51]

In the United States the Joint Commission for the Accreditation of Healthcare Organizations (JCAHO) revised standards for individual in-hospital resuscitation capabilities to include evaluation of resuscitation policies, procedures, processes, protocols, equipment, staff training, and outcome review.[52]

In 2000 the American Heart Association established the National Registry of Cardiopulmonary Resuscitation (NRCPR) to assist participating hospitals with systematic data collection on resuscitative efforts.[53] The objectives of the registry are to develop a well-defined database to document resuscitation performance of hospitals over time. This information can establish the baseline performance of a hospital, target its problem areas, and identify opportunities for improvement in data collection and the resuscitation program in general. The registry is also the largest repository of information on in-hospital cardiopulmonary arrest. For further information about the NRCPR, visit the website: *www.nrcpr.org.*

Medical Emergency Teams (METs)

The concept of Medical Emergency Teams (METs) has been explored as a method to identify patients at risk and intervene to prevent the development of cardiac arrest. METs studied generally consist of a physician and nurse with critical care training. The team is available at all times, with nurses and other hospital staff authorized to activate the team based on specific calling criteria, following implementation of an education and awareness program.

Three supportive before-and-after single center studies (LOE 3)[54–56] documented significant reductions in cardiac arrest rates and improved outcome following cardiac arrest. Two neutral studies (LOE 3)[57,58] documented a trend toward reduction in the rates of adult in-hospital cardiac arrest and improved outcome[57] and a reduction in unplanned ICU admissions.[58] The most recent study, a cluster-randomized controlled trial in 23 hospitals, documented no difference in the composite primary outcome (cardiac arrest, unexpected death, unplanned ICU admission) between 12 hospitals in which a MET system was introduced and 11 hospitals that had no MET system in place (LOE 2).[59]

Introduction of a MET system for adult in-hospital patients should be considered, with special attention to details of implementation (eg, composition and availability of the team, calling criteria, education and awareness of hospital staff, and method of team activation). There is insufficient evidence to make a recommendation on the use of a MET for children. Further research is needed about the critical details of implementation and the potential effectiveness of METs in preventing cardiac arrest or improving other important patient outcomes.

Summary

These guidelines provide simplified information and emphasize the importance and fundamentals of high-quality CPR.

The following chapters provide more detail about the role of CPR, coordination of CPR with defibrillation, the role of CPR in advanced life support, and basic and advanced life support in newborns, infants and children. We hope that with more people learning high-quality CPR technique, more victims of SCA will receive good bystander CPR and thousands of lives will be saved.

References

1. Zheng ZJ, Croft JB, Giles WH, Mensah GA. Sudden cardiac death in the United States, 1989 to 1998. *Circulation.* 2001;104:2158–2163.
2. Chugh SS, Jui J, Gunson K, Stecker EC, John BT, Thompson B, Ilias N, Vickers C, Dogra V, Daya M, Kron J, Zheng ZJ, Mensah G, McAnulty J. Current burden of sudden cardiac death: multiple source surveillance versus retrospective death certificate–based review in a large US community. *J Am Coll Cardiol.* 2004;44:1268–1275.
3. Vaillancourt C, Stiell IG. Cardiac arrest care and emergency medical services in Canada. *Can J Cardiol.* 2004;20:1081–1090.
4. Rea TD, Eisenberg MS, Sinibaldi G, White RD. Incidence of EMS-treated out-of-hospital cardiac arrest in the United States. *Resuscitation.* 2004;63:17–24.
5. Cobb LA, Fahrenbruch CE, Olsufka M, Copass MK. Changing incidence of out-of-hospital ventricular fibrillation, 1980–2000. *JAMA.* 2002;288: 3008–3013.
6. Centers for Disease Control and Prevention. Web-based Injury Statistics Query and Reporting System (WISQARS) [online]. National Center for Injury Prevention and Control, Centers for Disease Control and Prevention (producer). Available at: http://www.cdc.gov/ncipc/wisqars. Accessed February 3, 2005.
7. Weisfeldt ML, Becker LB. Resuscitation after cardiac arrest: a 3-phase time-sensitive model. *JAMA.* 2002;288:3035–3038.
8. Nichol G, Stiell IG, Laupacis A, Pham B, De Maio VJ, Wells GA. A cumulative meta-analysis of the effectiveness of defibrillator-capable emergency medical services for victims of out-of-hospital cardiac arrest. *Ann Emerg Med.* 1999;34(pt 1):517–525.
9. Caffrey SL, Willoughby PJ, Pepe PE, Becker LB. Public use of automated external defibrillators. *N Engl J Med.* 2002;347:1242–1247.
10. The Public Access Defibrillation Trial Investigators. Public-access defibrillation and survival after out-of-hospital cardiac arrest. *N Engl J Med.* 2004;351:637–646.
11. Page RL, Joglar JA, Kowal RC, Zagrodzky JD, Nelson LL, Ramaswamy K, Barbera SJ, Hamdan MH, McKenas DK. Use of automated external defibrillators by a US airline. *N Engl J Med.* 2000;343:1210–1216.
12. Valenzuela TD, Roe DJ, Nichol G, Clark LL, Spaite DW, Hardman RG. Outcomes of rapid defibrillation by security officers after cardiac arrest in casinos. *N Engl J Med.* 2000;343:1206–1209.
13. White RD, Bunch TJ, Hankins DG. Evolution of a community-wide early defibrillation programme experience over 13 years using police/fire personnel and paramedics as responders. *Resuscitation.* 2005;279–283.
14. Larsen MP, Eisenberg MS, Cummins RO, Hallstrom AP. Predicting survival from out-of-hospital cardiac arrest: a graphic model. *Ann Emerg Med.* 1993;22:1652–1658.
15. Valenzuela TD, Roe DJ, Cretin S, Spaite DW, Larsen MP. Estimating effectiveness of cardiac arrest interventions: a logistic regression survival model. *Circulation.* 1997;96:3308–3313.
16. Holmberg M, Holmberg S, Herlitz J. Factors modifying the effect of bystander cardiopulmonary resuscitation on survival in out-of-hospital cardiac arrest patients in Sweden. *Eur Heart J.* 2001;22:511–519.
17. Holmberg M, Holmberg S, Herlitz J, Gardelov B. Survival after cardiac arrest outside hospital in Sweden. Swedish Cardiac Arrest Registry. *Resuscitation.* 1998;36:29–36.
18. Cobb LA, Fahrenbruch CE, Walsh TR, Copass MK, Olsufka M, Breskin M, Hallstrom AP. Influence of cardiopulmonary resuscitation prior to defibrillation in patients with out-of-hospital ventricular fibrillation. *JAMA.* 1999;281:1182–1188.
19. Wik L, Hansen TB, Fylling F, Steen T, Vaagenes P, Auestad BH, Steen PA. Delaying defibrillation to give basic cardiopulmonary resuscitation to patients with out-of-hospital ventricular fibrillation: a randomized trial. *JAMA.* 2003;289:1389–1395.
20. White RD, Russell JK. Refibrillation, resuscitation and survival in out-of-hospital sudden cardiac arrest victims treated with biphasic automated external defibrillators. *Resuscitation.* 2002;55:17–23.
21. Carpenter J, Rea TD, Murray JA, Kudenchuk PJ, Eisenberg MS. Defibrillation waveform and post-shock rhythm in out-of-hospital ventricular fibrillation cardiac arrest. *Resuscitation.* 2003;59:189–196.
22. Berg MD, Clark LL, Valenzuela TD, Kern KB, Berg RA. Post-shock chest compression delays with automated external defibrillator use. *Resuscitation.* 2005;64:287–291.
23. Appleton GO, Cummins RO, Larson MP, Graves JR. CPR and the single rescuer: at what age should you "call first" rather than "call fast"? *Ann Emerg Med.* 1995;25:492–494.
24. Hickey RW, Cohen DM, Strausbaugh S, Dietrich AM. Pediatric patients requiring CPR in the prehospital setting. *Ann Emerg Med.* 1995;25:495–501.
25. Mogayzel C, Quan L, Graves JR, Tiedeman D, Fahrenbruch C, Herndon P. Out-of-hospital ventricular fibrillation in children and adolescents: causes and outcomes. *Ann Emerg Med.* 1995;25:484–491.
26. Berg RA, Hilwig RW, Kern KB, Babar I, Ewy GA. Simulated mouth-to-mouth ventilation and chest compressions (bystander cardiopulmonary resuscitation) improves outcome in a swine model of prehospital pediatric asphyxial cardiac arrest. *Crit Care Med.* 1999;27:1893–1899.
27. Berg RA, Hilwig RW, Kern KB, Ewy GA. "Bystander" chest compressions and assisted ventilation independently improve outcome from piglet asphyxial pulseless "cardiac arrest." *Circulation.* 2000;101:1743–1748.
28. American Heart Association in collaboration with International Liaison Committee on Resuscitation. Guidelines 2000 for Cardiopulmonary Resuscitation and Emergency Cardiovascular Care: International Consensus on Science. *Circulation.* 2000;102(suppl):I1-I384.
29. Samson R, Berg R, Bingham R, Pediatric Advanced Life Support Task Force ILCoR. Use of automated external defibrillators for children: an update. An advisory statement from the Pediatric Advanced Life Support Task Force, International Liaison Committee on Resuscitation. *Resuscitation.* 2003;57:237–243.
30. Cummins RO, Ornato JP, Thies WH, Pepe PE. Improving survival from sudden cardiac arrest: the "chain of survival" concept: a statement for health professionals from the Advanced Cardiac Life Support Subcommittee and the Emergency Cardiac Care Committee, American Heart Association. *Circulation.* 1991;83:1832–1847.
31. Herlitz J, Ekstrom L, Wennerblom B, Axelsson A, Bang A, Holmberg S. Effect of bystander initiated cardiopulmonary resuscitation on ventricular fibrillation and survival after witnessed cardiac arrest outside hospital. *Br Heart J.* 1994;72:408–412.
32. Stiell I, Nichol G, Wells G, De Maio V, Nesbitt L, Blackburn J, Spaite D, Group OS. Health-related quality of life is better for cardiac arrest survivors who received citizen cardiopulmonary resuscitation. *Circulation.* 2003;108:1939–1944.
33. Aufderheide TP, Sigurdsson G, Pirrallo RG, Yannopoulos D, McKnite S, von Briesen C, Sparks CW, Conrad CJ, Provo TA, Lurie KG. Hyperventilation-induced hypotension during cardiopulmonary resuscitation. *Circulation.* 2004;109:1960–1965.
34. Abella BS, Alvarado JP, Myklebust H, Edelson DP, Barry A, O'Hearn N, Vanden Hoek TL, Becker LB. Quality of cardiopulmonary resuscitation during in-hospital cardiac arrest. *JAMA.* 2005;293:305–310.
35. Wik L, Kramer-Johansen J, Myklebust H, Sorebo H, Svensson L, Fellows B, Steen PA. Quality of cardiopulmonary resuscitation during out-of-hospital cardiac arrest. *JAMA.* 2005;293:299–304.
36. Assar D, Chamberlain D, Colquhoun M, Donnelly P, Handley AJ, Leaves S, Kern KB. Randomised controlled trials of staged teaching for basic life support, 1: skill acquisition at bronze stage. *Resuscitation.* 2000;45:7–15.
37. Heidenreich JW, Higdon TA, Kern KB, Sanders AB, Berg RA, Niebler R, Hendrickson J, Ewy GA. Single-rescuer cardiopulmonary resuscitation: 'two quick breaths'—an oxymoron. *Resuscitation.* 2004;62:283–289.
38. Eftestol T, Sunde K, Steen PA. Effects of interrupting precordial compressions on the calculated probability of defibrillation success during out-of-hospital cardiac arrest. *Circulation.* 2002;105:2270–2273.
39. Yu T, Weil MH, Tang W, Sun S, Klouche K, Povoas H, Bisera J. Adverse outcomes of interrupted precordial compression during automated defibrillation. *Circulation.* 2002;106:368–372.
40. Abella BS, Sandbo N, Vassilatos P, Alvarado JP, O'Hearn N, Wigder HN, Hoffman P, Tynus K, Vanden Hoek TL, Becker LB. Chest compression rates during cardiopulmonary resuscitation are suboptimal: a prospective study during in-hospital cardiac arrest. *Circulation.* 2005;111:428–434.
41. Chamberlain DA, Hazinski MF. Education in resuscitation: an ILCOR symposium: Utstein Abbey: Stavanger, Norway: June 22–24, 2001. *Circulation.* 2003;108:2575–2594.
42. Locke CJ, Berg RA, Sanders AB, Davis MF, Milander MM, Kern KB, Ewy GA. Bystander cardiopulmonary resuscitation: concerns about mouth-to-mouth contact. *Arch Intern Med.* 1995;155:938–943.

43. Ornato JP, Hallagan LF, McMahan SB, Peeples EH, Rostafinski AG. Attitudes of BCLS instructors about mouth-to-mouth resuscitation during the AIDS epidemic. *Ann Emerg Med.* 1990;19:151–156.
44. Brenner BE, Kauffman J. Reluctance of internists and medical nurses to perform mouth-to-mouth resuscitation. *Arch Intern Med.* 1993;153: 1763–1769.
45. Brenner B, Stark B, Kauffman J. The reluctance of house staff to perform mouth-to-mouth resuscitation in the inpatient setting: what are the considerations? *Resuscitation.* 1994;28:185–193.
46. Mejicano GC, Maki DG. Infections acquired during cardiopulmonary resuscitation: estimating the risk and defining strategies for prevention. *Ann Intern Med.* 1998;129:813–828.
47. Simmons M, Deao D, Moon L, Peters K, Cavanaugh S. Bench evaluation: three face-shield CPR barrier devices. *Respir Care.* 1995;40:618–623.
48. Cummins RO. The Utstein style for uniform reporting of data from out-of-hospital cardiac arrest. *Ann Emerg Med.* 1993;22:37–40.
49. Zaritsky A, Nadkarni V, Hazinski M, Foltin G, Quan L, Wright J, Fiser D, Zideman D, O'Malley P, Chameides L, Cummins R. Recommended guidelines for uniform reporting of pediatric advanced life support: the pediatric Utstein style. *Circulation.* 1995;92:2006–2020.
50. Cummins RO, Chamberlain D, Hazinski MF, Nadkarni V, Kloeck W, Kramer E, Becker L, Robertson C, Koster R, Zaritsky A, Bossaert L, Ornato JP, Callanan V, Allen M, Steen P, Connolly B, Sanders A, Idris A, Cobbe S. Recommended guidelines for reviewing, reporting, and conducting research on in-hospital resuscitation: the in-hospital 'Utstein style.' *American* Heart Association. *Circulation.* 1997;95:2213–2239.
51. Jacobs I, Nadkarni V, Bahr J, Berg RA, Billi JE, Bossaert L, Cassan P, Coovadia A, D'Este K, Finn J, Halperin H, Handley A, Herlitz J, Hickey R, Idris A, Kloeck W, Larkin GL, Mancini ME, Mason P, Mears G, Monsieurs K, Montgomery W, Morley P, Nichol G, Nolan J, Okada K, Perlman J, Shuster M, Steen PA, Sterz F, Tibballs J, Timerman S, Truitt T, Zideman D; International Liason Committee on Resusitation. Cardiac arrest and cardiopulmonary resuscitation outcome reports: update and simplification of the Utstein templates for resuscitation registries. A statement for healthcare professionals from a task force of the international liaison committee on resuscitation (American Heart Association, European Resuscitation Council, Australian Resuscitation Council, New Zealand Resuscitation Council, Heart and Stroke Foundation of Canada, InterAmerican Heart Foundation, Resuscitation Council of Southern Africa). *Circulation.* 2004 Nov 23;110:3385–3397.
52. In-hospital resuscitation requirements reinstated for hospitals. *Jt Comm Perspect.* 1998;18:5.
53. Peberdy MA, Kaye W, Ornato JP, Larkin GL, Nadkarni V, Mancini ME, Berg RA, Nichol G, Lane-Trultt T. Cardiopulmonary resuscitation of adults in the hospital: a report of 14720 cardiac arrests from the National Registry of Cardiopulmonary Resuscitation. *Resuscitation.* 2003;58:297–308.
54. Bellomo R, Goldsmith D, Uchino S, Buckmaster J, Hart GK, Opdam H, Silvester W, Doolan L, Gutteridge G. A prospective before-and-after trial of a medical emergency team. *Med J Aust.* 2003;179:283–287.
55. Buist MD, Moore GE, Berenard SA, Waxman BP, Anderson JN, Nguyen TV. Effects of a medical emergency team on reduction of incidence of and mortality from unexpected cardiac arrests in hospital: preliminary study. *BMJ.* 2002;324:387–390.
56. Goldhill DR, Worthington L, Mulcahy A, Tarling M, Sumner A. The patient-at-risk team: identifying and managing seriously ill ward patients. *Anaesthesia.* 1999;54:853–860.
57. Kenwood G, Castle N, Hodgetts T, Shaikh L, Evaluation of a medical emergency team one year after implementation. *Resuscitation.* 2004;61: 257–263.
58. Bristow PJ, Hillman KM, Chey T, Daffurn K, Jacques TC, Normal SL, Bishop GF, Simmons EG. Rates of in-hospital arrests, deaths and intensive care admissions: the effect of a medical emergency team. *Med J Aust.* 2000;173:236–240.
59. MERIT trial investigators. Introduction of the medical emergency team (MET) system: a cluster-randomised controlled trial. *Lancet.* 2005;365: 2091–2097.

Part 4: Adult Basic Life Support

Basic life support (BLS) includes recognition of signs of sudden cardiac arrest (SCA), heart attack, stroke, and foreign-body airway obstruction (FBAO); cardiopulmonary resuscitation (CPR); and defibrillation with an automated external defibrillator (AED). This section summarizes BLS guidelines for lay rescuers and healthcare providers.

Introduction

As noted in Part 3: "Overview of CPR," SCA is a leading cause of death in the United States and Canada.[1–3] At the first analysis of heart rhythm, about 40% of victims of out-of-hospital SCA demonstrate ventricular fibrillation (VF).[3–5] VF is characterized by chaotic rapid depolarizations and repolarizations that cause the heart to quiver so that it is unable to pump blood effectively.[6] It is likely that an even larger number of SCA victims have VF or rapid ventricular tachycardia (VT) at the time of collapse, but by the time of first rhythm analysis the rhythm has deteriorated to asystole.[7]

Many SCA victims can survive if bystanders act immediately while VF is still present, but successful resuscitation is unlikely once the rhythm deteriorates to asystole.[8] Treatment for VF SCA is immediate bystander CPR plus delivery of a shock with a defibrillator. The mechanism of cardiac arrest in victims of trauma, drug overdose, drowning, and in many children is asphyxia. CPR with both compressions and rescue breaths is critical for resuscitation of these victims.

The American Heart Association uses 4 links in a chain (the "Chain of Survival") to illustrate the important time-sensitive actions for victims of VF SCA (Figure 1). Three and possibly all 4 of these links are also relevant for victims of asphyxial arrest.[9] These links are

- Early recognition of the emergency and activation of the emergency medical services (EMS) or local emergency response system: "phone 911."[10,11]
- Early bystander CPR: immediate CPR can double or triple the victim's chance of survival from VF SCA.[8,12–14]
- Early delivery of a shock with a defibrillator: CPR plus defibrillation within 3 to 5 minutes of collapse can produce survival rates as high as 49% to 75%.[15–23]
- Early advanced life support followed by postresuscitation care delivered by healthcare providers.

Bystanders can perform 3 of the 4 links in the Chain of Survival. When bystanders recognize the emergency and activate the EMS system, they ensure that basic and advanced life support providers are dispatched to the site of the emergency. In many communities the time interval from EMS call to EMS arrival is 7 to 8 minutes or longer.[24] This means that in the first minutes after collapse the victim's chance of survival is in the hands of bystanders.

Shortening the EMS response interval increases survival from SCA, but the effect is minimal once the EMS response interval (from the time of EMS call until arrival) exceeds 5 to 6 minutes (LOE 3).[25–31] EMS systems should evaluate their protocols for cardiac arrest patients and try to shorten response intervals when improvements are feasible and resources are available (Class I). Each EMS system should measure the rate of survival to hospital discharge for victims of VF SCA and use these measurements to document the impact of changes in procedures (Class IIa).[32–35]

Victims of cardiac arrest need immediate CPR. CPR provides a small but critical amount of blood flow to the heart and brain. CPR prolongs the time VF is present and increases the likelihood that a shock will terminate VF (defibrillate the heart) and allow the heart to resume an effective rhythm and effective systemic perfusion. CPR is especially important if a shock is not delivered for 4 (LOE 4),[36] 5 (LOE 2),[37] or more minutes after collapse. Defibrillation does not "restart" the heart; defibrillation "stuns" the heart, briefly stopping VF and other cardiac electrical activity. If the heart is still viable, its normal pacemakers may then resume firing and produce an effective ECG rhythm that may ultimately produce adequate blood flow.

In the first few minutes after successful defibrillation, asystole or bradycardia may be present and the heart may pump ineffectively. In one recent study of VF SCA, only 25% to 40% of victims demonstrated an organized rhythm 60 seconds after shock delivery; it is likely that even fewer had effective perfusion at that point.[38] Therefore, CPR may be needed for several minutes following defibrillation until adequate perfusion is present.[39]

Lay rescuers can be trained to use a computerized device called an AED to analyze the victim's rhythm and deliver a shock if the victim has VF or rapid VT. The AED uses audio and visual prompts to guide the rescuer. It analyzes the victim's rhythm and informs the rescuer if a shock is needed. AEDs are extremely accurate and will deliver a shock only when VF (or its precursor, rapid VT) is present.[40] AED function and operation are discussed in Part 5: "Electrical Therapies: Automated External Defibrillators, Defibrillation, Cardioversion, and Pacing."

Successful rescuer actions at the scene of an SCA are time critical. Several studies have shown the beneficial effects of immediate CPR and the detrimental impact of delays in defibrillation on survival from SCA. For every minute without CPR, survival from witnessed VF SCA decreases 7% to 10%.[8] When bystander CPR is provided, the decrease in survival is more gradual and averages 3% to 4% per minute from collapse to defibrillation.[8,12] CPR has been shown to double[8,12] or triple[41] survival from witnessed SCA at many intervals to defibrillation.[42]

(*Circulation*. 2005;112:IV-19-IV-34.)

This special supplement to *Circulation* is freely available at http://www.circulationaha.org

DOI: 10.1161/CIRCULATIONAHA.105.166553

Public access defibrillation and first-responder AED programs may increase the number of SCA victims who receive bystander CPR and early defibrillation, improving survival from out-of-hospital SCA.[43] These programs require an organized and practiced response with rescuers trained and equipped to recognize emergencies, activate the EMS system, provide CPR, and use the AED.[43] Lay rescuer AED programs in airports,[19] on airplanes,[20,21] in casinos,[22] and in first-responder programs with police officers[23,44–46] have achieved survival rates as high as 49% to 75%[19–23] from out-of-hospital witnessed VF SCA with provision of immediate bystander CPR and defibrillation within 3 to 5 minutes of collapse. These high survival rates, however, may not be attained in programs that fail to reduce time to defibrillation.[47–49]

Cardiopulmonary Emergencies

Emergency Medical Dispatch

Emergency medical dispatch is an integral component of the EMS response.[50–53] Dispatchers should receive appropriate training in providing prearrival telephone CPR instructions to callers (Class IIa).[10,54–57] Observational studies (LOE 4)[51,58] and a randomized trial (LOE 2)[57] documented that dispatcher CPR instructions increased the likelihood of bystander CPR being performed. It is not clear if prearrival instructions increase the rate of survival from SCA.[58,59]

Dispatchers who provide telephone CPR instructions to bystanders treating children and adult victims with a high likelihood of an asphyxial cause of arrest (eg, drowning) should give directions for rescue breathing followed by chest compressions. In other cases (eg, likely SCA) telephone instruction in chest compressions alone may be preferable (Class IIb). The EMS system's quality improvement program should include periodic review of the dispatcher CPR instructions provided to specific callers (Class IIa).

When dispatchers ask bystanders to determine if breathing is present, bystanders often misinterpret occasional gasps as indicating that the victim is breathing. This erroneous information can result in failure to initiate CPR for a victim of cardiac arrest (LOE 5).[60] Dispatcher CPR instruction programs should develop strategies to help bystanders identify patients with occasional gasps as likely victims of cardiac arrest and thus increase the likelihood of provision of bystander CPR for such victims (Class IIb).

Acute Coronary Syndromes

Coronary heart disease continues to be the nation's single leading cause of death, with >500 000 deaths and 1.2 million patients with an acute myocardial infarction (AMI) annually.[61] Approximately 52% of deaths from AMI occur out of the hospital, most within the first 4 hours after onset of symptoms.[62,63]

Early recognition, diagnosis, and treatment of AMI can improve outcome by limiting damage to the heart,[64,65] but treatment is most effective if provided within a few hours of the onset of symptoms.[66,67] Patients at risk for acute coronary syndromes (ACS) and their families should be taught to recognize the signs of ACS and immediately activate the EMS system rather than contact the family physician or drive to the hospital. The classic symptom associated with ACS is chest discomfort, but symptoms may also include discomfort in other areas of the upper body, shortness of breath, sweating, nausea, and lightheadedness. The symptoms of AMI characteristically last more than 15 minutes. Atypical symptoms of ACS are more common in the elderly, women, and diabetic patients.[68–71]

To improve ACS outcome, all dispatchers and EMS providers must be trained to recognize ACS symptoms. EMS providers should be trained to determine onset of ACS symptoms, stabilize the patient, and provide prearrival notification and transport to an appropriate medical care facility.

EMS providers can support the airway, administer oxygen (Class IIb), and administer aspirin and nitroglycerin. If the patient has not taken aspirin and has no history of aspirin allergy, EMS providers should give the patient 160 to 325 mg of aspirin to chew (Class I) and notify the receiving hospital before arrival.[72–75] Paramedics should be trained and equipped to obtain a 12-lead electrocardiogram (ECG) and transmit the ECG or their interpretation of it to the receiving hospital (Class IIa). More specifics on these topics are covered in Part 8: "Stabilization of the Patient With Acute Coronary Syndromes."

Stroke

Stroke is the nation's No. 3 killer and a leading cause of severe, long-term disability.[61] Fibrinolytic therapy administered within the first hours of the onset of symptoms limits neurologic injury and improves outcome in selected patients with acute ischemic stroke.[76–78] The window of opportunity is extremely limited, however. Effective therapy requires early

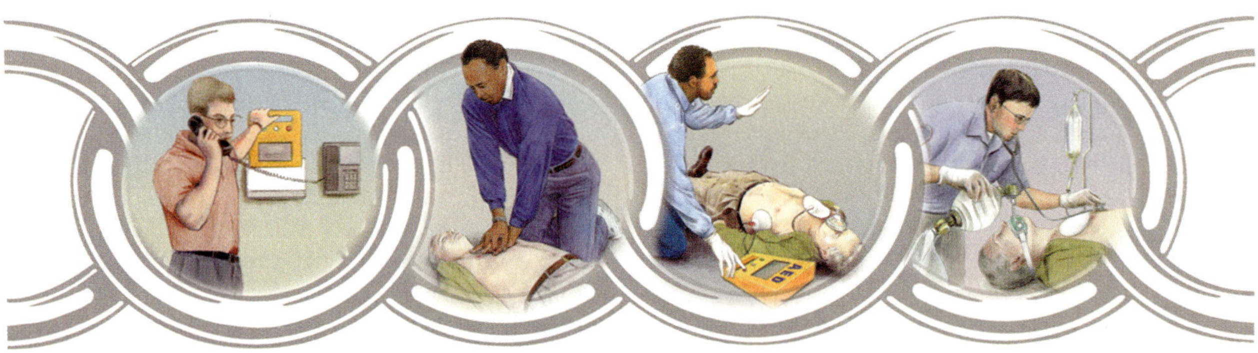

Figure 1. Adult Chain of Survival.

detection of the signs of stroke, prompt activation of the EMS system, prompt dispatch of EMS personnel, rapid delivery to a hospital capable of providing acute stroke care, prearrival notification, immediate and organized hospital care, appropriate evaluation and testing, and rapid delivery of fibrinolytic agents to eligible patients.[79,80]

Patients at high risk for a stroke and their family members must learn to recognize the signs and symptoms of stroke and to call EMS as soon as they detect any of them. The signs and symptoms of stroke are sudden numbness or weakness of the face, arm, or leg, especially on one side of the body; sudden confusion, trouble speaking or understanding; sudden trouble seeing in one or both eyes; sudden trouble walking, dizziness, loss of balance or coordination; and sudden severe headache with no known cause.[81,82]

EMS dispatchers should be trained to suspect stroke and rapidly dispatch responders[83] who should be able to perform an out-of-hospital stroke assessment (LOE 3 to 5; Class IIa),[84–87] establish the time the patient was last known to be "normal," support the ABCs, notify the receiving hospital that a patient with possible stroke is being transported there, and consider triaging the patient to a facility with a stroke unit (LOE 5 to 8; Class IIb).[88–91] It may be helpful for a family member to accompany the patient during transport to verify the time of symptom onset. If authorized by medical control, EMS providers should check the patient's glucose level during transport to rule out hypoglycemia as the cause of altered neurologic function and to give glucose if blood sugar is low.

When the stroke victim arrives at the emergency department (ED), the goal of care is to streamline evaluation so that initial assessment is performed within 10 minutes, a computed tomography (CT) scan is performed and interpreted within 25 minutes, and fibrinolytics are administered to selected patients within 60 minutes of arrival at the ED and within 3 hours of the onset of symptoms. Additional information about the assessment of stroke using stroke scales and the management of stroke is included in Part 9: "Adult Stroke."

Adult BLS Sequence

The steps of BLS consist of a series of sequential assessments and actions, which are illustrated in the BLS algorithm (Figure 2). The intent of the algorithm is to present the steps in a logical and concise manner that will be easy to learn, remember, and perform. The box numbers in the following section refer to the corresponding boxes in the Adult BLS Healthcare Provider Algorithm.

Safety during CPR training and performance, including the use of barrier devices, is discussed in Part 3. Before approaching the victim, the rescuer must ensure that the scene is safe. Lay rescuers should move trauma victims only if absolutely necessary (eg, the victim is in a dangerous location, such as a burning building).

Check for Response (Box 1)

Once the rescuer has ensured that the scene is safe, the rescuer should check for response. To check for response, tap the victim on the shoulder and ask, "Are you all right?" If the victim responds but is injured or needs medical assistance, leave the victim to phone 911. Then return as quickly as possible and recheck the victim's condition frequently.

Activate the EMS System (Box 2)

If a lone rescuer finds an unresponsive adult (ie, no movement or response to stimulation), the rescuer should activate the EMS system (phone 911), get an AED (if available), and return to the victim to provide CPR and defibrillation if needed. When 2 or more rescuers are present, one rescuer should begin the steps of CPR while a second rescuer activates the EMS system and gets the AED. If the emergency occurs in a facility with an established medical response system, notify that system instead of the EMS system.

Healthcare providers may tailor the sequence of rescue actions to the most likely cause of arrest.[92] If a lone healthcare provider sees an adult or child suddenly collapse, the collapse is likely to be cardiac in origin, and the provider should phone 911, get an AED, and return to the victim to provide CPR and use the AED. If a lone healthcare provider aids a drowning victim or other victim of likely asphyxial (primary respiratory) arrest of any age, the healthcare provider should give 5 cycles (about 2 minutes) of CPR before leaving the victim to activate the EMS system.

When phoning 911 for help, the rescuer should be prepared to answer the dispatcher's questions about location, what happened, number and condition of victims, and type of aid provided. The caller should hang up only when instructed to do so by the dispatcher and should then return to the victim to provide CPR and defibrillation if needed.

Open the Airway and Check Breathing (Box 3)

To prepare for CPR, place the victim on a hard surface in a face up (supine) position. If an unresponsive victim is face down (prone), roll the victim to a supine (face up) position. If a hospitalized patient with an advanced airway (eg, endotracheal tube, laryngeal mask airway [LMA], or esophageal-tracheal combitube [Combitube]) cannot be placed in the supine position (eg, during spinal surgery), the healthcare provider may attempt CPR with the patient in a prone position (Class IIb). See below.

Open the Airway: Lay Rescuer

The lay rescuer should open the airway using a head tilt–chin lift maneuver for both injured and noninjured victims (Class IIa). The jaw thrust is no longer recommended for lay rescuers because it is difficult for lay rescuers to learn and perform, is often not an effective way to open the airway, and may cause spinal movement (Class IIb).

Open the Airway: Healthcare Provider

A healthcare provider should use the head tilt–chin lift maneuver to open the airway of a victim without evidence of head or neck trauma. Although the head tilt–chin lift technique was developed using unconscious, paralyzed adult volunteers and has not been studied in victims with cardiac arrest, clinical[93] and radiographic (LOE 3) evidence[94,95] and a case series (LOE 5)[96] have shown it to be effective.

Approximately 2% of victims with blunt trauma have a spinal injury, and this risk is tripled if the victim has a

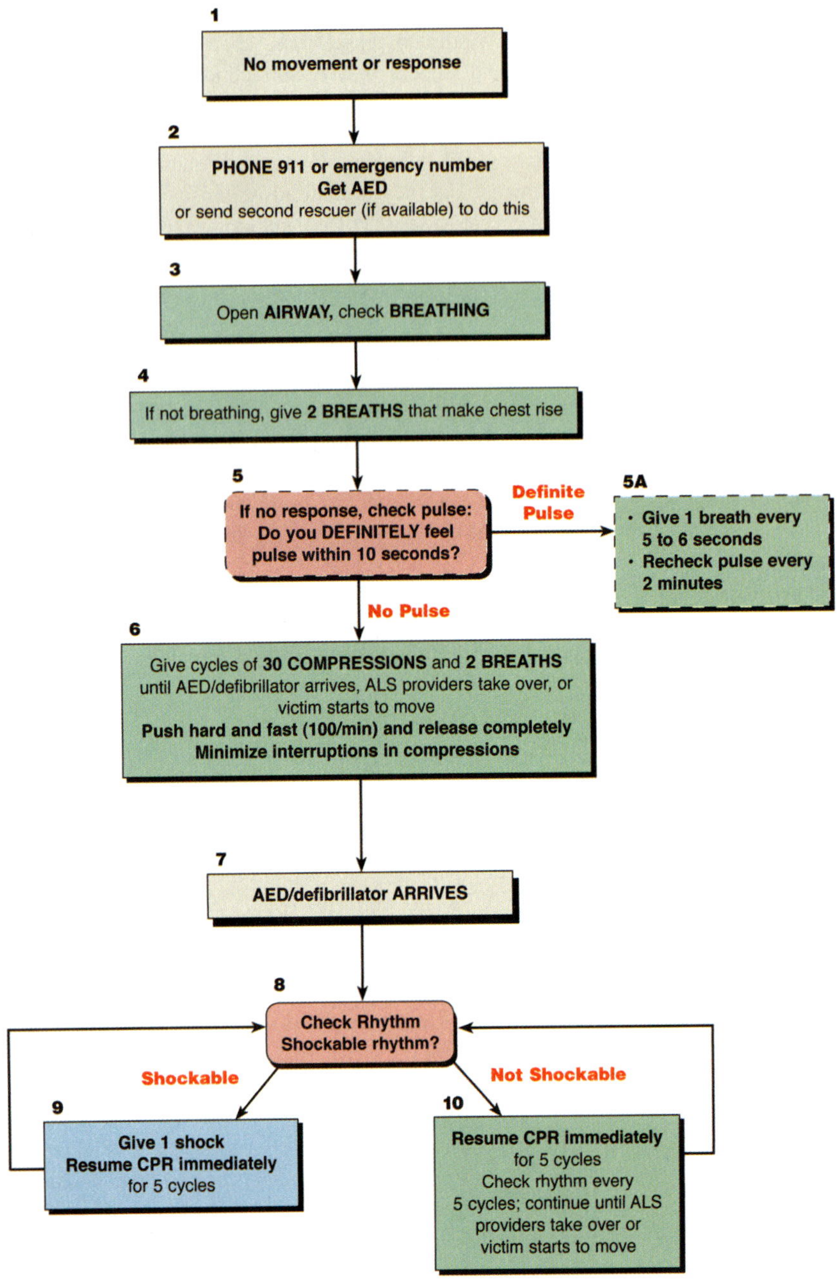

Figure 2. Adult BLS Healthcare Provider Algorithm. Boxes bordered with dotted lines indicate actions or steps performed by the healthcare provider but not the lay rescuer.

craniofacial injury,[97] a Glasgow Coma Scale score of <8,[98] or both.[97,99] If a healthcare provider suspects a cervical spine injury, open the airway using a jaw thrust without head extension (Class IIb).[96] Because maintaining a patent airway and providing adequate ventilation is a priority in CPR (Class I), use a head tilt–chin lift maneuver if the jaw thrust does not open the airway.

Use manual spinal motion restriction rather than immobilization devices for victims with suspected spinal injury (Class IIb).[100,101] Manual spinal motion restriction is safer, and immobilization devices may interfere with a patent airway (LOE 3 to 4).[102–104] Cervical collars may complicate airway management during CPR (LOE 4),[102] and they can cause increased intracranial pressure in a victim with a head injury (LOE 4 to 5; Class IIb).[105–108] Spine immobilization devices, however, are necessary during transport.

Check Breathing

While maintaining an open airway, look, listen, and feel for breathing. If you are a lay rescuer and do not confidently detect *normal* breathing or if you are a healthcare provider and do not detect *adequate* breathing within 10 seconds, give 2 breaths (see below). If you are a lay rescuer and you are unwilling or unable to give rescue breaths, begin chest compressions (Class IIa).

Professional as well as lay rescuers may be unable to accurately determine the presence or absence of adequate or normal breathing in unresponsive victims (LOE 7)[109–111] because the airway is not open[112] or the victim has occasional gasps, which can occur in the first minutes after SCA and may be confused with adequate breathing. Occasional gasps are not effective breaths. Treat the victim who has occasional gasps as if he or she is not breathing (Class I) and give rescue breaths. CPR training should emphasize how to recognize occasional gasps and should instruct rescuers to give rescue breaths and proceed with the steps of CPR when the unresponsive victim demonstrates occasional gasps (Class IIa).

Give Rescue Breaths (Boxes 4 and 5A)

Give 2 rescue breaths, each over 1 second, with enough volume to produce visible chest rise. This recommended 1-second duration to make the chest rise applies to all forms of ventilation during CPR, including mouth-to-mouth and bag-mask ventilation and ventilation through an advanced airway, with and without supplementary oxygen (Class IIa).

During CPR the purpose of ventilation is to maintain adequate oxygenation, but the optimal tidal volume, respiratory rate, and inspired oxygen concentration to achieve this are not known. The following general recommendations can be made:

1. During the first minutes of VF SCA, rescue breaths are probably not as important as chest compressions[113] because the oxygen level in the blood remains high for the first several minutes after cardiac arrest. In early cardiac arrest, myocardial and cerebral oxygen delivery is limited more by the diminished blood flow (cardiac output) than a lack of oxygen in the blood. During CPR blood flow is provided by chest compressions. Rescuers must be sure to provide effective chest compressions (see below) and minimize any interruption of chest compressions.
2. Both ventilations and compressions are important for victims of prolonged VF SCA, when oxygen in the blood is utilized. Ventilations and compressions are also important for victims of asphyxial arrest, such as children and drowning victims who are hypoxemic at the time of cardiac arrest.
3. During CPR blood flow to the lungs is substantially reduced, so an adequate ventilation-perfusion ratio can be maintained with lower tidal volumes and respiratory rates than normal.[114] Rescuers should not provide hyperventilation (too many breaths or too large a volume). Excessive ventilation is unnecessary and is harmful because it increases intrathoracic pressure, decreases venous return to the heart, and diminishes cardiac output and survival.[115]
4. Avoid delivering breaths that are too large or too forceful. Such breaths are not needed and may cause gastric inflation and its resultant complications.[116]

The *ECC Guidelines 2000*[117] recommended a variety of tidal volumes, respiratory rates, and breath delivery intervals. But it is unrealistic to expect the rescuer to distinguish half-second differences in inspiratory times or to judge tidal volumes delivered by mouth-to-mouth or bag-mask ventilation. So these guidelines provide simple recommendations for delivery of rescue breaths during cardiac arrest as follows:

- Deliver each rescue breath over 1 second (Class IIa).
- Give a sufficient tidal volume (by mouth-to-mouth/mask or bag mask with or without supplementary oxygen) to produce *visible chest rise* (Class IIa).
- Avoid rapid or forceful breaths.
- When an advanced airway (ie, endotracheal tube, Combitube, or LMA) is in place during 2-person CPR, ventilate at a rate of 8 to 10 breaths per minute without attempting to synchronize breaths between compressions. There should be no pause in chest compressions for delivery of ventilations (Class IIa).

Studies in anesthetized adults (with normal perfusion) suggest that a tidal volume of 8 to 10 mL/kg maintains normal oxygenation and elimination of CO_2. During CPR cardiac output is ≈25% to 33% of normal,[118] so oxygen uptake from the lungs and CO_2 delivery to the lungs are also reduced.[119] As a result, low minute ventilation (lower than normal tidal volume and respiratory rate) can maintain effective oxygenation and ventilation during CPR.[120–123] During adult CPR tidal volumes of approximately 500 to 600 mL (6 to 7 mL/kg) should suffice (Class IIa). Although a rescuer cannot estimate tidal volume, this guide may be useful for setting automatic transport ventilators and as a reference for manikin manufacturers.

If you are delivering ventilation with a bag and mask, use an adult ventilating bag (volume of 1 to 2 L); a pediatric bag delivers inadequate tidal volume for an adult.[124,125]

When giving rescue breaths, give sufficient volume to cause visible chest rise (LOE 6, 7; Class IIa). In 1 observational study trained BLS providers were able to detect "adequate" chest rise in anesthetized, intubated, and paralyzed adult patients when a tidal volume of approximately 400 mL was delivered.[114] It is likely, however, that a larger volume is required to produce chest rise in a victim with no advanced airway (eg, endotracheal tube, Combitube, LMA) in place. We therefore recommend a tidal volume of 500 to 600 mL but emphasize that *the volume delivered should produce visible chest rise* (Class IIa). It is reasonable to use the same tidal volume in patients with asphyxial and arrhythmic cardiac arrest (Class IIb).

Currently manikins show visible chest rise when tidal volumes reach about 700 to 1000 mL. To provide a realistic practice experience, manikins should be designed to achieve a visible chest rise at a tidal volume of 500 to 600 mL.[114] Automated and mechanical ventilators are discussed briefly at the end of this chapter and in Part 6: "CPR Techniques and Devices."

Gastric inflation often develops when ventilation is provided without an advanced airway. It can cause regurgitation and aspiration, and by elevating the diaphragm, it can restrict lung movement and decrease respiratory compliance.[117] Air delivered with each rescue breath can enter the stomach when pressure in the esophagus exceeds the lower esophageal sphincter opening pressure. Risk of gastric inflation is increased by high proximal airway pressure[114] and the reduced opening pressure of the lower esophageal sphincter.[126] High pressure can be created by a short inspiratory time, large tidal volume, high peak inspiratory pressure, incomplete airway opening, and decreased lung compliance.[127] To minimize the potential for gastric inflation and its complications, deliver each breath to patients with or without an advanced airway over 1 second and deliver a tidal volume that is sufficient to produce a visible chest rise (Class IIa). But do not deliver more volume or use more force than is needed to produce visible chest rise.

Mouth-to-Mouth Rescue Breathing

Mouth-to-mouth rescue breathing provides oxygen and ventilation to the victim.[128] To provide mouth-to-mouth rescue breaths, open the victim's airway, pinch the victim's nose, and create an airtight mouth-to-mouth seal. Give 1 breath over 1 second, take a "regular" (not a deep) breath, and give a second rescue breath over 1 second (Class IIb). Taking a regular rather than a deep breath prevents you from getting dizzy or lightheaded. The most common cause of ventilation difficulty is an improperly opened airway,[112] so if the victim's chest does not rise with the first rescue breath, perform the head tilt–chin lift and give the second rescue breath.[120,121]

Mouth-to–Barrier Device Breathing

Despite its safety,[129] some healthcare providers[130–132] and lay rescuers may hesitate to give mouth-to-mouth rescue breathing and prefer to use a barrier device. Barrier devices may not reduce the risk of infection transmission,[129] and some may increase resistance to air flow.[133,134] If you use a barrier device, do not delay rescue breathing.

Barrier devices are available in 2 types: face shields and face masks. Face shields are clear plastic or silicone sheets that reduce direct contact between the victim and rescuer but do not prevent contamination of the rescuer's side of the shield.[135–137]

A rescuer with a duty to respond should use a face shield only as a substitute for mouth-to-mouth breathing. These responders should switch to face mask or bag-mask ventilation as soon as possible.[137] Masks used for mouth-to-mask breathing should contain a 1-way valve that directs the rescuer's breath into the patient while diverting the patient's exhaled air away from the rescuer.[137]

Some masks include an oxygen inlet for administration of supplementary oxygen. When oxygen is available, healthcare providers should provide it at a minimum flow rate of 10 to 12 L/min.

Mouth-to-Nose and Mouth-to-Stoma Ventilation

Mouth-to-nose ventilation is recommended if it is impossible to ventilate through the victim's mouth (eg, the mouth is seriously injured), the mouth cannot be opened, the victim is in water, or a mouth-to-mouth seal is difficult to achieve (Class IIa). A case series suggests that mouth-to-nose ventilation in adults is feasible, safe, and effective (LOE 5).[138]

Give mouth-to-stoma rescue breaths to a victim with a tracheal stoma who requires rescue breathing. A reasonable alternative is to create a tight seal over the stoma with a round pediatric face mask (Class IIb). There is no published evidence on the safety, effectiveness, or feasibility of mouth-to-stoma ventilation. One study of patients with laryngectomies showed that a pediatric face mask created a better peristomal seal than a standard ventilation bag (LOE 4).[139]

Ventilation With Bag and Mask

Rescuers can provide bag-mask ventilation with room air or oxygen. A bag-mask device provides positive-pressure ventilation without an advanced airway and therefore may produce gastric inflation and its complications (see above). When using a bag-mask device, deliver each breath over a period of 1 second and provide sufficient tidal volume to cause visible chest rise.

The Bag-Mask Device

A bag-mask device should have the following[140]: a nonjam inlet valve; either no pressure relief valve or a pressure relief valve that can be bypassed; standard 15-mm/22-mm fittings; an oxygen reservoir to allow delivery of high oxygen concentrations; a nonrebreathing outlet valve that cannot be obstructed by foreign material and will not jam with an oxygen flow of 30 L/min; and the capability to function satisfactorily under common environmental conditions and extremes of temperature.

Masks should be made of transparent material to allow detection of regurgitation. They should be capable of creating a tight seal on the face, covering both mouth and nose. Masks should be fitted with an oxygen (insufflation) inlet, have a standard 15-mm/22-mm connector,[141] and should be available in one adult and several pediatric sizes.

Bag-Mask Ventilation

Bag-mask ventilation is a challenging skill that requires considerable practice for competency.[142,143] The lone rescuer using a bag-mask device should be able to simultaneously open the airway with a jaw lift, hold the mask tightly against the patient's face, and squeeze the bag. The rescuer must also watch to be sure the chest rises with each breath.

Bag-mask ventilation is most effective when provided by 2 trained and experienced rescuers. One rescuer opens the airway and seals the mask to the face while the other squeezes the bag. Both rescuers watch for visible chest rise.[142–144]

The rescuer should use an adult (1 to 2 L) bag to deliver a tidal volume sufficient to achieve visible chest rise (Class IIa). If the airway is open and there are no leaks (ie, there is a good seal between face and mask), this volume can be delivered by squeezing a 1-L adult bag about one half to two thirds of its volume or a 2-L adult bag about one-third its volume. As long as the patient does not have an advanced airway in place, the rescuer(s) should deliver cycles of 30 compressions and 2 breaths. The rescuer delivers the breaths during pauses in compressions and delivers each breath over 1 second (Class IIa).

The healthcare provider should use supplementary oxygen (O_2 >40%, a minimum flow rate of 10 to 12 L/min) when available. Ideally the bag should be attached to an oxygen reservoir to enable delivery of 100% oxygen.

Advanced airway devices such as the LMA[145,146] and the esophageal-tracheal combitube[147–149] are currently within the scope of BLS practice in a number of regions (with specific authorization from medical control). These devices may provide acceptable alternatives to bag-mask devices for healthcare providers who are well trained and have sufficient experience to use them (Class IIb). It is not clear that these devices are any more or less complicated to use than a bag and mask; training is needed for safe and effective use of both the bag-mask device and each of the advanced airways.

Ventilation With an Advanced Airway

When the victim has an advanced airway in place during CPR, 2 rescuers no longer deliver cycles of CPR (ie, compressions interrupted by pauses for ventilation). Instead, the compressing rescuer should give continuous chest compressions at a rate of 100 per minute without pauses for ventilation. The rescuer delivering ventilation provides 8 to 10 breaths per minute. The 2 rescuers should change compressor and ventilator roles approximately every 2 minutes to prevent compressor fatigue and deterioration in quality and rate of chest compressions. When multiple rescuers are present, they should rotate the compressor role about every 2 minutes.

Rescuers should avoid excessive ventilation by giving the recommended breaths per minute and limiting tidal volume to achieve chest rise (Class IIa).[115] A translational research study showed that delivery of >12 breaths per minute during CPR leads to increased intrathoracic pressure, impeding venous return to the heart during chest compressions.[115] Reduced venous return leads to diminished cardiac output during chest compressions and decreased coronary and cerebral perfusion.[150,151] It is critically important that rescuers maintain a ventilation rate of 8 to 10 breaths per minute during CPR and avoid excessive ventilation.[115,150]

Automatic Transport Ventilators and Manually Triggered, Flow-Limited Resuscitators

Automatic transport ventilators (ATVs) are useful for ventilation of adult patients with a pulse who have an advanced airway in place, both in and out of the hospital (Class IIa). For the adult cardiac arrest patient who does not have an advanced airway in place, the ATV may be useful if tidal volumes are delivered by a flow-controlled, time-cycled ventilator without positive end-expiratory pressure (PEEP).

Manually triggered, oxygen-powered, flow-limited resuscitators may be considered for mask ventilation of the patient who does not have an advanced airway in place during CPR. For further information about these devices see Part 6.

Cricoid Pressure

Pressure applied to the victim's cricoid cartilage pushes the trachea posteriorly, compresses the esophagus against the cervical vertebrae, and can prevent gastric inflation and reduce the risk of regurgitation and aspiration.[152,153] Application of cricoid pressure usually requires a third rescuer, one who is not responsible for chest compressions or ventilations. Cricoid pressure should be used only if the victim is deeply unconscious (ie, has no cough or gag reflex).

Pulse Check (for Healthcare Providers) (Box 5)

Lay rescuers fail to recognize the absence of a pulse in 10% of pulseless victims (poor sensitivity for cardiac arrest) and fail to detect a pulse in 40% of victims with a pulse (poor specificity). In the *ECC Guidelines 2000*[117] the pulse check was deleted from training for lay rescuers and deemphasized in training for healthcare providers. There is no evidence, however, that checking for breathing, coughing, or movement is superior for detection of circulation.[154] For ease of training, the lay rescuer will be taught to assume that cardiac arrest is present if the unresponsive victim is not breathing.

Healthcare providers also may take too long to check for a pulse[109,155] and have difficulty determining if a pulse is present or absent. The healthcare provider should take no more than 10 seconds to check for a pulse (Cla pulse is not definitely felt within 10 seconds, proceeu wi.. chest compressions (see below).

Rescue Breathing Without Chest Compressions (for Healthcare Providers Only—Box 5A)

If an adult victim with spontaneous circulation (ie, palpable pulses) requires support of ventilation, give rescue breaths at a rate of 10 to 12 breaths per minute, or about 1 breath every 5 to 6 seconds (Class IIb). Each breath should be given over 1 second regardless of whether an advanced airway is in place. Each breath should cause visible chest rise.

During delivery of rescue breaths, reassess the pulse approximately every 2 minutes (Class IIa), but spend no more than 10 seconds doing so.

Chest Compressions (Box 6)

Chest compressions consist of rhythmic applications of pressure over the lower half of the sternum. These compressions create blood flow by increasing intrathoracic pressure and directly compressing the heart. Although properly performed chest compressions can produce systolic arterial pressure peaks of 60 to 80 mm Hg, diastolic pressure is low[118] and mean arterial pressure in the carotid artery seldom exceeds 40 mm Hg.[118]

Blood flow generated by chest compressions delivers a small but critical amount of oxygen and substrate to the brain and myocardium. In victims of VF SCA, chest compressions increase the likelihood that a shock (ie, attempted defibrillation) will be successful. Chest compressions are especially important if the first shock is delivered ≥4 minutes after collapse.[36,37,156]

Much of the information about the physiology of chest compressions and the effect of varying compression rates, compression-ventilation ratios, and duty cycles (percent of time the chest is compressed versus time allowed for chest recoil) is derived from animal models. Researchers at the 2005 Consensus Conference,[157] however, reached several conclusions about chest compressions:

1. "Effective" chest compressions are essential for providing blood flow during CPR (Class I).
2. To give "effective" chest compressions, "push hard and push fast." Compress the adult chest at a rate of about 100 compressions per minute, with a compression depth of 1½ to 2 inches (approximately 4 to 5 cm). Allow the chest to recoil *completely* after each compression, and allow approximately equal compression and relaxation times.
3. Minimize interruptions in chest compressions.
4. Further studies are needed to define the best method for coordinating ventilations and chest compressions and to identify the best compression-ventilation ratio in terms of survival and neurologic outcome.

Technique

To maximize the effectiveness of compressions, the victim should lie supine on a hard surface (eg, backboard or floor),[158] with the rescuer kneeling beside the victim's thorax.[159] The safety and efficacy of over-the-head CPR (OTH-CPR) for lone rescuers and 2-person straddle CPR are unknown, but these techniques may be advantageous in confined spaces (LOE 6).[159,160] "CPR-friendly" deflatable mattresses have been studied, and they do not provide an adequate surface on which to perform chest compressions (LOE 6).[161,162]

The rescuer should compress the lower half of the victim's sternum in the center (middle) of the chest, between the nipples.[163] The rescuer should place the heel of the hand on the sternum in the center (middle) of the chest between the nipples and then place the heel of the second hand on top of the first so that the hands are overlapped and parallel (LOE 6; Class IIa).[163–165]

Depress the sternum approximately 1½ to 2 inches (approximately 4 to 5 cm) and then allow the chest to return to its normal position. Complete chest recoil allows venous return to the heart, is necessary for effective CPR, and should be emphasized in training (Class IIb).[166,167] Compression and chest recoil/relaxation times should be approximately equal (Class IIb).[168–171] In studies of chest compression in out-of-hospital[172] and in-hospital settings,[173] 40% of chest compressions were of insufficient depth. Rescuers should practice to ensure good chest compressions and should relieve one another every few minutes to reduce the contribution of fatigue to inadequate chest compression depth and rate (see below).

There is insufficient evidence from human studies to identify a single optimal chest compression rate. Animal[174] and human[175,176] studies support a chest compression rate of >80 compressions per minute to achieve optimal forward blood flow during CPR. We recommend a compression rate of about 100 compressions per minute (Class IIa).

Two human observational studies[172,173] showed that interruptions of chest compressions were common. In these studies of healthcare provider CPR, no chest compressions were provided for 24% to 49%[172,173,177] of total arrest time.

Interruption of chest compressions in animal models is associated with reduced coronary artery perfusion pressure, and the more frequent or prolonged the interruption, the lower the mean coronary perfusion pressure. In 3 animal studies frequent or prolonged interruptions in chest compressions were associated with reduced return of spontaneous circulation (ROSC), reduced survival rates, and reduced postresuscitation myocardial function (LOE 6).[113,174,178,179] Some animal studies suggest that continuous chest compressions with minimal or no interruptions produce higher survival rates than standard CPR (LOE 6).[151,179–181] These guidelines recommend that all rescuers minimize interruption of chest compressions for checking the pulse, analyzing rhythm, or performing other activities (Class IIa).

Lay rescuers should continue CPR until an AED arrives, the victim begins to move, or EMS personnel take over CPR (Class IIa). Lay rescuers should no longer interrupt chest compressions to check for signs of circulation or response. Healthcare providers should interrupt chest compressions as infrequently as possible and try to limit interruptions to no longer than 10 seconds except for specific interventions such as insertion of an advanced airway or use of a defibrillator (Class IIa).

We strongly recommend that patients not be moved while CPR is in progress unless the patient is in a dangerous environment or is a trauma patient in need of surgical intervention. CPR is better and has fewer interruptions when the resuscitation is conducted where the patient is found.

Allow the chest wall to recoil completely after each compression. In studies of CPR in humans[166] and pigs,[167] incomplete chest wall recoil was common, particularly when rescuers were fatigued.[182] Incomplete recoil during BLS CPR is associated with higher intrathoracic pressures, decreased coronary perfusion, and decreased cerebral perfusion (LOE 6).[167] CPR instruction should emphasize the importance of allowing complete chest recoil between compressions.[166]

Manikin[168] and animal studies[170,183] suggest that with duty cycles (the compression part of the cycle) of 20% to 50%, coronary and cerebral perfusion increase as the chest compression rate increases up to 130 to 150 compressions per minute (LOE 6).[170,183] A duty cycle of 50% is recommended because it is easy to achieve with practice.[168]

Rescuer fatigue may lead to inadequate compression rates or depth. Significant fatigue and shallow compressions are seen after 1 minute of CPR, although rescuers may deny that fatigue is present for ≥5 minutes (LOE 6).[182] When 2 or more rescuers are available, it is reasonable to switch the compressor about every 2 minutes (or after 5 cycles of compressions and ventilations at a ratio of 30:2). Every effort should be made to accomplish this switch in <5 seconds (Class IIb). If the 2 rescuers are positioned on either side of the patient, one rescuer will be ready and waiting to relieve the "working compressor" every 2 minutes.

In the past sternal compression force was gauged as adequate if it generated a palpable carotid or femoral pulse. But a venous pulse may be felt during CPR in the absence of effective arterial blood flow.[110,184] The available evidence suggests that blood flow is optimized by using the recommended chest compression force and duration and maintaining a chest compression rate of approximately 100 compressions per minute.[170]

Compression-Ventilation Ratio

A compression-ventilation ratio of 30:2 is recommended and further validation of this guideline is needed (Class IIa).[150,151,180,185–187] In infants and children (see Part 11: "Pediatric Basic Life Support"), 2 rescuers should use a ratio of 15:2 (Class IIb).

This 30:2 ratio is based on a consensus of experts rather than clear evidence. It is designed to increase the number of compressions, reduce the likelihood of hyperventilation, minimize interruptions in chest compressions for ventilation, and simplify instruction for teaching and skills retention. A manikin study suggests that rescuers may find a compression-ventilation ratio of 30:2 more tiring than a ratio of 15:2.[182] Further studies are needed to define the best method for coordinating chest compressions and ventilations during CPR and to define the best compression-ventilation ratio in terms of survival and neurologic outcome in patients with or without an advanced airway in place.

Once an advanced airway is in place, 2 rescuers no longer deliver cycles of CPR (ie, compressions interrupted by pauses for ventilation). Instead, the compressing rescuer should give continuous chest compressions at a rate of 100 per minute without pauses for ventilation. The rescuer delivering ventilation provides 8 to 10 breaths per minute. The 2 rescuers should change compressor and ventilator roles approximately every 2 minutes to prevent compressor fatigue and deterioration in quality and rate of chest compressions. When multiple rescuers are present, they should rotate the compressor role about every 2 minutes.

The compression rate refers to the *speed* of compressions, not the actual *number* of compressions delivered per minute. The actual number of chest compressions delivered per minute is determined by the rate of chest compressions and the number and duration of interruptions to open the airway, deliver rescue breaths, and allow AED analysis.[185,188] Rescuers must make every effort to minimize these interruptions in chest compressions. In 1 out-of-hospital study rescuers intermittently achieved compression rates of 100 to 121 compressions per minute, but the mean number of compressions delivered per minute was reduced to 64 compressions per minute by frequent interruptions.[172]

CPR Prompts

Evidence from 2 adult studies[172,173] show that the chest compression rate during unprompted CPR is frequently inadequate in both out-of-hospital and in-hospital settings. Human,[176,189] animal,[190,191] and manikin studies[37,192–196] showed consistent improvement in end-tidal CO_2 and/or quality of CPR in both the out-of-hospital and in-hospital settings when CPR prompt devices were used. A CPR prompt device may be useful in both out-of-hospital and in-hospital settings (Class IIb).

Compression-Only CPR

The outcome of chest compressions without ventilations is significantly better than the outcome of no CPR for adult cardiac arrest.[113,197–201] In surveys healthcare providers[130–132] as well as lay rescuers[132,202] were reluctant to perform mouth-to-mouth ventilation for unknown victims of cardiac arrest.

In observational studies of adults with cardiac arrest treated by lay rescuers, survival rates were better with chest compressions only than with no CPR but were best with compressions and ventilation (LOE 3[203]; 4[204]). Some animal studies (LOE 6)[113,197–200,205,206] and extrapolation from clinical evidence[207] suggest that rescue breathing is not essential during the first 5 minutes of adult CPR for VF SCA. If the airway is open, occasional gasps and passive chest recoil may provide some air exchange.[186,187,199] In addition, a low minute ventilation may be all that is necessary to maintain a normal ventilation-perfusion ratio during CPR.[208,209]

Laypersons should be encouraged to do compression-only CPR if they are unable or unwilling to provide rescue breaths (Class IIa), although the best method of CPR is compressions coordinated with ventilations.

Alternative Approaches to Chest Compressions

Additional information about alternative CPR techniques and devices can be found in Part 6.

"Cough" CPR

"Cough" CPR currently has no role when the victim is unresponsive,[210–215] so it has no role in lay rescuer CPR. So-called cough CPR has been reported only in awake monitored patients who develop VF or VT.[216] For more information see Part 6.

Prone CPR

When the patient cannot be placed in the supine position, rescuers may consider providing CPR with the patient in the prone position, particularly in hospitalized patients with an advanced airway in place (LOE 5; Class IIb). One crossover study of 6 patients (LOE 3)[217] and 3 case reports (LOE 5)[218–220] documented higher blood pressure in hospitalized intubated patients during CPR in the prone position when compared with patients who received CPR in the supine position. Six case series that included 22 intubated hospitalized patients documented survival to discharge in 10 patients who received CPR in the prone position (LOE 5).[219,220]

Defibrillation (Boxes 8, 9, 10)

All BLS providers should be trained to provide defibrillation because VF is the most common rhythm found in adults with witnessed, nontraumatic SCA.[7] For these victims survival rates are highest when immediate bystander CPR is provided and defibrillation occurs within 3 to 5 minutes.[8,12–14,19–23]

Immediate defibrillation is the treatment of choice for VF of short duration, such as witnessed SCA (Class I).

The effect of CPR before defibrillation for prolonged VF SCA has largely been positive. When EMS arrived more than 4[36] to 5[37] minutes after dispatch, a brief period of CPR (1½ to 3 minutes) before defibrillation improved ROSC and survival rates for adults with out-of-hospital VF/VT in a before-after study (LOE 3)[36] and a randomized trial (LOE 2).[37] But in another randomized trial in adults with out-of-hospital VF/VT, CPR before defibrillation did not improve ROSC or survival rates (LOE 2).[221]

Thus, for adult out-of-hospital cardiac arrest that is not witnessed by the EMS provider, rescuers may give a period of CPR (eg, about 5 cycles or about 2 minutes) before checking the rhythm and attempting defibrillation (Class IIb). In settings with lay rescuer AED programs (AED on-site and available) and for in-hospital environments or if the EMS rescuer witnesses the collapse, the rescuer should use the defibrillator as soon as it is available (Class IIa). Defibrillation is discussed in further detail in Part 5: Electrical Therapies.

Special Resuscitation Situations

Drowning

Drowning is a preventable cause of death. The duration and severity of hypoxia sustained as a result of drowning is the single most important determinant of outcome. Rescuers should provide CPR, particularly rescue breathing, as soon as an unresponsive submersion victim is removed from the water (Class IIa). When rescuing a drowning victim of any age, the lone healthcare provider should give 5 cycles (about 2 minutes) of CPR before leaving the victim to activate the EMS system.

Mouth-to-mouth ventilation in the water may be helpful when administered by a trained rescuer (LOE 5; Class IIb). Chest compressions are difficult to perform in water, may not be effective, and could potentially cause harm to both the rescuer and the victim.[222,223] There is no evidence that water acts as an obstructive foreign body. Maneuvers to relieve FBAO are not recommended for drowning victims because such maneuvers are not necessary and they can cause injury, vomiting, and aspiration and delay CPR.[224]

Rescuers should remove drowning victims from the water by the fastest means available and should begin resuscitation as quickly as possible (Class IIa). Only victims with obvious clinical signs of injury or alcohol intoxication or a history of diving, waterslide use, or trauma should be treated as a "potential spinal cord injury," with stabilization and possible immobilization of the cervical and thoracic spine.[225–231]

Hypothermia

In an unresponsive victim with hypothermia, a healthcare provider should assess breathing to confirm respiratory arrest and assess the pulse to confirm cardiac arrest or profound bradycardia for 30 to 45 seconds because heart rate and breathing may be very slow, depending on the degree of hypothermia. If the victim is not breathing, initiate rescue breathing immediately.

If the victim does not have a pulse, begin chest compressions immediately. Do not wait until the victim is rewarmed to start CPR. To prevent further heat loss, remove wet clothes from the victim; insulate or shield the victim from wind, heat, or cold; and if possible, ventilate the victim with warm, humidified oxygen.

Avoid rough movement, and transport the victim to a hospital as soon as possible. If VF is detected, emergency personnel should deliver shocks using the same protocols used for the normothermic cardiac arrest victim (see Part 10.4: "Hypothermia").

For the hypothermic patient in cardiac arrest, continue resuscitative efforts until the patient is evaluated by advanced care providers. In the out-of-hospital setting, passive warming can be used until active warming is available (Class Indeterminate).

Recovery Position

The recovery position is used for unresponsive adult victims who have normal breathing (Class IIb) and effective circulation. This position is designed to maintain a patent airway and reduce the risk of airway obstruction and aspiration. The victim is placed on his or her side with the lower arm in front of the body.

There are several variations of the recovery position, each with its own advantages. No single position is perfect for all victims.[232,233] The position should be stable, near a true lateral position, with the head dependent and no pressure on the chest to impair breathing. Although healthy volunteers report compression of vessels and nerves in the dependent limb when the lower arm is placed in front,[234,235] the ease of turning the victim into this position may outweigh the risk. Studies in normal volunteers[236] show that extension of the lower arm above the head and rolling the head onto the arm, while bending both legs, may be feasible for victims with known or suspected spinal injury (LOE 7; Class IIb).[236,237]

Foreign-Body Airway Obstruction (Choking)

Death from FBAO is an uncommon but preventable cause of death.[238] Most reported cases of FBAO in adults are caused by impacted food and occur while the victim is eating. Most reported episodes of choking in infants and children occur during eating or play, when parents or childcare providers are present. The choking event is therefore commonly witnessed, and the rescuer usually intervenes while the victim is still responsive.

Recognition of Foreign-Body Airway Obstruction

Because recognition of airway obstruction is the key to successful outcome, it is important to distinguish this emergency from fainting, heart attack, seizure, or other conditions that may cause sudden respiratory distress, cyanosis, or loss of consciousness.

Foreign bodies may cause either mild or severe airway obstruction. The rescuer should intervene if the choking victim has signs of severe airway obstruction. These include signs of poor air exchange and increased breathing difficulty, such as a silent cough, cyanosis, or inability to speak or breathe. The victim may clutch the neck, demonstrating the universal choking sign. Quickly ask, "Are you choking?" If the victim indicates "yes" by nodding his head without speaking, this will verify that the victim has severe airway obstruction.

Relief of Foreign-Body Airway Obstruction

When FBAO produces signs of severe airway obstruction, rescuers must act quickly to relieve the obstruction. If mild obstruction is present and the victim is coughing forcefully, do not interfere with the patient's spontaneous coughing and breathing efforts. Attempt to relieve the obstruction only if signs of severe obstruction develop: the cough becomes silent, respiratory difficulty increases and is accompanied by stridor, or the victim becomes unresponsive. Activate the EMS system quickly if the patient is having difficulty breathing. If more than one rescuer is present, one rescuer should phone 911 while the other rescuer attends to the choking victim.

The clinical data on choking is largely retrospective and anecdotal. For responsive adults and children >1 year of age with severe FBAO, case reports show the feasibility and effectiveness of back blows or "slaps,"[239–241] abdominal thrusts,[239,240,242–247] and chest thrusts.[239,248] Case reports (LOE 5)[242,249,250] and 1 large case series of 229 choking episodes (LOE 5)[239] report that approximately 50% of the episodes of airway obstruction were not relieved by a single technique. The likelihood of success was increased when combinations of back blows or slaps, abdominal thrusts, and chest thrusts were used.

Although chest thrusts, back slaps, and abdominal thrusts are feasible and effective for relieving severe FBAO in conscious (responsive) adults and children ≥1 year of age, for simplicity in training we recommend that the abdominal thrust be applied in rapid sequence until the obstruction is relieved (Class IIb). If abdominal thrusts are not effective, the rescuer may consider chest thrusts (Class IIb). It is important to note that abdominal thrusts are not recommended for infants <1 year of age because thrusts may cause injuries.

Chest thrusts should be used for obese patients if the rescuer is unable to encircle the victim's abdomen (Class Indeterminate). If the choking victim is in the late stages of pregnancy, the rescuer should use chest thrusts instead of abdominal thrusts (Class Indeterminate). Because abdominal thrusts can cause injury,[251–272] victims of FBAO who are treated with abdominal thrusts should be encouraged to undergo an examination by a physician for injury (Class IIb).

Epidemiologic data[238] does not distinguish between FBAO fatalities in which the victims were responsive when first encountered and those in which the victims were unresponsive when initially encountered. However, the likelihood that a cardiac arrest or unresponsiveness will be caused by an unsuspected FBAO is thought to be low.[238]

If the adult victim with FBAO becomes unresponsive, the rescuer should carefully support the patient to the ground, immediately activate EMS, and then begin CPR. A randomized trial of maneuvers to open the airway in cadavers[273] and 2 prospective studies in anesthetized volunteers[274,275] show that higher sustained airway pressures can be generated using the chest thrust rather than the abdominal thrust (LOE 7). Each time the airway is opened during CPR, the rescuer should look for an object in the victim's mouth and remove it. Simply looking into the mouth should not increase the time it takes to attempt the ventilations and proceed to the 30 chest compressions.

A healthcare provider should use a finger sweep only when the provider can see solid material obstructing the airway of an unresponsive patient (Class Indeterminate). No studies have evaluated the routine use of the finger sweep to clear an airway in the absence of visible airway obstruction.[95,276,277] The recommendation to use the finger sweep in past guidelines was based on anecdotal reports that suggested that it was helpful for relieving an airway obstruction.[240,250,251] But 4 case reports have documented harm to the victim[276,277] or rescuer (LOE 7).[95,96]

Summary: The Quality of BLS

Methods should be developed to improve the quality of CPR delivered at the scene of cardiac arrest by healthcare providers and lay rescuers (Class IIa). These may include education, training, assistance or feedback from biomedical devices, mechanical CPR, and electronic monitoring. Components of CPR known to affect hemodynamics include ventilation rate and duration, compression depth, compression rate and number, complete chest recoil, and hands-off time.

Systems that deliver professional CPR should implement processes of continuous quality improvement that include monitoring the quality of CPR delivered at the scene of cardiac arrest, other process-of-care measures (eg, initial rhythm, bystander CPR, and response intervals), and patient outcome up to hospital discharge. This evidence should be used to maximize the quality of CPR delivered (Class Indeterminate).

References

1. Zheng ZJ, Croft JB, Giles WH, Mensah GA. Sudden cardiac death in the United States, 1989 to 1998. *Circulation*. 2001;104:2158–2163.
2. Chugh SS, Jui J, Gunson K, Stecker EC, John BT, Thompson B, Ilias N, Vickers C, Dogra V, Daya M, Kron J, Zheng ZJ, Mensah G, McAnulty J. Current burden of sudden cardiac death: multiple source surveillance versus retrospective death certificate-based review in a large US community. *J Am Coll Cardiol*. 2004;44:1268–1275.
3. Vaillancourt C, Stiell IG. Cardiac arrest care and emergency medical services in Canada. *Can J Cardiol*. 2004;20:1081–1090.
4. Cobb LA, Fahrenbruch CE, Olsufka M, Copass MK. Changing incidence of out-of-hospital ventricular fibrillation, 1980–2000. *JAMA*. 2002;288:3008–3013.
5. Rea TD, Eisenberg MS, Sinibaldi G, White RD. Incidence of EMS-treated out-of-hospital cardiac arrest in the United States. *Resuscitation*. 2004;63:17–24.
6. Cummins RO. CPR and ventricular fibrillation: lasts longer, ends better. *Ann Emerg Med*. 1995;25:833–836.
7. Bayes de Luna A, Coumel P, Leclercq JF. Ambulatory sudden cardiac death: mechanisms of production of fatal arrhythmia on the basis of data from 157 cases. *Am Heart J*. 1989;117:151–159.
8. Larsen MP, Eisenberg MS, Cummins RO, Hallstrom AP. Predicting survival from out-of-hospital cardiac arrest: a graphic model. *Ann Emerg Med*. 1993;22:1652–1658.
9. Cummins RO, Ornato JP, Thies WH, Pepe PE. Improving survival from sudden cardiac arrest: the "chain of survival" concept. A statement for health professionals from the Advanced Cardiac Life Support Subcommittee and the Emergency Cardiac Care Committee, American Heart Association. *Circulation*. 1991;83:1832–1847.
10. Calle PA, Lagaert L, Vanhaute O, Buylaert WA. Do victims of an out-of-hospital cardiac arrest benefit from a training program for emergency medical dispatchers? *Resuscitation*. 1997;35:213–218.
11. Curka PA, Pepe PE, Ginger VF, Sherrard RC, Ivy MV, Zachariah BS. Emergency medical services priority dispatch. *Ann Emerg Med*. 1993; 22:1688–1695.
12. Valenzuela TD, Roe DJ, Cretin S, Spaite DW, Larsen MP. Estimating effectiveness of cardiac arrest interventions: a logistic regression survival model. *Circulation*. 1997;96:3308–3313.
13. Holmberg M, Holmberg S, Herlitz J. Factors modifying the effect of bystander cardiopulmonary resuscitation on survival in out-of-hospital cardiac arrest patients in Sweden. *Eur Heart J*. 2001;22:511–519.
14. Holmberg M, Holmberg S, Herlitz J, Gardelov B. Survival after cardiac arrest outside hospital in Sweden. Swedish Cardiac Arrest Registry. *Resuscitation*. 1998;36:29–36.
15. Weaver WD, Hill D, Fahrenbruch CE, Copass MK, Martin JS, Cobb LA, Hallstrom AP. Use of the automatic external defibrillator in the management of out-of-hospital cardiac arrest. *N Engl J Med*. 1988;319: 661–666.
16. Auble TE, Menegazzi JJ, Paris PM. Effect of out-of-hospital defibrillation by basic life support providers on cardiac arrest mortality: a metaanalysis. *Ann Emerg Med*. 1995;25:642–658.
17. Stiell IG, Wells GA, DeMaio VJ, Spaite DW, Field BJ III, Munkley DP, Lyver MB, Luinstra LG, Ward R. Modifiable factors associated with improved cardiac arrest survival in a multicenter basic life support/defibrillation system: OPALS Study Phase I results. Ontario Prehospital Advanced Life Support. *Ann Emerg Med*. 1999;33:44–50.
18. Stiell IG, Wells GA, Field BJ, Spaite DW, De Maio VJ, Ward R, Munkley DP, Lyver MB, Luinstra LG, Campeau T, Maloney J, Dagnone E. Improved out-of-hospital cardiac arrest survival through the inexpensive optimization of an existing defibrillation program: OPALS study phase II. Ontario Prehospital Advanced Life Support. *JAMA*. 1999;281:1175–1181.
19. Caffrey SL, Willoughby PJ, Pepe PE, Becker LB. Public use of automated external defibrillators. *N Engl J Med*. 2002;347:1242–1247.
20. O'Rourke MF, Donaldson E, Geddes JS. An airline cardiac arrest program. *Circulation*. 1997;96:2849–2853.
21. Page RL, Hamdan MH, McKenas DK. Defibrillation aboard a commercial aircraft. *Circulation*. 1998;97:1429–1430.
22. Valenzuela TD, Roe DJ, Nichol G, Clark LL, Spaite DW, Hardman RG. Outcomes of rapid defibrillation by security officers after cardiac arrest in casinos. *N Engl J Med*. 2000;343:1206–1209.
23. White RD, Bunch TJ, Hankins DG. Evolution of a community-wide early defibrillation programme experience over 13 years using police/fire personnel and paramedics as responders. *Resuscitation*. 2005;65:279–83.
24. Eisenberg MS, Horwood BT, Cummins RO, Reynolds-Haertle R, Hearne TR. Cardiac arrest and resuscitation: a tale of 29 cities. *Ann Emerg Med*. 1990;19:179–86.
25. Braun O, McCallion R, Fazackerley J. Characteristics of midsized urban EMS systems. *Ann Emerg Med*. 1990;19:536–546.
26. MacDonald RD, Mottley JL, Weinstein C. Impact of prompt defibrillation on cardiac arrest at a major international airport. *Prehosp Emerg Care*. 2002;6:1–5.

27. Nichol G, Detsky AS, Stiell IG, O'Rourke K, Wells G, Laupacis A. Effectiveness of emergency medical services for victims of out-of-hospital cardiac arrest: a metaanalysis. *Ann Emerg Med.* 1996;27: 700–710.
28. Nichol G, Laupacis A, Stiell IG, O'Rourke K, Anis A, Bolley H, Detsky AS. Cost-effectiveness analysis of potential improvements to emergency medical services for victims of out-of-hospital cardiac arrest. *Ann Emerg Med.* 1996;27:711–720.
29. Nichol G, Stiell IG, Laupacis A, Pham B, De Maio VJ, Wells GA. A cumulative meta-analysis of the effectiveness of defibrillator-capable emergency medical services for victims of out-of-hospital cardiac arrest. *Ann Emerg Med.* 1999;34:517–525.
30. Nichol G, Valenzuela T, Roe D, Clark L, Huszti E, Wells GA. Cost effectiveness of defibrillation by targeted responders in public settings. *Circulation.* 2003;108:697–703.
31. Sweeney TA, Runge JW, Gibbs MA, Raymond JM, Schafermeyer RW, Norton HJ, Boyle-Whitesel MJ. EMT defibrillation does not increase survival from sudden cardiac death in a two-tiered urban-suburban EMS system. *Ann Emerg Med.* 1998;31:234–240.
32. Cummins RO, Chamberlain DA. The Utstein Abbey and survival from cardiac arrest: what is the connection? *Ann Emerg Med.* 1991;20:918–919.
33. Cummins RO. The Utstein style for uniform reporting of data from out-of-hospital cardiac arrest. *Ann Emerg Med.* 1993;22:37–40.
34. Zaritsky A, Nadkarni V, Hazinski M, Foltin G, Quan L, Wright J, Fiser D, Zideman D, O'Malley P, Chameides L, Cummins R. Recommended guidelines for uniform reporting of pediatric advanced life support: the pediatric Utstein style. *Circulation.* 1995;92:2006–2020.
35. Jacobs I, Nadkarni V, Bahr J, Berg RA, Billi JE, Bossaert L, Cassan P, Coovadia A, D'Este K, Finn J, Halperin H, Handley A, Herlitz J, Hickey R, Idris A, Kloeck W, Larkin GL, Mancini ME, Mason P, Mears G, Monsieurs K, Montgomery W, Morley P, Nichol G, Nolan J, Okada K, Perlman J, Shuster M, Steen PA, Sterz F, Tibballs J, Timerman S, Truitt T, Zideman D. Cardiac arrest and cardiopulmonary resuscitation outcome reports: update and simplification of the Utstein templates for resuscitation registries: a statement for healthcare professionals from a task force of the International Liaison Committee on Resuscitation (American Heart Association, European Resuscitation Council, Australian Resuscitation Council, New Zealand Resuscitation Council, Heart and Stroke Foundation of Canada, InterAmerican Heart Foundation, Resuscitation Councils of Southern Africa). *Circulation.* 2004;110:3385–3397.
36. Cobb LA, Fahrenbruch CE, Walsh TR, Copass MK, Olsufka M, Breskin M, Hallstrom AP. Influence of cardiopulmonary resuscitation prior to defibrillation in patients with out-of-hospital ventricular fibrillation. *JAMA.* 1999;281:1182–1188.
37. Wik L, Hansen TB, Fylling F, Steen T, Vaagenes P, Auestad BH, Steen PA. Delaying defibrillation to give basic cardiopulmonary resuscitation to patients with out-of-hospital ventricular fibrillation: a randomized trial. *JAMA.* 2003;289:1389–1395.
38. Carpenter J, Rea TD, Murray JA, Kudenchuk PJ, Eisenberg MS. Defibrillation waveform and post-shock rhythm in out-of-hospital ventricular fibrillation cardiac arrest. *Resuscitation.* 2003;59:189–96.
39. White RD, Russell JK. Refibrillation, resuscitation and survival in out-of-hospital sudden cardiac arrest victims treated with biphasic automated external defibrillators. *Resuscitation.* 2002;55:17–23.
40. Kerber RE, Becker LB, Bourland JD, Cummins RO, Hallstrom AP, Michos MB, Nichol G, Ornato JP, Thies WH, White RD, Zuckerman BD. Automatic external defibrillators for public access defibrillation: recommendations for specifying and reporting arrhythmia analysis algorithm performance, incorporating new waveforms, and enhancing safety. A statement for health professionals from the American Heart Association Task Force on Automatic External Defibrillation, Subcommittee on AED Safety and Efficacy. *Circulation.* 1997;95:1677–1682.
41. Holmberg M, Holmberg S, Herlitz J. Effect of bystander cardiopulmonary resuscitation in out-of-hospital cardiac arrest patients in Sweden. *Resuscitation.* 2000;47:59–70.
42. Swor RA, Jackson RE, Cynar M, Sadler E, Basse E, Boji B, Rivera-Rivera EJ, Maher A, Grubb W, Jacobson R, et al. Bystander CPR, ventricular fibrillation, and survival in witnessed, unmonitored out-of-hospital cardiac arrest. *Ann Emerg Med.* 1995;25:780–784.
43. The Public Access Defibrillation Trial Investigators. Public-access defibrillation and survival after out-of-hospital cardiac arrest. *N Engl J Med.* 2004;351:637–646.
44. White RD, Asplin BR, Bugliosi TF, Hankins DG. High discharge survival rate after out-of-hospital ventricular fibrillation with rapid defibrillation by police and paramedics. *Ann Emerg Med.* 1996;28:480–485.
45. White RD, Hankins DG, Bugliosi TF. Seven years' experience with early defibrillation by police and paramedics in an emergency medical services system. *Resuscitation.* 1998;39:145–151.
46. Mosesso VN Jr, Davis EA, Auble TE, Paris PM, Yealy DM. Use of automated external defibrillators by police officers for treatment of out-of-hospital cardiac arrest. *Ann Emerg Med.* 1998;32:200–207.
47. Groh WJ, Newman MM, Beal PE, Fineberg NS, Zipes DP. Limited response to cardiac arrest by police equipped with automated external defibrillators: lack of survival benefit in suburban and rural Indiana–the police as responder automated defibrillation evaluation (PARADE). *Acad Emerg Med.* 2001;8:324–330.
48. van Alem AP, Waalewijn RA, Koster RW, de Vos R. Assessment of quality of life and cognitive function after out-of-hospital cardiac arrest with successful resuscitation. *Am J Cardiol.* 2004;93:131–135.
49. Sayre M, Evans J, White L, Brennan T. Providing automated external defibrillators to urban police officers in addition to fire department rapid defibrillation program is not effective. *Resuscitation.* In press.
50. Pepe PE, Zachariah BS, Sayre MR, Floccare D. Ensuring the chain of recovery for stroke in your community. Chain of Recovery Writing Group. *Prehosp Emerg Care.* 1998;2:89–95.
51. Bang A, Biber B, Isaksson L, Lindqvist J, Herlitz J. Evaluation of dispatcher-assisted cardiopulmonary resuscitation. *Eur J Emerg Med.* 1999;6:175–183.
52. Becker LB, Pepe PE. Ensuring the effectiveness of community-wide emergency cardiac care. *Ann Emerg Med.* 1993;22:354–365.
53. Zachariah BS, Pepe PE. The development of emergency medical dispatch in the USA: a historical perspective. *Eur J Emerg Med.* 1995; 2:109–112.
54. Emergency medical dispatching: rapid identification and treatment of acute myocardial infarction. National Heart Attack Alert Program Coordinating Committee Access to Care Subcommittee. *Am J Emerg Med.* 1995;13:67–73.
55. Nordberg M. Emergency medical dispatch: a changing profession. *Emerg Med Serv.* 1998;27:25–26, 28–34.
56. Nordberg M. NAEMD (National Academy of Emergency Medical Dispatch) strives for universal certification. *Emerg Med Serv.* 1999;28:45–46.
57. Hallstrom A, Cobb L, Johnson E, Copass M. Cardiopulmonary resuscitation by chest compression alone or with mouth-to-mouth ventilation. *N Engl J Med.* 2000;342:1546–1553.
58. Culley LL, Clark JJ, Eisenberg MS, Larsen MP. Dispatcher-assisted telephone CPR: common delays and time standards for delivery. *Ann Emerg Med.* 1991;20:362–366.
59. Bang A, Herlitz J, Holmberg S. Possibilities of implementing dispatcher-assisted cardiopulmonary resuscitation in the community: an evaluation of 99 consecutive out-of-hospital cardiac arrests. *Resuscitation.* 2000;44:19–26.
60. Hauff SR, Rea TD, Culley LL, Kerry F, Becker L, Eisenberg MS. Factors impeding dispatcher-assisted telephone cardiopulmonary resuscitation. *Ann Emerg Med.* 2003;42:731–737.
61. American Heart Association. Heart Disease and Stroke Statistics—2005 Update. *Dallas, Tex.: American Heart Association.* 2005.
62. American Heart Association in collaboration with International Liaison Committee on Resuscitation. Guidelines 2000 for Cardiopulmonary Resuscitation and Emergency Cardiovascular Care: International Consensus on Science, Part 7: the Era of Reperfusion: Section 1: Acute Coronary Syndromes (Acute Myocardial Infarction). *Circulation.* 2000; 102(suppl I):I-172–I-203.
63. Chiriboga D, Yarzebski J, Goldberg RJ, Gore JM, Alpert JS. Temporal trends (1975 through 1990) in the incidence and case-fatality rates of primary ventricular fibrillation complicating acute myocardial infarction: a communitywide perspective. *Circulation.* 1994;89:998–1003.
64. Anderson JL, Karagounis LA, Califf RM. Metaanalysis of five reported studies on the relation of early coronary patency grades with mortality and outcomes after acute myocardial infarction. *Am J Cardiol.* 1996;78:1–8.
65. Franzosi MG, Santoro E, De Vita C, Geraci E, Lotto A, Maggioni AP, Mauri F, Rovelli F, Santoro L, Tavazzi L, Tognoni G. Ten-year follow-up of the first megatrial testing thrombolytic therapy in patients with acute myocardial infarction: results of the Gruppo Italiano per lo Studio della Sopravvivenza nell'Infarto-1 study. The GISSI Investigators. *Circulation.* 1998;98:2659–2665.
66. Brouwer MA, Martin JS, Maynard C, Wirkus M, Litwin PE, Verheugt FW, Weaver WD. Influence of early prehospital thrombolysis on mortality and event-free survival (the Myocardial Infarction Triage and Intervention [MITI] Randomized Trial). MITI Project Investigators. *Am J Cardiol.* 1996;78:497–502.
67. Raitt MH, Maynard C, Wagner GS, Cerqueira MD, Selvester RH, Weaver WD. Relation between symptom duration before thrombolytic therapy and final myocardial infarct size. *Circulation.* 1996;93:48–53.
68. Douglas PS, Ginsburg GS. The evaluation of chest pain in women. *N Engl J Med.* 1996;334:1311–1315.
69. Solomon CG, Lee TH, Cook EF, Weisberg MC, Brand DA, Rouan GW, Goldman L. Comparison of clinical presentation of acute myocardial

infarction in patients older than 65 years of age to younger patients: the Multicenter Chest Pain Study experience. *Am J Cardiol*. 1989;63:772–776.
70. Peberdy MA, Ornato JP. Coronary artery disease in women. *Heart Dis Stroke*. 1992;1:315–319.
71. Sullivan AK, Holdright DR, Wright CA, Sparrow JL, Cunningham D, Fox KM. Chest pain in women: clinical, investigative, and prognostic features. *BMJ*. 1994;308:883–886.
72. Haynes BE, Pritting J. A rural emergency medical technician with selected advanced skills. *Prehosp Emerg Care*. 1999;3:343–346.
73. Funk D, Groat C, Verdile VP. Education of paramedics regarding aspirin use. *Prehosp Emerg Care*. 2000;4:62–64.
74. Freimark D, Matetzky S, Leor J, Boyko V, Barbash IM, Behar S, Hod H. Timing of aspirin administration as a determinant of survival of patients with acute myocardial infarction treated with thrombolysis. *Am J Cardiol*. 2002;89:381–385.
75. Verheugt FW, van der Laarse A, Funke-Kupper AJ, Sterkman LG, Galema TW, Roos JP. Effects of early intervention with low-dose aspirin (100 mg) on infarct size, reinfarction and mortality in anterior wall acute myocardial infarction. *Am J Cardiol*. 1990;66:267–270.
76. Grotta JC, Chiu D, Lu M, Patel S, Levine SR, Tilley BC, Brott TG, Haley EC Jr, Lyden PD, Kothari R, Frankel M, Lewandowski CA, Libman R, Kwiatkowski T, Broderick JP, Marler JR, Corrigan J, Huff S, Mitsias P, Talati S, Tanne D. Agreement and variability in the interpretation of early CT changes in stroke patients qualifying for intravenous rtPA therapy. *Stroke*. 1999;30:1528–1533.
77. Ingall TJ, O'Fallon WM, Asplund K, Goldfrank LR, Hertzberg VS, Louis TA, Christianson TJ. Findings from the reanalysis of the NINDS tissue plasminogen activator for acute ischemic stroke treatment trial. *Stroke*. 2004;35:2418–2424.
78. Kwiatkowski TG, Libman RB, Frankel M, Tilley BC, Morgenstern LB, Lu M, Broderick JP, Lewandowski CA, Marler JR, Levine SR, Brott T. Effects of tissue plasminogen activator for acute ischemic stroke at one year. National Institute of Neurological Disorders and Stroke Recombinant Tissue Plasminogen Activator Stroke Study Group. *N Engl J Med*. 1999;340:1781–1787.
79. A systems approach to immediate evaluation and management of hyperacute stroke: experience at eight centers and implications for community practice and patient care. The National Institute of Neurological Disorders and Stroke (NINDS) rt-PA Stroke Study Group. *Stroke*. 1997;28:1530–1540.
80. Broderick JP, Hacke W. Treatment of acute ischemic stroke, part II: neuroprotection and medical management. *Circulation*. 2002;106: 1736–1740.
81. Barsan WG, Brott TG, Olinger CP, Adams HP Jr, Haley EC Jr, Levy DE. Identification and entry of the patient with acute cerebral infarction. *Ann Emerg Med*. 1988;17:1192–1195.
82. Barsan WG, Brott TG, Broderick JP, Haley EC, Levy DE, Marler JR. Time of hospital presentation in patients with acute stroke. *Arch Intern Med*. 1993;153:2558–2561.
83. Zachariah B, Dunford J, Van Cott CC. Dispatch life support and the acute stroke patient: making the right call. In: *Proceedings of the National Institute of Neurological Disorders and Stroke*. Bethesda, Md: National Institute of Neurological Disorders and Stroke; 1991:29–33.
84. Smith WS, Isaacs M, Corry MD. Accuracy of paramedic identification of stroke and transient ischemic attack in the field. *Prehosp Emerg Care*. 1998;2:170–175.
85. Kidwell CS, Starkman S, Eckstein M, Weems K, Saver JL. Identifying stroke in the field: prospective validation of the Los Angeles prehospital stroke screen (LAPSS). *Stroke*. 2000;31:71–76.
86. Kothari R, Barsan W, Brott T, Broderick J, Ashbrock S. Frequency and accuracy of prehospital diagnosis of acute stroke. *Stroke*. 1995;26:937–941.
87. Smith WS, Corry MD, Fazackerley J, Isaacs SM. Improved paramedic sensitivity in identifying stroke victims in the prehospital setting. In: *Prehosp Emerg Care*; 1999:207–210.
88. Merino JG, Silver B, Wong E, Foell B, Demaerschalk B, Tamayo A, Poncha F, Hachinski V. Extending tissue plasminogen activator use to community and rural stroke patients. *Stroke*. 2002;33:141–146.
89. Chapman KM, Woolfenden AR, Graeb D, Johnston DC, Beckman J, Schulzer M, Teal PA. Intravenous tissue plasminogen activator for acute ischemic stroke: a Canadian hospital's experience. *Stroke*. 2000;31: 2920–2924.
90. Cross DT III, Tirschwell DL, Clark MA, Tuden D, Derdeyn CP, Moran CJ, Dacey RG Jr. Mortality rates after subarachnoid hemorrhage: variations according to hospital case volume in 18 states. *J Neurosurg*. 2003;99:810–817.
91. Riopelle RJ, Howse DC, Bolton C, Elson S, Groll DL, Holtom D, Brunet DG, Jackson AC, Melanson M, Weaver DF. Regional access to acute ischemic stroke intervention. *Stroke*. 2001;32:652–655.
92. Hazinski MF. Is pediatric resuscitation unique? Relative merits of early CPR and ventilation versus early defibrillation for young victims of prehospital cardiac arrest. *Ann Emerg Med*. 1995;25:540–543.
93. Guildner CW. Resuscitation: opening the airway. A comparative study of techniques for opening an airway obstructed by the tongue. *JACEP*. 1976;5:588–590.
94. Greene DG, Elam JO, Dobkin AB, Studley CL. Cinefluorographic study of hyperextension of the neck and upper airway patency. *JAMA*. 1961;176: 570–573.
95. Ruben HM, Elam JO, Ruben AM, Greene DG. Investigation of upper airway problems in resuscitation, 1: studies of pharyngeal x-rays and performance by laymen. *Anesthesiology*. 1961;22:271–279.
96. Elam JO, Greene DG, Schneider MA, Ruben HM, Gordon AS, Hustead RF, Benson DW, Clements JA, Ruben A. Head-tilt method of oral resuscitation. *JAMA*. 1960;172:812–815.
97. Hackl W, Hausberger K, Sailer R, Ulmer H, Gassner R. Prevalence of cervical spine injuries in patients with facial trauma. *Oral Surg Oral Med Oral Pathol Oral Radiol Endod*. 2001;92:370–376.
98. Demetriades D, Charalambides K, Chahwan S, Hanpeter D, Alo K, Velmahos G, Murray J, Asensio J. Nonskeletal cervical spine injuries: epidemiology and diagnostic pitfalls. *J Trauma*. 2000;48:724–727.
99. Holly LT, Kelly DF, Counelis GJ, Blinman T, McArthur DL, Cryer HG. Cervical spine trauma associated with moderate and severe head injury: incidence, risk factors, and injury characteristics. *J Neurosurg Spine*. 2002;96:285–291.
100. Majernick TG, Bieniek R, Houston JB, Hughes HG. Cervical spine movement during orotracheal intubation. *Ann Emerg Med*. 1986;15: 417–420.
101. Lennarson PJ, Smith DW, Sawin PD, Todd MM, Sato Y, Traynelis VC. Cervical spinal motion during intubation: efficacy of stabilization maneuvers in the setting of complete segmental instability. *J Neurosurg Spine*. 2001;94:265–270.
102. Heath KJ. The effect of laryngoscopy of different cervical spine immobilisation techniques. *Anaesthesia*. 1994;49:843–845.
103. Hastings RH, Wood PR. Head extension and laryngeal view during laryngoscopy with cervical spine stabilization maneuvers. *Anesthesiology*. 1994;80:825–831.
104. Gerling MC, Davis DP, Hamilton RS, Morris GF, Vilke GM, Garfin SR, Hayden SR. Effects of cervical spine immobilization technique and laryngoscope blade selection on an unstable cervical spine in a cadaver model of intubation. *Ann Emerg Med*. 2000;36:293–300.
105. Davies G, Deakin C, Wilson A. The effect of a rigid collar on intracranial pressure. *Injury*. 1996;27:647–649.
106. Kolb JC, Summers RL, Galli RL. Cervical collar-induced changes in intracranial pressure. *Am J Emerg Med*. 1999;17:135–137.
107. Mobbs RJ, Stoodley MA, Fuller J. Effect of cervical hard collar on intracranial pressure after head injury. *ANZ J Surg*. 2002;72:389–391.
108. Wechsler B, Kim H, Hunter J. Trampolines, children, and strokes. *Am J Phys Med Rehabil*. 2001;80:608–613.
109. Eberle B, Dick WF, Schneider T, Wisser G, Doetsch S, Tzanova I. Checking the carotid pulse check: diagnostic accuracy of first responders in patients with and without a pulse. *Resuscitation*. 1996;33: 107–116.
110. Bahr J, Klingler H, Panzer W, Rode H, Kettler D. Skills of lay people in checking the carotid pulse. *Resuscitation*. 1997;35:23–26.
111. Ruppert M, Reith MW, Widmann JH, Lackner CK, Kerkmann R, Schweiberer L, Peter K. Checking for breathing: evaluation of the diagnostic capability of emergency medical services personnel, physicians, medical students, and medical laypersons. *Ann Emerg Med*. 1999;34:720–729.
112. Safar P, Escarraga LA, Chang F. Upper airway obstruction in the unconscious patient. *J Appl Physiol*. 1959;14:760–764.
113. Kern KB, Hilwig RW, Berg RA, Sanders AB, Ewy GA. Importance of continuous chest compressions during cardiopulmonary resuscitation: improved outcome during a simulated single lay-rescuer scenario. *Circulation*. 2002;105:645–649.
114. Baskett P, Nolan J, Parr M. Tidal volumes which are perceived to be adequate for resuscitation. *Resuscitation*. 1996;31:231–234.
115. Aufderheide TP, Sigurdsson G, Pirrallo RG, Yannopoulos D, McKnite S, von Briesen C, Sparks CW, Conrad CJ, Provo TA, Lurie KG. Hyperventilation-induced hypotension during cardiopulmonary resuscitation. *Circulation*. 2004;109:1960–1965.
116. Garnett AR, Ornato JP, Gonzalez ER, Johnson EB. End-tidal carbon dioxide monitoring during cardiopulmonary resuscitation. *JAMA*. 1987; 257:512–515.
117. American Heart Association in collaboration with International Liaison Committee on Resuscitation. Guidelines 2000 for Cardiopulmonary Resuscitation and Emergency Cardiovascular Care: International Con-

sensus on Science, Part 3: adult basic life support. *Circulation*. 2000; 102(suppl I):I-22–I-59.

118. Paradis NA, Martin GB, Goetting MG, Rosenberg JM, Rivers EP, Appleton TJ, Nowak RM. Simultaneous aortic, jugular bulb, and right atrial pressures during cardiopulmonary resuscitation in humans: insights into mechanisms. *Circulation*. 1989;80:361–368.
119. Idris AH, Staples ED, O'Brien DJ, Melker RJ, Rush WJ, Del Duca KD, Falk JL. Effect of ventilation on acid-base balance and oxygenation in low blood-flow states. *Crit Care Med*. 1994;22:1827–1834.
120. Idris AH, Gabrielli A, Caruso L. Smaller tidal volume is safe and effective for bag-valve-ventilation, but not for mouth-to-mouth ventilation: an animal model for basic life support [abstract]. *Circulation*. 1999;100(suppl I):I-644.
121. Idris A, Wenzel V, Banner MJ, Melker RJ. Smaller tidal volumes minimize gastric inflation during CPR with an unprotected airway [abstract]. *Circulation*. 1995;92(suppl):I-759.
122. Dorph E, Wik L, Steen PA. Arterial blood gases with 700 ml tidal volumes during out-of-hospital CPR. *Resuscitation*. 2004;61:23–27.
123. Winkler M, Mauritz W, Hackl W, Gilly H, Weindlmayr-Goettel M, Steinbereithner K, Schindler I. Effects of half the tidal volume during cardiopulmonary resuscitation on acid-base balance and haemodynamics in pigs. *Eur J Emerg Med*. 1998;5:201–206.
124. Dorges V, Ocker H, Hagelberg S, Wenzel V, Idris AH, Schmucker P. Smaller tidal volumes with room-air are not sufficient to ensure adequate oxygenation during bag-valve-mask ventilation. *Resuscitation*. 2000;44:37–41.
125. Dorges V, Ocker H, Wenzel V, Sauer C, Schmucker P. Emergency airway management by non-anaesthesia house officers–a comparison of three strategies. *Emerg Med J*. 2001;18:90–94.
126. Bowman FP, Menegazzi JJ, Check BD, Duckett TM. Lower esophageal sphincter pressure during prolonged cardiac arrest and resuscitation. *Ann Emerg Med*. 1995;26:216–219.
127. Davis K Jr, Johannigman JA, Johnson RC Jr, Branson RD. Lung compliance following cardiac arrest [published correction appears in *Acad Emerg Med*. 1995;2:1115]. *Acad Emerg Med*. 1995;2:874–878.
128. Wenzel V, Idris AH, Banner MJ, Fuerst RS, Tucker KJ. The composition of gas given by mouth-to-mouth ventilation during CPR. *Chest*. 1994;106:1806–1810.
129. Mejicano GC, Maki DG. Infections acquired during cardiopulmonary resuscitation: estimating the risk and defining strategies for prevention. *Ann Intern Med*. 1998;129:813–828.
130. Ornato JP, Hallagan LF, McMahan SB, Peeples EH, Rostafinski AG. Attitudes of BCLS instructors about mouth-to-mouth resuscitation during the AIDS epidemic. *Ann Emerg Med*. 1990;19:151–156.
131. Brenner BE, Van DC, Cheng D, Lazar EJ. Determinants of reluctance to perform CPR among residents and applicants: the impact of experience on helping behavior. *Resuscitation*. 1997;35:203–211.
132. Hew P, Brenner B, Kaufman J. Reluctance of paramedics and emergency medical technicians to perform mouth-to-mouth resuscitation. *J Emerg Med*. 1997;15:279–284.
133. Terndrup TE, Warner DA. Infant ventilation and oxygenation by basic life support providers: comparison of methods. *Prehospital Disaster Med*. 1992;7:35–40.
134. Hess D, Ness C, Oppel A, Rhoads K. Evaluation of mouth-to-mask ventilation devices. *Respir Care*. 1989;34:191–195.
135. Figura N. Mouth-to-mouth resuscitation and *Helicobacter pylori* infection. *Lancet*. 1996;347:1342.
136. Heilman KM, Muschenheim C. Primary cutaneous tuberculosis resulting from mouth-to-mouth respiration. *N Engl J Med*. 1965;273: 1035–1036.
137. Simmons M, Deao D, Moon L, Peters K, Cavanaugh S. Bench evaluation: three face-shield CPR barrier devices. *Respir Care*. 1995;40: 618–623.
138. Ruben H. The immediate treatment of respiratory failure. *Br J Anaesth*. 1964;36:542–549.
139. Bhalla RK, Corrigan A, Roland NJ. Comparison of two face masks used to deliver early ventilation to laryngectomized patients. *Ear Nose Throat J*. 2004;83:414–416.
140. Barnes TA. Emergency ventilation techniques and related equipment. *Respir Care*. 1992;37:673–694.
141. Johannigman JA, Branson RD, Davis K Jr, Hurst JM. Techniques of emergency ventilation: a model to evaluate tidal volume, airway pressure, and gastric insufflation. *J Trauma*. 1991;31:93–98.
142. Elam JO. Bag-valve-mask O_2 ventilation. In: Safar P, Elam JO, eds. *Advances in Cardiopulmonary Resuscitation: The Wolf Creek Conference on Cardiopulmonary Resuscitation*. New York, NY: Springer-Verlag, Inc;1977:73–79.
143. Dailey RH. *The Airway: Emergency Management*. St Louis, Mo: Mosby Year Book; 1992.
144. Elling R, Politis J. An evaluation of emergency medical technicians' ability to use manual ventilation devices. *Ann Emerg Med*. 1983;12: 765–768.
145. Wakeling HG, Butler PJ, Baxter PJC. The laryngeal mask airway: a comparison between two insertion techniques. *Anesth Analg*. 1997;85: 687–690.
146. Voyagis GS, Photakis D, Kellari A, Kostanti E, Kaklis S, Secha-Dousaitou PN, Tsakiropoulou-Alexiou H. The laryngeal mask airway: a survey of its usage in 1,096 patients. *Minerva Anestesiol*. 1996;62: 277–280.
147. Baraka A, Salem R. The Combitube oesophageal-tracheal double lumen airway for difficult intubation [letter]. *Can J Anaesth*. 1993;40: 1222–1223.
148. Frass M, Frenzer R, Rauscha F, Schuster E, Glogar D. Ventilation with the esophageal tracheal combitube in cardiopulmonary resuscitation: promptness and effectiveness. *Chest*. 1988;93:781–784.
149. Frass M, Rodler S, Frenzer R, Ilias W, Leithner C, Lackner F. Esophageal tracheal combitube, endotracheal airway, and mask: comparison of ventilatory pressure curves. *J Trauma*. 1989;29:1476–1479.
150. Dorph E, Wik L, Stromme TA, Eriksen M, Steen PA. Oxygen delivery and return of spontaneous circulation with ventilation:compression ratio 2:30 versus chest compressions only CPR in pigs. *Resuscitation*. 2004; 60:309–318.
151. Berg RA, Sanders AB, Kern KB, Hilwig RW, Heidenreich JW, Porter ME, Ewy GA. Adverse hemodynamic effects of interrupting chest compressions for rescue breathing during cardiopulmonary resuscitation for ventricular fibrillation cardiac arrest. *Circulation*. 2001;104: 2465–2470.
152. Sellick BA. Cricoid pressure to control regurgitation of stomach contents during induction of anaesthesia. *Lancet*. 1961;2:404–406.
153. Petito SP, Russell WJ. The prevention of gastric inflation—a neglected benefit of cricoid pressure. *Anaesth Intensive Care*. 1988;16:139–143.
154. Perkins GD, Stephenson B, Hulme J, Monsieurs KG. Birmingham assessment of breathing study (BABS). *Resuscitation*. 2005;64: 109–113.
155. Moule P. Checking the carotid pulse: diagnostic accuracy in students of the healthcare professions. *Resuscitation*. 2000;44:195–201.
156. Stiell I, Nichol G, Wells G, De Maio V, Nesbitt L, Blackburn J, Spaite D, Group OS. Health-related quality of life is better for cardiac arrest survivors who received citizen cardiopulmonary resuscitation. *Circulation*. 2003;108:1939–1944.
157. International Liaison Committee on Resuscitation. 2005 International Consensus on Cardiopulmonary Resuscitation and Emergency Cardiovascular Care Science With Treatment Recommendations. *Circulation*. 2005;112:III-1–III-136.
158. Kouwenhoven WB, Jude JR, Knickerbocker GG. Closed-chest cardiac massage. *JAMA*. 1960;173:1064–1067.
159. Handley AJ, Handley JA. Performing chest compressions in a confined space. *Resuscitation*. 2004;61:55–61.
160. Perkins GD, Stephenson BT, Smith CM, Gao F. A comparison between over-the-head and standard cardiopulmonary resuscitation. *Resuscitation*. 2004;61:155–161.
161. Perkins GD, Benny R, Giles S, Gao F, Tweed MJ. Do different mattresses affect the quality of cardiopulmonary resuscitation? *Intensive Care Med*. 2003;29:2330–2335.
162. Tweed M, Tweed C, Perkins GD. The effect of differing support surfaces on the efficacy of chest compressions using a resuscitation manikin model. *Resuscitation*. 2001;51:179–183.
163. Handley AJ. Teaching hand placement for chest compression–a simpler technique. *Resuscitation*. 2002;53:29–36.
164. Liberman M, Lavoie A, Mulder D, Sampalis J. Cardiopulmonary resuscitation: errors made by pre-hospital emergency medical personnel. *Resuscitation*. 1999;42:47–55.
165. Kundra P, Dey S, Ravishankar M. Role of dominant hand position during external cardiac compression. *Br J Anaesth*. 2000;84:491–493.
166. Aufderheide TP, Pirrallo RG, Yannopoulos D, Klein JP, von Briesen C, Sparks CW, Deja KA, Conrad CJ, Kitscha DJ, Provo TA, Lurie KG. Incomplete chest wall decompression: a clinical evaluation of CPR performance by EMS personnel and assessment of alternative manual chest compression-decompression techniques. *Resuscitation*. 2005;64: 353–362.
167. Yannopoulos D, McKnite S, Aufderheide TP, Sigurdsson G, Pirrallo RG, Benditt D, Lurie KG. Effects of incomplete chest wall decompression during cardiopulmonary resuscitation on coronary and cerebral perfusion pressures in a porcine model of cardiac arrest. *Resuscitation*. 2005;64:363–372.
168. Handley AJ, Handley JA. The relationship between rate of chest compression and compression:relaxation ratio. *Resuscitation*. 1995;30: 237–241.

169. Fitzgerald KR, Babbs CF, Frissora HA, Davis RW, Silver DI. Cardiac output during cardiopulmonary resuscitation at various compression rates and durations. *Am J Physiol*. 1981;241:H442–H448.
170. Halperin HR, Tsitlik JE, Guerci AD, Mellits ED, Levin HR, Shi AY, Chandra N, Weisfeldt ML. Determinants of blood flow to vital organs during cardiopulmonary resuscitation in dogs. *Circulation*. 1986;73: 539–550.
171. Swart GL, Mateer JR, DeBehnke DJ, Jameson SJ, Osborn JL. The effect of compression duration on hemodynamics during mechanical high-impulse CPR. *Acad Emerg Med*. 1994;1:430–437.
172. Wik L, Kramer-Johansen J, Myklebust H, Sorebo H, Svensson L, Fellows B, Steen PA. Quality of cardiopulmonary resuscitation during out-of-hospital cardiac arrest. *JAMA*. 2005;293:299–304.
173. Abella BS, Alvarado JP, Myklebust H, Edelson DP, Barry A, O'Hearn N, Vanden Hoek TL, Becker LB. Quality of cardiopulmonary resuscitation during in-hospital cardiac arrest. *JAMA*. 2005;293:305–310.
174. Yu T, Weil MH, Tang W, Sun S, Klouche K, Povoas H, Bisera J. Adverse outcomes of interrupted precordial compression during automated defibrillation. *Circulation*. 2002;106:368–372.
175. Swenson RD, Weaver WD, Niskanen RA, Martin J, Dahlberg S. Hemodynamics in humans during conventional and experimental methods of cardiopulmonary resuscitation. *Circulation*. 1988;78:630–639.
176. Kern KB, Sanders AB, Raife J, Milander MM, Otto CW, Ewy GA. A study of chest compression rates during cardiopulmonary resuscitation in humans: the importance of rate-directed chest compressions. *Arch Intern Med*. 1992;152:145–149.
177. Abella BS, Sandbo N, Vassilatos P, Alvarado JP, O'Hearn N, Wigder HN, Hoffman P, Tynus K, Vanden Hoek TL, Becker LB. Chest compression rates during cardiopulmonary resuscitation are suboptimal: a prospective study during in-hospital cardiac arrest. *Circulation*. 2005; 111:428–434.
178. Berg RA, Cobb LA, Doherty A, Ewy GA, Gerardi MJ, Handley AJ, Kinney S, Phillips B, Sanders A, Wyllie J. Chest compressions and basic life support-defibrillation. *Ann Emerg Med*. 2001;37:S26–S35.
179. Berg RA, Hilwig RW, Kern KB, Sanders AB, Xavier LC, Ewy GA. Automated external defibrillation versus manual defibrillation for prolonged ventricular fibrillation: lethal delays of chest compressions before and after countershocks. *Ann Emerg Med*. 2003;42:458–467.
180. Berg RA, Hilwig RW, Kern KB, Ewy GA. "Bystander" chest compressions and assisted ventilation independently improve outcome from piglet asphyxial pulseless "cardiac arrest." *Circulation*. 2000;101: 1743–1748.
181. Berg RA, Kern KB, Hilwig RW, Ewy GA. Assisted ventilation during 'bystander' CPR in a swine acute myocardial infarction model does not improve outcome. *Circulation*. 1997;96:4364–4371.
182. Greingor JL. Quality of cardiac massage with ratio compression-ventilation 5/1 and 15/2. *Resuscitation*. 2002;55:263–267.
183. Feneley MP, Maier GW, Kern KB, Gaynor JW, Gall SA Jr, Sanders AB, Raessler K, Muhlbaier LH, Rankin JS, Ewy GA. Influence of compression rate on initial success of resuscitation and 24 hour survival after prolonged manual cardiopulmonary resuscitation in dogs. *Circulation*. 1988;77:240–250.
184. Ochoa FJ, Ramalle-Gomara E, Carpintero JM, Garcia A, Saralegui I. Competence of health professionals to check the carotid pulse. *Resuscitation*. 1998;37:173–175.
185. Babbs CF, Kern KB. Optimum compression to ventilation ratios in CPR under realistic, practical conditions: a physiological and mathematical analysis. *Resuscitation*. 2002;54:147–157.
186. Berg RA, Kern KB, Hilwig RW, Berg MD, Sanders AB, Otto CW, Ewy GA. Assisted ventilation does not improve outcome in a porcine model of single-rescuer bystander cardiopulmonary resuscitation. *Circulation*. 1997;95:1635–1641.
187. Berg RA, Kern KB, Hilwig RW, Ewy GA. Assisted ventilation during 'bystander' CPR in a swine acute myocardial infarction model does not improve outcome. *Circulation*. 1997;96:4364–4371.
188. Kern KB, Hilwig RW, Berg RA, Ewy GA. Efficacy of chest compression-only BLS CPR in the presence of an occluded airway. *Resuscitation*. 1998;39:179–188.
189. Berg RA, Sanders AB, Milander M, Tellez D, Liu P, Beyda D. Efficacy of audio-prompted rate guidance in improving resuscitator performance of cardiopulmonary resuscitation on children. *Acad Emerg Med*. 1994; 1:35–40.
190. Barsan WG. Experimental design for study of cardiopulmonary resuscitation in dogs. *Ann Emerg Med*. 1981;10:135–137.
191. Milander MM, Hiscok PS, Sanders AB, Kern KB, Berg RA, Ewy GA. Chest compression and ventilation rates during cardiopulmonary resuscitation: the effects of audible tone guidance. *Acad Emerg Med*. 1995; 2:708–713.
192. Thomas SH, Stone CK, Austin PE, March JA, Brinkley S. Utilization of a pressure-sensing monitor to improve in-flight chest compressions. *Am J Emerg Med*. 1995;13:155–157.
193. Wik L, Thowsen J, Steen PA. An automated voice advisory manikin system for training in basic life support without an instructor: a novel approach to CPR training. *Resuscitation*. 2001;50:167–172.
194. Elding C, Baskett P, Hughes A. The study of the effectiveness of chest compressions using the CPR-plus. *Resuscitation*. 1998;36:169–173.
195. Handley AJ, Handley SA. Improving CPR performance using an audible feedback system suitable for incorporation into an automated external defibrillator. *Resuscitation*. 2003;57:57–62.
196. Wik L, Myklebust H, Auestad BH, Steen PA. Retention of basic life support skills 6 months after training with an automated voice advisory manikin system without instructor involvement. *Resuscitation*. 2002;52: 273–279.
197. Berg RA, Kern KB, Sanders AB, Otto CW, Hilwig RW, Ewy GA. Bystander cardiopulmonary resuscitation: is ventilation necessary? *Circulation*. 1993;88:1907–1915.
198. Chandra NC, Gruben KG, Tsitlik JE, Brower R, Guerci AD, Halperin HH, Weisfeldt ML, Permutt S. Observations of ventilation during resuscitation in a canine model. *Circulation*. 1994;90:3070–3075.
199. Tang W, Weil MH, Sun S, Kette D, Gazmuri RJ, O'Connell F, Bisera J. Cardiopulmonary resuscitation by precordial compression but without mechanical ventilation. *Am J Respir Crit Care Med*. 1994;150: 1709–1713.
200. Berg RA, Wilcoxson D, Hilwig RW, Kern KB, Sanders AB, Otto CW, Eklund DK, Ewy GA. The need for ventilatory support during bystander CPR. *Ann Emerg Med*. 1995;26:342–350.
201. Becker LB, Berg RA, Pepe PE, Idris AH, Aufderheide TP, Barnes TA, Stratton SJ, Chandra NC. A reappraisal of mouth-to-mouth ventilation during bystander-initiated cardiopulmonary resuscitation. A statement for healthcare professionals from the Ventilation Working Group of the Basic Life Support and Pediatric Life Support Subcommittees, American Heart Association. *Resuscitation*. 1997;35:189–201.
202. Sirbaugh PE, Pepe PE, Shook JE, Kimball KT, Goldman MJ, Ward MA, Mann DM. A prospective, population-based study of the demographics, epidemiology, management, and outcome of out-of-hospital pediatric cardiopulmonary arrest [published correction appears in *Ann Emerg Med*. 1999;33:358]. *Ann Emerg Med*. 1999;33:174–184.
203. Waalewijn RA, Tijssen JGP, Koster RW. Bystander initiated actions in out-of-hospital cardiopulmonary resuscitation: results from the Amsterdam Resuscitation Study (ARREST).*Resuscitation*. 2001;50: 273–279.
204. Van Hoeyweghen RJ, Bossaert LL, Mullie A, Calle P, Martens P, Buylaert WA, Delooz H. Quality and efficiency of bystander CPR. Belgian Cerebral Resuscitation Study Group. *Resuscitation*. 1993;26: 47–52.
205. Berg RA, Hilwig RW, Kern KB, Babar I, Ewy GA. Simulated mouth-to-mouth ventilation and chest compressions (bystander cardiopulmonary resuscitation) improves outcome in a swine model of prehospital pediatric asphyxial cardiac arrest. *Crit Care Med*. 1999;27:1893–1899.
206. Berg RA. Role of mouth-to-mouth rescue breathing in bystander cardiopulmonary resuscitation for asphyxial cardiac arrest. *Crit Care Med*. 2000;28(suppl):N193–N195.
207. Hallstrom AP. Dispatcher-assisted "phone" cardiopulmonary resuscitation by chest compression alone or with mouth-to-mouth ventilation. *Crit Care Med*. 2000;28:N190–N192.
208. Weil MH, Rackow EC, Trevino R, Grundler W, Falk JL, Griffel MI. Difference in acid-base state between venous and arterial blood during cardiopulmonary resuscitation. *N Engl J Med*. 1986;315:153–156.
209. Sanders AB, Otto CW, Kern KB, Rogers JN, Perrault P, Ewy GA. Acid-base balance in a canine model of cardiac arrest. *Ann Emerg Med*. 1988;17:667–671.
210. Criley JM, Blaufuss AH, Kissel GL. Cough-induced cardiac compression: self-administered from of cardiopulmonary resuscitation. *JAMA*. 1976;236:1246–1250.
211. Niemann JT, Rosborough JP, Niskanen RA, Alferness C, Criley JM. Mechanical "cough" cardiopulmonary resuscitation during cardiac arrest in dogs. *Am J Cardiol*. 1985;55:199–204.
212. Miller B, Cohen A, Serio A, Bettock D. Hemodynamics of cough cardiopulmonary resuscitation in a patient with sustained torsades de pointes/ventricular flutter. *J Emerg Med*. 1994;12:627–632.
213. Rieser MJ. The use of cough-CPR in patients with acute myocardial infarction. *J Emerg Med*. 1992;10:291–293.
214. Miller B, Lesnefsky E, Heyborne T, Schmidt B, Freeman K, Breckinridge S, Kelley K, Mann D, Reiter M. Cough-cardiopulmonary resuscitation in the cardiac catheterization laboratory: hemodynamics during an episode of prolonged hypotensive ventricular tachycardia. *Cathet Cardiovasc Diagn*. 1989;18:168–171.

215. Bircher N, Safar P, Eshel G, Stezoski W. Cerebral and hemodynamic variables during cough-induced CPR in dogs. *Crit Care Med*. 1982;10: 104–107.
216. Saba SE, David SW. Sustained consciousness during ventricular fibrillation: case report of cough cardiopulmonary resuscitation. *Cathet Cardiovasc Diagn*. 1996;37:47–48.
217. Mazer SP, Weisfeldt M, Bai D, Cardinale C, Arora R, Ma C, Sciacca RR, Chong D, Rabbani LE. Reverse CPR: a pilot study of CPR in the prone position. *Resuscitation*. 2003;57:279–285.
218. Sun WZ, Huang FY, Kung KL, Fan SZ, Chen TL. Successful cardiopulmonary resuscitation of two patients in the prone position using reversed precordial compression. *Anesthesiology*. 1992;77:202–204.
219. Tobias JD, Mencio GA, Atwood R, Gurwitz GS. Intraoperative cardiopulmonary resuscitation in the prone position. *J Pediatr Surg*. 1994;29: 1537–1538.
220. Brown J, Rogers J, Soar J. Cardiac arrest during surgery and ventilation in the prone position: a case report and systematic review. *Resuscitation*. 2001;50:233–238.
221. Jacobs IG, Finn JC, Oxer HF, Jelinek GA. CPR before defibrillation in out-of-hospital cardiac arrest: a randomized trial. *Emerg Med Australas*. 2005;17:39–45.
222. Perkins GD. In-water resuscitation: a pilot evaluation. *Resuscitation*. 2005;65:321–324.
223. March NF, Matthews RC. New techniques in external cardiac compressions: aquatic cardiopulmonary resuscitation. *JAMA*. 1980;244: 1229–1232.
224. Rosen P, Stoto M, Harley J. The use of the Heimlich maneuver in near-drowning: Institute of Medicine report. *J Emerg Med*. 1995;13: 397–405.
225. Watson RS, Cummings P, Quan L, Bratton S, Weiss NS. Cervical spine injuries among submersion victims. *J Trauma*. 2001;51:658–662.
226. Kewalramani LS, Kraus JF. Acute spinal-cord lesions from diving–epidemiological and clinical features. *West J Med*. 1977;126:353–361.
227. Hwang V, Shofer FS, Durbin DR, Baren JM. Prevalence of traumatic injuries in drowning and near drowning in children and adolescents. *Arch Pediatr Adolesc Med*. 2003;157:50–53.
228. Green BA, Gabrielsen MA, Hall WJ, O'Heir J. Analysis of swimming pool accidents resulting in spinal cord injury. *Paraplegia*. 1980;18: 94–100.
229. Good RP, Nickel VL. Cervical spine injuries resulting from water sports. *Spine*. 1980;5:502–506.
230. Goh SH, Low BY. Drowning and near-drowning–some lessons learnt. *Ann Acad Med Singapore*. 1999;28:183–188.
231. Branche CM, Sniezek JE, Sattin RW, Mirkin IR. Water recreation-related spinal injuries: risk factors in natural bodies of water. *Accid Anal Prev*. 1991;23:13–17.
232. Handley AJ. Recovery position. *Resuscitation*. 1993;26:93–95.
233. Turner S, Turner I, Chapman D, Howard P, Champion P, Hatfield J, James A, Marshall S, Barber S. A comparative study of the 1992 and 1997 recovery positions for use in the UK. *Resuscitation*. 1998;39: 153–160.
234. Fulstow R, Smith GB. The new recovery position, a cautionary tale. *Resuscitation*. 1993;26:89–91.
235. Rathgeber J, Panzer W, Gunther U, Scholz M, Hoeft A, Bahr J, Kettler D. Influence of different types of recovery positions on perfusion indices of the forearm. *Resuscitation*. 1996;32:13–17.
236. Gunn BD, Eizenberg N, Silberstein M, McMeeken JM, Tully EA, Stillman BC, Brown DJ, Gutteridge GA. How should an unconscious person with a suspected neck injury be positioned? *Prehosp Disaster Med*. 1995;10:239–244.
237. Blake WE, Stillman BC, Eizenberg N, Briggs C, McMeeken JM. The position of the spine in the recovery position–an experimental comparison between the lateral recovery position and the modified HAINES position. *Resuscitation*. 2002;53:289–297.
238. Fingerhut LA, Cox CS, Warner M. International comparative analysis of injury mortality: findings from the ICE on injury statistics. International Collaborative Effort on Injury Statistics. *Adv Data*. 1998:1–20.
239. Redding JS. The choking controversy: critique of evidence on the Heimlich maneuver. *Crit Care Med*. 1979;7:475–479.
240. Vilke GM, Smith AM, Ray LU, Steen PJ, Murrin PA, Chan TC. Airway obstruction in children aged less than 5 years: the prehospital experience. *Prehosp Emerg Care*. 2004;8:196–199.
241. Ingalls TH. Heimlich versus a slap on the back. *N Engl J Med*. 1979; 300:990.
242. Heimlich HJ. First aid for choking children: back blows and chest thrusts cause complications and death. *Pediatrics*. 1982;70:120–125.
243. Heimlich HJ. A life-saving maneuver to prevent food choking. *JAMA*. 1975;234:398–401.
244. Heimlich HJ, Hoffmann KA, Canestri FR. Food-choking and drowning deaths prevented by external subdiaphragmatic compression: physiological basis. *Ann Thorac Surg*. 1975;20:188–195.
245. Nelson KR. Heimlich maneuver for esophageal obstruction. *N Engl J Med*. 1989;320:1016.
246. Penny RW. The Heimlich manoeuvre. *BMJ (Clin Res Ed)*. 1983;286: 1145–1146.
247. Lapostolle F, Desmaizieres M, Adnet F, Minadeo J. Telephone-assisted Heimlich maneuver. *Ann Emerg Med*. 2000;36:171.
248. Skulberg A. Chest compression–an alternative to the Heimlich manoeuver? [letter]. *Resuscitation*. 1992;24:91.
249. Heimlich HJ. Death from food-choking prevented by a new life-saving maneuver. *Heart Lung*. 1976;5:755–758.
250. Brauner DJ. The Heimlich maneuver: procedure of choice? *J Am Geriatr Soc*. 1987;35:78.
251. Gallardo A, Rosado R, Ramirez D, Medina P, Mezquita S, Sanchez J. Rupture of the lesser gastric curvature after a Heimlich maneuver. *Surg Endosc*. 2003;17:1495.
252. Ayerdi J, Gupta SK, Sampson LN, Deshmukh N. Acute abdominal aortic thrombosis following the Heimlich maneuver. *Cardiovasc Surg*. 2002;10:154–156.
253. Tung PH, Law S, Chu KM, Law WL, Wong J. Gastric rupture after Heimlich maneuver and cardiopulmonary resuscitation. *Hepatogastroenterology*. 2001;48:109–111.
254. Majumdar A, Sedman PC. Gastric rupture secondary to successful Heimlich manoeuvre. *Postgrad Med J*. 1998;74:609–610.
255. Bintz M, Cogbill TH. Gastric rupture after the Heimlich maneuver. *J Trauma*. 1996;40:159–160.
256. Dupre MW, Silva E, Brotman S. Traumatic rupture of the stomach secondary to Heimlich maneuver. *Am J Emerg Med*. 1993;11:611–612.
257. van der Ham AC, Lange JF. Traumatic rupture of the stomach after Heimlich maneuver. *J Emerg Med*. 1990;8:713–715.
258. Cowan M, Bardole J, Dlesk A. Perforated stomach following the Heimlich maneuver. *Am J Emerg Med*. 1987;5:121–122.
259. Croom DW. Rupture of stomach after attempted Heimlich maneuver. *JAMA*. 1983;250:2602–2603.
260. Visintine RE, Baick CH. Ruptured stomach after Heimlich maneuver. *JAMA*. 1975;234:415.
261. Mack L, Forbes TL, Harris KA. Acute aortic thrombosis following incorrect application of the Heimlich maneuver. *Ann Vasc Surg*. 2002; 16:130–133.
262. Roehm EF, Twiest MW, Williams RC Jr. Abdominal aortic thrombosis in association with an attempted Heimlich maneuver. *JAMA*. 1983;249: 1186–1187.
263. Kirshner RL, Green RM. Acute thrombosis of abdominal aortic aneurysm subsequent to Heimlich maneuver: a case report. *J Vasc Surg*. 1985;2:594–596.
264. Rakotoharinandrasana H, Petit E, Dumas P, Vandermarcq P, Gil R, Neau JP. [Internal carotid artery dissection after Heimlich maneuver]. *Ann Fr Anesth Reanim*. 2003;22:43–45.
265. Wolf DA. Heimlich trauma: a violent maneuver. *Am J Forensic Med Pathol*. 2001;22:65–67.
266. Valero V. Mesenteric laceration complicating a Heimlich maneuver. *Ann Emerg Med*. 1986;15:105–106.
267. Ujjin V, Ratanasit S, Nagendran T. Diaphragmatic hernia as a complication of the Heimlich maneuver. *Int Surg*. 1984;69:175–176.
268. Rich GH. Pneumomediastinum following the Heimlich maneuver. *Ann Emerg Med*. 1980;9:279–280.
269. Agia GA, Hurst DJ. Pneumomediastinum following the Heimlich maneuver. *JACEP*. 1979;8:473–475.
270. Meredith MJ, Liebowitz R. Rupture of the esophagus caused by the Heimlich maneuver. *Ann Emerg Med*. 1986;15:106–107.
271. Chapman JH, Menapace FJ, Howell RR. Ruptured aortic valve cusp: a complication of the Heimlich maneuver. *Ann Emerg Med*. 1983;12: 446–448.
272. Orlowski JP. Vomiting as a complication of the Heimlich maneuver. *JAMA*. 1987;258:512–513.
273. Langhelle A, Sunde K, Wik L, Steen PA. Airway pressure with chest compressions versus Heimlich manoeuvre in recently dead adults with complete airway obstruction. *Resuscitation*. 2000;44:105–108.
274. Guildner CW, Williams D, Subitch T. Airway obstructed by foreign material: the Heimlich maneuver. *JACEP*. 1976;5:675–677.
275. Ruben H, Macnaughton FI. The treatment of food-choking. *Practitioner*. 1978;221:725–729.
276. Hartrey R, Bingham RM. Pharyngeal trauma as a result of blind finger sweeps in the choking child. *J Accid Emerg Med*. 1995;12:52–54.
277. Kabbani M, Goodwin SR. Traumatic epiglottis following blind finger sweep to remove a pharyngeal foreign body. *Clin Pediatr (Phila)*. 1995;34:495–497.

Part 5: Electrical Therapies

Automated External Defibrillators, Defibrillation, Cardioversion, and Pacing

This chapter presents guidelines for defibrillation with automated external defibrillators (AEDs) and manual defibrillators, synchronized cardioversion, and pacing. AEDs may be used by lay rescuers and healthcare providers as part of basic life support. Manual defibrillation, cardioversion, and pacing are advanced life support therapies.

Defibrillation Plus CPR: A Critical Combination

Early defibrillation is critical to survival from sudden cardiac arrest (SCA) for several reasons: (1) the most frequent initial rhythm in witnessed SCA is ventricular fibrillation (VF), (2) the treatment for VF is electrical defibrillation, (3) the probability of successful defibrillation diminishes rapidly over time, and (4) VF tends to deteriorate to asystole within a few minutes.[1]

Several studies have documented the effects of time to defibrillation and the effects of bystander CPR on survival from SCA. For every minute that passes between collapse and defibrillation, survival rates from witnessed VF SCA decrease 7% to 10% if no CPR is provided.[1] When bystander CPR is provided, the decrease in survival rates is more gradual and averages 3% to 4% per minute from collapse to defibrillation.[1,2] CPR can double[1–3] or triple[4] survival from witnessed SCA at most intervals to defibrillation.

If bystanders provide immediate CPR, many adults in VF can survive with intact neurologic function, especially if defibrillation is performed within about 5 minutes after SCA.[5,6] CPR prolongs VF[7–9] (ie, the window of time during which defibrillation can occur) and provides a small amount of blood flow that may maintain some oxygen and substrate delivery to the heart and brain.[10] Basic CPR alone, however, is unlikely to eliminate VF and restore a perfusing rhythm.

New Recommendations to Integrate CPR and AED Use

To treat VF SCA, rescuers must be able to rapidly integrate CPR with use of the AED. To give the victim the best chance of survival, 3 actions must occur within the first moments of a cardiac arrest: (1) activation of the emergency medical services (EMS) system or emergency medical response system, (2) provision of CPR, and (3) operation of an AED. When 2 or more rescuers are present, activation of EMS and initiation of CPR can occur simultaneously.

(*Circulation*. **2005;112:IV-35-IV-46.**)

This special supplement to *Circulation* is freely available at http://www.circulationaha.org

DOI: 10.1161/CIRCULATIONAHA.105.166554

Delays to either start of CPR or defibrillation can reduce survival from SCA. In the 1990s some predicted that CPR could be rendered obsolete by the widespread development of community AED programs. Cobb[6] noted, however, that as more Seattle first responders were equipped with AEDs, survival rates from SCA unexpectedly fell. He attributed this decline to reduced emphasis on CPR, and there is growing evidence to support this view. Part 4: "Adult Basic Life Support" summarizes the evidence on the importance of effective chest compressions and minimizing interruptions in providing compressions.

Two critical questions about integration of CPR with defibrillation were evaluated during the 2005 Consensus Conference.[11] The first question concerns whether CPR should be provided before defibrillation is attempted. The second question concerns the number of shocks to be delivered in a sequence before the rescuer resumes CPR.

Shock First Versus CPR First

When any rescuer witnesses an out-of-hospital arrest and an AED is immediately available on-site, the rescuer should use the AED as soon as possible. Healthcare providers who treat cardiac arrest in hospitals and other facilities with AEDs on-site should provide immediate CPR and should use the AED/defibrillator as soon as it is available. These recommendations are designed to support early CPR and early defibrillation, particularly when an AED is available within moments of the onset of SCA.

When an out-of-hospital cardiac arrest is not witnessed by EMS personnel, they may give about 5 cycles of CPR before checking the ECG rhythm and attempting defibrillation (Class IIb). One cycle of CPR consists of 30 compressions and 2 breaths. When compressions are delivered at a rate of about 100 per minute, 5 cycles of CPR should take roughly 2 minutes (range: about 1½ to 3 minutes). This recommendation regarding CPR prior to attempted defibrillation is supported by 2 clinical studies (LOE 2[5]; LOE 3[6]) of adult out-of-hospital VF SCA. In those studies when EMS call-to-arrival intervals were 4[6] to 5[5] minutes or longer, victims who received 1½ to 3 minutes of CPR before defibrillation showed an increased rate of initial resuscitation, survival to hospital discharge,[5,6] and 1-year survival[5] when compared with those who received immediate defibrillation for VF SCA. One randomized study,[12] however, found no benefit to CPR before defibrillation for non–paramedic-witnessed SCA.

EMS system medical directors may consider implementing a protocol that would allow EMS responders to provide about 5 cycles (about 2 minutes) of CPR before defibrillation of patients found by EMS personnel to be in VF, particularly when the EMS system call-to-response interval is >4 to 5 minutes. There is insufficient evidence to support or refute CPR before defibrillation for in-hospital cardiac arrest.

1-Shock Protocol Versus 3-Shock Sequence

At the time of the 2005 Consensus Conference, no published human or animal studies were found that compared a 1-shock protocol with a 3-stacked shock protocol for treatment of VF cardiac arrest. In animal studies, however, frequent or long interruptions in precordial chest compressions for rhythm analysis[13] or rescue breathing[14,15] were associated with post-resuscitation myocardial dysfunction and reduced survival rates. Secondary analyses of 2 randomized trials[16,17] showed that interruption in chest compressions is associated with a decreased probability of conversion of VF to another rhythm. In 2 recent clinical observational studies (LOE 4) of out-of-hospital[18] and in-hospital[19] CPR by healthcare providers, chest compressions were performed only 51%[18] to 76%[19] of total CPR time.

In 2005 the rhythm analysis for a 3-shock sequence performed by commercially available AEDs resulted in delays of up to 37 seconds between delivery of the first shock and delivery of the first post-shock compression.[13] This delay is difficult to justify in light of the first-shock efficacy of >90% reported by current biphasic defibrillators.[20–25] If 1 shock fails to eliminate VF, the incremental benefit of another shock is low, and resumption of CPR is likely to confer a greater value than another shock. This fact, combined with the data from animal studies documenting harmful effects from interruptions to chest compressions, suggests that a 1-shock scenario plus immediate CPR is reasonable.

When VF/pulseless ventricular tachycardia (VT) is present, the rescuer should deliver 1 shock and should then immediately resume CPR, beginning with chest compressions (Class IIa). The rescuer should not delay resumption of chest compressions to recheck the rhythm or pulse. After 5 cycles (about 2 minutes) of CPR, the AED should then analyze the cardiac rhythm and deliver another shock if indicated (Class IIb). If a nonshockable rhythm is detected, the AED should instruct the rescuer to resume CPR immediately, beginning with chest compressions (Class IIb). Concern that chest compressions might provoke recurrent VF in the presence of a post-shock organized rhythm does not appear to be warranted.[25]

AED voice prompts should not instruct the lay user to reassess the patient at any time. AED manufacturers should seek innovative methods to decrease the amount of time chest compressions are withheld for AED operation. Training materials for lay rescuers should emphasize the importance of continued CPR until basic or advanced life support personnel take over CPR or the victim begins to move.

First-shock efficacy for monophasic shocks is lower than first-shock efficacy for biphasic shocks.[17,26,27] Although the optimal energy level for defibrillation using any of the monophasic or biphasic waveforms has not been determined, a recommendation for higher initial energy when using a monophasic waveform was weighed by expert consensus with consideration of the potential negative effects of a high first-shock energy versus the negative effects of prolonged VF. The consensus was that rescuers using monophasic AEDs should give an initial shock of 360 J; if VF persists after the first shock, second and subsequent shocks of 360 J should be given. This single dose for monophasic shocks is designed to simplify instructions to rescuers but is not a mandate to recall monophasic AEDs for reprogramming. If the monophasic AED being used is programmed to deliver a different first or subsequent dose, that dose is acceptable.

One study compared the effectiveness of 175 J versus 320 J monophasic waveform shocks for out-of-hospital VF cardiac arrest.[28] Approximately 61% of patients who received shocks with either 175 J or 320 J monophasic damped sine waveform were defibrillated with the first shock, which was delivered an average of 10.6 minutes after the call to EMS. There was no significant difference in the percentage of patients who developed advanced atrioventricular (AV) block after 1 shock. AV block was more likely to develop after 2 or 3 shocks of 320 J than after 2 or 3 shocks of 175 J, but the block was transient and did not affect survival to hospital discharge.[28]

Healthcare providers must practice efficient coordination between CPR and defibrillation. When VF is present for more than a few minutes, the myocardium is depleted of oxygen and metabolic substrates. A brief period of chest compressions can deliver oxygen and energy substrates, increasing the likelihood that a perfusing rhythm will return after defibrillation (elimination of VF).[29] Analyses of VF waveform characteristics predictive of shock success have documented that the shorter the time between a chest compression and delivery of a shock, the more likely the shock will be successful.[29,30] Reduction in the interval from compression to shock delivery by even a few seconds can increase the probability of shock success.[16]

The rescuer providing chest compressions should minimize interruptions in chest compressions for rhythm analysis and shock delivery and should be prepared to resume CPR, beginning with chest compressions, as soon as a shock is delivered. When 2 rescuers are present, the rescuer operating the AED should be prepared to deliver a shock as soon as the compressor removes his or her hands from the victim's chest and all rescuers are "clear" of contact with the victim. The lone rescuer should practice coordination of CPR with efficient AED operation.

Defibrillation Waveforms and Energy Levels

Defibrillation involves delivery of current through the chest and to the heart to depolarize myocardial cells and eliminate VF. The energy settings for defibrillators are designed to provide the lowest effective energy needed to terminate VF. Because defibrillation is an electrophysiologic event that occurs in 300 to 500 milliseconds after shock delivery, the term *defibrillation* (shock success) is typically defined as termination of VF for at least 5 seconds following the shock.[31,32] VF frequently recurs after successful shocks, but this recurrence should not be equated with shock failure.[17,25]

Shock success using the typical definition of *defibrillation* should not be confused with resuscitation outcomes such as restoration of a perfusing rhythm, survival to hospital admission, or survival to hospital discharge.[31,33] Although resuscitation outcomes including survival may be affected by many variables in addition to shock delivery, defibrillation programs must strive to improve patient survival, not just shock success.

Modern defibrillators are classified according to 2 types of waveforms: monophasic and biphasic. Monophasic waveform defibrillators were introduced first, but biphasic waveforms are used in almost all AEDs and manual defibrillators sold today. Energy levels vary by type of device. No specific waveform (either monophasic or biphasic) is consistently associated with a higher rate of return of spontaneous circulation (ROSC) or rates of survival to hospital discharge after cardiac arrest.

Monophasic Waveform Defibrillators

Monophasic waveforms deliver current of one polarity (ie, direction of current flow). Monophasic waveforms can be further categorized by the rate at which the current pulse decreases to zero. The monophasic damped sinusoidal waveform (MDS) returns to zero gradually, whereas the monophasic truncated exponential waveform (MTE) current is abruptly returned to baseline (truncated) to zero current flow.

Few monophasic waveform defibrillators are being manufactured but many are still in use. Most of these use MDS waveforms. As noted above, no specific waveform (either monophasic or biphasic) is consistently associated with a greater incidence of ROSC or survival to hospital discharge rates after cardiac arrest than any other specific waveform. Research indicates, however, that when doses equivalent to or lower than monophasic doses are used, biphasic waveform shocks are safe and effective for termination of VF.

Biphasic Waveform Defibrillators

Researchers have collected data from both out-of-hospital[34–36] and in-hospital studies (electrophysiologic studies and implantable cardioverter-defibrillator [ICD] testing and evaluation).[37] Overall this research indicates that lower-energy biphasic waveform shocks have equivalent or higher success for termination of VF than either damped sinusoidal or truncated exponential monophasic waveform shocks delivering escalating energy (200 J, 300 J, 360 J) with successive shocks. No direct comparison of the different biphasic waveforms has been made.

The optimal energy for first-shock biphasic waveform defibrillation yielding the highest termination rate for VF has not been determined. Several randomized (LOE 2)[17,24,27] and observational studies (LOE 5)[26,38] have shown that defibrillation with biphasic waveforms of relatively low energy (≤200 J) is safe and has equivalent or higher efficacy for termination of VF than monophasic waveform shocks of equivalent or higher energy (Class IIa).[32,39–41]

Compensation for patient-to-patient differences in impedance may be achieved by changes in duration and voltage of shocks or by releasing the residual membrane charge (called *burping*). Whether there is an optimal ratio of first-phase to second-phase duration and leading-edge amplitude is unclear. It is unknown whether a waveform more effective for *immediate outcomes* (defibrillation) and *short-term outcomes* (ROSC, survival to hospital admission) results in better *long-term outcomes* (survival to hospital discharge, survival for 1 year). Given the high efficacy of all biphasic waveforms, other determinants of survival (eg, interval from collapse to CPR or defibrillation) are likely to supersede the impact of specific biphasic waveforms or energies.

Fixed and Escalating Energy

Commercially available biphasic AEDs provide either fixed or escalating energy levels.

Multiple prospective human clinical studies (LOE 2)[27,42] and retrospective[17,24,26,38,43,44] studies have failed to identify an optimal biphasic energy level for first or subsequent shocks. Therefore, it is not possible to make a definitive recommendation for the selected energy for the first or subsequent biphasic defibrillation attempts.

Biphasic defibrillators use one of two waveforms, and each waveform has been shown to be effective in terminating VF over a specific dose range. The ideal shock dose for a biphasic device is one that falls within the range that has been documented to be effective using that specific device. Current research confirms that it is reasonable to use selected energies of 150 J to 200 J with a biphasic truncated exponential waveform or 120 J with a rectilinear biphasic waveform for the initial shock. For second and subsequent biphasic shocks, use the same or higher energy (Class IIa). In this context "selected" refers to the energy dose selected by the operator (or programmed by the AED manufacturer). With the rectilinear biphasic waveform device, selected and delivered energies usually differ; delivered energy is typically higher in the usual range of impedance. For example, in a patient with 80 Ω impedance, a selected energy of 120 J will deliver 150 J.

None of the available evidence has shown superiority of either nonescalating or escalating energy biphasic waveform defibrillation for termination of VF. Nonescalating and escalating energy biphasic waveform shocks can be used safely and effectively to terminate short-duration and long-duration VF (Class IIa). The safety and efficacy data related to specific biphasic waveforms, the most effective initial shock, and whether to use escalating sequences require additional studies in both the in-hospital and out-of-hospital settings.

Automated External Defibrillators

AEDs are sophisticated, reliable computerized devices that use voice and visual prompts to guide lay rescuers and healthcare providers to safely defibrillate VF SCA.[34,36,45,46] In recent clinical trials,[18,19] modified prototype AEDs recorded information about frequency and depth of chest compressions during CPR. If such devices become commercially available, AEDs may one day prompt rescuers to improve CPR performance.

Lay Rescuer AED Programs

Since 1995 the American Heart Association (AHA) has recommended the development of lay rescuer AED programs to improve survival rates from out-of-hospital SCA.[47–49] These programs are also known as public access defibrillation, or PAD, programs. The goal of these programs is to shorten the time from onset of VF until CPR and shock delivery by ensuring that AEDs and trained lay rescuers are available in public areas where SCA is likely to occur. To maximize the effectiveness of these programs, the AHA has emphasized the importance of organization, planning, training, linking with the EMS system, and establishing a process of continuous quality improvement.[50,51]

Studies of lay rescuer AED programs in airports[52] and casinos[53,54] and first-responder programs with police officers[26,34,36,44,55–57] have shown a survival rate of 41% to 74% from out-of-hospital witnessed VF SCA when immediate bystander CPR is provided and defibrillation occurs within about 3 to 5 minutes of collapse. These high survival rates, however, are not attained in programs that fail to reduce time to defibrillation.[58–60]

In a large prospective randomized trial (LOE 1)[61] funded by the AHA, the National Heart, Lung, and Blood Institute (NHLBI), and several AED manufacturers, lay rescuer CPR + AED programs in targeted public settings doubled the number of survivors from out-of-hospital VF SCA when compared with programs that provided early EMS call and early CPR. The programs included a planned response, lay rescuer training, and frequent retraining/practice. The following elements are recommended for community lay rescuer AED programs[50,51]:

- A planned and practiced response; typically this requires oversight by a healthcare provider
- Training of anticipated rescuers in CPR and use of the AED
- Link with the local EMS system
- Process of ongoing quality improvement

More information is available on the AHA website: *www.americanheart.org/cpr*. Under the topic "Links on this site," select "Have a question?" and then select "AED."

Lay rescuer AED programs will have the greatest potential impact on survival from SCA if the programs are created in locations where SCA is likely to occur. In the NHLBI trial, programs were established at sites with a history of at least 1 out-of-hospital cardiac arrest every 2 years or where at least 1 out-of-hospital SCA was predicted during the study period (ie, sites having >250 adults over 50 years of age present for >16 h/d).[61]

To be effective, AED programs should be integrated into an overall EMS strategy for treating patients in cardiac arrest. CPR and AED use by public safety first responders (traditional and nontraditional) are recommended to increase survival rates for SCA (Class I). AED programs in public locations where there is a relatively high likelihood of witnessed cardiac arrest (eg, airports, casinos, sports facilities) are recommended (Class I). Because the improvement in survival rates in AED programs is affected by the time to CPR and to defibrillation, sites that deploy AEDs should establish a response plan, train likely responders in CPR and AED use, maintain equipment, and coordinate with local EMS systems.[50,51]

Approximately 80% of out-of-hospital cardiac arrests occur in private or residential settings (LOE 4).[62] Reviewers found no studies that documented the effectiveness of home AED deployment, so there is no recommendation for or against personal or home deployment of AEDs (Class Indeterminate).

AEDs are of no value for arrest not caused by VF/pulseless VT, and they are not effective for treatment of nonshockable rhythms that may develop after termination of VF. Nonperfusing rhythms are present in most patients after shock delivery,[25,26,28,44] and CPR is required until a perfusing rhythm returns. Therefore, the AED rescuer should be trained not only to recognize emergencies and use the AED but also to support ventilation and circulation with CPR as needed.

The mere presence of an AED does not ensure that it will be used when SCA occurs. Even in the NHLBI trial, in which almost 20 000 rescuers were trained to respond to SCA, lay rescuers attempted resuscitation before EMS arrival for only half of the victims of witnessed SCA, and the on-site AED was used for only 34% of the victims who experienced an arrest at locations with AED programs.[61] These findings suggest that lay rescuers need frequent practice to optimize response to emergencies.

It is reasonable for lay rescuer AED programs to implement processes of continuous quality improvement (Class IIa). These quality improvement efforts should use both routine inspections and postevent data (from AED recordings and responder reports) to evaluate the following[50,51]:

- Performance of the emergency response plan, including accurate time intervals for key interventions (such as collapse to shock or no shock advisory to initiation of CPR), and patient outcome
- Responder performance
- AED function, including accuracy of the ECG rhythm analysis
- Battery status and function
- Electrode pad function and readiness, including expiration date

Automated Rhythm Analysis

AEDs have microprocessors that analyze multiple features of the surface ECG signal, including frequency, amplitude, and some integration of frequency and amplitude, such as slope or wave morphology. Filters check for QRS-like signals, radio transmission, or 50- or 60-cycle interference as well as loose electrodes and poor electrode contact. Some devices are programmed to detect spontaneous movement by the patient or others. Prototype defibrillators were used in 2 recent clinical trials evaluating quality of CPR in the out-of-hospital and hospital settings, and they hold promise for future AEDs that may prompt rescuers to improve the quality of CPR provided.[18,19]

AEDs have been tested extensively, both in vitro against libraries of recorded cardiac rhythms and clinically in many field trials in adults[63,64] and children.[65,66] They are extremely accurate in rhythm analysis. Although AEDs are not designed to deliver synchronized shocks (ie, cardioversion for VT with pulses), AEDs will recommend a (nonsynchronized) shock for monomorphic and polymorphic VT if the rate and R-wave morphology exceed preset values.

Electrode Placement

Rescuers should place AED electrode pads on the victim's bare chest in the conventional sternal-apical (anterolateral) position (Class IIa). The right (sternal) chest pad is placed on the victim's right superior-anterior (infraclavicular) chest and the apical (left) pad is placed on the victim's inferior-lateral left chest, lateral to the left breast (Class IIa). Other acceptable pad positions are placement on the lateral chest wall on the right and left sides (biaxillary) or the left pad in the standard apical position and the other pad on the right or left upper back (Class IIa).

When an implantable medical device is located in an area where a pad would normally be placed, position the pad at least 1 inch (2.5 cm) away from the device (Class Indeterminate). If the victim has an ICD that is delivering shocks (ie, the patient's muscles contract in a manner similar to that observed during external defibrillation), allow 30 to 60 seconds for the ICD to complete the treatment cycle before attaching an AED. Occasionally the analysis and shock cycles of automatic ICDs and AEDs will conflict.[67]

Do not place AED electrode pads directly on top of a transdermal medication patch (eg, patch containing nitroglycerin, nicotine, analgesics, hormone replacements, antihypertensives) because the patch may block delivery of energy from the electrode pad to the heart and may cause small burns to the skin.[68] Remove medication patches and wipe the area before attaching the electrode pad.

If an unresponsive victim is lying in water or if the victim's chest is covered with water or the victim is extremely diaphoretic, remove the victim from water and briskly wipe the chest before attaching electrode pads and attempting defibrillation. AEDs can be used when the victim is lying on snow or ice. Most victims do not need any special preparation of the chest other than removal of the clothes from the chest. If the victim has a very hairy chest, it may be necessary to remove some hair so that the electrode pads will adhere to the chest. This may be accomplished by briskly removing an electrode pad (which will remove some hair), or it may be necessary to shave the chest in that area.

AED Use in Children

Cardiac arrest is less common in children than adults, and its causes are more diverse.[69–71] Although VF is not a common arrhythmia in children, it is observed in 5% to 15% of pediatric and adolescent arrests.[71–75] In these patients rapid defibrillation may improve outcomes.[75,76]

The lowest energy dose for effective defibrillation in infants and children is not known. The upper limit for safe defibrillation is also not known, but doses >4 J/kg (as high as 9 J/kg) have effectively defibrillated children[77,78] and pediatric animal models[79] with no significant adverse effects. Based on adult clinical data[17,24] and pediatric animal models,[79–81] biphasic shocks appear to be at least as effective as monophasic shocks and less harmful. Recommended manual defibrillation (monophasic or biphasic) doses are 2 J/kg for the first attempt (Class IIa; LOE 5[82] and 6[79]) and 4 J/kg for subsequent attempts (Class Indeterminate).

Many AEDs can accurately detect VF in children of all ages[65,66] and differentiate shockable from nonshockable rhythms with a high degree of sensitivity and specificity.[65,66] Some are equipped with pediatric attenuator systems (eg, pad-cable systems or a key), to reduce the delivered energy to a dose suitable for children.

For children 1 to 8 years of age the rescuer should use a pediatric dose-attenuator system if one is available.[78,83,84] If the rescuer provides CPR to a child in cardiac arrest and does not have an AED with a pediatric attenuator system, the rescuer should use a standard AED.

There is insufficient data to make a recommendation for or against the use of AEDs for infants <1 year of age (Class Indeterminate). During infancy the risk of VF SCA is unknown, and most cardiac arrest is thought to be related to progression of respiratory failure or shock. As a result there is concern that repeated interruption of CPR to try to detect and treat a rhythm uncommon in that age group may introduce more risk than benefit.[83]

If an AED program is established in systems or institutions that routinely provide care to children, the program should be equipped with AEDs with a high specificity for pediatric shockable rhythms and with a pediatric attenuator system (eg, pediatric pad-cable system or other method of attenuating the shock dose). This statement, however, should not be interpreted as a recommendation for or against AED placement in specific locations where children are present. Ideally healthcare systems that routinely provide care to children at risk for cardiac arrest should have available manual defibrillators capable of dose adjustment.[83]

In-Hospital Use of AEDs

At the time of the 2005 Consensus Conference, there were no published in-hospital randomized trials of AEDs versus manual defibrillators. Evidence from 1 study of fair quality (LOE 4)[85] and a case series (LOE 5)[86] indicated higher rates of survival to hospital discharge when AEDs were used to treat adult VF or pulseless VT in the hospital.

Defibrillation may be delayed when patients develop SCA in unmonitored hospital beds and in outpatient and diagnostic facilities. In such areas several minutes may elapse before centralized response teams arrive with the defibrillator, attach it, and deliver shocks.[87] Despite limited evidence, AEDs should be considered for the hospital setting as a way to facilitate early defibrillation (a goal of ≤3 minutes from collapse), especially in areas where staff have no rhythm recognition skills or defibrillators are used infrequently. An effective system for training and retraining should be in place.

When hospitals deploy AEDs, first-responding personnel should also receive authorization and training to use an AED, with the goal of providing the first shock for any SCA within 3 minutes of collapse. The objective is to make goals for in-hospital use of AEDs consistent with goals established in the out-of-hospital setting.[88] Early defibrillation capability should be available in ambulatory care facilities as well as throughout hospital inpatient areas. Hospitals should monitor collapse-to–first shock intervals and resuscitation outcomes (see Part 3: "Overview of CPR").

Manual Defibrillation

Shock Energies

At present it is clear that both low-energy and high-energy biphasic waveform shocks are effective, but definitive recommendations for the first and subsequent energy levels for all devices cannot be made because devices vary in waveform and reported shock success. Although both escalating-energy and nonescalating-energy defibrillators are available, there is insufficient data to recommend one approach over another. Any claim of superiority at this time is unsupported.

As noted, biphasic defibrillators use one of two waveforms, and each waveform has been shown to be effective in terminating VF over a specific dose range. The ideal shock dose with a biphasic device is one that falls within the range that has been documented to be effective using that specific device. Manufacturers should display the device-specific effective waveform dose range on the face of the device, and providers should use that dose range when attempting defibrillation with that device. Providers should be aware of the range of energy levels at which the specific waveform they use has been shown to be effective for terminating VF, and they should use that device-specific dose for attempted defibrillation. At this time there is no evidence that one biphasic waveform is more effective than another.

With a biphasic defibrillator it is reasonable to use selected energies of 150 J to 200 J with a biphasic truncated exponential waveform or 120 J with a rectilinear biphasic waveform for the initial shock. For second and subsequent shocks, use the same or higher energy (Class IIa). In this context "selected" refers to the energy dose selected by the operator (or programmed by the AED manufacturer). With the rectilinear biphasic waveform device, selected and delivered energies usually differ; delivered energy is typically higher in the usual range of impedance. For example, in a patient with 80 Ω impedance, a selected energy of 120 J will deliver 150 J.

If a provider is operating a manual biphasic defibrillator and is unaware of the effective dose range for that device to terminate VF, the rescuer may use a selected dose of 200 J for the first shock and an equal or higher dose for the second and subsequent shocks. The 200-J "default" energy level is not necessarily an optimal dose, but it was selected because it falls within the reported range of doses effective for first and subsequent biphasic shocks. In addition, this dose can be provided by every biphasic manual defibrillator available in 2005. Thus, it is a consensus default dose and not a recommended ideal dose. If devices are clearly labeled and providers are familiar with the devices they will use for clinical care, the device-specific dose will be used and there will be no need for the "default" 200-J dose.

If a monophasic defibrillator is used, select a dose of 360 J for all shocks. If VF is initially terminated by a shock but then recurs later in the arrest, deliver subsequent shocks at the previously successful energy level.

Defibrillation is achieved by generating amplitude of current flow and sustaining that flow for a time interval. Although the defibrillator operator selects the shock energy (in joules), it is the current flow (in amperes) that actually depolarizes the myocardium. Current depends in part on the selected shock dose and is affected by the thoracic pathway between the 2 defibrillator electrodes and the position of the heart in that pathway and impedance to current flow between the electrodes. The complexity of thoracic current flow has been observed experimentally.[89]

The most important determinant of survival in adult VF SCA is rapid defibrillation by either a monophasic or biphasic device. Thus, in the hospital it is acceptable to deliver 1 shock with a monophasic or biphasic defibrillator followed by immediate initiation of CPR, beginning with compressions. The goal is to minimize the time between chest compressions and shock delivery and between shock delivery and resumption of chest compressions. In specific settings (eg, critical care units with hemodynamic monitoring in place), this sequence may be modified at the physician's discretion (see Part 7.2: "Management of Cardiac Arrest" and Part 12: "Pediatric Advanced Life Support").

Transthoracic Impedance

The average adult human impedance is ≈70 to 80 Ω.[90–92] When transthoracic impedance is too high, a low-energy shock will not generate sufficient current to achieve defibrillation.[91,93,94] To reduce transthoracic impedance, the defibrillator operator should use conductive materials. This is accomplished with the use of gel pads or electrode paste with paddles or through the use of self-adhesive pads. No existing data suggests that one of these modalities is better than the others in decreasing impedance (Class Indeterminate).

In a male patient with a hairy chest, electrode-to-chest contact may be poor, and the hair may cause air trapping between the electrode and skin. This, as well as improper use of paddles, may result in high impedance, with occasional current arcing. Although extremely rare, in oxygen-rich environments such as critical care units, this arcing has been known to cause fires if an accelerant is present (see below). When using paddles, rescuers should apply them firmly to gel pads on the chest wall, avoiding contact with ECG leads. Use of self-adhesive pads will reduce the risk of arcing. It may be necessary to shave the area of intended pad placement.

Electrode Position

An overview of adhesive pad placement was provided in the AED section above. If electrode paddles are used instead of pads, the paddles should be well separated, and the paste or gel used to create the interface between the paddles and the skin should not be smeared on the chest between the paddles. Smearing of the paste or gel may allow current to follow a superficial pathway (arc) along the chest wall, "missing" the heart. Self-adhesive monitor/defibrillator electrode pads are as effective as gel pads or paste (LOE 3[95–97]), and they can be placed before cardiac arrest to allow for monitoring and then rapid administration of a shock when necessary.[98] Consequently, self-adhesive pads should be used routinely instead of standard paddles (Class IIa; LOE 2, 4).

When providing cardioversion or defibrillation for patients with permanent pacemakers or ICDs, do not place the electrodes over or close to the device generator, because defibrillation can cause the pacemaker to malfunction. A pacemaker or ICD also may block some current to the myocardium during defibrillation attempts, resulting in suboptimal energy delivery to the heart. Because some of the defibrillation current flows down the pacemaker leads, permanent pacemakers and ICDs should be reevaluated after the patient receives a shock.[99]

Electrode Size

In 1993 the Association for the Advancement of Medical Instrumentation recommended a minimum electrode size of 50 cm^2 for individual electrodes.[100] However, advances in electrode design and chemical composition may soon require modification of this recommendation.

For adult defibrillation, both handheld paddle electrodes and self-adhesive pad electrodes 8 to 12 cm in diameter perform well, although defibrillation success may be higher with electrodes 12 cm in diameter rather than with those 8 cm in diameter.[90,95] Small electrodes (4.3 cm) may be harmful and may cause myocardial necrosis.[101] When using handheld paddles and gel or pads, rescuers must ensure that the paddle is in full contact with the skin. Even smaller pads have been found to be effective[102] in VF of brief duration. Use of the smallest (pediatric) pads, however, can result in unacceptably high transthoracic impedance in larger children.[103] It is best to use the largest pads that can fit on the chest without overlap.

Fibrillation Waveform Analysis

Several retrospective case series, animal studies, and theoretical models (LOE 4[29,30,104–110] and LOE 6[111–121]) suggest that it is possible to predict, with varying reliability, the success of attempted defibrillation by analyzing the VF waveform. If prospective studies can select optimal defibrillation waveforms and optimal timing of shock delivery (eg, before or after a period of CPR), shock delivery may be more likely to result in return of spontaneous perfusion, and the delivery of unsuccessful high-energy shocks may be prevented. At present there is insufficient evidence to recommend for or against analysis of VF ECG characteristics (Class Indeterminate).

At issue is whether analysis of the VF waveform is useful in predicting therapeutic outcome and modifying therapy prospectively. Potential applications include prediction of success of cardioversion, selection of appropriate waveform type, and optimization of timing of defibrillation relative to CPR and medication delivery.

Current-Based Defibrillation

Because it is accepted that defibrillation is accomplished by the passage of sufficient current through the heart, the concept of current-based defibrillation is appealing. Energy is a nonphysiologic descriptor of defibrillation despite its entrenchment in traditional jargon. Current-based defibrillation has been assessed[92,122] but has not yet been used clinically as a better physiologic descriptor of defibrillation dose. This concept merits exploration in light of the variety of biphasic waveforms available that deliver current in different ways. Peak current amplitude, average current, phasic duration, and phasic current flow need to be examined as determinants of shock efficacy. Another difficulty with using energy as a descriptor was described earlier with regard to differences between operator-selected energy and that delivered with the rectilinear biphasic waveform. Transition to current-based description is timely and should be encouraged.

Clinical studies using MDS waveform shocks have tried to identify the range of current necessary to achieve defibrillation and cardioversion. The optimal current for ventricular defibrillation appears to be 30 to 40 A MDS.[92] Comparable information on current dosage for biphasic waveform shocks is under investigation.

"Occult" Versus "False" Asystole

There is no evidence that attempting to "defibrillate" asystole is beneficial. In 1989 Losek[123] published a retrospective review of initial shock delivery for 49 children (infants through 19 years of age) in asystole compared with no shock delivery for 41 children in asystole and found no improvement in rhythm change, ROSC, or survival in the group that received the shocks. In 1993 the Nine City High-Dose Epinephrine Study Group published an analysis of 77 asystolic patients who received initial shock compared with 117 who received standard therapy.[124] There was no benefit from shock delivery for asystole. In fact, in all outcomes studied, including ROSC and survival, the group that received shocks showed a trend toward a *worse* outcome than the group that did not receive shocks. With recent recognition of the importance of minimizing interruptions in chest compressions, it is difficult to justify any interruption in chest compressions to attempt shock delivery for asystole.

Fire Hazard

Several case reports have described fires ignited by sparks from poorly applied defibrillator paddles in the presence of an oxygen-enriched atmosphere (LOE 5).[125–130] Severe fires have been reported when ventilator tubing is disconnected from the tracheal tube and then left adjacent to the patient's head, blowing oxygen across the chest during attempted defibrillation (LOE 5).[126,128,130]

The use of self-adhesive defibrillation pads is probably the best way to minimize the risk of sparks igniting during defibrillation. If manual paddles are used, gel pads are preferable to electrode pastes and gels because the pastes and gels can spread between the 2 paddles, creating the potential for a spark (Class IIb). Do not use medical gels or pastes with poor electrical conductivity, such as ultrasound gel.

Rescuers should take precautions to minimize sparking during attempted defibrillation; try to ensure that defibrillation is not attempted in an oxygen-enriched atmosphere (Class IIa). When ventilation is interrupted for shock delivery, rescuers should try to ensure that oxygen does not flow across the patient's chest during defibrillation attempts.

Synchronized Cardioversion

Synchronized cardioversion is shock delivery that is timed (synchronized) with the QRS complex. This synchronization avoids shock delivery during the relative refractory portion of the cardiac cycle, when a shock could produce VF.[131] The energy (shock dose) used for a synchronized shock is lower than that used for unsynchronized shocks (defibrillation). These low-energy shocks should always be delivered as synchronized shocks because if they are delivered as *unsynchronized* shocks they are likely to induce VF. If cardioversion is needed and it is impossible to synchronize a shock (eg, the patient's rhythm is irregular), use high-energy unsynchronized shocks.

Delivery of synchronized shocks (cardioversion) is indicated to treat unstable tachyarrhythmias associated with an organized QRS complex and a perfusing rhythm (pulses). The unstable patient demonstrates signs of poor perfusion, including altered mental status, ongoing chest pain, hypotension, or other signs of shock (eg, pulmonary edema).

Synchronized cardioversion is recommended to treat unstable supraventricular tachycardia due to reentry, atrial fibrillation, and atrial flutter. These arrhythmias are all caused by reentry, an abnormal rhythm circuit that allows a wave of depolarization to travel in a circle. The delivery of a shock can stop these rhythms because it interrupts the circulating (reentry) pattern. Synchronized cardioversion is also recommended to treat unstable monomorphic VT. For additional information see Part 7.3: "Management of Symptomatic Bradycardia and Tachycardia."

Cardioversion will not be effective for treatment of junctional tachycardia or ectopic or multifocal atrial tachycardia because these rhythms have an automatic focus. Automatic rhythms are created when local cells are stimulated to spontaneously depolarize at a rapid rate. Sinus tachycardia is a good example of an automatic rhythm. It results when the cells in the sinus node are stimulated (eg, by catecholamines) to depolarize at a rapid rate. Junctional tachycardia and ectopic or multifocal atrial tachycardia also result when cells are stimulated to depolarize at a rapid rate. Delivery of a shock cannot stop these rhythms. In fact, shock delivery to a heart with a rapid automatic focus may increase the rate of the tachyarrhythmia.

Synchronized cardioversion is not used for treatment of VF, pulseless VT, or unstable polymorphic (irregular) VT. These rhythms require delivery of high-energy *unsynchronized* shocks (ie, defibrillation doses). Electrical therapy for VT is discussed further below. For additional information see Part 7.2: "Management of Cardiac Arrest."

Supraventricular Tachycardias (Reentry SVT)

The recommended initial monophasic energy dose for cardioversion of atrial fibrillation is 100 J to 200 J. Cardioversion of atrial flutter and other supraventricular tachycardias generally requires less energy; an initial energy of 50 J to 100 J MDS waveform is often sufficient. If the initial 50-J shock fails, providers should increase the dose in a stepwise fashion.[93] These recommendations are consistent with those contained in the *ECC Guidelines 2000.*[50] Cardioversion with biphasic waveforms is now available,[132] but the optimal doses for cardioversion with biphasic waveforms have not been established with certainty. Extrapolation from published experience with elective cardioversion of atrial fibrillation using rectilinear and truncated exponential waveforms supports an initial dose of 100 J to 120 J with escalation as needed.[133,134] This initial dose has been shown to be 80% to 85% effective in terminating atrial fibrillation. Until further evidence becomes available, this information can be used to extrapolate biphasic cardioversion doses to other tachyarrhythmias.[135–138]

A recent prospective randomized study that compared the rectilinear biphasic waveform (200 J maximum selected energy) with a biphasic truncated exponential waveform (360 J maximum energy) for elective cardioversion found no significant differences in efficacy between the 2 waveforms.[134]

Ventricular Tachycardia

The amount of energy and timing of shocks for treatment of VT with pulses are determined by the patient's condition and the morphologic characteristics of the VT.[139] Pulseless VT is treated as VF (see Part 7.2: "Management of Cardiac Arrest"). Management of stable VT is summarized in Part 7.3: "Management of Symptomatic Bradycardia and Tachycardia." Unstable monomorphic (regular) VT with pulses is treated with synchronized cardioversion. Unstable polymorphic (irregular) VT with or without pulses is treated as VF using *unsynchronized* high-energy shocks (ie, defibrillation doses).

Monomorphic VT (regular form and rate) with a pulse responds well to monophasic waveform cardioversion (synchronized) shocks at initial energies of 100 J. If there is no response to the first shock, increase the dose in a stepwise fashion (eg, 100 J, 200 J, 300 J, 360 J). These recommendations are consistent with the recommendations in the *ECC Guidelines 2000.*[50]

Although synchronized cardioversion is preferred for treatment of an organized ventricular rhythm, for some arrhythmias synchronization is not possible. The many QRS configurations and irregular rates that comprise polymorphic ventricular tachycardia make it difficult or impossible to reliably synchronize to a QRS complex. In addition, the patient with persistent polymorphic VT will probably not maintain perfusion/pulses for very long, so any attempt to distinguish between polymorphic VT with or without pulses quickly becomes moot. A good rule of thumb is that if your eye cannot synchronize to each QRS complex, neither can the defibrillator/cardioverter. If there is any doubt whether monomorphic or polymorphic VT is present in the *unstable* patient, do not delay shock delivery to perform detailed rhythm analysis—provide high energy unsynchronized shocks (ie, defibrillation doses).

The recommended shock doses for high-energy, *unsynchronized* shocks (defibrillation) with a biphasic or monophasic device are those presented earlier in this section (see "Manual Defibrillation, Shock Energies"). After shock delivery the healthcare provider should be prepared to provide immediate CPR (beginning with chest compressions) and follow the ACLS Pulseless Arrest Algorithm if pulseless arrest develops (for further information see Part 7.2: "Management of Cardiac Arrest").

There is limited data about the treatment of polymorphic (irregular) VT. Providers should consider consultation with an expert in arrhythmia management. Treatment of the patient with polymorphic VT is presented in section 7.3: "Management of Symptomatic Bradycardia and Tachycardia."

Pacing

Pacing is not recommended for patients in asystolic cardiac arrest. Pacing can be considered in patients with symptomatic bradycardia.

Three randomized controlled trials (LOE 2)[140–142] of fair quality and additional studies (LOE 3 to 7)[143–149] indicate no improvement in the rate of admission to hospital or survival to hospital discharge when paramedics or physicians attempted to provide pacing in asystolic patients in the prehospital or hospital (emergency department) setting. Given the recent recognition of the importance of maximizing chest compressions as well as the lack of demonstrated benefit of pacing for asystole, withholding chest compressions to attempt pacing for patients with asystole is not recommended (Class III).

Transcutaneous pacing is recommended for treatment of symptomatic bradycardia when a pulse is present. Healthcare providers should be prepared to initiate pacing in patients who do not respond to atropine (or second-line drugs if these do not delay definitive management). Immediate pacing is indicated if the patient is severely symptomatic, especially when the block is at or below the His Purkinje level. If the patient does not respond to transcutaneous pacing, transvenous pacing is needed. For further information see Part 7.3: "Management of Symptomatic Bradycardia and Tachycardia."

Maintaining Devices in a State of Readiness

User checklists have been developed to reduce equipment malfunction and operator errors. Failure to properly maintain the defibrillator or power supply is responsible for the majority of reported malfunctions. Checklists are useful when designed to identify and prevent such deficiencies.

Summary

The new recommendations for electrical therapies described in this section are designed to improve survival from SCA and life-threatening arrhythmias. For any victim of cardiac arrest, good CPR—push hard, push fast, allow complete chest recoil, and minimize interruptions in chest compressions—is essential. Some victims of VF SCA may benefit from a short period of CPR before attempted defibrillation. Whenever defibrillation is attempted, rescuers must coordinate good CPR with defibrillation to minimize interruptions in chest compressions and to ensure immediate resumption of chest compressions after shock delivery. The high first-shock efficacy of newer biphasic defibrillators led to the recommendation of single shocks plus immediate CPR instead of 3-shock sequences that were formerly recommended to treat VF. Further data is needed to refine recommendations for use of electrical therapies, particularly for the use of biphasic waveforms.

References

1. Larsen MP, Eisenberg MS, Cummins RO, Hallstrom AP. Predicting survival from out-of-hospital cardiac arrest: a graphic model. *Ann Emerg Med.* 1993;22:1652–1658.
2. Valenzuela TD, Roe DJ, Cretin S, Spaite DW, Larsen MP. Estimating effectiveness of cardiac arrest interventions: a logistic regression survival model. *Circulation.* 1997;96:3308–3313.
3. Swor RA, Jackson RE, Cynar M, Sadler E, Basse E, Boji B, Rivera-Rivera EJ, Maher A, Grubb W, Jacobson R, et al. Bystander CPR, ventricular fibrillation, and survival in witnessed, unmonitored out-of-hospital cardiac arrest. *Ann Emerg Med.* 1995;25:780–784.
4. Holmberg M, Holmberg S, Herlitz J. Incidence, duration and survival of ventricular fibrillation in out-of-hospital cardiac arrest patients in Sweden. *Resuscitation.* 2000;44:7–17.
5. Wik L, Hansen TB, Fylling F, Steen T, Vaagenes P, Auestad BH, Steen PA. Delaying defibrillation to give basic cardiopulmonary resuscitation to patients with out-of-hospital ventricular fibrillation: a randomized trial. *JAMA.* 2003;289:1389–1395.
6. Cobb LA, Fahrenbruch CE, Walsh TR, Copass MK, Olsufka M, Breskin M, Hallstrom AP. Influence of cardiopulmonary resuscitation prior to defibrillation in patients with out-of-hospital ventricular fibrillation. *JAMA.* 1999;281:1182–1188.
7. Cummins, RO, Eisenberg, MS, Hallstrom, AP, Litwin, PE. Survival of out-of-hospital cardiac arrest with early initiation of cardiopulmonary resuscitation. *Am J Emerg Med.* 1985;3:114–119.
8. Holmberg S, Holmberg M, Herlitz J, Effect of bystander cardiopulmonary resuscitation in out-of-hospital cardiac arrest patients in Sweden. *Resuscitation.* 2000; 47:59–70.
9. Waalewijn RA, Tijssen JG, Koster RW. Bystander initiated actions in out-of-hospital cardiopulmonary resuscitation: results from the Amsterdam Resuscitation Study (ARRESUST). *Resuscitation.* 2001;50: 273–279.
10. Weaver WD, Copass MK, Bufi D, Ray R, Hallstrom AP, Cobb LA. Improved neurologic recovery and survival after early defibrillation. *Circulation.* 1984;69:943–948.
11. International Liaison Committee on Resuscitation. 2005 International Consensus on Cardiopulmonary Resuscitation and Emergency Cardiovascular Care With Treatment Recommendations. *Circulation.* 2005; 112:III-1–III-136.
12. Jacobs IG, Finn JC, Oxer HF, Jelinek GA. CPR before defibrillation in out-of-hospital cardiac arrest: a randomized trial. *Emerg Med Australas.* 2005;17:39–45.
13. Yu T, Weil MH, Tang W, Sun S, Klouche K, Povoas H, Bisera J. Adverse outcomes of interrupted precordial compression during automated defibrillation. *Circulation.* 2002;106:368–372.
14. Berg RA, Sanders AB, Kern KB, Hilwig RW, Heidenreich JW, Porter ME, Ewy GA. Adverse hemodynamic effects of interrupting chest compressions for rescue breathing during cardiopulmonary resuscitation for ventricular fibrillation cardiac arrest. *Circulation.* 2001;104: 2465–2470.
15. Kern K, Hilwig R, Berb R, Sanders A, Ewy G. Importance of continuous chest compressions during CPR. *Circulation.* 2002;105:645–649.
16. Eftestol T, Sunde K, Steen PA. Effects of interrupting precordial compressions on the calculated probability of defibrillation success during out-of-hospital cardiac arrest. *Circulation.* 2002;105:2270–2273.
17. van Alem AP, Chapman FW, Lank P, Hart AA, Koster RW. A prospective, randomised and blinded comparison of first shock success of monophasic and biphasic waveforms in out-of-hospital cardiac arrest. *Resuscitation.* 2003;58:17–24.
18. Wik L, Kramer-Johansen J, Myklebust H, Sorebo H, Svensson L, Fellows B, Steen PA. Quality of cardiopulmonary resuscitation during out-of-hospital cardiac arrest. *JAMA.* 2005;293:299–304.
19. Abella BS, Alvarado JP, Myklebust H, Edelson DP, Barry A, O'Hearn N, Vanden Hoek TL, Becker LB. Quality of cardiopulmonary resuscitation during in-hospital cardiac arrest. *JAMA.* 2005;293:305–310.
20. Bain AC, Swerdlow CD, Love CJ, Ellenbogen KA, Deering TF, Brewer JE, Augostini RS, Tchou PJ. Multicenter study of principles-based waveforms for external defibrillation. *Ann Emerg Med.* 2001;37:5–12.
21. Poole JE, White RD, Kanz KG, Hengstenberg F, Jarrard GT, Robinson JC, Santana V, McKenas DK, Rich N, Rosas S, Merritt S, Magnotto L, Gallagher JV III, Gliner BE, Jorgenson DB, Morgan CB, Dillon SM, Kronmal RA, Bardy GH. Low-energy impedance-compensating biphasic waveforms terminate ventricular fibrillation at high rates in victims of out-of-hospital cardiac arrest. LIFE Investigators. *J Cardiovasc Electrophysiol.* 1997;8:1373–1385.
22. White RD, Blackwell TH, Russell JK, Snyder DE, Jorgenson DB. Transthoracic impedance does not affect defibrillation, resuscitation or survival in patients with out-of-hospital cardiac arrest treated with a non-escalating biphasic waveform defibrillator. *Resuscitation.* 2005;64: 63–69.
23. Mittal S, Ayati S, Stein KM, Knight BP, Morady F, Schwartzman D, Cavlovich D, Platia EV, Calkins H, Tchou PJ, Miller JM, Wharton JM, Sung RJ, Slotwiner DJ, Markowitz SM, Lerman BB. Comparison of a novel rectilinear biphasic waveform with a damped sine wave monophasic waveform for transthoracic ventricular defibrillation. ZOLL Investigators. *J Am Coll Cardiol.* 1999;34:1595–1601.
24. Schneider T, Martens PR, Paschen H, Kuisma M, Wolcke B, Gliner BE, Russell JK, Weaver WD, Bossaert L, Chamberlain D. Multicenter, randomized, controlled trial of 150-J biphasic shocks compared with 200- to 360-J monophasic shocks in the resuscitation of out-of-hospital cardiac arrest victims. *Circulation.* 2000;102:1780–1787.
25. Hess EP, White RD. Ventricular fibrillation is not provoked by chest compression during post-shock organized rhythms in out-of-hospital cardiac arrest. *Resuscitation* 2005;66:7–11.

26. Carpenter J, Rea TD, Murray JA, Kudenchuk PJ, Eisenberg MS. Defibrillation waveform and post-shock rhythm in out-of-hospital ventricular fibrillation cardiac arrest. *Resuscitation.* 2003;59:189–196.
27. Morrison LJ, Dorian P, Long J, Vermeulen M, Scwartz B, Sawadsky B, et al. Out-of-hospital Cardiac Arrest Rectilinear Biphasic to Monophasic Damped Sine Defibrillation Waveforms with Advanced Life Support Intervention Trial (ORBIT). *Resuscitation.* 2005;66:149–157.
28. Weaver WD, Cobb LA, Copass MK, Hallstrom AP. Ventricular defibrillation: a comparative trial using 175-J and 320-J shocks. *N Engl J Med.* 1982;307:1101–1106.
29. Eftestol T, Wik L, Sunde K, Steen PA. Effects of cardiopulmonary resuscitation on predictors of ventricular fibrillation defibrillation success during out-of-hospital cardiac arrest. *Circulation.* 2004;110: 10–15.
30. Eftestol T, Sunde K, Aase SO, Husoy JH, Steen PA. Predicting outcome of defibrillation by spectral characterization and nonparametric classification of ventricular fibrillation in patients with out-of-hospital cardiac arrest. *Circulation.* 2000;102:1523–1529.
31. White RD. External defibrillation: the need for uniformity in analyzing and reporting results [editorial]. *Ann Emerg Med.* 1998;32:234–236.
32. Gliner BE, White RD. Electrocardiographic evaluation of defibrillation shocks delivered to out-of-hospital sudden cardiac arrest patients. *Resuscitation.* 1999;41:133–144.
33. Cummins RO, Chamberlain DA, Abramson NS, Allen M, Baskett P, Becker L, Bossaert L, Delooz L, Dick W, Eisenberg M, et al. Recommended guidelines for uniform reporting of data from out-of-hospital cardiac arrest: the Utstein style. A statement for health professionals from a task force of the American Heart Association, the European Resuscitation Council, the Heart and Stroke Foundation of Canada, and the Australian Resuscitation Council. Circulation. 1991;84:960–975.
34. White RD, Hankins DG, Bugliosi TF. Seven years' experience with early defibrillation by police and paramedics in an emergency medical services system. *Resuscitation.* 1998;39:145–151.
35. Cummins RO, Eisenberg MS, Bergner L, Hallstrom A, Hearne T, Murray JA. Automatic external defibrillation: evaluations of its role in the home and in emergency medical services. *Ann Emerg Med.* 1984; 13:798–801.
36. White RD, Vukov LF, Bugliosi TF. Early defibrillation by police: initial experience with measurement of critical time intervals and patient outcome. *Ann Emerg Med.* 1994;23:1009–1013.
37. Faddy SC, Powell J, Craig J. Biphasic and monophasic shocks for transthoracic defibrillation: a metaanalysis of randomized controlled trials. *Resuscitation.* 2000;58:9–16.
38. Stothert JC, Hatcher TS, Gupton CL, Love JE, Brewer JE. Rectilinear biphasic waveform defibrillation of out-of-hospital cardiac arrest. *Prehosp Emerg Care.* 2004;8:388–392.
39. Schwarz B, Bowdle TA, Jett GK, Mair P, Lindner KH, Aldea GS, Lazzara RG, O'Grady SG, Schmitt PW, Walker RG, Chapman FW, Tacker WA. Biphasic shocks compared with monophasic damped sine wave shocks for direct ventricular defibrillation during open heart surgery. *Anesthesiology.* 2003;98:1063–1069.
40. Higgins SL, Herre JM, Epstein AE, Greer GS, Friedman PL, Gleva ML, Porterfield JG, Chapman FW, Finkel ES, Schmitt PW, Nova RC, Greene HL. A comparison of biphasic and monophasic shocks for external defibrillation. Physio-Control Biphasic Investigators. *Prehosp Emerg Care.* 2000;4:305–313.
41. Martens PR, Russell JK, Wolcke B, Paschen H, Kuisma M, Gliner BE, Weaver WD, Bossaert L, Chamberlain D, Schneider T. Optimal response to cardiac arrest study: defibrillation waveform effects. *Resuscitation.* 2001;49:233–243.
42. Walsh SJ, McClelland AJ, Owens CG, Allen J, Anderson JM, Turner C, Adgey AA. Efficacy of distinct energy delivery protocols comparing two biphasic defibrillators for cardiac arrest. *Am J Cardiol.* 2004;94: 378–380.
43. Gliner BE, Jorgenson DB, Poole JE, White RD, Kanz KG, Lyster TD, Leyde KW, Powers DJ, Morgan CB, Kronmal RA, Bardy GH. Treatment of out-of-hospital cardiac arrest with a low-energy impedance-compensating biphasic waveform automatic external defibrillator. The LIFE Investigators. *Biomed Instrum Technol.* 1998;32: 631–644.
44. White RD, Russell JK. Refibrillation, resuscitation and survival in out-of-hospital sudden cardiac arrest victims treated with biphasic automated external defibrillators. *Resuscitation.* 2002;55:17–23.
45. Cummins RO, Eisenberg M, Bergner L, Murray JA. Sensitivity, accuracy, and safety of an automatic external defibrillator. *Lancet.* 1984;2:318–320.
46. Davis EA, Mosesso VN Jr. Performance of police first responders in utilizing automated external defibrillation on victims of sudden cardiac arrest. *Prehosp Emerg Care.* 1998;2:101–107.
47. Weisfeldt ML, Kerber RE, McGoldrick RP, Moss AJ, Nichol G, Ornato JP, Palmer DG, Riegel B, Smith SCJ. American Heart Association Report on the Public Access Defibrillation Conference, December 8–10, 1994. Automatic External Defibrillation Task Force. *Circulation.* 1995; 92:2740–2747.
48. Weisfeldt ML, Kerber RE, McGoldrick RP, Moss AJ, Nichol G, Ornato JP, Palmer DG, Riegel B, Smith SC Jr. Public access defibrillation: a statement for healthcare professionals from the American Heart Association Task Force on Automatic External Defibrillation. *Circulation.* 1995;92:2763.
49. Nichol G, Hallstrom AP, Ornato JP, Riegel B, Stiell IG, Valenzuela T, Wells GA, White RD, Weisfeldt ML. Potential cost-effectiveness of public access defibrillation in the United States. *Circulation.* 1998;97: 1315–1320.
50. American Heart Association in collaboration with International Liaison Committee on Resuscitation. Guidelines 2000 for Cardiopulmonary Resuscitation and Emergency Cardiovascular Care: International Consensus on Science. *Circulation.* 2000;102(suppl):I1-I384.
51. Hazinski MF, Idris AH, Kerber RE, Epstein A, Atkins D, Tang W, Lurie K. Lay rescuer automated external defibrillator ("Public Access Defibrillation") Programs; lessons learned from an international multicenter trial. Advisory statement from the American Heart Association Emergency Cardiovascular Care Committee; the Council on Cardiopulmonary, Perioperative and Critical Care; and the Council on Clinical Cardiology. *Circulation.* 2005;111:3336–3340.
52. Caffrey SL, Willoughby PJ, Pepe PE, Becker LB. Public use of automated external defibrillators. *N Engl J Med.* 2002;347:1242–1247.
53. Valenzuela TD, Bjerke HS, Clark LL, et al. Rapid defibrillation by nontraditional responders: the Casino Project. *Acad Emerg Med.* 1998; 5:414–415.
54. Valenzuela TD, Roe DJ, Nichol G, Clark LL, Spaite DW, Hardman RG. Outcomes of rapid defibrillation by security officers after cardiac arrest in casinos. *N Engl J Med.* 2000;343:1206–1209.
55. White RD, Asplin BR, Bugliosi TF, Hankins DG. High discharge survival rate after out-of-hospital ventricular fibrillation with rapid defibrillation by police and paramedics. *Ann Emerg Med.* 1996;28: 480–485.
56. White RD. Early out-of-hospital experience with an impedance-compensating low-energy biphasic waveform automatic external defibrillator. *J Interv Card Electrophysiol.* 1997;1:203–208.
57. White RD, Bunch TJ, Hankins DG. Evolution of a community-wide early defibrillation programme Experience over 13 years using police/fire personnel and paramedics as responders. *Resuscitation.* 2005; 279–283
58. Groh WJ, Newman MM, Beal PE, Fineberg NS, Zipes DP. Limited response to cardiac arrest by police equipped with automated external defibrillators: lack of survival benefit in suburban and rural Indiana—the police as responder automated defibrillation evaluation (PARADE). *Acad Emerg Med.* 2001;8:324–330.
59. de Vries W, van Alem AP, de Vos R, van Oostrom J, Koster RW. Trained first-responders with an automated external defibrillator: how do they perform in real resuscitation attempts? *Resuscitation.* 2005;64: 157–161.
60. Sayre M, Evans J, White L, Brennan T. Providing automated external defibrillators to urban police officers in addition to fire department rapid defibrillation program is not effective. *Resuscitation.* 2005;66:189–196.
61. The Public Access Defibrillation Trial Investigators. Public-access defibrillation and survival after out-of-hospital cardiac arrest. *N Engl J Med.* 2004;351:637–646.
62. Becker L, Eisenberg M, Fahrenbruch C, Cobb L. Public locations of cardiac arrest: implications for public access defibrillation. *Circulation.* 1998;97:2106–2109.
63. Kerber RE, Becker LB, Bourland JD, Cummins RO, Hallstrom AP, Michos MB, Nichol G, Ornato JP, Thies WH, White RD, Zuckerman BD. Automatic external defibrillators for public access defibrillation: recommendations for specifying and reporting arrhythmia analysis algorithm performance, incorporating new waveforms, and enhancing safety. A statement for health professionals from the American Heart

Association Task Force on Automatic External Defibrillation, Subcommittee on AED Safety and Efficacy. *Circulation*. 1997;95:1677–1682.
64. Dickey W, Dalzell GW, Anderson JM, Adgey AA. The accuracy of decision-making of a semi-automatic defibrillator during cardiac arrest. *Eur Heart J*. 1992;13:608–615.
65. Atkinson E, Mikysa B, Conway JA, Parker M, Christian K, Deshpande J, Knilans TK, Smith J, Walker C, Stickney RE, Hampton DR, Hazinski MF. Specificity and sensitivity of automated external defibrillator rhythm analysis in infants and children. *Ann Emerg Med*. 2003;42: 185–196.
66. Cecchin F, Jorgenson DB, Berul CI, Perry JC, Zimmerman AA, Duncan BW, Lupinetti FM, Snyder D, Lyster TD, Rosenthal GL, Cross B, Atkins DL. Is arrhythmia detection by automatic external defibrillator accurate for children? Sensitivity and specificity of an automatic external defibrillator algorithm in 696 pediatric arrhythmias. *Circulation*. 2001;103:2483–2488.
67. Monsieurs KG, Conraads VM, Goethals MP, Snoeck JP, Bossaert LL. Semi-automatic external defibrillation and implanted cardiac pacemakers: understanding the interactions during resuscitation. *Resuscitation*. 1995;30:127–131.
68. Panacek EA, Munger MA, Rutherford WF, Gardner SF. Report of nitropatch explosions complicating defibrillation. *Am J Emerg Med*. 1992;10:128–129.
69. Kuisma M, Suominen P, Korpela R. Paediatric out-of-hospital cardiac arrests: epidemiology and outcome. *Resuscitation*. 1995;30:141–150.
70. Sirbaugh PE, Pepe PE, Shook JE, Kimball KT, Goldman MJ, Ward MA, Mann DM. A prospective, population-based study of the demographics, epidemiology, management, and outcome of out-of-hospital pediatric cardiopulmonary arrest [published correction appears in *Ann Emerg Med*. 1999;33:358]. *Ann Emerg Med*. 1999;33:174–184.
71. Hickey RW, Cohen DM, Strausbaugh S, Dietrich AM. Pediatric patients requiring CPR in the prehospital setting. *Ann Emerg Med*. 1995;25: 495–501.
72. Appleton GO, Cummins RO, Larson MP, Graves JR. CPR and the single rescuer: at what age should you "call first" rather than "call fast"? *Ann Emerg Med*. 1995;25:492–494.
73. Ronco R, King W, Donley DK, Tilden SJ. Outcome and cost at a children's hospital following resuscitation for out-of-hospital cardiopulmonary arrest. *Arch Pediatr Adolesc Med*. 1995;149:210–214.
74. Losek JD, Hennes H, Glaeser P, Hendley G, Nelson DB. Prehospital care of the pulseless, nonbreathing pediatric patient. *Am J Emerg Med*. 1987;5:370–374.
75. Mogayzel C, Quan L, Graves JR, Tiedeman D, Fahrenbruch C, Herndon P. Out-of-hospital ventricular fibrillation in children and adolescents: causes and outcomes. *Ann Emerg Med*. 1995;25:484–491.
76. Safranek DJ, Eisenberg MS, Larsen MP. The epidemiology of cardiac arrest in young adults. *Ann Emerg Med*. 1992;21:1102–1106.
77. Gurnett CA, Atkins DL. Successful use of a biphasic waveform automated external defibrillator in a high-risk child. *Am J Cardiol*. 2000;86:1051–1053.
78. Atkins D, Jorgenson D. Attenuated pediatric electrode pads for automated external defibrillator use in children. *Resuscitation*. 2005;66: 31–37.
79. Berg RA, Chapman FW, Berg MD, Hilwig RW, Banville I, Walker RG, Nova RC, Sherrill D, Kern KB. Attenuated adult biphasic shocks compared with weight-based monophasic shocks in a swine model of prolonged pediatric ventricular fibrillation. *Resuscitation*. 2004;61: 189–197.
80. Tang W, Weil MH, Jorgenson D, Klouche K, Morgan C, Yu T, Sun S, Snyder D. Fixed-energy biphasic waveform defibrillation in a pediatric model of cardiac arrest and resuscitation. *Crit Care Med*. 2002;30: 2736–2741.
81. Clark CB, Zhang Y, Davies LR, Karlsson G, Kerber RE. Pediatric transthoracic defibrillation: biphasic versus monophasic waveforms in an experimental model. *Resuscitation*. 2001;51:159–163.
82. Gutgesell HP, Tacker WA, Geddes LA, Davis S, Lie JT, McNamara DG. Energy dose for ventricular defibrillation of children. *Pediatrics*. 1976;58:898–901.
83. Samson RA, Berg RA, Bingham R, Biarent D, Coovadia A, Hazinski MF, Hickey RW, Nadkarni V, Nichol G, Tibballs J, Reis AG, Tse S, Zideman D, Potts J, Uzark K, Atkins D. Use of automated external defibrillators for children: an update: an advisory statement from the pediatric advanced life support task force, International Liaison Committee on Resuscitation. *Circulation*. 2003;107:3250–3255.
84. Jorgenson D, Morgan C, Snyder D, Griesser H, Solosko T, Chan K, Skarr T. Energy attenuator for pediatric application of an automated external defibrillator. *Crit Care Med*. 2002;30:S145–S147.
85. Zafari AM, Zarter SK, Heggen V, Wilson P, Taylor RA, Reddy K, Backscheider AG, Dudley SC Jr. A program encouraging early defibrillation results in improved in-hospital resuscitation efficacy. *J Am Coll Cardiol*. 2004;44:846–852.
86. Destro A, Marzaloni M, Sermasi S, Rossi F. Automatic external defibrillators in the hospital as well? *Resuscitation*. 1996;31:39–43.
87. Kaye W, Mancini M, Richards N. Organizing and implementing a hospital-wide first-responder automated external defibrillation program: strengthening the in-hospital chain of survival. *Resuscitation*. 1995;30: 151–156.
88. Peberdy MA, Kaye W, Ornato JP, Larkin GL, Nadkarni V, Mancini ME, Berg RA, Nichol G, Lane-Trultt T. Cardiopulmonary resuscitation of adults in the hospital: a report of 14720 cardiac arrests from the National Registry of Cardiopulmonary Resuscitation. *Resuscitation*. 2003;58: 297–308.
89. Yoon RS, DeMonte TP, Hasanov KF, Jorgenson DB, Joy ML. Measurement of thoracic current flow in pigs for the study of defibrillation and cardioversion. *IEEE Trans Biomed Eng*. 2003;50:1167–1173.
90. Kerber RE, Grayzel J, Hoyt R, Marcus M, Kennedy J. Transthoracic resistance in human defibrillation: influence of body weight, chest size, serial shocks, paddle size and paddle contact pressure. *Circulation*. 1981;63:676–682.
91. Kerber RE, Kouba C, Martins J, Kelly K, Low R, Hoyt R, Ferguson D, Bailey L, Bennett P, Charbonnier F. Advance prediction of transthoracic impedance in human defibrillation and cardioversion: importance of impedance in determining the success of low-energy shocks. *Circulation*. 1984;70:303–308.
92. Lerman BB, DiMarco JP, Haines DE. Current-based versus energy-based ventricular defibrillation: a prospective study. *J Am Coll Cardiol*. 1988;12:1259–1264.
93. Kerber RE, Martins JB, Kienzle MG, Constantin L, Olshansky B, Hopson R, Charbonnier F. Energy, current, and success in defibrillation and cardioversion: clinical studies using an automated impedance-based method of energy adjustment. *Circulation*. 1988;77:1038–1046.
94. Dalzell GW, Cunningham SR, Anderson J, Adgey AA. Electrode pad size, transthoracic impedance and success of external ventricular defibrillation. *Am J Cardiol*. 1989;64:741–744.
95. Stults KR, Brown DD, Cooley F, Kerber RE. Self-adhesive monitor/defibrillation pads improve prehospital defibrillation success. *Ann Emerg Med*. 1987;16:872–877.
96. Kerber RE, Martins JB, Kelly KJ, Ferguson DW, Kouba C, Jensen SR, Newman B, Parke JD, Kieso R, Melton J. Self-adhesive preapplied electrode pads for defibrillation and cardioversion. *J Am Coll Cardiol*. 1984;3:815–820.
97. Kerber RE, Martins JB, Ferguson DW, Jensen SR, Parke JD, Kieso R, Melton J. Experimental evaluation and initial clinical application of new self-adhesive defibrillation electrodes. *Int J Cardiol*. 1985;8:57–66.
98. Perkins GD, Roberts C, Gao F. Delays in defibrillation: influence of different monitoring techniques. *Br J Anaesth*. 2002;89:405–408.
99. Levine PA, Barold SS, Fletcher RD, Talbot P. Adverse acute and chronic effects of electrical defibrillation and cardioversion on implanted unipolar cardiac pacing systems. *J Am Coll Cardiol*. 1983;1: 1413–1422.
100. *American National Standard: Automatic External Defibrillators and Remote Controlled Defibrillators (DF39)*. Arlington, Va: Association for the Advancement of Medical Instrumentation; 1993.
101. Dahl CF, Ewy GA, Warner ED, Thomas ED. Myocardial necrosis from direct current countershock: effect of paddle electrode size and time interval between discharges. *Circulation*. 1974;50:956–961.
102. Wilson RF, Sirna S, White CW, Kerber RE. Defibrillation of high-risk patients during coronary angiography using self-adhesive, preapplied electrode pads. *Am J Cardiol*. 1987;60:380–382.
103. Samson RA, Atkins DL, Kerber RE. Optimal size of self-adhesive preapplied electrode pads in pediatric defibrillation. *Am J Cardiol*. 1995;75:544–545.
104. Callaway CW, Sherman LD, Mosesso VN Jr, Dietrich TJ, Holt E, Clarkson MC. Scaling exponent predicts defibrillation success for out-of-hospital ventricular fibrillation cardiac arrest. *Circulation*. 2001;103: 1656–1661.
105. Weaver WD, Cobb LA, Dennis D, Ray R, Hallstrom AP, Copass MK. Amplitude of ventricular fibrillation waveform and outcome after cardiac arrest. *Ann Intern Med*. 1985;102:53–55.

106. Brown CG, Dzwonczyk R. Signal analysis of the human electrocardiogram during ventricular fibrillation: frequency and amplitude parameters as predictors of successful countershock. *Ann Emerg Med.* 1996;27: 184–188.
107. Callaham M, Braun O, Valentine W, Clark DM, Zegans C. Prehospital cardiac arrest treated by urban first-responders: profile of patient response and prediction of outcome by ventricular fibrillation waveform. *Ann Emerg Med.* 1993;22:1664–1677.
108. Strohmenger HU, Lindner KH, Brown CG. Analysis of the ventricular fibrillation ECG signal amplitude and frequency parameters as predictors of countershock success in humans. *Chest.* 1997;111:584–589.
109. Strohmenger HU, Eftestol T, Sunde K, Wenzel V, Mair M, Ulmer H, Lindner KH, Steen PA. The predictive value of ventricular fibrillation electrocardiogram signal frequency and amplitude variables in patients with out-of-hospital cardiac arrest. *Anesth Analg.* 2001;93:1428–1433.
110. Podbregar M, Kovacic M, Podbregar-Mars A, Brezocnik M. Predicting defibrillation success by 'genetic' programming in patients with out-of-hospital cardiac arrest. *Resuscitation.* 2003;57:153–159.
111. Menegazzi JJ, Callaway CW, Sherman LD, Hostler DP, Wang HE, Fertig KC, Logue ES. Ventricular fibrillation scaling exponent can guide timing of defibrillation and other therapies. *Circulation.* 2004;109: 926–931.
112. Povoas HP, Weil MH, Tang W, Bisera J, Klouche K, Barbatsis A. Predicting the success of defibrillation by electrocardiographic analysis. *Resuscitation.* 2002;53:77–82.
113. Noc M, Weil MH, Tang W, Sun S, Pernat A, Bisera J. Electrocardiographic prediction of the success of cardiac resuscitation. *Crit Care Med.* 1999;27:708–714.
114. Strohmenger HU, Lindner KH, Keller A, Lindner IM, Pfenninger EG. Spectral analysis of ventricular fibrillation and closed-chest cardiopulmonary resuscitation. *Resuscitation.* 1996;33:155–161.
115. Noc M, Weil MH, Gazmuri RJ, Sun S, Biscera J, Tang W. Ventricular fibrillation voltage as a monitor of the effectiveness of cardiopulmonary resuscitation. *J Lab Clin Med.* 1994;124:421–426.
116. Lightfoot CB, Nremt P, Callaway CW, Hsieh M, Fertig KC, Sherman LD, Menegazzi JJ. Dynamic nature of electrocardiographic waveform predicts rescue shock outcome in porcine ventricular fibrillation. *Ann Emerg Med.* 2003;42:230–241.
117. Marn-Pernat A, Weil MH, Tang W, Pernat A, Bisera J. Optimizing timing of ventricular defibrillation. *Crit Care Med.* 2001;29:2360–2365.
118. Hamprecht FA, Achleitner U, Krismer AC, Lindner KH, Wenzel V, Strohmenger HU, Thiel W, van Gunsteren WF, Amann A. Fibrillation power, an alternative method of ECG spectral analysis for prediction of countershock success in a porcine model of ventricular fibrillation. *Resuscitation.* 2001;50:287–296.
119. Amann A, Achleitner U, Antretter H, Bonatti JO, Krismer AC, Lindner KH, Rieder J, Wenzel V, Voelckel WG, Strohmenger HU. Analysing ventricular fibrillation ECG-signals and predicting defibrillation success during cardiopulmonary resuscitation employing N(alpha)-histograms. *Resuscitation.* 2001;50:77–85.
120. Brown CG, Griffith RF, Van Ligten P, Hoekstra J, Nejman G, Mitchell L, Dzwonczyk R. Median frequency—a new parameter for predicting defibrillation success rate. *Ann Emerg Med.* 1991;20:787–789.
121. Amann A, Rheinberger K, Achleitner U, Krismer AC, Lingnau W, Lindner KH, Wenzel V. The prediction of defibrillation outcome using a new combination of mean frequency and amplitude in porcine models of cardiac arrest. *Anesth Analg.* 2002;95:716–722.
122. Kerber RE, McPherson D, Charbonnier F, Kieso R, Hite P. Automated impedance-based energy adjustment for defibrillation: experimental studies. *Circulation.* 1985;71:136–140.
123. Losek JD, Hennes H, Glaeser PW, Smith DS, Hendley G. Prehospital countershock treatment of pediatric asystole. *Am J Emerg Med.* 1989; 7:571–575.
124. Martin DR, Gavin T, Bianco J, Brown CG, Stueven H, Pepe PE, Cummins RO, Gonzalez E, Jastremski M. Initial countershock in the treatment of asystole. *Resuscitation.* 1993;26:63–68.
125. Miller PH. Potential fire hazard in defibrillation. *JAMA.* 1972;221:192.
126. Hummel RS III, Ornato JP, Weinberg SM, Clarke AM. Spark-generating properties of electrode gels used during defibrillation: a potential fire hazard. *JAMA.* 1988;260:3021–3024.
127. Fires from defibrillation during oxygen administration. *Health Devices.* 1994;23:307–309.
128. Lefever J, Smith A. Risk of fire when using defibrillation in an oxygen enriched atmosphere. *Med Devices Agency Safety Notices.* 1995;3:1–3.
129. Ward ME. Risk of fires when using defibrillators in an oxygen enriched atmosphere. *Resuscitation.* 1996;31:173.
130. Theodorou AA, Gutierrez JA, Berg RA. Fire attributable to a defibrillation attempt in a neonate. *Pediatrics.* 2003;112:677–679.
131. Lown B. Electrical reversion of cardiac arrhythmias. *Br Heart J.* 1967; 29:469–489.
132. Page RL, Kerber R, Russell JK, et al. Biphasic vs. monophasic shock waveform for conversion of atrial fibrillation: the results of an international randomized, double-blind multicenter trial. *Circulation.* 2000; 102:II-574.
133. Mittal S, Ayati S, Stein KM, Schwartzman D, Cavlovich D, Tchou PJ, Markowitz SM, Slotwiner DJ, Scheiner MA, Lerman BB. Transthoracic cardioversion of atrial fibrillation: comparison of rectilinear biphasic versus damped sine wave monophasic shocks. *Circulation.* 2000;101: 1282–1287.
134. Alatawi F, Gurevitz O, White R. Prospective, randomized comparison of two biphasic waveforms for the efficacy and safety of transthoracic biphasic cardioversion of atrial fibrillation. *Heart Rhythm.* 2005;2: 382–387.
135. Adgey AA, Walsh SJ. Theory and practice of defibrillation: (1) atrial fibrillation and DC conversion. *Heart.* 2004;90:1493–1498.
136. Koster RW, Dorian P, Chapman FW, Schmitt PW, O'Grady SG, Walker RG. A randomized trial comparing monophasic and biphasic waveform shocks for external cardioversion of atrial fibrillation. *Am Heart J.* 2004;147:e20.
137. Neal S, Ngarmukos T, Lessard D, Rosenthal L. Comparison of the efficacy and safety of two biphasic defibrillator waveforms for the conversion of atrial fibrillation to sinus rhythm. *Am J Cardiol.* 2003;92: 810–814.
138. Kim ML, Kim SG, Park DS, Gross JN, Ferrick KJ, Palma EC, Fisher JD. Comparison of rectilinear biphasic waveform energy versus truncated exponential biphasic waveform energy for transthoracic cardioversion of atrial fibrillation. *Am J Cardiol.* 2004;94:1438–1440.
139. Kerber RE, Kienzle MG, Olshansky B, Waldo AL, Wilber D, Carlson MD, Aschoff AM, Birger S, Fugatt L, Walsh S, et al. Ventricular tachycardia rate and morphology determine energy and current requirements for transthoracic cardioversion. *Circulation.* 1992;85: 158–163.
140. Hedges JR, Syverud SA, Dalsey WC, Feero S, Easter R, Shultz B. Prehospital trial of emergency transcutaneous cardiac pacing. *Circulation.* 1987;76:1337–1343.
141. Barthell E, Troiano P, Olson D, Stueven HA, Hendley G. Prehospital external cardiac pacing: a prospective, controlled clinical trial. *Ann Emerg Med.* 1988;17:1221–1226.
142. Cummins RO, Graves JR, Larsen MP, Hallstrom AP, Hearne TR, Ciliberti J, Nicola RM, Horan S. Out-of-hospital transcutaneous pacing by emergency medical technicians in patients with asystolic cardiac arrest. *N Engl J Med.* 1993;328:1377–1382.
143. Ornato JP, Peberdy MA. The mystery of bradyasystole during cardiac arrest. *Ann Emerg Med.* 1996;27:576–587.
144. Niemann JT, Adomian GE, Garner D, Rosborough JP. Endocardial and transcutaneous cardiac pacing, calcium chloride, and epinephrine in postcountershock asystole and bradycardias. *Crit Care Med.* 1985;13: 699–704.
145. Quan L, Graves JR, Kinder DR, Horan S, Cummins RO. Transcutaneous cardiac pacing in the treatment of out-of-hospital pediatric cardiac arrests. *Ann Emerg Med.* 1992;21:905–909.
146. Dalsey WC, Syverud SA, Hedges JR. Emergency department use of transcutaneous pacing for cardiac arrests. *Crit Care Med.* 1985;13: 399–401.
147. Knowlton AA, Falk RH. External cardiac pacing during in-hospital cardiac arrest. *Am J Cardiol.* 1986;57:1295–1298.
148. Ornato JP, Carveth WL, Windle JR. Pacemaker insertion for prehospital bradyasystolic cardiac arrest. *Ann Emerg Med.* 1984;13:101–103.
149. White JD. Transthoracic pacing in cardiac asystole. *Am J Emerg Med.* 1983;1:264–266.

Part 6: CPR Techniques and Devices

Over the past 25 years a variety of alternatives to standard manual CPR have been developed in an effort to improve ventilation or perfusion during cardiac arrest and ultimately to improve survival. Compared with standard CPR, these techniques and devices typically require more personnel, training, or equipment, or they apply to a specific setting. Maximum benefits are reported when adjuncts are begun early in the treatment of cardiac arrest, so that the use of these alternatives to CPR is often limited to the hospital setting. To date no adjunct has consistently been shown to be superior to standard manual CPR for out-of-hospital basic life support, and no device other than a defibrillator has consistently improved long-term survival from out-of-hospital cardiac arrest. The data reported here is limited to clinical trials, so most animal data is excluded from this section.

CPR Techniques

High-Frequency Chest Compressions

High-frequency (>100 per minute) manual or mechanical chest compressions have been studied as a technique for improving resuscitation from cardiac arrest.[1–4] The sparse animal and human data available show mixed results. One clinical trial of 9 patients showed that high-frequency (120 per minute) chest compressions improved hemodynamics over standard CPR (LOE 4).[5] The use of high-frequency chest compressions for cardiac arrest by adequately trained rescue personnel can be considered, but there is insufficient evidence to recommend for or against its use (Class Indeterminate).

Open-Chest CPR

No prospective randomized studies of open-chest CPR for resuscitation have been published. Four relevant human studies were reviewed: 2 were performed to treat in-hospital cardiac arrest following cardiac surgery (LOE 4[6]; LOE 5[7]), and 2 were performed after out-of-hospital cardiac arrest (LOE 4[8]; LOE 5[9]). The observed benefits of open-chest cardiac massage were improved coronary perfusion pressure[9] and increased return of spontaneous circulation (ROSC).[8]

Open-chest CPR should be considered (Class IIa) for patients with cardiac arrest in the early postoperative period after cardiothoracic surgery or when the chest or abdomen is already open (eg, in trauma surgery). For further information about trauma resuscitation, see Part 10.7: "Special Resuscitation Situations: Cardiac Arrest Associated With Trauma."

Interposed Abdominal Compression

The interposed abdominal compression (IAC)-CPR technique uses a dedicated rescuer to provide manual compression of the abdomen (midway between the xiphoid and the umbilicus) during the relaxation phase of chest compression. The purpose is to enhance venous return during CPR.[10,11] When IAC-CPR performed by trained providers was compared with standard CPR for cardiac arrest in the in-hospital setting, IAC-CPR improved ROSC and short-term survival in 2 randomized trials (LOE 1)[12,13] and improved survival to hospital discharge in 1 study.[13] The data from these studies was combined in 2 positive meta-analyses (LOE 1).[14,15] Evidence from 1 randomized controlled trial of out-of-hospital cardiac arrest (LOE 2),[16] however, did not show any survival advantage to IAC-CPR. Although there is 1 pediatric case report[17] of complications, no harm was reported in the other studies, which involved a total of 426 patients.

IAC-CPR may be considered during in-hospital resuscitation when sufficient personnel trained in its use are available (Class IIb). There is insufficient evidence to recommend for or against the use of IAC-CPR in the out-of-hospital setting (Class Indeterminate).

"Cough" CPR

"Cough" CPR is not useful for the treatment of an unresponsive victim,[18–23] and it should not be taught to lay rescuers. Human "cough" CPR has been reported only in awake, monitored patients who developed ventricular fibrillation (VF) or rapid ventricular tachycardia (VT).[20,22,24] Several small case series (LOE 5)[18,20,22,24] reporting experiences in the cardiac catheterization suite suggest that repeated coughing every 1 to 3 seconds during episodes of VF or rapid VT by conscious, supine, monitored patients trained in the technique can maintain a mean arterial pressure >100 mm Hg and can maintain consciousness for up to 90 seconds.

The increase in intrathoracic pressure that occurs with coughing generates blood flow to the brain and helps maintain consciousness. Coughing every 1 to 3 seconds for up to 90 seconds after the onset of VF or pulseless VT is safe and effective only in conscious, supine, monitored patients previously trained to perform this maneuver (Class IIb). Defibrillation remains the treatment of choice for VF or pulseless VT.

CPR Devices

Devices to Assist Ventilation

Automatic and Mechanical Transport Ventilators

Automatic transport ventilators (ATVs). One prospective cohort study of 73 intubated patients, most of whom were in cardiac arrest, in an out-of-hospital urban setting showed no difference in arterial blood gas parameters between those ventilated with an ATV and those ventilated with a bag-mask device (LOE 4).[25] Disadvantages of ATVs include the need for an oxygen source and electric power. Thus, providers should always have a bag-mask device available for manual backup. Some ATVs may be inappropriate for use in children <5 years of age.

(*Circulation*. 2005;112:IV-47-IV-50.)

DOI: 10.1161/CIRCULATIONAHA.105.166555

In both the out-of-hospital and in-hospital settings, ATVs are useful for ventilation of adult patients with a pulse who have an advanced airway (eg, endotracheal tube, esophageal-tracheal combitube [Combitube], or laryngeal mask airway [LMA]) in place (Class IIa). For the adult cardiac arrest patient who does not have an advanced airway in place, the ATV may be useful if tidal volumes are delivered by a flow-controlled, time-cycled ventilator without positive end-expiratory pressure (PEEP). If the ATV has adjustable output control valves, tidal volume should be adjusted to make the chest rise (approximately 6 to 7 mL/kg or 500 to 600 mL), with breaths delivered over 1 second. Until an advanced airway is in place, an additional rescuer should provide cricoid pressure to reduce the risk of gastric inflation. Once an advanced airway is in place, the ventilation rate should be 8 to 10 breaths per minute during CPR.

Manually triggered, oxygen-powered, flow-limited resuscitators. In a study of 104 anesthetized nonarrest patients without an advanced airway in place (ie, no endotracheal tube; patients were ventilated through a mask), patients ventilated by firefighters with manually triggered, oxygen-powered, flow-limited resuscitators had less gastric inflation than those ventilated with a bag-mask device (LOE 5).[26] Manually triggered, oxygen-powered, flow-limited resuscitators may be considered for the management of patients who do not have an advanced airway in place and for whom a mask is being used for ventilation during CPR. Rescuers should avoid using the automatic mode of the oxygen-powered, flow-limited resuscitator because it applies continuous PEEP that is likely to impede cardiac output during chest compressions (Class III).

Devices to Support Circulation

Active Compression-Decompression CPR

Active compression-decompression CPR (ACD-CPR) is performed with a hand-held device equipped with a suction cup to actively lift the anterior chest during decompression. It is thought that decreasing intrathoracic pressure during the decompression phase enhances venous return to the heart. As of 2005 no ACD-CPR devices have been cleared by the Food and Drug Administration for sale in the United States.

Results from the use of ACD-CPR have been mixed. In 4 randomized studies (LOE 1[27,28]; LOE 2[29,30]) ACD-CPR improved long-term survival rates when it was used by adequately trained providers for patients with cardiac arrest in the out-of-hospital[27,28] and in-hospital[29,30] settings. In 5 other randomized studies (LOE 1[31–34]; LOE 2[35]), however, no positive or negative effects were observed. In 4 clinical studies (LOE 3)[30,36–38] ACD-CPR improved hemodynamics over standard CPR, and in 1 clinical study (LOE 3)[39] did not. Frequent training seems to be a significant factor in achieving efficacy.[28]

A meta-analysis of 10 trials involving 4162 patients in the out-of-hospital setting (LOE 1)[40] and a meta-analysis of 2 trials in the in-hospital setting (826 patients)[40] failed to document any early or late survival benefit of ACD-CPR over conventional CPR. The out-of-hospital meta-analysis found a large but nonsignificant worsening in neurologic outcome in survivors in the ACD-CPR group, and 1 small study[41] showed increased incidence of sternal fractures in the ACD-CPR group.

ACD-CPR may be considered for use in the in-hospital setting when providers are adequately trained (Class IIb). There is insufficient evidence to recommend for or against the use of ACD-CPR in the prehospital setting (Class Indeterminate).

Impedance Threshold Device

The impedance threshold device (ITD) is a valve that limits air entry into the lungs during chest recoil between chest compressions. It is designed to reduce intrathoracic pressure and enhance venous return to the heart. In initial studies the ITD was used with a cuffed endotracheal tube during bag-tube ventilation and ACD-CPR.[42–44] The ITD and ACD device are thought to act synergistically to enhance venous return during active decompression.

In recent reports the ITD has been used during conventional CPR[45,46] with an endotracheal tube or face mask. Studies suggest that when the ITD is used with a face mask, it may create the same negative intratracheal pressure as use of the ITD with an endotracheal tube if rescuers can maintain a tight face mask seal.[43,45,46]

In 2 randomized studies (LOE 1)[44,47] of 610 adults in cardiac arrest in the out-of-hospital setting, use of ACD-CPR plus the ITD was associated with improved ROSC and 24-hour survival rates when compared with use of standard CPR alone. A randomized study of 230 adults documented increased admission to the intensive care unit and 24-hour survival (LOE 2)[45] when an ITD was used during standard CPR in patients in cardiac arrest (pulseless electrical activity only) in the out-of-hospital setting. The addition of the ITD was associated with improved hemodynamics during standard CPR in 1 clinical study (LOE 2).[46]

Although increased long-term survival rates have not been documented, when the ITD is used by trained personnel as an adjunct to CPR in intubated adult cardiac arrest patients, it can improve hemodynamic parameters and ROSC (Class IIa).

Mechanical Piston Device

The mechanical piston device depresses the sternum via a compressed gas-powered plunger mounted on a backboard. In 1 prospective randomized study and 2 prospective randomized crossover studies in adults (LOE 2),[48–50] mechanical piston CPR used by medical and paramedical personnel improved end-tidal CO_2 and mean arterial pressure in patients in cardiac arrest in both the out-of-hospital and in-hospital settings.

Mechanical piston CPR may be considered for patients in cardiac arrest in circumstances that make manual resuscitation difficult (Class IIb). The device should be programmed to deliver standard CPR with adequate compression depth at the rate of 100 compressions per minute with a compression-ventilation ratio of 30:2 (until an advanced airway is in place) and a compression duration that is 50% of the compression-decompression cycle length. The device should allow complete chest wall recoil.

Load-Distributing Band CPR or Vest CPR

The load-distributing band (LDB) is a circumferential chest compression device composed of a pneumatically or electrically actuated constricting band and backboard. Evidence from a case control study of 162 adults (LOE 4)[51] documented improvement in survival to the emergency department when LDB-CPR was administered by adequately trained rescue personnel to patients with cardiac arrest in the out-of-hospital setting. The use of LDB-CPR improved hemodynamics in 1 in-hospital study of end-stage patients (LOE 3)[52] and 2 laboratory studies (LOE 6).[53,54] LDB-CPR may be considered for use by properly trained personnel as an adjunct to CPR for patients with cardiac arrest in the out-of-hospital or in-hospital setting (Class IIb).

Phased Thoracic-Abdominal Compression-Decompression CPR With a Hand-Held Device

Phased thoracic-abdominal compression-decompression CPR (PTACD-CPR) combines the concepts of IAC-CPR and ACD-CPR. A hand-held device alternates chest compression and abdominal decompression with chest decompression and abdominal compression. Evidence from 1 prospective randomized clinical study of adults in cardiac arrest (LOE 2)[55] documented no improvement in survival rates with use of PTACD-CPR for assistance of circulation during advanced cardiovascular life support (ACLS) in the out-of-hospital and in-hospital settings. Thus, there is insufficient evidence to support the use of PTACD-CPR outside the research setting (Class Indeterminate).

Extracorporeal Techniques and Invasive Perfusion Devices

Much of the literature showing the effectiveness of extracorporeal CPR (ECPR) includes patients with cardiac disease. ECPR is more successful in postcardiotomy patients than in those with cardiac arrest from other causes (LOE 5).[56] ECPR may be particularly effective for these patients because they are more likely to have a reversible (ie, surgically correctable or short-term) cause of cardiac arrest, and typically they suffer cardiac arrest without preceding multisystem organ failure.

ECPR for induction of hypothermia has been shown to improve survival rates in a small study of patients who arrived at the ED in cardiac arrest and failed to respond to standard ACLS techniques (LOE 5).[57]

ECPR should be considered for in-hospital patients in cardiac arrest when the duration of the no-flow arrest is brief and the condition leading to the cardiac arrest is reversible (eg, hypothermia or drug intoxication) or amenable to heart transplantation or revascularization (Class IIb).[58,59]

Summary

A variety of CPR techniques and devices may improve hemodynamics or short-term survival when used by well-trained providers in selected patients. To date no adjunct has consistently been shown to be superior to standard manual CPR for out-of-hospital basic life support, and no device other than a defibrillator has consistently improved long-term survival from out-of-hospital cardiac arrest.

References

1. Feneley MP, Maier GW, Kern KB, Gaynor JW, Gall SA Jr, Sanders AB, Raessler K, Muhlbaier LH, Rankin JS, Ewy GA. Influence of compression rate on initial success of resuscitation and 24 hour survival after prolonged manual cardiopulmonary resuscitation in dogs. *Circulation*. 1988;77:240–250.
2. Halperin HR, Tsitlik JE, Guerci AD, Mellits ED, Levin HR, Shi AY, Chandra N, Weisfeldt ML. Determinants of blood flow to vital organs during cardiopulmonary resuscitation in dogs. *Circulation*. 1986;73:539–550.
3. Kern KB, Sanders AB, Raife J, Milander MM, Otto CW, Ewy GA. A study of chest compression rates during cardiopulmonary resuscitation in humans: the importance of rate-directed chest compressions. *Arch Intern Med*. 1992;152:145–149.
4. Ornato JP, Gonzalez ER, Garnett AR, Levine RL, McClung BK. Effect of cardiopulmonary resuscitation compression rate on end-tidal carbon dioxide concentration and arterial pressure in man. *Crit Care Med*. 1988;16:241–245.
5. Swenson RD, Weaver WD, Niskanen RA, Martin J, Dahlberg S. Hemodynamics in humans during conventional and experimental methods of cardiopulmonary resuscitation. *Circulation*. 1988;78:630–639.
6. Anthi A, Tzelepis GE, Alivizatos P, Michalis A, Palatianos GM, Geroulanos S. Unexpected cardiac arrest after cardiac surgery: incidence, predisposing causes, and outcome of open chest cardiopulmonary resuscitation. *Chest*. 1998;113:15–19.
7. Pottle A, Bullock I, Thomas J, Scott L. Survival to discharge following open chest cardiac compression (OCCC): a 4-year retrospective audit in a cardiothoracic specialist centre—Royal Brompton and Harefield NHS Trust, United Kingdom. *Resuscitation*. 2002;52:269–272.
8. Takino M, Okada Y. The optimum timing of resuscitative thoracotomy for non-traumatic out-of-hospital cardiac arrest. *Resuscitation*. 1993;26:69–74.
9. Boczar ME, Howard MA, Rivers EP, Martin GB, Horst HM, Lewandowski C, Tomlanovich MC, Nowak RM. A technique revisited: hemodynamic comparison of closed- and open-chest cardiac massage during human cardiopulmonary resuscitation. *Crit Care Med*. 1995;23:498–503.
10. Beyar R, Kishon Y, Kimmel E, Neufeld H, Dinnar U. Intrathoracic and abdominal pressure variations as an efficient method for cardiopulmonary resuscitation: studies in dogs compared with computer model results. *Cardiovasc Res*. 1985;19:335–342.
11. Voorhees WD, Niebauer MJ, Babbs CF. Improved oxygen delivery during cardiopulmonary resuscitation with interposed abdominal compressions. *Ann Emerg Med*. 1983;12:128–135.
12. Sack JB, Kesselbrenner MB, Jarrad A. Interposed abdominal compression-cardiopulmonary resuscitation and resuscitation outcome during asystole and electromechanical dissociation. *Circulation*. 1992;86:1692–1700.
13. Sack JB, Kesselbrenner MB, Bregman D. Survival from in-hospital cardiac arrest with interposed abdominal counterpulsation during cardiopulmonary resuscitation. *JAMA*. 1992;267:379–385.
14. Babbs CF. Interposed abdominal compression CPR: a comprehensive evidence based review. *Resuscitation*. 2003;59:71–82.
15. Babbs CF. Simplified meta-analysis of clinical trials in resuscitation. *Resuscitation*. 2003;57:245–255.
16. Mateer JR, Stueven HA, Thompson BM, Aprahamian C, Darin JC. Pre-hospital IAC-CPR versus standard CPR: paramedic resuscitation of cardiac arrests. *Am J Emerg Med*. 1985;3:143–146.
17. Waldman PJ, Walters BL, Grunau CF. Pancreatic injury associated with interposed abdominal compressions in pediatric cardiopulmonary resuscitation. *Am J Emerg Med*. 1984;2:510–512.
18. Criley JM, Blaufuss AH, Kissel GL. Cough-induced cardiac compression: self-administered from of cardiopulmonary resuscitation. *JAMA*. 1976;236:1246–1250.
19. Niemann JT, Rosborough JP, Niskanen RA, Alferness C, Criley JM. Mechanical "cough" cardiopulmonary resuscitation during cardiac arrest in dogs. *Am J Cardiol*. 1985;55:199–204.
20. Miller B, Cohen A, Serio A, Bettock D. Hemodynamics of cough cardiopulmonary resuscitation in a patient with sustained torsades de pointes/ventricular flutter. *J Emerg Med*. 1994;12:627–632.
21. Rieser MJ. The use of cough-CPR in patients with acute myocardial infarction. *J Emerg Med*. 1992;10:291–293.
22. Miller B, Lesnefsky E, Heyborne T, Schmidt B, Freeman K, Breckinridge S, Kelley K, Mann D, Reiter M. Cough-cardiopulmonary resuscitation in the cardiac catheterization laboratory: hemodynamics during an episode of prolonged hypotensive ventricular tachycardia. *Cathet Cardiovasc Diagn*. 1989;18:168–171.

23. Bircher N, Safar P, Eshel G, Stezoski W. Cerebral and hemodynamic variables during cough-induced CPR in dogs. *Crit Care Med.* 1982;10: 104–107.
24. Saba SE, David SW. Sustained consciousness during ventricular fibrillation: case report of cough cardiopulmonary resuscitation. *Cathet Cardiovasc Diagn.* 1996;37:47–48.
25. Johannigman JA, Branson RD, Johnson DJ, Davis K Jr, Hurst JM. Out-of-hospital ventilation: bag–valve device vs transport ventilator. *Acad Emerg Med.* 1995;2:719–724.
26. Noordergraaf GJ, van Dun PJ, Kramer BP, Schors MP, Hornman HP, de Jong W, Noordergraaf A. Can first responders achieve and maintain normocapnia when sequentially ventilating with a bag-valve device and two oxygen-driven resuscitators? A controlled clinical trial in 104 patients. *Eur J Anaesthesiol.* 2004;21:367–372.
27. Lurie KG, Shultz JJ, Callaham ML, Schwab TM, Gisch T, Rector T, Frascone RJ, Long L. Evaluation of active compression-decompression CPR in victims of out-of-hospital cardiac arrest. *JAMA.* 1994;271: 1405–1411.
28. Plaisance P, Lurie KG, Vicaut E, Adnet F, Petit JL, Epain D, Ecollan P, Gruat R, Cavagna P, Biens J, Payen D. A comparison of standard cardiopulmonary resuscitation and active compression-decompression resuscitation for out-of-hospital cardiac arrest. French Active Compression-Decompression Cardiopulmonary Resuscitation Study Group. *N Engl J Med.* 1999;341:569–575.
29. Cohen TJ, Goldner BG, Maccaro PC, Ardito AP, Trazzera S, Cohen MB, Dibs SR. A comparison of active compression-decompression cardiopulmonary resuscitation with standard cardiopulmonary resuscitation for cardiac arrests occurring in the hospital. *N Engl J Med.* 1993;329: 1918–1921.
30. Tucker KJ, Galli F, Savitt MA, Kahsai D, Bresnahan L, Redberg RF. Active compression-decompression resuscitation: effect on resuscitation success after in-hospital cardiac arrest. *J Am Coll Cardiol.* 1994;24: 201–209.
31. Schwab TM, Callaham ML, Madsen CD, Utecht TA. A randomized clinical trial of active compression-decompression CPR vs standard CPR in out-of-hospital cardiac arrest in two cities. *JAMA.* 1995;273: 1261–1268.
32. Stiell I, H'ebert P, Well G, Laupacis A, Vandemheen K, Dreyer J, Eisenhauer M, Gibson J, Higginson L, Kirby A, Mahon J, Maloney J, Weitzman B. The Ontario trial of active compression-decompression cardiopulmonary resuscitation for in-hospital and prehospital cardiac arrest. *JAMA.* 1996;275:1417–1423.
33. Mauer D, Schneider T, Dick W, Withelm A, Elich D, Mauer M. Active compression-decompression resuscitation: a prospective, randomized study in a two-tiered EMS system with physicians in the field. *Resuscitation.* 1996;33:125–134.
34. Nolan J, Smith G, Evans R, McCusker K, Lubas P, Parr M, Baskett P. The United Kingdom pre-hospital study of active compression-decompression resuscitation. *Resuscitation.* 1998;37:119–125.
35. Luiz T, Ellinger K, Denz C. Active compression-decompression cardiopulmonary resuscitation does not improve survival in patients with prehospital cardiac arrest in a physician-manned emergency medical system. *J Cardiothorac Vasc Anesth.* 1996;10:178–186.
36. Guly UM and Robertson CE. Active decompression improves the haemodynamic state during cardiopulmonary resuscitation. *Br Heart J*.1995; 73(4):372–6.
37. Orliaguet GA, Carli PA, Rozenberg A, Janniere D, Sauval P, Delpech P. End-tidal carbon dioxide during out-of-hospital cardiac arrest resuscitation: comparison of active compression-decompression and standard CPR. *Ann Emerg Med.* 1995;25:48–51.
38. Shultz JJ, Coffeen P, Sweeney M, Detloff B, Kehler C, Pineda E, Yakshe P, Adler SW, Chang M, Lurie KG. Evaluation of standard and active compression-decompression CPR in an acute human model of ventricular fibrillation. *Circulation.* 1994;89:684–693.
39. Malzer R, Zeiner A, Binder M, Domanovits H, Knappitsch G, Sterz F, Laggner AN. Hemodynamic effects of active compression-decompression after prolonged CPR. *Resuscitation.* 1996;31:243–253.
40. Lafuente-Lafuente C, Melero-Bascones M. Active chest compression-decompression for cardiopulmonary resuscitation. *Cochrane Database Syst Rev.* 2004:CD002751.
41. Baubin M, Rabl W, Pfeiffer KP, Benzer A, Gilly H. Chest injuries after active compression-decompression cardiopulmonary resuscitation (ACD-CPR) in cadavers. *Resuscitation.* 1999;43:9–15.
42. Plaisance P, Lurie KG, Payen D. Inspiratory impedance during active compression-decompression cardiopulmonary resuscitation: a randomized evaluation in patients in cardiac arrest. *Circulation.* 2000;101: 989–994.
43. Plaisance P, Soleil C, Lurie KG, Vicaut E, Ducros L, Payen D. Use of an inspiratory impedance threshold device on a facemask and endotracheal tube to reduce intrathoracic pressures during the decompression phase of active compression-decompression cardiopulmonary resuscitation. *Crit Care Med.* 2005;33:990–994.
44. Wolcke BB, Mauer DK, Schoefmann MF, Teichmann H, Provo TA, Lindner KH, Dick WF, Aeppli D, Lurie KG. Comparison of standard cardiopulmonary resuscitation versus the combination of active compression-decompression cardiopulmonary resuscitation and an inspiratory impedance threshold device for out-of-hospital cardiac arrest. *Circulation.* 2003;108:2201–2205.
45. Aufderheide TP, Pirrallo RG, Provo TA, Lurie KG. Clinical evaluation of an inspiratory impedance threshold device during standard cardiopulmonary resuscitation in patients with out-of-hospital cardiac arrest. *Crit Care Med.* 2005;33:734–740.
46. Pirrallo RG, Aufderheide TP, Provo TA, Lurie KG. Effect of an inspiratory impedance threshold device on hemodynamics during conventional manual cardiopulmonary resuscitation. *Resuscitation.* 2005;66: 13–20.
47. Plaisance P, Lurie KG, Vicaut E, Martin D, Gueugniaud PY, Petit JL, Payen D. Evaluation of an impedance threshold device in patients receiving active compression-decompression cardiopulmonary resuscitation for out of hospital cardiac arrest. *Resuscitation.* 2004;61:265–271.
48. Dickinson ET, Verdile VP, Schneider RM, Salluzzo RF. Effectiveness of mechanical versus manual chest compressions in out-of-hospital cardiac arrest resuscitation: a pilot study. *Am J Emerg Med.* 1998;16:289–292.
49. McDonald JL. Systolic and mean arterial pressures during manual and mechanical CPR in humans. *Ann Emerg Med.* 1982;11:292–295.
50. Ward KR, Menegazzi JJ, Zelenak RR, Sullivan RJ, McSwain N Jr. A comparison of chest compressions between mechanical and manual CPR by monitoring end-tidal PCO2 during human cardiac arrest. *Ann Emerg Med.* 1993;22:669–674.
51. Casner M, Anderson D, et al. Preliminary report of the impact of a new CPR assist device on the rate of return of spontaneous circulation in out of hospital cardiac arrest. *Prehosp Emerg Med.* 2005;9:61–67.
52. Timerman S, Cardoso LF, Ramires JA, Halperin H. Improved hemodynamic performance with a novel chest compression device during treatment of in-hospital cardiac arrest. *Resuscitation.* 2004;61:273–280.
53. Halperin H, Berger R, Chandra N, Ireland M, Leng C, Lardo A, Paradis N. Cardiopulmonary resuscitation with a hydraulic-pneumatic band. *Crit Care Med.* 2000;28:N203–N206.
54. Halperin HR, Paradis N, Ornato JP, Zviman M, Lacorte J, Lardo A, Kern KB. Cardiopulmonary resuscitation with a novel chest compression device in a porcine model of cardiac arrest: improved hemodynamics and mechanisms. *J Am Coll Cardiol.* 2004;44:2214–2220.
55. Arntz HR, Agrawal R, Richter H, Schmidt S, Rescheleit T, Menges M, Burbach H, Schroder J, Schultheiss HP. Phased chest and abdominal compression-decompression versus conventional cardiopulmonary resuscitation in out-of-hospital cardiac arrest. *Circulation.* 2001;104:768–772.
56. Chen Y-S, Chao A, Yu H-Y, Ko W-J, Wu I-H, Chen RJ-C, Huang S-C, Lin F-Y, Wang S-S. Analysis and results of prolonged resuscitation in cardiac arrest patients rescued by extracorporeal membrane oxygenation. *J Am Coll Cardiol.* 2003;41:197–203.
57. Nagao K, Hayashi N, Kanmatsuse K, Arima K, Ohtsuki J, Kikushima K, Watanabe I. Cardiopulmonary cerebral resuscitation using emergency cardiopulmonary bypass, coronary reperfusion therapy and mild hypothermia in patients with cardiac arrest outside the hospital. *J Am Coll Cardiol.* 2000;36:776–783.
58. Younger JG, Schreiner RJ, Swaniker F, Hirschl RB, Chapman RA, Bartlett RH. Extracorporeal resuscitation of cardiac arrest. *Acad Emerg Med.* 1999;6:700–707.
59. Martin GB, Rivers EP, Paradis NA, Goetting MG, Morris DC, Nowak RM. Emergency department cardiopulmonary bypass in the treatment of human cardiac arrest. *Chest.* 1998;113:743–751.

Part 7.1: Adjuncts for Airway Control and Ventilation

This section highlights recommendations for the support of ventilation and oxygenation during resuscitation and the periarrest period. The purpose of ventilation during CPR is to maintain adequate oxygenation and sufficient elimination of carbon dioxide, but research has not identified the optimal tidal volume, respiratory rate, and inspired oxygen concentration required to do so. During the first minutes of ventricular fibrillation sudden cardiac arrest (VF SCA), rescue breaths are probably not as important as chest compressions, because oxygen delivery to the tissues, including the heart and brain, appears to be limited more by blood flow than by arterial oxygen content. Thus, during the first minutes of VF SCA the lone rescuer should attempt to limit interruptions in chest compressions for ventilation. The advanced provider must be careful to limit interruptions in chest compressions for attempts to insert an advanced airway or check the rhythm.

Ventilation and compressions are both thought to be important for victims of prolonged VF SCA and for all victims of asphyxial arrest (eg, drowning victims and victims of drug overdose with primary respiratory arrest) because these victims are hypoxemic before arrest.

Because systemic and, therefore, lung perfusion is substantially reduced during CPR, rescuers can support a normal ventilation-perfusion match with a minute ventilation that is much lower than normal. During CPR with an advanced airway in place we now recommend a lower rate of rescue breathing (see Part 4: "Adult Basic Life Support") than that recommended in the *ECC Guidelines 2000*.[1] During the prearrest and postarrest periods, the patient will require support of oxygenation and ventilation with tidal volumes and respiratory rates that more closely approximate normal.

Beyond the first minutes of cardiac arrest, tissue hypoxia develops. CPR provides approximately 25% to 33% of normal cardiac output. This low-flow state maintains a small but critical amount of blood flow to the heart and brain, but tissue hypoxia will persist until restoration of effective spontaneous perfusion. Additional factors that contribute to hypoxia include intrapulmonary shunting with microcirculatory dysfunction and attendant ventilation-perfusion abnormalities. Some patients may also have underlying respiratory disease. Tissue hypoxia leads to anaerobic metabolism and metabolic acidosis. Acid-base imbalance occasionally blunts the beneficial effects of chemical and electrical therapy.

To improve oxygenation, healthcare providers should give 100% inspired oxygen ($Fio_2 = 1.0$) during basic life support and advanced cardiovascular life support as soon as it becomes available. High inspired oxygen tension will tend to maximize arterial oxygen saturation and, in turn, arterial oxygen content. This will help support oxygen delivery (cardiac output × arterial oxygen content) when cardiac output is limited. This short-term oxygen therapy does not produce oxygen toxicity.

(*Circulation*. 2005;112:IV-51-IV-57.)

DOI: 10.1161/CIRCULATIONAHA.105.166556

Bag-Mask Ventilation

All healthcare providers should be familiar with the use of the bag-mask device for support of oxygenation and ventilation.[2–4] Bag-mask ventilation is particularly helpful during the first few minutes of resuscitation or when placement of an advanced airway is delayed or unsuccessful. Effective bag-mask ventilation requires adequate training and frequent practice.

The desirable components of a bag-mask device are listed in Part 4: "Adult Basic Life Support." When using a bag-mask device (ie, no advanced airway is in place), the rescuer should deliver a tidal volume sufficient to produce chest rise (approximately 6 to 7 mL/kg or 500 to 600 mL) over 1 second.[5] This volume of ventilation minimizes the risk of gastric inflation. The rescuer should be sure to open the airway adequately with a chin lift, lifting the jaw against the mask and holding the mask against the face, creating a tight seal. During CPR, give 2 breaths during a brief (about 3 to 4 seconds) pause after every 30 chest compressions. When an advanced airway (eg, endotracheal tube, esophageal-tracheal combitube [Combitube], or laryngeal mask airway [LMA]) replaces the face mask, rescuers should deliver 8 to 10 breaths per minute during CPR. Deliver each breath over about 1 second while chest compressions are delivered at a rate of 100 per minute, and do not attempt to synchronize the compressions with the ventilations.

For ventilation of patients with a perfusing rhythm (ie, better pulmonary blood flow than is present during CPR), deliver approximately 10 to 12 breaths per minute (1 breath every 6 to 7 seconds). Deliver these breaths over 1 second when using a mask or an advanced airway.

In patients with severe obstructive pulmonary disease and increased resistance to exhalation, providers should try to prevent air trapping that may result in inadvertent generation of intrinsic positive end-expiratory pressure (PEEP), so-called "auto-PEEP." In patients with hypovolemia, auto-PEEP may substantially reduce cardiac output and blood pressure. To prevent this, use lower respiratory rates (eg, 6 to 8 breaths per minute) in these patients, allowing more time for complete exhalation.

Bag-mask ventilation can produce gastric inflation with complications, including regurgitation, aspiration, and pneumonia. Gastric inflation can elevate the diaphragm, restrict lung movement, and decrease respiratory system compliance.[4,6–9]

Airway Adjuncts

Oropharyngeal Airways

Oropharyngeal airways should be reserved for use in unconscious (unresponsive) patients with no cough or gag reflex and should be inserted only by persons trained in their use (Class IIa). Incorrect insertion of an airway can displace the tongue into the hypopharynx, causing airway obstruction. Although studies have not specifically considered the use of advanced airways in arrest, airways may aid in the delivery of adequate ventilation with a bag-mask device by preventing the tongue from occluding the airway.

Nasopharyngeal Airways

Nasopharyngeal airways are useful in patients with airway obstruction or those at risk for development of airway obstruction, particularly when conditions such as a clenched jaw prevent placement of an oral airway. Nasopharyngeal airways are better tolerated than oral airways in patients who are not deeply unconscious. Airway bleeding can occur in up to 30% of patients following insertion of a nasopharyngeal airway (LOE 5).[10] Two case reports of inadvertent intracranial placement of a nasopharyngeal airway in patients with basilar skull fractures (LOE 7)[11,12] suggest that nasopharyngeal airways should be used with caution in patients with severe craniofacial injury.

As with all adjunctive equipment, safe use of the nasopharyngeal airway requires adequate training, practice, and retraining. No studies on the use of this device in patients in cardiac arrest have been found. The nasopharyngeal airway may be used in patients with an obstructed airway to facilitate delivery of ventilations with a bag-mask device.

Advanced Airways

Rescuers must be aware of the risks and benefits of insertion of an advanced airway during a resuscitation attempt. Such risks are affected by the condition of the patient and the rescuer's expertise in airway control. Because insertion of an advanced airway may require interruption of chest compressions for many seconds, the rescuer should weigh the need for compressions against the need for insertion of an advanced airway. Rescuers may defer insertion of an advanced airway until the patient fails to respond to initial CPR and defibrillation attempts or demonstrates return of spontaneous circulation (Class IIb). To use any of the advanced airways effectively, healthcare providers must maintain knowledge and skills through frequent practice with these devices. It may be helpful for providers to train in one primary method of airway control and gain experience and expertise in that method. Providers should have a second (backup) strategy for airway management and ventilation if they are unable to establish the first-choice airway adjunct. Bag-mask ventilation may provide that backup strategy.

Once an advanced airway is in place, 2 rescuers no longer deliver cycles of CPR (ie, compressions interrupted by pauses for ventilation). Instead, the compressing rescuer should give continuous chest compressions at a rate of 100 per minute, without pauses for ventilation. The rescuer delivering ventilation provides 8 to 10 breaths per minute. The 2 rescuers should change compressor and ventilator roles approximately every 2 minutes to prevent compressor fatigue and deterioration in quality and rate of chest compressions. When multiple rescuers are present, they should rotate the compressor role about every 2 minutes.

Bag-Mask Ventilation Versus the Advanced Airway

Bag-mask ventilation or ventilation with a bag through an advanced airway (eg, endotracheal tube, Combitube, or LMA) is acceptable for ventilation during CPR. As noted above, all healthcare providers should be trained in delivering effective oxygenation and ventilation with a bag and mask. Because there are times when ventilation with a bag-mask device is inadequate or transport times are prolonged, advanced care providers should also be trained and experienced in insertion of an advanced airway.

The endotracheal tube was once considered the optimal method of managing the airway during cardiac arrest. It is now clear, however, that the incidence of complications is unacceptably high when intubation is performed by inexperienced providers or monitoring of tube placement is inadequate. The optimal method of managing the airway during cardiac arrest will vary based on provider experience, emergency medical services (EMS) or healthcare system characteristics, and the patient's condition.

No prospective randomized trials have directly assessed the outcome of adult victims of cardiac arrest with provision of bag-mask ventilation compared with endotracheal intubation. Studies comparing outcomes of out-of-hospital cardiac arrest in adults treated by either emergency medical technicians or paramedics failed to show a link between long-term survival rates and paramedic skills such as intubation, intravenous cannulation, and drug administration.[13–15] One prospective randomized controlled trial in an EMS system with short out-of-hospital transport intervals[16] showed no survival advantage for endotracheal intubation over bag-mask ventilation in children. In this study providers had limited training and experience in intubation.

In retrospective (LOE 5) studies, endotracheal intubation has been associated with a 6%[17–19] to 14%[20] incidence of unrecognized tube misplacement or displacement. This may reflect inadequate initial training or experience on the part of the provider who performed intubation, or it may result from displacement of a correctly positioned tube during movement of the patient. To reduce the risk of unrecognized tube misplacement or displacement, providers should use a device such as an exhaled CO_2 detector or an esophageal detector device to confirm endotracheal tube placement in the field, in the transport vehicle, on arrival at the hospital, and after any subsequent movement of the patient. These devices are described below.

When prehospital providers are trained in the use of advanced airways such as the Combitube and LMA, they appear to be able to use these devices safely, and they can provide ventilation that is as effective as that provided with a bag and mask (Class IIa).[2,21,22] However, advanced airway interventions are technically complicated, failure can occur, and maintenance of skills through frequent experience or practice is essential.[23] It is important to remember that there is no evidence that advanced airway measures improve survival rates in the setting of prehospital cardiac arrest.

Esophageal-Tracheal Combitube

The advantages of the Combitube compared with the face mask are similar to those of the endotracheal tube: isolation of the airway, reduced risk of aspiration, and more reliable ventilation. The advantages of the Combitube over the endotracheal tube are related chiefly to ease of training.[2,24] Ventilation and oxygenation with the Combitube compare favorably with those achieved with the endotracheal tube.[25]

In 5 randomized controlled trials involving both in-hospital and out-of-hospital adult resuscitation, providers with all levels of experience were able to insert the Combitube and deliver ventilation that was comparable to that achieved with endotracheal intubation (LOE 2).[21,26–29] Thus, it is acceptable for healthcare professionals to use the Combitube as an alternative to the endotracheal tube for airway management in cardiac arrest (Class IIa).

Fatal complications may occur with use of the Combitube if the position of the distal lumen of the Combitube in the esophagus or trachea is identified incorrectly. For this reason confirmation of tube placement is essential. Other possible complications related to the use of the Combitube are esophageal trauma, including lacerations, bruising, and subcutaneous emphysema (LOE 2[30]; LOE 5[25,31]).

Laryngeal Mask Airway

The LMA provides a more secure and reliable means of ventilation than the face mask.[32,33] Although the LMA does not ensure absolute protection against aspiration, studies have shown that regurgitation is less likely with the LMA than with the bag-mask device and that aspiration is uncommon. When compared with the endotracheal tube, the LMA provides equivalent ventilation[33,34]; successful ventilation during CPR is reported in 71.5% to 97% of patients.[22,25,35–38]

Training in the placement and use of an LMA is simpler than that for endotracheal intubation because insertion of the LMA does not require laryngoscopy and visualization of the vocal cords. The LMA may also have advantages over the endotracheal tube when access to the patient is limited,[39,40] there is a possibility of unstable neck injury,[41] or appropriate positioning of the patient for endotracheal intubation is impossible.

Results from multiple high-level studies in anesthetized patients that compared the LMA with endotracheal intubation (LOE 2)[39,42–46] and multiple additional studies that compared the LMA with other airways or ventilation techniques (LOE 2)[2,47–52] support the use of the LMA in controlling the airway in a variety of settings by nurses, respiratory therapists, and EMS personnel, many of whom had not previously used this device.

After successful insertion a small proportion of patients cannot be ventilated with the LMA.[2,25,33] With this in mind, it is important for providers to have an alternative strategy for management of the airway. Providers who insert the LMA should receive adequate initial training and should practice insertion of the device regularly. Success rates and the occurrence of complications should be monitored closely. It is acceptable for healthcare professionals to use the LMA as an alternative to the endotracheal tube for airway management in cardiac arrest (Class IIa).

Endotracheal Intubation

The endotracheal tube keeps the airway patent, permits suctioning of airway secretions, enables delivery of a high concentration of oxygen, provides an alternative route for the administration of some drugs, facilitates delivery of a selected tidal volume, and with use of a cuff may protect the airway from aspiration.[53]

Endotracheal intubation attempts by unskilled providers can produce complications, such as trauma to the oropharynx, interruption of compressions and ventilations for unacceptably long periods, and hypoxemia from prolonged intubation attempts or failure to recognize tube misplacement or displacement. Providers who perform endotracheal intubation require adequate initial training and either frequent experience or frequent retraining (Class I). EMS systems that provide prehospital intubation should establish a process for ongoing quality improvement to minimize complications (Class IIa).

Indications for emergency endotracheal intubation are (1) the inability of the rescuer to adequately ventilate the unconscious patient with a bag and mask and (2) the absence of airway protective reflexes (coma or cardiac arrest). The rescuer must have appropriate training and experience in endotracheal intubation.

During CPR we recommend that rescuers minimize the number and duration of interruptions in chest compressions, with a goal to limit interruptions to no more than 10 seconds except as needed for interventions such as placement of an advanced airway. Interruptions needed for intubation can be minimized if the intubating rescuer is prepared to begin the intubation attempt (ie, insert the laryngoscope blade with the tube ready at hand) as soon as the compressing rescuer pauses compressions. The compressions should be interrupted only as long as the intubating rescuer needs to visualize the vocal cords and insert the tube. The compressing rescuer should be prepared to resume chest compressions immediately after the tube is passed through the vocal cords. If more than one intubation attempt is required, the rescuers should provide a period of adequate ventilation and oxygenation and chest compressions between attempts.

If endotracheal intubation is performed for the patient with a perfusing rhythm, use pulse oximetry and ECG monitoring continuously during intubation attempts and interrupt the attempt to provide oxygenation and ventilation if needed.

Even when the endotracheal tube is seen to pass through the vocal cords and tube position is verified by chest expansion and auscultation during positive-pressure ventilation, rescuers should obtain additional confirmation of placement using an end-tidal CO_2 or esophageal detection device (Class IIa).[54] There is a high risk of tube misplacement, displacement, or obstruction,[16,20] especially when the patient is moved.[55] No single confirmation technique, including clinical signs[56] or the presence of water vapor in the tube,[57] is completely reliable. Techniques to confirm endotracheal tube placement are discussed further below. The provider should use both clinical assessment and confirmation devices to verify tube placement immediately after insertion and when the patient is moved.

Clinical Assessment to Confirm Tube Placement

Providers should perform a thorough assessment of endotracheal tube position immediately after placement. This assessment should not require interruption of chest compressions. Assessment by physical examination consists of visualizing chest expansion bilaterally and listening over the epigastrium (breath sounds should not be heard) and the lung fields bilaterally (breath sounds should be equal and adequate). A device should also be used to confirm correct placement in the trachea (see below). If there is doubt about correct tube placement, use the laryngoscope to visualize the tube passing through the vocal cords. If still in doubt, remove the tube and provide bag-mask ventilation until the tube can be replaced.

Use of Devices to Confirm Tube Placement

Providers should always use both clinical assessment and devices to confirm endotracheal tube location immediately after placement and each time the patient is moved. No study, however, has identified a single device as both sensitive and specific for endotracheal tube placement in the trachea or esophagus. All confirmation devices should be considered adjuncts to other confirmation techniques. There is no data to quantify the capability of devices to monitor tube position after initial placement.

Exhaled CO_2 Detectors

Detection of exhaled CO_2 is one of several independent methods of confirming endotracheal tube position. Given the simplicity of the exhaled CO_2 detector, it can be used as the initial method for detecting correct tube placement even in the victim of cardiac arrest (Class IIa). Detection of exhaled CO_2, however, is not infallible as a means of confirming tube placement, particularly during cardiac arrest. Evidence from 1 meta-analysis in adults (LOE 1),[58] 1 prospective controlled cohort study (LOE 3),[59] and several case series and reports (LOE 5)[60–68] indicate that exhaled CO_2 detectors (waveform, colorimetry, or digital) may be useful as adjuncts to confirm endotracheal tube placement during cardiac arrest. The range of results obtained from the reviewed papers is as follows:

- Sensitivity (percentage of correct endotracheal placement detected when CO_2 is detected): 33% to 100%
- Specificity (percentage of incorrect esophageal placement detected when no CO_2 is detected): 97% to 100%
- Positive predictive value (probability of endotracheal placement if CO_2 is detected): 100%
- Negative predictive value (probability of esophageal placement if no CO_2 is detected): 20% to 100%

When exhaled CO_2 is detected (positive reading for CO_2) in cardiac arrest, it is usually a reliable indicator of tube position in the trachea. False-positive readings (CO_2 is detected but the tube is located in the esophagus) have been observed in animals that ingested large amounts of carbonated liquids before the arrest.[69]

False-negative readings (in this context defined as failure to detect CO_2 despite tube placement in the trachea) may be present during cardiac arrest for several reasons. The most common explanation for false-negative readings during CPR is that blood flow and delivery of CO_2 to the lungs is low. False-negative results have also been reported in association with pulmonary embolus because pulmonary blood flow and carbon dioxide delivery to the lungs are reduced. If the detector is contaminated with gastric contents or acidic drugs (eg, endotracheally administered epinephrine), a colorimetric device may display a constant color rather than breath-to-breath color change. In addition, elimination and detection of CO_2 can be drastically reduced following an intravenous bolus of epinephrine[70] or with severe airway obstruction (eg, status asthmaticus) and pulmonary edema.[65,71–73] For these reasons, if CO_2 is not detected, we recommend that a second method be used to confirm endotracheal tube placement, such as direct visualization or the esophageal detector device.

Use of CO_2 detecting devices to determine the correct placement of other advanced airways (eg, Combitube, LMA) has not been adequately studied (Class Indeterminate).

Esophageal Detector Devices

The esophageal detector device (EDD) consists of a bulb that is compressed and attached to the endotracheal tube. If the tube is in the esophagus (positive result for an EDD), the suction created by the EDD will collapse the lumen of the esophagus or pull the esophageal tissue against the tip of the tube, and the bulb will not reexpand. The EDD may also consist of a syringe that is attached to the endotracheal tube; the rescuer attempts to pull the barrel of the syringe. If the tube is in the esophagus, it will not be possible to pull the barrel (aspirate air) with the syringe.

Eight studies of at least fair quality evaluated the accuracy of the EDD (self-inflating bulb or syringe) (LOE 3[18,66,74]; LOE 5[75]; LOE 7 [noncardiac arrest setting][76–79]), but many suffer from small numbers and lack of a control group.

The EDD was highly sensitive for detection of endotracheal tubes that were misplaced in the esophagus (sensitive for esophageal placement) in 5 case series (LOE 5[75]; LOE 7[76–79]). But in 2 studies (LOE 3)[66,74] involving patients in cardiac arrest, the EDD had poor specificity for indicating tracheal placement of an endotracheal tube. In these studies up to 30% of correctly placed tubes may have been removed because the EDD suggested esophageal placement (LOE 3).[67] In the operating room the EDD had poor sensitivity and specificity in 20 children <1 year of age (LOE 2).[80] With these findings in mind, use of the EDD should be considered as just one of several independent methods for confirmation of correct endotracheal tube placement.

The EDD may yield misleading results in patients with morbid obesity, late pregnancy, or status asthmaticus, or when there are copious endotracheal secretions,[81,82] because with these conditions the trachea tends to collapse. There is no evidence that the EDD is accurate for the continued monitoring of endotracheal tube placement.

Postintubation Care

After inserting the advanced airway and confirming correct placement, the rescuer should record the depth of the tube as marked at the front teeth and secure it. Because there is significant potential for endotracheal tube movement with head flexion and extension,[83–85] we recommend ongoing monitoring of endotracheal tube placement during transport and particularly when the patient is moved from one location to another.[86,87] Providers should verify correct placement of all advanced airways immediately after insertion and whenever the patient is moved.

Secure the endotracheal tube with tape or a commercial device (Class I). Two studies in the intensive care setting (LOE 7)[88,89] indicate that backboards, commercial devices for securing the endotracheal tube, and other strategies provide an equivalent method for preventing accidental tube displacement when compared with traditional methods of securing the tube (tape). These devices may be considered during patient transport (Class IIb). After tube confirmation and fixation, obtain a chest x-ray (when feasible) to confirm that the end of the endotracheal tube is properly positioned above the carina.

The 3 most important caveats for rescuers performing CPR after insertion of the advanced airway are

- Be sure the advanced airway is correctly placed (verify).
- Two rescuers no longer deliver "cycles" of CPR (ie, compressions interrupted by pauses for ventilation). Instead, the compressing rescuer should give continuous chest compressions at a rate of 100 per minute without pauses for ventilation. The rescuer delivering ventilation provides 8 to 10 breaths per minute. The 2 rescuers should change compressor and ventilator roles approximately every 2 minutes to prevent compressor fatigue and deterioration in quality and rate of chest compressions. When multiple rescuers are present, they should rotate the compressor role about every 2 minutes.
- Rescuers should avoid delivering an excessive ventilation rate because it can compromise venous return and cardiac output during CPR.

Suction Devices

Both portable and installed suction devices should be available for resuscitation emergencies. Portable units should provide adequate vacuum and flow for pharyngeal suction. The suction device should be fitted with large-bore, nonkinking suction tubing and semirigid pharyngeal tips. Several sterile suction catheters of various sizes should be available for suctioning the lumen of the advanced airway, along with a nonbreakable collection bottle and sterile water for cleaning tubes and catheters. The installed suction unit should be powerful enough to provide an airflow of >40 L/min at the end of the delivery tube and a vacuum of >300 mm Hg when the tube is clamped. The amount of suction should be adjustable for use in children and intubated patients.

Automatic Transport Ventilators

See Part 6: "CPR Techniques and Devices."

Summary

All basic and advanced healthcare providers should be able to provide ventilation with a bag-mask device during CPR or when the patient demonstrates cardiorespiratory compromise. Airway control with an advanced airway is a fundamental ACLS skill. All providers should be able to confirm correct placement of endotracheal tubes and other advanced airways. This key skill is required for safe and effective use of these devices. Training, frequency of use, and monitoring of success and complications affect the long-term impact of any device more than choice of a specific device.

References

1. American Heart Association in collaboration with International Liaison Committee on Resuscitation. Guidelines 2000 for Cardiopulmonary Resuscitation and Emergency Cardiovascular Care: International Consensus on Science, Part 3: Adult Basic Life Support. *Circulation*. 2000; 102(suppl I):I22–I59.
2. Dorges V, Wenzel V, Knacke P, Gerlach K. Comparison of different airway management strategies to ventilate apneic, nonpreoxygenated patients. *Crit Care Med*. 2003;31:800–804.
3. Bailey AR, Hett DA. The laryngeal mask airway in resuscitation. *Resuscitation*. 1994;28:107–110.
4. Doerges V, Sauer C, Ocker H, Wenzel V, Schmucker P. Airway management during cardiopulmonary resuscitation—a comparative study of bag-valve-mask, laryngeal mask airway and combitube in a bench model. *Resuscitation*. 1999;41:63–69.
5. Dorges V, Ocker H, Hagelberg S, Wenzel V, Idris AH, Schmucker P. Smaller tidal volumes with room-air are not sufficient to ensure adequate oxygenation during bag-valve-mask ventilation. *Resuscitation*. 2000;44: 37–41.
6. Bowman FP, Menegazzi JJ, Check BD, Duckett TM. Lower esophageal sphincter pressure during prolonged cardiac arrest and resuscitation. *Ann Emerg Med*. 1995;26:216–219.
7. Weiler N, Heinrichs W, Dick W. Assessment of pulmonary mechanics and gastric inflation pressure during mask ventilation. *Prehospital Disaster Med*. 1995;10:101–105.
8. Ocker H, Wenzel V, Schmucker P, Dorges V. Effectiveness of various airway management techniques in a bench model simulating a cardiac arrest patient. *J Emerg Med*. 2001;20:7–12.
9. Kurola J, Harve H, Kettunen T, Laakso JP, Gorski J, Paakkonen H, Silfvast T. Airway management in cardiac arrest—comparison of the laryngeal tube, tracheal intubation and bag-valve mask ventilation in emergency medical training. *Resuscitation*. 2004;61:149–153.
10. Stoneham MD. The nasopharyngeal airway: assessment of position by fibreoptic laryngoscopy. *Anaesthesia*. 1993;48:575–580.
11. Schade K, Borzotta A, Michaels A. Intracranial malposition of nasopharyngeal airway. *J Trauma*. 2000;49:967–968.
12. Muzzi DA, Losasso TJ, Cucchiara RF. Complication from a nasopharyngeal airway in a patient with a basilar skull fracture. *Anesthesiology*. 1991;74:366–368.
13. Guly UM, Mitchell RG, Cook R, Steedman DJ, Robertson CE. Paramedics and technicians are equally successful at managing cardiac arrest outside hospital. *BMJ*. 1995;310:1091–1094.
14. Updike G, Mosesso VNJ, Auble TE, Delgado E. Comparison of bag-valve-mask, manually triggered ventilator, and automated ventilator devices used while ventilating a nonintubated mannikin model. *Prehosp Emerg Care*. 1998;2:52–55.
15. Stiell IG, Wells GA, Field B, Spaite DW, Nesbitt LP, De Maio VJ, Nichol G, Cousineau D, Blackburn J, Munkley D, Luinstra-Toohey L, Campeau T, Dagnone E, Lyver M. Advanced cardiac life support in out-of-hospital cardiac arrest. *N Engl J Med*. 2004;351:647–656.
16. Gausche M, Lewis RJ, Stratton SJ, Haynes BE, Gunter CS, Goodrich SM, Poore PD, McCollough MD, Henderson DP, Pratt FD, Seidel JS. Effect of out-of-hospital pediatric endotracheal intubation on survival and neurological outcome: a controlled clinical trial. *JAMA*. 2000;283:783–790.
17. Jones JH, Murphy MP, Dickson RL, Somerville GG, Brizendine EJ. Emergency physician-verified out-of-hospital intubation: miss rates by paramedics. *Acad Emerg Med*. 2004;11:707–709.
18. Pelucio M, Halligan L, Dhindsa H. Out-of-hospital experience with the syringe esophageal detector device. *Acad Emerg Med*. 1997;4:563–568.
19. Sayre MR, Sakles JC, Mistler AF, Evans JL, Kramer AT, Pancioli AM. Field trial of endotracheal intubation by basic EMTs. *Ann Emerg Med*. 1998;31:228–233.
20. Katz SH, Falk JL. Misplaced endotracheal tubes by paramedics in an urban emergency medical services system. *Ann Emerg Med*. 2001;37: 32–37.

21. Rabitsch W, Schellongowski P, Staudinger T, Hofbauer R, Dufek V, Eder B, Raab H, Thell R, Schuster E, Frass M. Comparison of a conventional tracheal airway with the Combitube in an urban emergency medical services system run by physicians. *Resuscitation.* 2003;57:27–32.
22. Rumball CJ, MacDonald D. The PTL, Combitube, laryngeal mask, and oral airway: a randomized prehospital comparative study of ventilatory device effectiveness and cost-effectiveness in 470 cases of cardiorespiratory arrest. *Prehosp Emerg Care.* 1997;1:1–10.
23. Vertongen VM, Ramsay MP, Herbison P. Skills retention for insertion of the Combitube and laryngeal mask airway. *Emerg Med.* 2003;15: 459–464.
24. Lefrancois DP, Dufour DG. Use of the esophageal tracheal combitube by basic emergency medical technicians. *Resuscitation.* 2002;52:77–83.
25. Tanigawa K, Shigematsu A. Choice of airway devices for 12,020 cases of nontraumatic cardiac arrest in Japan. *Prehosp Emerg Care.* 1998;2: 96–100.
26. Atherton GL, Johnson JC. Ability of paramedics to use the Combitube in prehospital cardiac arrest. *Ann Emerg Med.* 1993;22:1263–1268.
27. Frass M, Frenzer R, Rauscha F, Schuster E, Glogar D. Ventilation with the esophageal tracheal combitube in cardiopulmonary resuscitation: promptness and effectiveness. *Chest.* 1988;93:781–784.
28. Rumball C, Macdonald D, Barber P, Wong H, Smecher C. Endotracheal intubation and esophageal tracheal combitube insertion by regular ambulance attendants: a comparative trial. *Prehosp Emerg Care.* 2004; 8:15–22.
29. Staudinger T, Brugger S, Roggla M, Rintelen C, Atherton GL, Johnson JC, Frass M. [Comparison of the Combitube with the endotracheal tube in cardiopulmonary resuscitation in the prehospital phase.] *Wien Klin Wochenschr.* 1994;106:412–415.
30. Rabitsch W, Krafft P, Lackner FX, Frenzer R, Hofbauer R, Sherif C, Frass M. [Evaluation of the oesophageal-tracheal double-lumen tube (Combitube) during general anaesthesia.] *Wien Klin Wochenschr.* 2004; 116:90–93.
31. Vezina D, Lessard MR, Bussieres J, Topping C, Trepanier CA. Complications associated with the use of the esophageal-tracheal Combitube. *Can J Anaesth.* 1998;45:76–80.
32. Stone BJ, Chantler PJ, Baskett PJ. The incidence of regurgitation during cardiopulmonary resuscitation: a comparison between the bag valve mask and laryngeal mask airway. *Resuscitation.* 1998;38:3–6.
33. The use of the laryngeal mask airway by nurses during cardiopulmonary resuscitation: results of a multicentre trial. *Anesthesia.* 1994;49:3–7.
34. Samarkandi AH, Seraj MA, el Dawlatly A, Mastan M, Bakhamees HB. The role of laryngeal mask airway in cardiopulmonary resuscitation. *Resuscitation.* 1994;28:103–106.
35. Verghese C, Prior-Willeard PF, Baskett PJ. Immediate management of the airway during cardiopulmonary resuscitation in a hospital without a resident anaesthesiologist. *Eur J Emerg Med.* 1994;1:123–125.
36. Grantham H, Phillips G, Gilligan JE. The laryngeal mask in prehospital emergency care. *Emerg Med Clin North Am.* 1994;6:193–197.
37. Kokkinis K. The use of the laryngeal mask airway in CPR. *Resuscitation.* 1994;27:9–12.
38. Leach A, Alexander CA, Stone B. The laryngeal mask in cardiopulmonary resuscitation in a district general hospital: a preliminary communication. *Resuscitation.* 1993;25:245–248.
39. Flaishon R, Sotman A, Ben-Abraham R, Rudick V, Varssano D, Weinbroum AA. Antichemical protective gear prolongs time to successful airway management: a randomized, crossover study in humans. *Anesthesiology.* 2004;100:260–266.
40. Goldik Z, Bornstein J, Eden A, Ben-Abraham R. Airway management by physicians wearing anti-chemical warfare gear: comparison between laryngeal mask airway and endotracheal intubation. *Eur J Anaesthesiol.* 2002;19:166–169.
41. Pennant JH, Pace NA, Gajraj NM. Role of the laryngeal mask airway in the immobile cervical spine. *J Clin Anesth.* 1993;5:226–230.
42. Davies PR, Tighe SQ, Greenslade GL, Evans GH. Laryngeal mask airway and tracheal tube insertion by unskilled personnel. *Lancet.* 1990;336: 977–979.
43. Ho BY, Skinner HJ, Mahajan RP. Gastro-oesophageal reflux during day case gynaecological laparoscopy under positive pressure ventilation: laryngeal mask vs. tracheal intubation. *Anaesthesia.* 1998;53:921–924.
44. Reinhart DJ, Simmons G. Comparison of placement of the laryngeal mask airway with endotracheal tube by paramedics and respiratory therapists. *Ann Emerg Med.* 1994;24:260–263.
45. Rewari W, Kaul HL. Regurgitation and aspiration during gynaecological laparoscopy: comparison between laryngeal mask airway and tracheal intubation. *J Anaesthesiol Clin Pharmacol.* 1999;15:67–70.
46. Pennant JH, Walker MB. Comparison of the endotracheal tube and laryngeal mask in airway management by paramedical personnel. *Anesth Analg.* 1992;74:531–534.
47. Alexander R, Hodgson P, Lomax D, Bullen C. A comparison of the laryngeal mask airway and Guedel airway, bag and face mask for manual ventilation following formal training. *Anaesthesia.* 1993;48:231–234.
48. Burgoyne L, Cyna A. Laryngeal mask vs intubating laryngeal mask: insertion and ventilation by inexperienced resuscitators. *Anaesth Intensive Care.* 2001;29:604–608.
49. Coulson A, Brimacombe J, Keller C, Wiseman L, Ingham T, Cheung D, Popwycz L, Hall B. A comparison of the ProSeal and classic laryngeal mask airways for airway management by inexperienced personnel after manikin-only training. *Anaesth Intensive Care.* 2003;31:286–289.
50. Dingley J, Baynham P, Swart M, Vaughan RS. Ease of insertion of the laryngeal mask airway by inexperienced personnel when using an introducer. *Anaesthesia.* 1997;52:756–760.
51. Roberts I, Allsop P, Dickinson M, Curry P, Eastwick-Field P, Eyre G. Airway management training using the laryngeal mask airway: a comparison of two different training programmes. Resuscitation. 1997;33: 211–214.
52. Yardy N, Hancox D, Strang T. A comparison of two airway aids for emergency use by unskilled personnel: the Combitube and laryngeal mask. Anaesthesia. 1999;54:181–183.
53. Pepe PE, Copass MK, Joyce TH. Prehospital endotracheal intubation: rationale for training emergency medical personnel. Ann Emerg Med. 1985;14:1085–1092.
54. White SJ, Slovis CM. Inadvertent esophageal intubation in the field: reliance on a fool's "gold standard." Acad Emerg Med. 1997;4:89–91.
55. Beyer AJ III, Land G, Zaritsky A. Nonphysician transport of intubated pediatric patients: a system evaluation. Crit Care Med. 1992;20:961–966.
56. Andersen KH, Schultz-Lebahn T. Oesophageal intubation can be undetected by auscultation of the chest. Acta Anaesthesiol Scand. 1994;38: 580–582.
57. Kelly JJ, Eynon CA, Kaplan JL, de Garavilla L, Dalsey WC. Use of tube condensation as an indicator of endotracheal tube placement. Ann Emerg Med. 1998;31:575–578.
58. Li J. Capnography alone is imperfect for endotracheal tube placement confirmation during emergency intubation. J Emerg Med. 2001;20: 223–229.
59. Grmec S. Comparison of three different methods to confirm tracheal tube placement in emergency intubation. Intensive Care Med. 2002;28: 701–704.
60. Anton WR, Gordon RW, Jordan TM, Posner KL, Cheney FW. A disposable end-tidal CO_2 detector to verify endotracheal intubation. Ann Emerg Med. 1991;20:271–275.
61. Bhende MS, Thompson AE, Cook DR, Saville AL. Validity of a disposable end-tidal CO2 detector in verifying endotracheal tube placement in infants and children. Ann Emerg Med. 1992;21:142–145.
62. Bhende MS, Thompson AE. Evaluation of an end-tidal CO2 detector during pediatric cardiopulmonary resuscitation. Pediatrics. 1995;95: 395–399.
63. Hayden SR, Sciammarella J, Viccellio P, Thode H, Delagi R. Colorimetric end-tidal CO_2 detector for verification of endotracheal tube placement in out-of-hospital cardiac arrest. Acad Emerg Med. 1995;2:499–502.
64. MacLeod BA, Heller MB, Gerard J, Yealy DM, Menegazzi JJ. Verification of endotracheal tube placement with colorimetric end-tidal CO2 detection. Ann Emerg Med. 1991;20:267–270.
65. Ornato JP, Shipley JB, Racht EM, Slovis CM, Wrenn KD, Pepe PE, Almeida SL, Ginger VF, Fotre TV. Multicenter study of a portable, hand-size, colorimetric end-tidal carbon dioxide detection device. Ann Emerg Med. 1992;21:518–523.
66. Takeda T, Tanigawa K, Tanaka H, Hayashi Y, Goto E, Tanaka K. The assessment of three methods to verify tracheal tube placement in the emergency setting. Resuscitation. 2003;56:153–157.
67. Tanigawa K, Takeda T, Goto E, Tanaka K. The efficacy of esophageal detector devices in verifying tracheal tube placement: a randomized cross-over study of out-of-hospital cardiac arrest patients. Anesth Analg. 2001;92:375–378.
68. Varon AJ, Morrina J, Civetta JM. Clinical utility of a colorimetric end-tidal CO2 detector in cardiopulmonary resuscitation and emergency intubation. J Clin Monit. 1991;7:289–293.

69. Sum Ping ST, Mehta MP, Symreng T. Accuracy of the FEF CO2 detector in the assessment of endotracheal tube placement. Anesth Analg. 1992; 74:415–419.
70. Cantineau JP, Merckx P, Lambert Y, Sorkine M, Bertrand C, Duvaldestin P. Effect of epinephrine on end-tidal carbon dioxide pressure during prehospital cardiopulmonary resuscitation. Am J Emerg Med. 1994;12: 267–270.
71. Ward KR, Yealy DM. End-tidal carbon dioxide monitoring in emergency medicine, part 2: clinical applications. Acad Emerg Med. 1998;5: 637–646.
72. Hand IL, Shepard EK, Krauss AN, Auld PA. Discrepancies between transcutaneous and end-tidal carbon dioxide monitoring in the critically ill neonate with respiratory distress syndrome. Crit Care Med. 1989;17: 556–559.
73. Tobias JD, Meyer DJ. Noninvasive monitoring of carbon dioxide during respiratory failure in toddlers and infants: end-tidal versus transcutaneous carbon dioxide. Anesth Analg. 1997;85:55–58.
74. Tanigawa K, Takeda T, Goto E, Tanaka K. Accuracy and reliability of the self-inflating bulb to verify tracheal intubation in out-of-hospital cardiac arrest patients. Anesthesiology. 2000;93:1432–1436.
75. Bozeman WP, Hexter D, Liang HK, Kelen GD. Esophageal detector device versus detection of end-tidal carbon dioxide level in emergency intubation. Ann Emerg Med. 1996;27:595–599.
76. Sharieff GQ, Rodarte A, Wilton N, Bleyle D. The self-inflating bulb as an airway adjunct: is it reliable in children weighing less than 20 kilograms? Acad Emerg Med. 2003;10:303–308.
77. Wee MY, Walker AK. The oesophageal detector device: an assessment with uncuffed tubes in children. Anaesthesia. 1991;46:869–871.
78. Williams KN, Nunn JF. The oesophageal detector device: a prospective trial on 100 patients. Anaesthesia. 1989;44:412–424.
79. Zaleski L, Abello D, Gold MI. The esophageal detector device. Does it work? Anesthesiology. 1993;79:244–247.
80. Haynes SR, Morton NS. Use of the oesophageal detector device in children under one year of age. Anaesthesia. 1990;45:1067–1069.
81. Baraka A, Khoury PJ, Siddik SS, Salem MR, Joseph NJ. Efficacy of the self-inflating bulb in differentiating esophageal from tracheal intubation in the parturient undergoing cesarean section. Anesth Analg. 1997;84: 533–537.
82. Davis DP, Stephen KA, Vilke GM. Inaccuracy in endotracheal tube verification using a Toomey syringe. J Emerg Med. 1999;17:35–38.
83. Yap SJ, Morris RW, Pybus DA. Alterations in endotracheal tube position during general anaesthesia. Anaesth Intensive Care. 1994;22:586–588.
84. Sugiyama K, Yokoyama K. Displacement of the endotracheal tube caused by change of head position in pediatric anesthesia: evaluation by fiberoptic bronchoscopy. Anesth Analg. 1996;82:251–253.
85. King HK. A new device: Tube Securer. An endotracheal tube holder with integrated bite-block. Acta Anaesthesiol Sin. 1997;35:257–259.
86. Falk JL, Sayre MR. Confirmation of airway placement. Prehosp Emerg Care. 1999;3:273–278.
87. Wang HE, Kupas DF, Paris PM, Bates RR, Yealy DM. Preliminary experience with a prospective, multi-center evaluation of out-of-hospital endotracheal intubation. Resuscitation. 2003;58:49–58.
88. Levy H, Griego L. A comparative study of oral endotracheal tube securing methods. Chest. 1993;104:1537–1540.
89. Tasota FJ, Hoffman LA, Zullo TG, Jamison G. Evaluation of two methods used to stabilize oral endotracheal tubes. Heart Lung. 1987;16: 140–146.

Part 7.2: Management of Cardiac Arrest

Four rhythms produce pulseless cardiac arrest: ventricular fibrillation (VF), rapid ventricular tachycardia (VT), pulseless electrical activity (PEA), and asystole. Survival from these arrest rhythms requires both basic life support (BLS) and advanced cardiovascular life support (ACLS).

The foundation of ACLS care is good BLS care, beginning with prompt high-quality bystander CPR and, for VF/pulseless VT, attempted defibrillation within minutes of collapse. For victims of witnessed VF arrest, prompt bystander CPR and early defibrillation can significantly increase the chance for survival to hospital discharge. In comparison, typical ACLS therapies, such as insertion of advanced airways and pharmacologic support of the circulation, have not been shown to increase rate of survival to hospital discharge. This section details the general care of a patient in cardiac arrest and provides an overview of the ACLS Pulseless Arrest Algorithm.

Access for Medications: Correct Priorities

During cardiac arrest, basic CPR and early defibrillation are of primary importance, and drug administration is of secondary importance. Few drugs used in the treatment of cardiac arrest are supported by strong evidence. After beginning CPR and attempting defibrillation, rescuers can establish intravenous (IV) access, consider drug therapy, and insert an advanced airway.

Central Versus Peripheral Infusions

Central line access is not needed in most resuscitation attempts. If IV access has not been established, the provider should insert a large peripheral venous catheter. Although in adults peak drug concentrations are lower and circulation times longer when drugs are administered via peripheral sites rather than central sites, the establishment of peripheral access does not require interruption of CPR.[1,2] Drugs typically require 1 to 2 minutes to reach the central circulation when given via a peripheral vein but require less time when given via central venous access.

If a resuscitation drug is administered by a peripheral venous route, administer the drug by bolus injection and follow with a 20-mL bolus of IV fluid. Elevate the extremity for 10 to 20 seconds to facilitate drug delivery to the central circulation.[3]

Intraosseous (IO) cannulation provides access to a noncollapsible venous plexus, enabling drug delivery similar to that achieved by central venous access. Two prospective (LOE 3) trials, in children[4] and adults,[5] and 6 other studies (LOE 4[6]; LOE 5[7–9]; LOE 7[10,11]) documented that IO access is safe and effective for fluid resuscitation, drug delivery, and blood sampling for laboratory evaluation, and is attainable in all age groups. Providers may establish IO access if IV access is unavailable (Class IIa). Commercially available kits can facilitate IO access in adults.

If spontaneous circulation does not return after defibrillation and peripheral venous or IO drug administration, the provider may consider placement of a central line (unless there are contraindications). Note that central venous catheterization is a relative (not absolute) contraindication for fibrinolytic therapy in patients with stroke or acute coronary syndromes.

If IV and IO access cannot be established, some resuscitation drugs may be administered by the endotracheal route. One study in children (LOE 2),[12] 5 studies in adults (LOE 2[13–15]; LOE 3[16,17]), as well as multiple animal studies (LOE 6),[18–20] showed that lidocaine,[14,21] epinephrine,[22] atropine,[23] naloxone, and vasopressin[20] are absorbed via the trachea. Administration of resuscitation drugs into the trachea, however, results in lower blood concentrations than the same dose given intravascularly. Furthermore, recent animal studies[24–27] suggest that the lower epinephrine concentrations achieved when the drug is delivered by the endotracheal route may produce transient β-adrenergic effects. These effects can be detrimental, causing hypotension, lower coronary artery perfusion pressure and flow, and reduced potential for return of spontaneous circulation (ROSC). Thus, although endotracheal administration of some resuscitation drugs is possible, IV or IO drug administration is preferred because it will provide more predictable drug delivery and pharmacologic effect.

In one nonrandomized cohort study of out-of-hospital cardiac arrest in adults (LOE 4)[28] using a randomized control, administration of atropine and epinephrine by the IV route was associated with a higher rate of ROSC and survival to hospital admission than administration of the drugs by the endotracheal route. Five percent of those who received IV drugs survived to hospital discharge, but no patient survived in the group receiving drugs by the endotracheal route.

The optimal endotracheal dose of most drugs is unknown, but typically the dose given by the endotracheal route is 2 to 2½ times the recommended IV dose. In 2 CPR studies the equipotent epinephrine dose given endotracheally was approximately 3 to 10 times higher than the IV dose (LOE 5[29]; LOE 6[30]). Providers should dilute the recommended dose in 5 to 10 mL of water or normal saline and inject the drug directly into the endotracheal tube.[22] Studies with epinephrine[31] and lidocaine[17] showed that dilution with water instead of 0.9% saline may achieve better drug absorption.

Arrest Rhythms

The management of pulseless arrest is highlighted in the ACLS Pulseless Arrest Algorithm (Figure). Box numbers in the text refer to the numbered boxes in the algorithm.

(*Circulation*. 2005;112:IV-58-IV-66.)

This special supplement to *Circulation* is freely available at http://www.circulationaha.org

DOI: 10.1161/CIRCULATIONAHA.105.166557

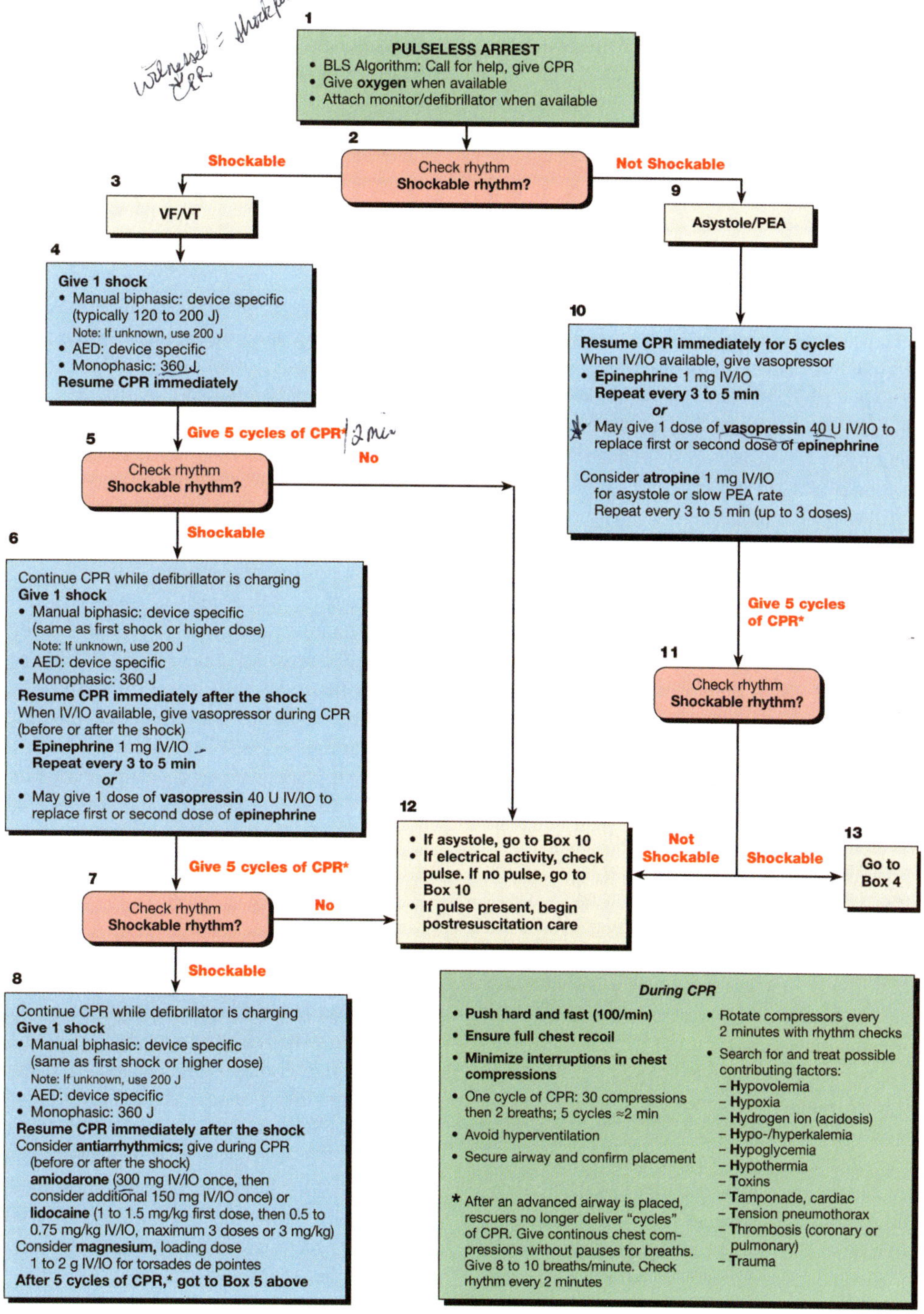

ACLS Pulseless Arrest Algorithm.

Ventricular Fibrillation/Pulseless Ventricular Tachycardia

The most critical interventions during the first minutes of VF or pulseless VT are immediate bystander CPR (Box 1) with minimal interruption in chest compressions and defibrillation as soon as it can be accomplished (Class I). In cases of witnessed arrest with a defibrillator on-site, after delivery of 2 rescue breaths the healthcare provider should check for a pulse. If the provider definitely does not feel a pulse within 10 seconds, the provider should turn on the defibrillator, place adhesive pads or paddles, and check the rhythm (Box 2).

If the healthcare provider does not witness the arrest in the out-of-hospital setting (eg, the emergency medical services [EMS] provider arrives at the scene of an arrest), the provider may give 5 cycles of CPR before attempting defibrillation. In adults with a prolonged arrest, shock delivery may be more successful after a period of effective chest compressions.[32–34] For further information about the sequence of CPR first versus shock first, see Part 5: "Electrical Therapies: Automated External Defibrillators, Defibrillation, Cardioversion, and Pacing."

If VF/pulseless VT is present (Box 3), providers should deliver 1 shock (Box 4) and then resume CPR immediately, beginning with chest compressions. If a biphasic defibrillator is available, providers should use the dose at which that defibrillator has been shown to be effective for terminating VF (typically a selected energy of 120 J to 200 J). If the provider is unaware of the effective dose range of the device, the rescuer may use a dose of 200 J for the first shock and an equal or higher shock dose for the second and subsequent shocks. If a monophasic defibrillator is used, providers should deliver an initial shock of 360 J and use that dose for subsequent shocks. If VF is initially terminated by a shock but then recurs later in the arrest, deliver subsequent shocks at the previously successful energy level.

Biphasic defibrillators use a variety of waveforms, and each waveform has been shown to be effective in terminating VF over a specific dose range. Manufacturers should display this effective waveform dose range on the face of the biphasic device, and providers should use that dose range to attempt defibrillation with that device. The 200-J "default" energy level was selected because it falls within the reported range of selected doses that are effective for first and subsequent biphasic shocks and can be provided by every biphasic manual defibrillator available in 2005. This is a consensus default dose and not a recommended ideal dose. If biphasic devices are clearly labeled and providers are familiar with the devices they use in clinical care, there will be no need for the default 200-J dose. Ongoing research is necessary to firmly establish the most appropriate initial settings for both monophasic and biphasic defibrillators.

Providers should give 1 shock rather than the 3 successive ("stacked") shocks recommended in previous versions of the ECC guidelines[35] for the treatment of VF/pulseless VT because the first-shock success rate for biphasic defibrillators is high[36] and it is important to minimize interruptions in chest compressions. Although the 1-shock strategy has not been directly studied against a 3-shock strategy, the evidence is compelling that interruption of chest compressions reduces coronary perfusion pressure. The time required to charge a defibrillator, deliver a shock, and check a pulse can interrupt compressions for 37 seconds or longer[37] (for further information see Part 5: "Electrical Therapies: Automated External Defibrillators, Defibrillation, Cardioversion, and Pacing").

When a rhythm check reveals VF/VT, rescuers should provide CPR while the defibrillator charges (when possible), until it is time to "clear" the victim for shock delivery. Give the shock as quickly as possible. Immediately after shock delivery, resume CPR (beginning with chest compressions) without delay and continue for 5 cycles (or about 2 minutes if an advanced airway is in place), and then check the rhythm (Box 5). In in-hospital units with continuous monitoring (eg, electrocardiography, hemodynamics), this sequence may be modified at the physician's discretion (see Part 5).

The management strategy depicted in the ACLS Pulseless Arrest Algorithm is designed to minimize the number of times that chest compressions are interrupted and to enable rescuers to deliver shocks as efficiently as possible. Pulse and rhythm checks are limited and are not recommended immediately after shock delivery; instead healthcare providers give 5 cycles (about 2 minutes of CPR) immediately after the shock and then check the rhythm. Ideally, compression should be interrupted only for ventilation (until an advanced airway is placed), rhythm check, or shock delivery.

Once an advanced airway (eg, endotracheal tube, esophageal-tracheal combitube [Combitube], laryngeal mask airway [LMA]) is placed, 2 rescuers no longer deliver cycles of compressions interrupted with pauses for ventilation. Instead, the compressing rescuer should deliver 100 compressions per minute continuously, without pauses for ventilation. The rescuer delivering the ventilations should give 8 to 10 breaths per minute and should be careful to avoid delivering an excessive number of ventilations. Two or more rescuers should rotate the compressor role approximately every 2 minutes (when the victim's rhythm is checked). This change should prevent compressor fatigue and deterioration in quality and rate of chest compressions.

Establishing IV access is important (see below), but it should not interfere with CPR and delivery of shocks. As always, the provider should recall the H's and T's to identify a factor that may have caused the arrest or may be complicating the resuscitative effort (see the green box, "During CPR," at the bottom of the algorithm).

There is inadequate evidence to identify an optimal number of CPR cycles and defibrillation shocks that should be given before pharmacologic therapy is initiated. The recommended sequence depicted in the algorithm is based on expert consensus. If VF/VT persists after delivery of 1 or 2 shocks plus CPR, give a vasopressor (epinephrine every 3 to 5 minutes during cardiac arrest; one dose of vasopressin may replace either the first or second dose of epinephrine—see Box 6). Do not interrupt CPR to give medications.

The drug should be administered during CPR and as soon as possible after the rhythm is checked. It can be administered before or after shock delivery, in a CPR–RHYTHM CHECK–CPR (while drug administered and defibrillator charged)–SHOCK sequence (repeated as needed). This sequence differs from the one recommended in 2000[35]: it is designed to minimize interruptions in chest compressions. The 2000 recommendations resulted in too many interruptions in chest compressions.

In these 2005 recommendations, during treatment of cardiac arrest the drug doses should be prepared *before* the rhythm check so they can be administered as soon as possible after the rhythm check, but the timing of drug delivery is less important than the need to minimize interruptions in chest compressions. Rhythm checks should be very brief (see below). If a drug is administered immediately after the rhythm check (before or after the shock) it will be circulated by the CPR given before and after the shock. After 5 cycles (or about 2 minutes) of CPR, analyze the rhythm again (Box 7) and be prepared to deliver another shock immediately if indicated.

When VF/pulseless VT persists after 2 to 3 shocks plus CPR and administration of a vasopressor, consider administering an antiarrhythmic such as amiodarone (Box 8). If amiodarone is unavailable, lidocaine may be considered. Consider magnesium for torsades de pointes associated with a long QT interval (see below). You should administer the drug during CPR, as soon as possible after rhythm analysis. If a nonshockable rhythm is present and the rhythm is organized (complexes appear regular or narrow), try to palpate a pulse (see Box 12).

Rhythm checks should be brief, and pulse checks should generally be performed only if an organized rhythm is observed. If there is any doubt about the presence of a pulse, resume CPR. If the patient has ROSC, begin postresuscitation care. If the patient's rhythm changes to asystole or PEA, see "Asystole and Pulseless Electrical Activity" below (Boxes 9 and 10).

If a perfusing rhythm is transiently restored but not successfully maintained between repeated shocks (recurrent VF/VT), the patient may be a candidate for early treatment with antiarrhythmic medications (see Part 7.3: "Management of Symptomatic Bradycardia and Tachycardia").

During treatment of VF/pulseless VT, healthcare providers must practice efficient coordination between CPR and shock delivery. When VF is present for more than a few minutes, the myocardium is depleted of oxygen and metabolic substrates. A brief period of chest compressions can deliver oxygen and energy substrates, increasing the likelihood that a perfusing rhythm will return after shock delivery.[38] Analyses of VF waveform characteristics predictive of shock success have documented that the shorter the time between chest compression and shock delivery, the more likely the shock will be successful.[38,39] Reduction in the interval from compression to shock delivery by even a few seconds can increase the probability of shock success.[40]

Asystole and Pulseless Electrical Activity (Box 9)

PEA encompasses a heterogeneous group of pulseless rhythms that includes pseudo-electromechanical dissociation (pseudo-EMD), idioventricular rhythms, ventricular escape rhythms, postdefibrillation idioventricular rhythms, and bradyasystolic rhythms. Research with cardiac ultrasonography and indwelling pressure catheters has confirmed that pulseless patients with electrical activity have associated mechanical contractions, but these contractions are too weak to produce a blood pressure detectable by palpation or noninvasive blood pressure monitoring. PEA is often caused by reversible conditions and can be treated if those conditions are identified and corrected.

The survival rate from cardiac arrest with asystole is dismal. During a resuscitation attempt, brief periods of an organized complex may appear on the monitor screen, but spontaneous circulation rarely emerges. As with PEA, the hope for resuscitation is to identify and treat a reversible cause.

Because of the similarity in causes and management of these two arrest rhythms, their treatment has been combined in the second part of the ACLS Pulseless Arrest Algorithm.

Patients who have either asystole or PEA will not benefit from defibrillation attempts. The focus of resuscitation is to perform high-quality CPR with minimal interruptions and to identify reversible causes or complicating factors. Providers should insert an advanced airway (eg, endotracheal tube, Combitube, LMA). Once the airway is in place, 2 rescuers should no longer deliver cycles of CPR (ie, compressions interrupted by pauses when breaths are delivered). Instead the compressing rescuer should give continuous chest compressions at a rate of 100 per minute without pauses for ventilation. The rescuer delivering ventilation provides 8 to 10 breaths per minute. The 2 rescuers should change compressor and ventilator roles approximately every 2 minutes (when the rhythm is checked) to prevent compressor fatigue and deterioration in quality and rate of chest compressions. When multiple rescuers are present, they should rotate the compressor role about every 2 minutes. Rescuers should minimize interruptions in chest compressions while inserting the airway and should not interrupt CPR while establishing IV or IO access.

If the rhythm check confirms asystole or PEA, resume CPR immediately. A vasopressor (epinephrine or vasopressin) may be administered at this time. Epinephrine can be administered approximately every 3 to 5 minutes during cardiac arrest; one dose of vasopressin may be substituted for either the first or second epinephrine dose (Box 10). For a patient in asystole or slow PEA, consider atropine (see below). Do not interrupt CPR to deliver any medication. Give the drug as soon as possible after the rhythm check.

After drug delivery and approximately 5 cycles (or about 2 minutes) of CPR, recheck the rhythm (Box 11). If a shockable rhythm is present, deliver a shock (go to Box 4). If no rhythm is present or if there is no change in the appearance of the electrocardiogram, immediately resume CPR (Box 10). If an organized rhythm is present (Box 12), try to palpate a pulse. If no pulse is present (or if there is any doubt about the presence of a pulse), continue CPR (Box 10). If a pulse is present the provider should identify the rhythm and treat appropriately (see Part 7.3: "Management of Symptomatic Bradycardia and Tachycardia"). If the patient appears to have an organized rhythm with a good pulse, begin postresuscitative care.

When Should Resuscitative Efforts Stop?

The resuscitation team must make a conscientious and competent effort to give patients a trial of CPR and ACLS, provided that the patient has not expressed a decision to forego resuscitative efforts. The final decision to stop efforts can never be as simple as an isolated time interval. Clinical judgment and respect for human dignity must enter into decision making. There is little data to guide this decision.

Emergency medical response systems should not require field personnel to transport every victim of cardiac arrest to a hospital or emergency department (ED). Transportation with continuing CPR is justified if interventions are available in the ED that cannot be performed in the field, such as cardiopulmonary bypass or extracorporeal circulation for victims of severe hypothermia (Class IIb).

Unless special situations are present (eg, hypothermia), for nontraumatic and blunt traumatic out-of-hospital cardiac arrest, evidence confirms that ACLS care in the ED offers no advantage over ACLS care in the field. Stated succinctly, if ACLS care in the field cannot resuscitate the victim, ED care will not resuscitate the victim. Civil rules, administrative concerns, medical insurance requirements, and even reimbursement enhancement have frequently led to requirements to transport all cardiac arrest victims to a hospital or ED. If these requirements are nonselective, they are inappropriate, futile, and ethically unacceptable. Cessation of efforts in the out-of-hospital setting, following system-specific criteria and under direct medical control, should be standard practice in all EMS systems.

Medications for Arrest Rhythms

Vasopressors

To date no placebo-controlled trials have shown that administration of any vasopressor agent at any stage during management of pulseless VT, VF, PEA, or asystole increases the rate of neurologically intact survival to hospital discharge. There is evidence, however, that the use of vasopressor agents favors initial ROSC.

Epinephrine and Vasopressin

VF and Pulseless VT

Epinephrine

Epinephrine hydrochloride produces beneficial effects in patients during cardiac arrest, primarily because of its α-adrenergic receptor-stimulating (ie, vasoconstrictor) properties.[41] The α-adrenergic effects of epinephrine can increase coronary and cerebral perfusion pressure during CPR.[42] The value and safety of the β-adrenergic effects of epinephrine are controversial because they may increase myocardial work and reduce subendocardial perfusion.[43]

Although epinephrine has been used universally in resuscitation, there is a paucity of evidence to show that it improves survival in humans. Both beneficial and toxic physiologic effects of epinephrine administration during CPR have been shown in animal and human studies.[44–50] Initial or escalating high-dose epinephrine has occasionally improved initial ROSC and early survival rates. But in 8 randomized clinical studies involving >9000 cardiac arrest patients, high-dose epinephrine produced no improvement in survival to hospital discharge rates or neurologic outcomes when compared with standard doses, even in subgroups given initial high-dose epinephrine.[50–57]

It is appropriate to administer a 1-mg dose of epinephrine IV/IO every 3 to 5 minutes during adult cardiac arrest (Class IIb). Higher doses may be indicated to treat specific problems, such as β-blocker or calcium channel blocker overdose. If IV/IO access is delayed or cannot be established, epinephrine may be given by the endotracheal route at a dose of 2 to 2.5 mg.

Vasopressin

Vasopressin is a nonadrenergic peripheral vasoconstrictor that also causes coronary and renal vasoconstriction.[58,59] Despite 1 promising randomized study (LOE 2),[60] additional lower-level studies (LOE 5),[61–63] and multiple well-performed animal studies, 2 large randomized controlled human trials (LOE 1)[64,65] failed to show an increase in rates of ROSC or survival when vasopressin (40 U, with the dose repeated in 1 study) was compared with epinephrine (1 mg, repeated) as the initial vasopressor for treatment of cardiac arrest. In the large multicenter trial involving 1186 out-of-hospital cardiac arrests with all rhythms (LOE 1),[65] a post-hoc analysis of the subset of patients with asystole showed significant improvement in survival to hospital discharge but not neurologically intact survival when 40 U (repeated once if necessary) of vasopressin was used as the initial vasopressor compared with epinephrine (1 mg, repeated if necessary).

A meta-analysis of 5 randomized trials (LOE 1)[66] showed no statistically significant differences between vasopressin and epinephrine for ROSC, 24-hour survival, or survival to hospital discharge. The subgroup analysis based on initial cardiac rhythm did not show any statistically significant difference in survival to hospital discharge (LOE 1).[66]

In a large in-hospital study of cardiac arrest, 200 patients were randomly assigned to receive either 1 mg of epinephrine (initial rhythm: 16% VF, 3% VT, 54% PEA, 27% asystole) or 40 U of vasopressin (initial rhythm: 20% VF, 3% VT, 41% PEA, 34% asystole). There was no difference in survival to 1 hour (epinephrine: 35%, vasopressin: 39%) or to hospital discharge (epinephrine: 14%, vasopressin: 12%) between groups or subgroups.[64]

A retrospective analysis documented the effects of epinephrine alone (231 patients) compared with a combination of vasopressin and epinephrine (37 patients) in out-of-hospital cardiac arrest with VF/VT, PEA, or asystole. There was no difference in survival or ROSC when VF or PEA was the presenting rhythm, but ROSC was increased in the epinephrine plus vasopressin group among patients presenting with asystole.[67]

Because vasopressin effects have not been shown to differ from those of epinephrine in cardiac arrest, one dose of vasopressin 40 U IV/IO may replace either the first or second dose of epinephrine in the treatment of pulseless arrest (Class Indeterminate).

Asystole and Pulseless Electrical Activity

Vasopressors

The studies described above enrolled patients with PEA and asystole and failed to show that either vasopressin or epinephrine is superior for treatment of PEA regardless of the order of administration. In the case of asystole, a single post-hoc analysis of a larger study found a survival benefit of vasopressin over epinephrine but did not find an increase in intact neurologic survival.

On the basis of these findings, providers may consider vasopressin for treatment of asystole, but there is insufficient evidence to recommend for or against its use in PEA. Further studies are required. Epinephrine may be administered every 3 to 5 minutes during the attempted resuscitation; vasopressin may be substituted for the first or second epinephrine dose.

Atropine

Atropine sulfate reverses cholinergic-mediated decreases in heart rate, systemic vascular resistance, and blood pressure. No prospective controlled studies support the use of atropine in asystole or slow PEA arrest. Administration of atropine for asystole is supported by a retrospective review (LOE 4)[68] of intubated patients with refractory asystole who showed improved survival to hospital admission with atropine. A case series (LOE 5)[69] of adults in cardiac arrest documented conversion from asystole to sinus rhythm in 7 of 8 patients.

Literature to refute the use of atropine is equally sparse and of limited quality. A small prospective controlled nonrandomized study (LOE 3)[70] of patients with out-of-hospital cardiac arrest found no difference versus control when atropine 1 to 2 mg was given as the initial resuscitation medication, but subtherapeutic dosing and delay to epinephrine administration may have had an impact on survival in the study. In an animal model of PEA (LOE 6),[71] no difference was noted in resuscitation outcome between standard-dose atropine and placebo groups.

Asystole can be precipitated or exacerbated by excessive vagal tone, and administration of a vagolytic medication is consistent with a physiologic approach. Atropine is inexpensive, easy to administer, and has few side effects and therefore can be considered for asystole or PEA. The recommended dose of atropine for cardiac arrest is 1 mg IV, which can be repeated every 3 to 5 minutes (maximum total of 3 doses or 3 mg) if asystole persists (Class Indeterminate).

Antiarrhythmics

There is no evidence that any antiarrhythmic drug given routinely during human cardiac arrest increases survival to hospital discharge. Amiodarone, however, has been shown to increase short-term survival to hospital admission when compared with placebo or lidocaine.

VF and Pulseless VT

Amiodarone

IV amiodarone affects sodium, potassium, and calcium channels as well as α- and β-adrenergic blocking properties. It can be considered for the treatment of VF or pulseless VT unresponsive to shock delivery, CPR, and a vasopressor.

In blinded randomized controlled clinical trials in adults with refractory VF/pulseless VT in the out-of-hospital setting (LOE 1),[72,73] paramedic administration of amiodarone (300 mg[72] or 5 mg/kg[73]) improved survival to hospital admission rates when compared with administration of placebo[72] or 1.5 mg/kg of lidocaine.[73] Additional studies (LOE 7)[74–78] documented consistent improvement in defibrillation response when amiodarone was given to humans or animals with VF or hemodynamically unstable VT.

Amiodarone produced vasodilation and hypotension in 1 of the out-of-hospital studies.[72] A canine study (LOE 6)[79] noted that administration of a vasoconstrictor before amiodarone prevented hypotension. A new aqueous formulation of amiodarone does not contain the vasoactive solvents (polysorbate 80 and benzyl alcohol) of the standard formulation. In an analysis of the combined data of 4 prospective clinical trials of patients with VT (some included hemodynamically unstable patients), aqueous amiodarone produced no more hypotension than lidocaine.[77]

In summary, amiodarone may be administered for VF or pulseless VT unresponsive to CPR, shock, and a vasopressor (Class IIb). An initial dose of 300 mg IV/IO can be followed by one dose of 150 mg IV/IO.

Lidocaine

The use of lidocaine for ventricular arrhythmias was supported by initial studies in animals (LOE 6)[80,81] and extrapolation from the historic use of the drug to suppress premature ventricular contractions and prevent VF after acute myocardial infarction.[82] Although lidocaine improved short-term survival in 1 prehospital study (LOE 4),[83] 3 randomized trials comparing amiodarone and lidocaine found lower rates of ROSC[73,84] and a higher incidence of asystole[85] with use of lidocaine. The out-of-hospital double-blind randomized controlled trial (LOE 1)[73] that compared amiodarone with lidocaine found that amiodarone improved rate of survival to hospital admission and that lidocaine was associated with more asystole after defibrillation.

In summary, lidocaine is an alternative antiarrhythmic of long standing and widespread familiarity with fewer immediate side effects than may be encountered with other antiarrhythmics. Lidocaine, however, has no proven short-term or long-term efficacy in cardiac arrest. Lidocaine should be considered an alternative treatment to amiodarone (Class Indeterminate). The initial dose is 1 to 1.5 mg/kg IV. If VF/pulseless VT persists, additional doses of 0.5 to 0.75 mg/kg IV push may be administered at 5- to 10-minute intervals, to a maximum dose of 3 mg/kg. This is the same dose that was recommended in the *ECC Guidelines 2000.*

Magnesium

Two observational studies (LOE 5)[86,87] showed that IV magnesium can effectively terminate torsades de pointes (irregular/polymorphic VT associated with prolonged QT interval). One small adult case series in adults (LOE 5)[88] showed that isoproterenol or ventricular pacing can be effective in terminating torsades de pointes associated with bradycardia and drug-induced QT prolongation. Magnesium is not likely to be effective in terminating irregular/polymorphic VT in patients with a normal QT interval.[87]

When VF/pulseless VT cardiac arrest is associated with torsades de pointes, providers may administer magnesium sulfate at a dose of 1 to 2 g diluted in 10 mL D_5W IV/IO push, typically over 5 to 20 minutes (Class IIa for torsades). When torsades is present in the patient *with pulses*, the same 1 to 2 g is mixed in 50 to 100 mL of D_5W and given as a loading dose. It can be given more slowly (eg, over 5 to 60 minutes IV) under these conditions. See Part 7.3: "Management of Symptomatic Bradycardia and Tachycardia" for additional information about management of torsades de pointes not associated with cardiac arrest.

Potentially Beneficial Therapies

Fibrinolysis

Adults have been successfully resuscitated following administration of fibrinolytics (tPA) after initial failure of standard CPR techniques, particularly when the condition leading to the arrest was acute pulmonary embolism or other presumed cardiac cause (LOE 3[89]; LOE 4[90–92]; LOE 5[93–97]). Evidence from 1 large clinical trial (LOE 2),[98] however, failed to show any significant treatment effect when a fibrinolytic (tPA) was given to out-of-hospital patients with undifferentiated PEA cardiac arrest unresponsive to initial interventions.

There is insufficient evidence to recommend for or against the routine use of fibrinolysis for cardiac arrest. It may be considered on a case-by-case basis when pulmonary embolus is suspected (Class IIa). Ongoing CPR is not a contraindication to fibrinolysis.

Interventions Not Supported by Outcome Evidence

Pacing in Arrest

Several randomized controlled trials (LOE 2)[99–101] failed to show benefit from attempted pacing for asystole. At this time use of pacing for patients with asystolic cardiac arrest is not recommended.

Procainamide in VF and Pulseless VT

Use of procainamide in cardiac arrest is supported by 1 retrospective comparison study of 20 patients.[102] Administration of procainamide in cardiac arrest is limited by the need for slow infusion and by uncertain efficacy in emergent circumstances.

Norepinephrine

Norepinephrine has been studied in only a limited fashion for treatment of cardiac arrest. Human data is limited, but it suggests that norepinephrine produces effects equivalent to epinephrine in the initial resuscitation of cardiac arrest.[53,103] In the only prospective human trial comparing standard-dose epinephrine, high-dose epinephrine, and high-dose norepinephrine, the norepinephrine was associated with no benefit and a trend toward worse neurologic outcome (LOE 1).[53]

Precordial Thump for VF or Pulseless VT

There are no prospective studies that evaluated the use of precordial (chest) thump. In 3 case series (LOE 5),[104–106] VF or pulseless VT was converted to a perfusing rhythm by a precordial thump. In contrast, other case series documented deterioration in cardiac rhythm, such as rate acceleration of VT, conversion of VT to VF, or development of complete heart block or asystole following the use of the thump (LOE 5[105,107–111]; LOE 6[112]).

The precordial thump is not recommended for BLS providers. In light of the limited evidence in support of its efficacy and reports of potential harm, no recommendation can be made for or against its use by ACLS providers (Class Indeterminate).

Electrolyte Therapies in Arrest Rhythms

Magnesium

In-hospital and out-of-hospital studies in adult cardiac arrest (LOE 2[113–116]; LOE 3[117]; LOE 7[118]) and animal studies (LOE 6)[119–122] showed no increase in the rate of ROSC when magnesium was routinely given during CPR. Administration of magnesium can be considered for treatment of torsades de pointes (Class IIa—see above), but it is not effective for treatment of cardiac arrest from other causes.

Routine Administration of IV Fluids During Cardiac Arrest

There were no published human studies evaluating the effect of routine fluid administration during normovolemic cardiac arrest, and the results of 4 animal studies (LOE 6)[123–126] were neutral. There is insufficient evidence to recommend routine administration of fluids to treat cardiac arrest (Class Indeterminate). Fluids should be infused if hypovolemia is suspected.

Summary

Ideally ACLS providers will prevent pulseless arrest if they are able to intervene in the prearrest period. If arrest occurs, good ACLS begins with high-quality BLS. During resuscitation rescuers must provide good chest compressions (adequate rate and depth), allow complete recoil of the chest between compressions, and minimize interruptions in chest compressions. Rescuers should be careful to avoid provision of excessive ventilation, particularly once an advanced airway is in place. Resuscitation drugs have not been shown to increase rate of survival to hospital discharge, and none has the impact of early and effective CPR and prompt defibrillation.

References

1. Barsan WG, Levy RC, Weir H. Lidocaine levels during CPR: differences after peripheral venous, central venous, and intracardiac injections. *Ann Emerg Med.* 1981;10:73–78.
2. Kuhn GJ, White BC, Swetnam RE, Mumey JF, Rydesky MF, Tintinalli JE, Krome RL, Hoehner PJ. Peripheral vs central circulation times during CPR: a pilot study. *Ann Emerg Med.* 1981;10:417–419.
3. Emerman CL, Pinchak AC, Hancock D, Hagen JF. Effect of injection site on circulation times during cardiac arrest. *Crit Care Med.* 1988;16: 1138–1141.
4. Banerjee S, Singhi SC, Singh S, Singh M. The intraosseous route is a suitable alternative to intravenous route for fluid resuscitation in severely dehydrated children. *Indian Pediatr.* 1994;31:1511–1520.
5. Brickman KR, Krupp K, Rega P, Alexander J, Guinness M. Typing and screening of blood from intraosseous access. *Ann Emerg Med.* 1992;21: 414–417.
6. Fiser RT, Walker WM, Seibert JJ, McCarthy R, Fiser DH. Tibial length following intraosseous infusion: a prospective, radiographic analysis. *Pediatr Emerg Care.* 1997;13:186–188.
7. Ummenhofer W, Frei FJ, Urwyler A, Drewe J. Are laboratory values in bone marrow aspirate predictable for venous blood in paediatric patients? *Resuscitation.* 1994;27:123–128.
8. Glaeser PW, Hellmich TR, Szewczuga D, Losek JD, Smith DS. Five-year experience in prehospital intraosseous infusions in children and adults. *Ann Emerg Med.* 1993;22:1119–1124.
9. Guy J, Haley K, Zuspan SJ. Use of intraosseous infusion in the pediatric trauma patient. *J Pediatr Surg.* 1993;28:158–161.
10. Macnab A, Christenson J, Findlay J, Horwood B, Johnson D, Jones L, Phillips K, Pollack C Jr, Robinson DJ, Rumball C, Stair T, Tiffany B, Whelan M. A new system for sternal intraosseous infusion in adults. *Prehosp Emerg Care.* 2000;4:173–177.
11. Ellemunter H, Simma B, Trawoger R, Maurer H. Intraosseous lines in preterm and full term neonates. *Arch Dis Child Fetal Neonatal Ed.* 1999; 80:F74–F75.
12. Howard RF, Bingham RM. Endotracheal compared with intravenous administration of atropine. *Arch Dis Child.* 1990;65:449–450.
13. Lee PL, Chung YT, Lee BY, Yeh CY, Lin SY, Chao CC. The optimal dose of atropine via the endotracheal route. *Ma Zui Xue Za Zhi.* 1989;27:35–38.
14. Prengel AW, Lindner KH, Hahnel J, Ahnefeld FW. Endotracheal and endobronchial lidocaine administration: effects on plasma lidocaine concentration and blood gases. *Crit Care Med.* 1991;19:911–915.
15. Schmidbauer S, Kneifel HA, Hallfeldt KK. Endobronchial application of high dose epinephrine in out of hospital cardiopulmonary resuscitation. *Resuscitation.* 2000;47:89.
16. Raymondos K, Panning B, Leuwer M, Brechelt G, Korte T, Niehaus M, Tebbenjohanns J, Piepenbrock S. Absorption and hemodynamic effects of airway administration of adrenaline in patients with severe cardiac disease. *Ann Intern Med.* 2000;132:800–803.
17. Hahnel JH, Lindner KH, Schurmann C, Prengel A, Ahnefeld FW. Plasma lidocaine levels and PaO2 with endobronchial administration: dilution with normal saline or distilled water? *Ann Emerg Med.* 1990;19:1314–1317.
18. Brown LK, Diamond J. The efficacy of lidocaine in ventricular fibrillation due to coronary artery ligation: endotracheal vs intravenous use. *Proc West Pharmacol Soc.* 1982;25:43–45.
19. Jasani MS, Nadkarni VM, Finkelstein MS, Hofmann WT, Salzman SK. Inspiratory-cycle instillation of endotracheal epinephrine in porcine arrest. *Acad Emerg Med.* 1994;1:340–345.
20. Wenzel V, Lindner KH, Prengel AW, Lurie KG, Strohmenger HU. Endobronchial vasopressin improves survival during cardiopulmonary resuscitation in pigs. *Anesthesiology.* 1997;86:1375–1381.

21. Prengel AW, Rembecki M, Wenzel V, Steinbach G. A comparison of the endotracheal tube and the laryngeal mask airway as a route for endobronchial lidocaine administration. *Anesth Analg*. 2001;92:1505–1509.
22. Jasani MS, Nadkarni VM, Finkelstein MS, Mandell GA, Salzman SK, Norman ME. Effects of different techniques of endotracheal epinephrine administration in pediatric porcine hypoxic-hypercarbic cardiopulmonary arrest. *Crit Care Med*. 1994;22:1174–1180.
23. Johnston C. Endotracheal drug delivery. *Pediatr Emerg Care*. 1992;8: 94–97.
24. Vaknin Z, Manisterski Y, Ben-Abraham R, Efrati O, Lotan D, Barzilay Z, Paret G. Is endotracheal adrenaline deleterious because of the beta adrenergic effect? *Anesth Analg*. 2001;92:1408–1412.
25. Manisterski Y, Vaknin Z, Ben-Abraham R, Efrati O, Lotan D, Berkovitch M, Barak A, Barzilay Z, Paret G. Endotracheal epinephrine: a call for larger doses. *Anesth Analg*. 2002;95:1037–1041.
26. Efrati O, Ben-Abraham R, Barak A, Modan-Moses D, Augarten A, Manisterski Y, Barzilay Z, Paret G. Endobronchial adrenaline: should it be reconsidered? Dose response and haemodynamic effect in dogs. *Resuscitation*. 2003;59:117–122.
27. Elizur A, Ben-Abraham R, Manisterski Y, Barak A, Efrati O, Lotan D, Barzilay Z, Paret G. Tracheal epinephrine or norepinephrine preceded by beta blockade in a dog model: can beta blockade bestow any benefits? *Resuscitation*. 2003;59:271–276.
28. Niemann JT, Stratton SJ, Cruz B, Lewis RJ. Endotracheal drug administration during out-of-hospital resuscitation: where are the survivors? *Resuscitation*. 2002;53:153–157.
29. Schuttler J, Bartsch A, Ebeling BJ, Hornchen U, Kulka P, Suhling B, Stoeckel H. [Endobronchial administration of adrenaline in preclinical cardiopulmonary resuscitation.] *Anasth Intensivther Notfallmed*. 1987;22: 63–68.
30. Hornchen U, Schuttler J, Stoeckel H, Eichelkraut W, Hahn N. Endobronchial instillation of epinephrine during cardiopulmonary resuscitation. *Crit Care Med*. 1987;15:1037–1039.
31. Naganobu K, Hasebe Y, Uchiyama Y, Hagio M, Ogawa H. A comparison of distilled water and normal saline as diluents for endobronchial administration of epinephrine in the dog. *Anesth Analg*. 2000;91:317–321.
32. Cobb LA, Fahrenbruch CE, Walsh TR, Copass MK, Olsufka M, Breskin M, Hallstrom AP. Influence of cardiopulmonary resuscitation prior to defibrillation in patients with out-of-hospital ventricular fibrillation. *JAMA*. 1999;281:1182–1188.
33. Yakaitis RW, Ewy GA, Otto CW, Taren DL, Moon TE. Influence of time and therapy on ventricular defibrillation in dogs. *Crit Care Med*. 1980;8: 157–163.
34. Wik L, Hansen TB, Fylling F, Steen T, Vaagenes P, Auestad BH, Steen PA. Delaying defibrillation to give basic cardiopulmonary resuscitation to patients with out-of-hospital ventricular fibrillation: a randomized trial. *JAMA*. 2003;289:1389–1395.
35. American Heart Association in collaboration with the International Liaison Committee on Resuscitation. Guidelines 2000 for Cardiopulmonary Resuscitation and Emergency Cardiovascular Care: International Consensus on Science. *Circulation*. 2000;102:I1–I384.
36. Martens PR, Russell JK, Wolcke B, Paschen H, Kuisma M, Gliner BE, Weaver WD, Bossaert L, Chamberlain D, Schneider T. Optimal Response to Cardiac Arrest study: defibrillation waveform effects. *Resuscitation*. 2001;49:233–243.
37. Yu T, Weil MH, Tang W, Sun S, Klouche K, Povoas H, Bisera J. Adverse outcomes of interrupted precordial compression during automated defibrillation. *Circulation*. 2002;106:368–372.
38. Eftestol T, Wik L, Sunde K, Steen PA. Effects of cardiopulmonary resuscitation on predictors of ventricular fibrillation defibrillation success during out-of-hospital cardiac arrest. *Circulation*. 2004;110:10–15.
39. Eftestol T, Sunde K, Aase SO, Husoy JH, Steen PA. Predicting outcome of defibrillation by spectral characterization and nonparametric classification of ventricular fibrillation in patients with out-of-hospital cardiac arrest. *Circulation*. 2000;102:1523–1529.
40. Eftestol T, Sunde K, Steen PA. Effects of interrupting precordial compressions on the calculated probability of defibrillation success during out-of-hospital cardiac arrest. *Circulation*. 2002;105:2270–2273.
41. Yakaitis RW, Otto CW, Blitt CD. Relative importance of α and β adrenergic receptors during resuscitation. *Crit Care Med*. 1979;7:293–296.
42. Michael JR, Guerci AD, Koehler RC, Shi AY, Tsitlik J, Chandra N, Niedermeyer E, Rogers MC, Traystman RJ, Weisfeldt ML. Mechanisms by which epinephrine augments cerebral and myocardial perfusion during cardiopulmonary resuscitation in dogs. *Circulation*. 1984;69:822–835.
43. Ditchey RV, Lindenfeld J. Failure of epinephrine to improve the balance between myocardial oxygen supply and demand during closed-chest resuscitation in dogs. *Circulation*. 1988;78:382–389.
44. Berg RA, Otto CW, Kern KB, Hilwig RW, Sanders AB, Henry CP, Ewy GA. A randomized, blinded trial of high-dose epinephrine versus standard-dose epinephrine in a swine model of pediatric asphyxial cardiac arrest. *Crit Care Med*. 1996;24:1695–1700.
45. Hoekstra JW, Griffith R, Kelley R, Cody RJ, Lewis D, Scheatzle M, Brown CG. Effect of standard-dose versus high-dose epinephrine on myocardial high-energy phosphates during ventricular fibrillation and closed-chest CPR. *Ann Emerg Med*. 1993;22:1385–1391.
46. Hornchen U, Lussi C, Schuttler J. Potential risks of high-dose epinephrine for resuscitation from ventricular fibrillation in a porcine model. *J Cardiothorac Vasc Anesth*. 1993;7:184–187.
47. Niemann JT, Cairns CB, Sharma J, Lewis RJ. Treatment of prolonged ventricular fibrillation: immediate countershock versus high-dose epinephrine and CPR preceding countershock. *Circulation*. 1992;85:281–287.
48. Tang W, Weil MH, Sun S, Noc M, Yang L, Gazmuri RJ. Epinephrine increases the severity of postresuscitation myocardial dysfunction. *Circulation*. 1995;92:3089–3093.
49. Rivers EP, Wortsman J, Rady MY, Blake HC, McGeorge FT, Buderer NM. The effect of the total cumulative epinephrine dose administered during human CPR on hemodynamic, oxygen transport, and utilization variables in the postresuscitation period. *Chest*. 1994;106:1499–1507.
50. Lindner KH, Ahnefeld FW, Prengel AW. Comparison of standard and high-dose adrenaline in the resuscitation of asystole and electromechanical dissociation. *Acta Anaesthesiol Scand*. 1991;35:253–256.
51. Brown CG, Martin DR, Pepe PE, Stueven H, Cummins RO, Gonzalez E, Jastremski M. A comparison of standard-dose and high-dose epinephrine in cardiac arrest outside the hospital: the Multicenter High-Dose Epinephrine Study Group. *N Engl J Med*. 1992;327:1051–1055.
52. Stiell IG, Hebert PC, Weitzman BN, Wells GA, Raman S, Stark RM, Higginson LA, Ahuja J, Dickinson GE. High-dose epinephrine in adult cardiac arrest. *N Engl J Med*. 1992;327:1045–1050.
53. Callaham M, Madsen CD, Barton CW, Saunders CE, Pointer J. A randomized clinical trial of high-dose epinephrine and norepinephrine vs standard-dose epinephrine in prehospital cardiac arrest. *JAMA*. 1992;268: 2667–2672.
54. Lipman J, Wilson W, Kobilski S, Scribante J, Lee C, Kraus P, Cooper J, Barr J, Moyes D. High-dose adrenaline in adult in-hospital asystolic cardiopulmonary resuscitation: a double-blind randomised trial. *Anaesth Intensive Care*. 1993;21:192–196.
55. Choux C, Gueugniaud PY, Barbieux A, Pham E, Lae C, Dubien PY, Petit P. Standard doses versus repeated high doses of epinephrine in cardiac arrest outside the hospital. *Resuscitation*. 1995;29:3–9.
56. Sherman BW, Munger MA, Foulke GE, Rutherford WF, Panacek EA. High-dose versus standard-dose epinephrine treatment of cardiac arrest after failure of standard therapy. *Pharmacotherapy*. 1997;17:242–247.
57. Gueugniaud PY, Mols P, Goldstein P, Pham E, Dubien PY, Deweerdt C, Vergnion M, Petit P, Carli P. A comparison of repeated high doses and repeated standard doses of epinephrine for cardiac arrest outside the hospital. European Epinephrine Study Group. *N Engl J Med*. 1998;339: 1595–1601.
58. Oyama H, Suzuki Y, Satoh S, Kajita Y, Takayasu M, Shibuya M, Sugita K. Role of nitric oxide in the cerebral vasodilatory responses to vasopressin and oxytocin in dogs. *J Cereb Blood Flow Metab*. 1993;13:285–290.
59. Lindner KH, Strohmenger HU, Ensinger H, Hetzel WD, Ahnefeld FW, Georgieff M. Stress hormone response during and after cardiopulmonary resuscitation. *Anesthesiology*. 1992;77:662–668.
60. Lindner KH, Dirks B, Strohmenger HU, Prengel AW, Lindner IM, Lurie KG. Randomised comparison of epinephrine and vasopressin in patients with out-of-hospital ventricular fibrillation. *Lancet*. 1997;349:535–537.
61. Lindner KH, Prengel AW, Brinkmann A, Strohmenger HU, Lindner IM, Lurie KG. Vasopressin administration in refractory cardiac arrest. *Ann Intern Med*. 1996;124:1061–1064.
62. Mann K, Berg RA, Nadkarni V. Beneficial effects of vasopressin in prolonged pediatric cardiac arrest: a case series. *Resuscitation*. 2002;52: 149–156.
63. Morris DC, Dereczyk BE, Grzybowski M, Martin GB, Rivers EP, Wortsman J, Amico JA. Vasopressin can increase coronary perfusion pressure during human cardiopulmonary resuscitation. *Acad Emerg Med*. 1997;4:878–883.
64. Stiell IG, Hebert PC, Wells GA, Vandemheen KL, Tang AS, Higginson LA, Dreyer JF, Clement C, Battram E, Watpool I, Mason S, Klassen T, Weitzman BN. Vasopressin versus epinephrine for inhospital cardiac arrest: a randomised controlled trial. *Lancet*. 2001;358:105–109.
65. Wenzel V, Krismer AC, Arntz HR, Sitter H, Stadlbauer KH, Lindner KH. A comparison of vasopressin and epinephrine for out-of-hospital cardiopulmonary resuscitation. *N Engl J Med*. 2004;350:105–113.
66. Aung K, Htay T. Vasopressin for cardiac arrest: a systematic review and meta-analysis. *Arch Intern Med*. 2005;165:17–24.
67. Guyette FX, Guimond GE, Hostler D, Callaway CW. Vasopressin administered with epinephrine is associated with a return of a pulse in out-of-hospital cardiac arrest. *Resuscitation*. 2004;63:277–282.
68. Stueven HA, Tonsfeldt DJ, Thompson BM, Whitcomb J, Kastenson E, Aprahamian C. Atropine in asystole: human studies. *Ann Emerg Med*. 1984;13:815–817.
69. Brown DC, Lewis AJ, Criley JM. Asystole and its treatment: the possible role of the parasympathetic nervous system in cardiac arrest. *JACEP*. 1979;8:448–452.
70. Coon GA, Clinton JE, Ruiz E. Use of atropine for bradyasystolic prehospital cardiac arrest. *Ann Emerg Med*. 1981;10:462–467.
71. DeBehnke DJ, Swart GL, Spreng D, Aufderheide TP. Standard and higher doses of atropine in a canine model of pulseless electrical activity. *Acad Emerg Med*. 1995;2:1034–1041.
72. Kudenchuk PJ, Cobb LA, Copass MK, Cummins RO, Doherty AM, Fahrenbruch CE, Hallstrom AP, Murray WA, Olsufka M, Walsh T. Amiodarone for resuscitation after out-of-hospital cardiac arrest due to ventricular fibrillation. *N Engl J Med*. 1999;341:871–878.
73. Dorian P, Cass D, Schwartz B, Cooper R, Gelaznikas R, Barr A. Amiodarone as compared with lidocaine for shock-resistant ventricular fibrillation. *N Engl J Med*. 2002;346:884–890.
74. Skrifvars MB, Kuisma M, Boyd J, Maatta T, Repo J, Rosenberg PH, Castren M. The use of undiluted amiodarone in the management of out-of-hospital cardiac arrest. *Acta Anaesthesiol Scand*. 2004;48:582–587.
75. Petrovic T, Adnet F, Lapandry C. Successful resuscitation of ventricular fibrillation after low-dose amiodarone. *Ann Emerg Med*. 1998;32:518–519.
76. Levine JH, Massumi A, Scheinman MM, Winkle RA, Platia EV, Chilson DA, Gomes A, Woosley RL. Intravenous amiodarone for recurrent sus-

tained hypotensive ventricular tachyarrhythmias. Intravenous Amiodarone Multicenter Trial Group. *J Am Coll Cardiol.* 1996;27:67–75.
77. Somberg JC, Bailin SJ, Haffajee CI, Paladino WP, Kerin NZ, Bridges D, Timar S, Molnar J. Intravenous lidocaine versus intravenous amiodarone (in a new aqueous formulation) for incessant ventricular tachycardia. *Am J Cardiol.* 2002;90:853–859.
78. Somberg JC, Timar S, Bailin SJ, Lakatos F, Haffajee CI, Tarjan J, Paladino WP, Sarosi I, Kerin NZ, Borbola J, Bridges DE, Molnar J. Lack of a hypotensive effect with rapid administration of a new aqueous formulation of intravenous amiodarone. *Am J Cardiol.* 2004;93:576–581.
79. Paiva EF, Perondi MB, Kern KB, Berg RA, Timerman S, Cardoso LF, Ramirez JA. Effect of amiodarone on haemodynamics during cardiopulmonary resuscitation in a canine model of resistant ventricular fibrillation. *Resuscitation.* 2003;58:203–208.
80. Borer JS, Harrison LA, Kent KM, Levy R, Goldstein RE, Epstein SE. Beneficial effect of lidocaine on ventricular electrical stability and spontaneous ventricular fibrillation during experimental myocardial infarction. *Am J Cardiol.* 1976;37:860–863.
81. Spear JF, Moore EN, Gerstenblith G. Effect of lidocaine on the ventricular fibrillation threshold in the dog during acute ischemia and premature ventricular contractions. *Circulation.* 1972;46:65–73.
82. Lie KI, Wellens HJ, van Capelle FJ, Durrer D. Lidocaine in the prevention of primary ventricular fibrillation: a double-blind, randomized study of 212 consecutive patients. *N Engl J Med.* 1974;291:1324–1326.
83. Herlitz J, Bang A, Holmberg M, Axelsson A, Lindkvist J, Holmberg S. Rhythm changes during resuscitation from ventricular fibrillation in relation to delay until defibrillation, number of shocks delivered and survival. *Resuscitation.* 1997;34:17–22.
84. Kentsch M, Berkel H, Bleifeld W. Intravenose Amiodaron-Applikation bei therapierefraktarem Kammerflimmern. *Intensivmedizin.* 1988;25:70–74.
85. Weaver WD, Fahrenbruch CE, Johnson DD, Hallstrom AP, Cobb LA, Copass MK. Effect of epinephrine and lidocaine therapy on outcome after cardiac arrest due to ventricular fibrillation. *Circulation.* 1990;82: 2027–2034.
86. Manz M, Pfeiffer D, Jung W, Lueritz B. Intravenous treatment with magnesium in recurrent persistent ventricular tachycardia. *New Trends in Arrhythmias.* 1991;7:437–442.
87. Tzivoni D, Banai S, Schuger C, Benhorin J, Keren A, Gottlieb S, Stern S. Treatment of torsade de pointes with magnesium sulfate. *Circulation.* 1988;77:392–397.
88. Keren A, Tzivoni D, Gavish D, Levi J, Gottlieb S, Benhorin J, Stern S. Etiology, warning signs and therapy of torsade de pointes: a study of 10 patients. *Circulation.* 1981;64:1167–1174.
89. Bottiger BW, Bode C, Kern S, Gries A, Gust R, Glatzer R, Bauer H, Motsch J, Martin E. Efficacy and safety of thrombolytic therapy after initially unsuccessful cardiopulmonary resuscitation: a prospective clinical trial. *Lancet.* 2001;357:1583–1585.
90. Lederer W, Lichtenberger C, Pechlaner C, Kroesen G, Baubin M. Recombinant tissue plasminogen activator during cardiopulmonary resuscitation in 108 patients with out-of-hospital cardiac arrest. *Resuscitation.* 2001;50: 71–76.
91. Lederer W, Lichtenberger C, Pechlaner C, Kinzl J, Kroesen G, Baubin M. Long-term survival and neurological outcome of patients who received recombinant tissue plasminogen activator during out-of-hospital cardiac arrest. *Resuscitation.* 2004;61:123–129.
92. Janata K, Holzer M, Kurkciyan I, Losert H, Riedmuller E, Pikula B, Laggner AN, Laczika K. Major bleeding complications in cardiopulmonary resuscitation: the place of thrombolytic therapy in cardiac arrest due to massive pulmonary embolism. *Resuscitation.* 2003;57:49–55.
93. Scholz KH, Hilmer T, Schuster S, Wojcik J, Kreuzer H, Tebbe U. Thrombolysis in resuscitated patients with pulmonary embolism. *Dtsch Med Wochenschr.* 1990;115:930–935.
94. Klefisch F, et al. Praklinische ultima-ratio thrombolyse bei therapierefraktarer kardiopulmonaler reanimation. *Intensivmedizin.* 1995;32: 155–162.
95. Tiffany PA, Schultz M, Stueven H. Bolus thrombolytic infusions during CPR for patients with refractory arrest rhythms: outcome of a case series. *Ann Emerg Med.* 1998;31:124–126.
96. Gramann J, Lange-Braun P, Bodemann T, Hochrein H. Der Einsatz von Thrombolytika in der Reanimation als Ultima ratio zur Überwindung des Herztodes. *Intensiv-und Notfallbehandlung.* 1991;16:134–137.
97. Ruiz-Bailen M, Aguayo de Hoyos E, Serrano-Corcoles MC, Diaz-Castellanos MA, Ramos-Cuadra JA, Reina-Toral A. Efficacy of thrombolysis in patients with acute myocardial infarction requiring cardiopulmonary resuscitation. *Intensive Care Med.* 2001;27:1050–1057.
98. Abu-Laban RB, Christenson JM, Innes GD, van Beek CA, Wanger KP, McKnight RD, MacPhail IA, Puskaric J, Sadowski RP, Singer J, Schechter MT, Wood VM. Tissue plasminogen activator in cardiac arrest with pulseless electrical activity. *N Engl J Med.* 2002;346:1522–1528.
99. Hedges JR, Syverud SA, Dalsey WC, Feero S, Easter R, Shultz B. Prehospital trial of emergency transcutaneous cardiac pacing. *Circulation.* 1987;76:1337–1343.
100. Barthell E, Troiano P, Olson D, Stueven HA, Hendley G. Prehospital external cardiac pacing: a prospective, controlled clinical trial. *Ann Emerg Med.* 1988;17:1221–1226.
101. Cummins RO, Graves JR, Larsen MP, Hallstrom AP, Hearne TR, Ciliberti J, Nicola RM, Horan S. Out-of-hospital transcutaneous pacing by emergency medical technicians in patients with asystolic cardiac arrest. *N Engl J Med.* 1993;328:1377–1382.
102. Stiell IG, Wells GA, Hebert PC, Laupacis A, Weitzman BN. Association of drug therapy with survival in cardiac arrest: limited role of advanced cardiac life support drugs. *Acad Emerg Med.* 1995;2:264–273.
103. Lindner KH, Ahnefeld FW, Bowdler IM. Comparison of different doses of epinephrine on myocardial perfusion and resuscitation success during cardiopulmonary resuscitation in a pig model. *Am J Emerg Med.* 1991;9: 27–31.
104. Befeler B. Mechanical stimulation of the heart; its therapeutic value in tachyarrhythmias. *Chest.* 1978;73:832–838.
105. Volkmann HK, Klumbies A, Kühnert H, Paliege R, Dannberg G, Siegert K. [Terminating ventricular tachycardias by mechanical heart stimulation with precordial thumps.] *Z Kardiol.* 1990;79:717–724.
106. Caldwell G, Millar G, Quinn E. Simple mechanical methods for cardioversion: defence of the precordial thump and cough version. *BMJ.* 1985; 291:627–630.
107. Morgera T, Baldi N, Chersevani D, Medugno G, Camerini F. Chest thump and ventricular tachycardia. *Pacing Clin Electrophysiol.* 1979;2:69–75.
108. Rahner E, Zeh E. Die Regularisierung von Kammertachykardien durch präkordialen Faustschlag [The regularization of ventricular tachycardias by precordial thumping]. *Medizinsche Welt.* 1978;29:1659–1663.
109. Gertsch M, Hottinger S, Hess T. Serial chest thumps for the treatment of ventricular tachycardia in patients with coronary artery disease. *Clin Cardiol.* 1992;15:181–188.
110. Krijne R. Rate acceleration of ventricular tachycardia after a precordial chest thump. *Am J Cardiol.* 1984;53:964–965.
111. Sclarovsky S, Kracoff OH, Agmon J. Acceleration of ventricular tachycardia induced by a chest thump. *Chest.* 1981;80:596–599.
112. Yakaitis RW, Redding JS. Precordial thumping during cardiac resuscitation. *Crit Care Med.* 1973;1:22–26.
113. Thel MC, Armstrong AL, McNulty SE, Califf RM, O'Connor CM. Randomised trial of magnesium in in-hospital cardiac arrest. Duke Internal Medicine Housestaff. *Lancet.* 1997;350:1272–1276.
114. Allegra J, Lavery R, Cody R, Birnbaum G, Brennan J, Hartman A, Horowitz M, Nashed A, Yablonski M. Magnesium sulfate in the treatment of refractory ventricular fibrillation in the prehospital setting. *Resuscitation.* 2001;49:245–249.
115. Fatovich D, Prentice D, Dobb G. Magnesium in in-hospital cardiac arrest. *Lancet.* 1998;351:446.
116. Hassan TB, Jagger C, Barnett DB. A randomised trial to investigate the efficacy of magnesium sulphate for refractory ventricular fibrillation. *Emerg Med J.* 2002;19:57–62.
117. Miller B, Craddock L, Hoffenberg S, Heinz S, Lefkowitz D, Callender ML, Battaglia C, Maines C, Masick D. Pilot study of intravenous magnesium sulfate in refractory cardiac arrest: safety data and recommendations for future studies. *Resuscitation.* 1995;30:3–14.
118. Longstreth WT Jr, Fahrenbruch CE, Olsufka M, Walsh TR, Copass MK, Cobb LA. Randomized clinical trial of magnesium, diazepam, or both after out-of-hospital cardiac arrest. *Neurology.* 2002;59:506–514.
119. Siemkowicz E. Magnesium sulfate solution dramatically improves immediate recovery of rats from hypoxia. *Resuscitation.* 1997;35:53–59.
120. Brown CG, Griffith RF, Neely D, Hobson J, Miller B. The effect of intravenous magnesium administration on aortic, right atrial and coronary perfusion pressures during CPR in swine. *Resuscitation.* 1993;26:3–12.
121. Seaberg DC, Menegazzi JJ, Check B, MacLeod BA, Yealy DM. Use of a cardiocerebral-protective drug cocktail prior to countershock in a porcine model of prolonged ventricular fibrillation. *Resuscitation.* 2001;51: 301–308.
122. Zhang Y, Davies LR, Martin SM, Bawaney IM, Buettner GR, Kerber RE. Magnesium reduces free radical concentration and preserves left ventricular function after direct current shocks. *Resuscitation.* 2003;56:199–206.
123. Ditchey RV, Lindenfeld J. Potential adverse effects of volume loading on perfusion of vital organs during closed-chest resuscitation. *Circulation.* 1984;69:181–189.
124. Gentile NT, Martin GB, Appleton TJ, Moeggenberg J, Paradis NA, Nowak RM. Effects of arterial and venous volume infusion on coronary perfusion pressures during canine CPR. *Resuscitation.* 1991;22:55–63.
125. Jameson SJ, Mateer JR, DeBehnke DJ. Early volume expansion during cardiopulmonary resuscitation. *Resuscitation.* 1993;26:243–250.
126. Voorhees WD, Ralston SH, Kougias C, Schmitz PM. Fluid loading with whole blood or Ringer's lactate solution during CPR in dogs. *Resuscitation.* 1987;15:113–123.

Part 7.3: Management of Symptomatic Bradycardia and Tachycardia

Cardiac arrhythmias are a common cause of sudden death. ECG monitoring should be established as soon as possible for all patients who collapse suddenly or have symptoms of coronary ischemia or infarction. To avoid delay, apply adhesive electrodes with a conventional or automated external defibrillator (AED) or use the "quick-look" paddles feature on conventional defibrillators. For patients with acute coronary ischemia, the greatest risk for serious arrhythmias occurs during the first 4 hours after the onset of symptoms (see Part 8: "Stabilization of the Patient With Acute Coronary Syndromes").[1]

Principles of Arrhythmia Recognition and Management

The ECG and rhythm information should be interpreted within the context of total patient assessment. Errors in diagnosis and treatment are likely to occur if ACLS providers base treatment decisions solely on rhythm interpretation and neglect clinical evaluation. Providers must evaluate the patient's symptoms and clinical signs, including ventilation, oxygenation, heart rate, blood pressure, and level of consciousness, and look for signs of inadequate organ perfusion. These guidelines emphasize the importance of clinical evaluation and highlight principles of therapy with algorithms that have been refined and streamlined since the 2000 edition of the guidelines.[2] The principles of arrhythmia recognition and management in adults are as follows:

- If bradycardia produces signs and symptoms (eg, acute altered mental status, ongoing severe ischemic chest pain, congestive heart failure, hypotension, or other signs of shock) that persist despite adequate airway and breathing, prepare to provide pacing. For symptomatic high-degree (second-degree or third-degree) atrioventricular (AV) block, provide transcutaneous pacing without delay.
- If the tachycardic patient is unstable with severe signs and symptoms related to tachycardia, prepare for immediate cardioversion.
- If the patient with tachycardia is stable, determine if the patient has a narrow-complex or wide-complex tachycardia and then tailor therapy accordingly.
- You must understand the initial diagnostic electrical and drug treatment options for rhythms that are unstable or immediately life-threatening.
- Know when to call for expert consultation regarding complicated rhythm interpretation, drugs, or management decisions.

(*Circulation*. 2005;112:IV-67-IV-77.)

This special supplement to *Circulation* is freely available at http://www.circulationaha.org

DOI: 10.1161/CIRCULATIONAHA.105.166558

A comprehensive presentation of the evaluation and management of bradyarrhythmias and tachyarrhythmias is beyond the scope of these guidelines. For further information see the following sources:

- American College of Cardiology/American Heart Association/European Society of Cardiology Guidelines for the Management of Patients With Supraventricular Arrhythmias,[3] available at the following sites: *www.acc.org*, *www.americanheart.org*, and *www.escardio.org*.
- *ACLS: Principles and Practice*, Chapters 12 through 16.[4]

There are 3 major sections in Part 7.3. The first 2 sections, "Bradycardia" and "Tachycardia," begin with evaluation and treatment and provide an overview of the information summarized in the ACLS bradycardia and tachycardia algorithms. To simplify these algorithms, we have included some recommended drugs but not all possible useful drugs. The overview presents information about the drugs cited in the algorithms. The third section, "Antiarrhythmic Drugs," provides more detailed information about a wider selection of drug therapies.

Bradycardia

See the Bradycardia Algorithm, Figure 1. Box numbers in the text refer to the numbered boxes in the algorithm.

Evaluation

Bradycardia is generally defined as a heart rate of <60 beats per minute (Box 1). A slow heart rate may be physiologically normal for some patients, and heart rates >60 beats per minute may be inadequate for others. This bradycardia algorithm focuses on management of clinically significant bradycardia (ie, bradycardia that is inadequate for clinical condition).

Initial treatment of any patient with bradycardia should focus on support of airway and breathing (Box 2). Provide supplementary oxygen, place the patient on a monitor, evaluate blood pressure and oxyhemoglobin saturation, and establish intravenous (IV) access. Obtain an ECG to better define the rhythm. While initiating treatment, evaluate the clinical status of the patient and identify potential reversible causes.

The provider must identify signs and symptoms of poor perfusion and determine if those signs are likely to be caused by the bradycardia (Box 3). Signs and symptoms of bradycardia may be mild, and asymptomatic patients do not require treatment. They should be monitored for signs of deterioration (Box 4A). Provide immediate therapy for patients with hypotension, acute altered mental status, chest pain, congestive heart failure, seizures, syncope, or other signs of shock related to the bradycardia (Box 4).

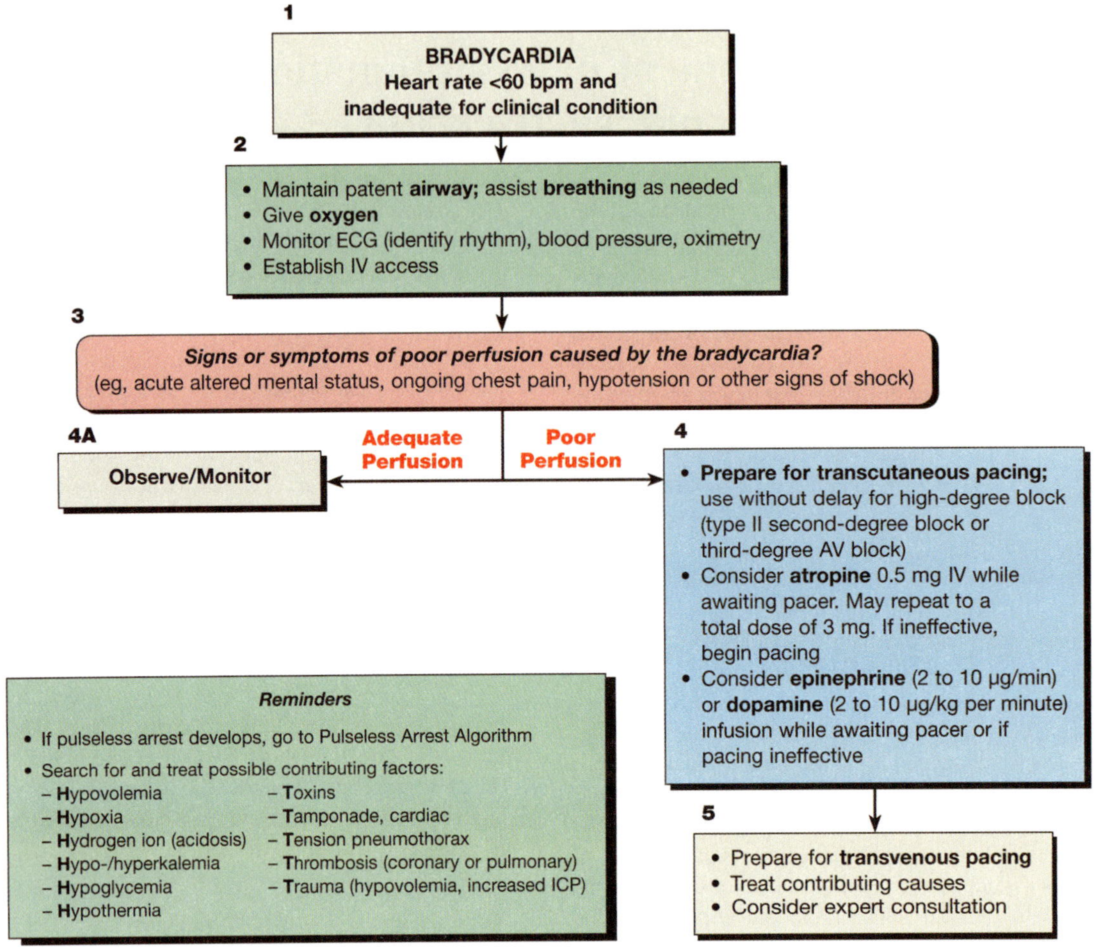

Figure 1. Bradycardia Algorithm.

AV blocks are classified as first, second, and third degree. They may be caused by medications or electrolyte disturbances, as well as structural problems resulting from acute myocardial infarction and myocarditis. A first-degree AV block is defined by a prolonged PR interval (>0.20 second) and is usually benign. Second-degree AV block is divided into Mobitz types I and II. In Mobitz type I block, the block is at the AV node; the block is often transient and may be asymptomatic. In Mobitz type II block, the block is most often below the AV node at the bundle of His or at the bundle branches; the block is often symptomatic, with the potential to progress to complete (third-degree) AV block. Third-degree heart block may occur at the AV node, bundle of His, or bundle branches. When third-degree AV block is present, no impulses pass between the atria and ventricles. Third-degree heart block can be permanent or transient, depending on the underlying cause.

Therapy (Box 4)

Be prepared to initiate transcutaneous pacing quickly in patients who do not respond to atropine (or second-line drugs if these do not delay definitive management). Pacing is also recommended for severely symptomatic patients, especially when the block is at or below the His-Purkinje level (ie, type II second-degree or third-degree AV block).

Atropine

In the absence of reversible causes, atropine remains the first-line drug for acute symptomatic bradycardia (Class IIa). In 1 randomized clinical trial in adults (LOE 2)[5] and additional lower-level studies (LOE 4),[6,7] IV atropine improved heart rate and signs and symptoms associated with bradycardia. An initial dose of 0.5 mg, repeated as needed to a total of 1.5 mg, was effective in both in-hospital and out-of-hospital treatment of symptomatic bradycardia.[5–7] Transcutaneous pacing is usually indicated if the patient fails to respond to atropine, although second-line drug therapy with drugs such as dopamine or epinephrine may be successful (see below).

Use transcutaneous pacing without delay for symptomatic high-degree (second-degree or third-degree) block. Atropine sulfate reverses cholinergic-mediated decreases in heart rate and should be considered a temporizing measure while awaiting a transcutaneous pacemaker for patients with symptomatic high-degree AV block. Atropine is useful for treating symptomatic sinus bradycardia and may be beneficial for any type of AV block at the nodal level.[7]

The recommended atropine dose for bradycardia is 0.5 mg IV every 3 to 5 minutes to a maximum total dose of 3 mg. Doses of atropine sulfate of <0.5 mg may paradoxically result in further slowing of the heart rate.[8] Atropine administration should not delay implementation of external pacing for patients with poor perfusion.

Use atropine cautiously in the presence of acute coronary ischemia or myocardial infarction; increased heart rate may worsen ischemia or increase the zone of infarction.

Atropine may be used with caution and appropriate monitoring following cardiac transplantation. It will likely be ineffective because the transplanted heart lacks vagal innervation. One small uncontrolled study (LOE 5)[9] documented paradoxical slowing of the heart rate and high-degree AV block when atropine was administered to patients after cardiac transplantation.

Avoid relying on atropine in type II second-degree or third-degree AV block or in patients with third-degree AV block with a new wide-QRS complex. These patients require immediate pacing.

Pacing

Transcutaneous pacing is a Class I intervention for symptomatic bradycardias. It should be started immediately for patients who are unstable, particularly those with high-degree (Mobitz type II second-degree or third-degree) block. Some limitations apply. Transcutaneous pacing can be painful and may fail to produce effective mechanical capture. If cardiovascular symptoms are not caused by the bradycardia, the patient may not improve despite effective pacing.

Transcutaneous pacing is noninvasive and can be performed by ECC providers at the bedside. Initiate transcutaneous pacing immediately if there is no response to atropine, if atropine is unlikely to be effective, or if the patient is severely symptomatic. Verify mechanical capture and reassess the patient's condition. Use analgesia and sedation for pain control, and try to identify the cause of the bradyarrhythmia.

If transcutaneous pacing is ineffective (eg, inconsistent capture), prepare for transvenous pacing and consider obtaining expert consultation.

Alternative Drugs to Consider

These drugs are not first-line agents for treatment of symptomatic bradycardia. They may be considered when the bradycardia is unresponsive to atropine and as temporizing measures while awaiting the availability of a pacemaker. To simplify the algorithm, we have listed epinephrine and dopamine as alternative drugs to consider (Class IIb); they are widely available and familiar to ACLS clinicians. In this section we also summarize evidence in support of other drugs that may be considered.

Epinephrine

Epinephrine infusion may be used for patients with symptomatic bradycardia or hypotension after atropine or pacing fails (Class IIb). Begin the infusion at 2 to 10 μg/min and titrate to patient response. Assess intravascular volume and support as needed.

Dopamine

Dopamine hydrochloride has both α- and β-adrenergic actions. Dopamine infusion (at rates of 2 to 10 μg/kg per minute) can be added to epinephrine or administered alone. Titrate the dose to patient response. Assess intravascular volume and support as needed.

Glucagon

One case series (LOE 5)[10] documented improvement in heart rate, symptoms, and signs associated with bradycardia when IV glucagon (3 mg initially, followed by infusion at 3 mg/h if necessary) was given to in-hospital patients with drug-induced (eg, β-blocker or calcium channel blocker overdose) symptomatic bradycardia not responding to atropine.

Tachycardia

This section summarizes the management of a wide variety of tachyarrhythmias. Following the overview of tachyarrhythmias and summary of the initial evaluation and treatment of tachycardia, common antiarrhythmic drugs used in the treatment of tachycardia are presented.

Classification of Tachyarrhythmias

The tachycardias can be classified in several ways based on the appearance of the QRS complex. Professionals at the ACLS level should be able to recognize and differentiate between sinus tachycardia, narrow-complex supraventricular tachycardia (SVT), and wide-complex tachycardia. Because ACLS providers may be unable to distinguish between supraventricular and ventricular rhythms, they should be aware that most wide-complex (broad-complex) tachycardias are *ventricular* in origin.

- Narrow–QRS-complex (SVT) tachycardias (QRS <0.12 second) in order of frequency
  - Sinus tachycardia
  - Atrial fibrillation
  - Atrial flutter
  - AV nodal reentry
  - Accessory pathway–mediated tachycardia
  - Atrial tachycardia (ectopic and reentrant)
  - Multifocal atrial tachycardia (MAT)
  - Junctional tachycardia
- Wide–QRS-complex tachycardias (QRS ≥0.12 second)
  - Ventricular tachycardia (VT)
  - SVT with aberrancy
  - Pre-excited tachycardias (*advanced* recognition rhythms using an accessory pathway)

Irregular narrow-complex tachycardias are probably atrial fibrillation or possibly atrial flutter or MAT. The management of atrial fibrillation and flutter is discussed in the section "Irregular Tachycardias," below.

Initial Evaluation and Treatment of Tachyarrhythmias

The evaluation and management of tachyarrhythmias is depicted in the ACLS Tachycardia Algorithm (Figure 2). Box numbers in the text refer to numbered boxes in this algorithm. Note that the "screened" boxes (boxes with text that is noticeably lighter, ie, Boxes 9, 10, 11, 13, and 14) indicate therapies that are intended for in-hospital use or with expert consultation available.

This algorithm summarizes the management of the tachycardic patient with pulses (Box 1). If pulseless arrest develops at any time, see the ACLS Pulseless Arrest Algorithm in Part 7.2: "Management of Cardiac Arrest."

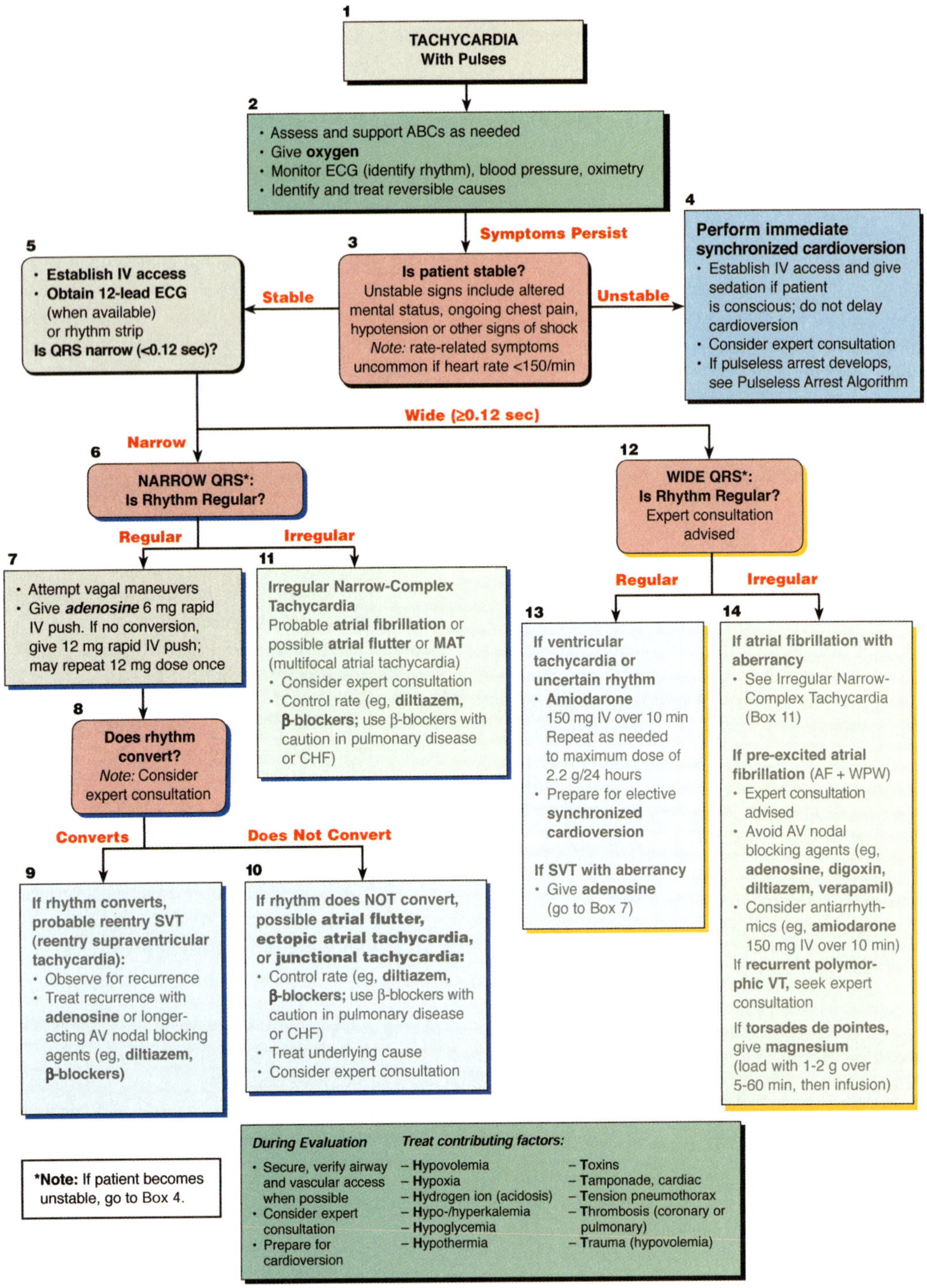

Figure 2. ACLS Tachycardia Algorithm.

The provider must assess the patient while supporting the airway and breathing, administering oxygen (Box 2), obtaining an ECG to identify the rhythm, and monitoring blood pressure and oxyhemoglobin saturation. The provider should establish IV access when possible and identify and treat reversible causes of the tachycardia.

If signs and symptoms persist despite provision of supplementary oxygen and support of airway and ventilation, the provider should determine if the patient is unstable and if signs of cardiovascular compromise are related to the tachycardia (Box 3). If the patient demonstrates rate-related cardiovascular compromise, with signs and symptoms such as altered mental status, ongoing chest pain, hypotension, or other signs of shock, provide immediate synchronized cardioversion (Box 4—see below). Serious signs and symptoms are uncommon if the ventricular rate is <150 beats per minute in patients with a healthy heart. Patients with impaired cardiac function or significant comorbid conditions may become symptomatic at lower heart rates. If the patient is unstable with narrow-complex reentry SVT, you may administer adenosine while preparations are made for synchronized cardioversion (Class IIb), but do not delay cardioversion to administer the drug or to establish IV access.

If the patient with tachycardia is stable (ie, no serious signs or symptoms related to the tachycardia), the provider has time to obtain a 12-lead ECG and evaluate the rhythm (Box 5) and determine treatment options. Stable patients may await expert consultation because treatment has the potential for harm.

Synchronized Cardioversion and Unsynchronized Shocks (Box 4)

Synchronized cardioversion is shock delivery that is timed (synchronized) with the QRS complex. This synchronization avoids shock delivery during the relative refractory period of the cardiac cycle (some call it the "vulnerable period"), when a shock could produce VF.[11] The energy (shock dose) used for synchronized cardioversion is lower than the doses used for unsynchronized shocks (ie, doses for attempted defibrillation). Low-energy shocks should always be delivered as *synchronized* shocks because delivery of low energy unsynchronized shocks is likely to induce VF. If cardioversion is needed and it is impossible to synchronize a shock (eg, the patient's rhythm is irregular), use high-energy unsynchronized shocks (defibrillation doses).

Synchronized cardioversion is recommended to treat (1) unstable SVT due to reentry, (2) unstable atrial fibrillation, and (3) unstable atrial flutter. These arrhythmias are caused by reentry, an abnormal rhythm circuit that allows a wave of depolarization to travel in a circle. Delivery of a shock can stop these rhythms because it interrupts the circulating (reentry) pattern. Synchronized cardioversion is also recommended to treat unstable monomorphic (regular) VT.

If possible, establish IV access before cardioversion and administer sedation if the patient is conscious. But do not delay cardioversion. Consider expert consultation. For further information about defibrillation and cardioversion, see Part 5: "Electrical Therapies."

The recommended initial dose for cardioversion of atrial fibrillation is 100 J to 200 J with a monophasic waveform. A dose of 100 J to 120 J is reasonable with a biphasic waveform. Escalate the second and subsequent shock doses as needed.

Cardioversion of atrial flutter and other SVTs generally requires less energy. An initial energy of 50 J to 100 J monophasic damped sine (MDS) waveform is often sufficient. If the initial 50-J shock fails, increase the dose in a stepwise fashion.[12] More data is needed before detailed comparative dosing recommendations for cardioversion with biphasic waveforms can be made.

Cardioversion is not likely to be effective for treatment of junctional tachycardia or ectopic or multifocal atrial tachycardia because these rhythms have an automatic focus, arising from cells that are spontaneously depolarizing at a rapid rate. Delivery of a shock generally cannot stop these rhythms. In fact, shock delivery to a heart with a rapid automatic focus may increase the rate of the tachyarrhythmia.

The amount of energy required for cardioversion of VT is determined by the morphologic characteristics and the rate of the VT.[13] If the patient with monomorphic VT (regular form and rate) is unstable but has a pulse, treat with synchronized cardioversion. To treat monomorphic VT using a monophasic waveform, provide an initial shock of 100 J. If there is no response to the first shock, increase the dose in a stepwise fashion (eg, 100 J, 200 J, 300 J, 360 J). These recommendations are consistent with the recommendations in the *ECC Guidelines 2000*.[2] There is insufficient data to recommend specific biphasic energy doses for treatment of VT.

If a patient has polymorphic VT and is unstable, treat the rhythm as VF and deliver high-energy *unsynchronized* shocks (ie, defibrillation doses). Although synchronized cardioversion is preferred for treatment of an organized ventricular rhythm, for some irregular rhythms, such as polymorphic VT, synchronization is not possible. If there is any doubt whether monomorphic or polymorphic VT is present in the *unstable* patient, do not delay shock delivery to perform detailed rhythm analysis—provide high-energy unsynchronized shocks (ie, defibrillation doses). Use the ACLS Pulseless Arrest Algorithm (see Part 7.2: "Management of Cardiac Arrest").

Regular Narrow-Complex Tachycardia (Boxes 7, 8, 9, 10)

Sinus Tachycardia

Sinus tachycardia is common and usually results from a physiologic stimulus, such as fever, anemia, or shock. Sinus tachycardia occurs when the sinus node discharge rate is >100 times per minute in response to a variety of stimuli or sympathomimetic agents. No specific drug treatment is required. Therapy is directed toward identification and treatment of the underlying cause. When cardiac function is poor, cardiac output can be dependent on a rapid heart rate. In such compensatory tachycardias, stroke volume is limited, so "normalizing" the heart rate can be detrimental.

Supraventricular Tachycardia (Reentry SVT)

Evaluation

Reentry SVT is a regular tachycardia that is caused by reentry, an abnormal rhythm circuit that allows a wave of depolarization to travel in a circle. The often abrupt onset and termination of this tachyarrhythmia led to its original name, paroxysmal supraventricular tachycardia (PSVT). The rate of reentry SVT exceeds the typical upper limits of sinus tachycardia at rest (>120 beats per minute) with or without discernible P waves. The rhythm is considered to be of supraventricular origin if the QRS complex is narrow (<120 milliseconds or <0.12 second) or if the QRS complex is wide (broad) and bundle branch aberrancy is *known* to be present. Reentry SVT may include AV nodal reentrant tachycardia or AV reentry tachycardia.

Therapy

Vagal Maneuvers. Vagal maneuvers and adenosine are the preferred initial therapeutic choices for the termination of stable reentry SVT (Box 7). Vagal maneuvers alone (Valsalva maneuver or carotid sinus massage) will terminate about 20% to 25% of reentry SVT[14]; adenosine treatment is required for the remainder. In 1 study (LOE 4)[15] of stable reentry SVT in younger patients, vagal maneuvers were often unsuccessful.

Adenosine. If reentry SVT does not respond to vagal maneuvers, give 6 mg of IV adenosine as a rapid IV push (Class I). Give adenosine rapidly over 1 to 3 seconds through a large (eg, antecubital) vein followed by a 20-mL saline flush and elevation of the arm. If the rate does not convert within 1 to 2 minutes, give a 12-mg bolus. Give a second 12-mg bolus if the rate fails to convert within 1 to 2 minutes after the first 12-mg bolus.

Five prospective controlled nonrandomized cohort studies (LOE 2[16]; LOE 3[17–20]) showed that adenosine is safe and effective in converting SVT in both the in-hospital and out-of-hospital settings. Although 2 randomized clinical trials (LOE 3)[17,21] documented a similar SVT conversion rate between adenosine and calcium channel blockers, adenosine was more rapid with fewer severe side effects than verapamil. Amiodarone can achieve nearly 100% efficacy in the inhibition of induced sustained reentrant SVT (LOE 6).[22]

Adenosine is safe and effective in pregnancy.[23] Adenosine, however, does have several important drug interactions. Larger doses may be required for patients with a significant blood level of theophylline, caffeine, or theobromine. The initial dose should be reduced to 3 mg in patients taking dipyridamole or carbamazepine, those with transplanted hearts, or if given by central venous access. Side effects with adenosine are common but transient; flushing, dyspnea, and chest pain are the most frequently observed.[24]

If the rhythm does convert (Box 9), it was probably reentry SVT. Monitor the patient for recurrence and treat any recurrence with adenosine or control the rate with a longer-acting AV nodal blocking agent (eg, diltiazem or β-blocker).

Calcium Channel Blockers and β-Blockers. If adenosine fails to convert reentry SVT (Box 10), attempt rate control with a nondihydropyridine calcium channel blocker (ie, verapamil or diltiazem) or β-blocker as a second-line agent (Class IIa).[25–27] These drugs act primarily on nodal tissue either to slow the ventricular response to atrial arrhythmias by blocking conduction through the AV node or to terminate the reentry SVT that depends on conduction through the AV node.

Verapamil and, to a lesser extent, diltiazem may decrease myocardial contractility and critically reduce cardiac output in patients with severe left ventricular dysfunction. Calcium channel blockers that affect the AV node (including verapamil and diltiazem) are considered harmful when given to patients with atrial fibrillation or atrial flutter associated with known pre-excitation (Wolff-Parkinson-White [WPW]) syndrome. β-Blockers should be used with caution in patients with pulmonary disease or congestive heart failure.

For verapamil, give a 2.5 to 5 mg IV bolus over 2 minutes (over 3 minutes in older patients). If there is no therapeutic response and no drug-induced adverse event, repeated doses of 5 to 10 mg may be administered every 15 to 30 minutes to a total dose of 20 mg. An alternative dosing regimen is to give a 5-mg bolus every 15 minutes to a total dose of 30 mg. Verapamil should be given *only* to patients with narrow-complex reentry SVT or arrhythmias known with certainty to be of supraventricular origin. It should not be given to patients with impaired ventricular function or heart failure.

For diltiazem, give a dose of 15 to 20 mg (0.25 mg/kg) IV over 2 minutes; if needed, in 15 minutes give an IV dose of 20 to 25 mg (0.35 mg/kg). The maintenance infusion dose is 5 to 15 mg/h, titrated to heart rate.

A wide variety of β-blockers may be given for treatment of supraventricular tachyarrhythmias. More detailed information is provided below. Side effects of β-blockers can include bradycardias, AV conduction delays, and hypotension.

Wide- (Broad-) Complex Tachycardia (Boxes 12, 13, 14)

Evaluation

The first step in the management of any tachycardia is to determine if the patient's condition is stable or unstable (Box 3). An unstable patient with wide-complex tachycardia is presumed to have VT, and immediate cardioversion is performed (Box 4 and see above).

If the patient is stable, the second step in management is to obtain a 12-lead ECG (Box 5) to evaluate the QRS duration (ie, narrow or wide). At this point the provider should consider the need to obtain expert consultation. If the patient becomes unstable at any time, proceed with synchronized cardioversion. If the patient develops pulseless arrest or is unstable with polymorphic VT, treat as VF and deliver high-energy unsynchronized shocks (ie, defibrillation doses).

Wide-complex tachycardias are defined as those with a QRS $\geq$0.12 second. The most common forms of wide-complex tachycardia are

- VT
- SVT with aberrancy
- Pre-excited tachycardias (associated with or mediated by an accessory pathway)

The third step in management of a tachycardia is to determine if the rhythm is regular or irregular (Box 12). A *regular* wide-complex tachycardia is likely to be VT or SVT with aberrancy. An irregular wide-complex tachycardia may be atrial fibrillation with aberrancy, pre-excited atrial fibrillation (ie, atrial fibrillation with WPW syndrome), or polymorphic VT. Polymorphic VT may represent torsades de pointes (see below). Providers should consider the need for expert consultation when treating wide-complex tachycardias.

Therapy for Regular Wide-Complex Tachycardias (Box 13)

If the wide-complex regular tachycardia is thought to be SVT, adenosine is recommended. The dose used (6 mg rapid IV push; providers may follow the first dose with a 12-mg bolus and a second 12-mg bolus if the rate fails to convert) is the same as that for reentry SVT (see above for more information).

Synchronized cardioversion is appropriate for treatment of monomorphic (regular) wide-complex tachycardia, particularly if the patient is symptomatic (eg, signs of altered level of consciousness). If the rhythm is identified as likely VT in a stable patient, IV antiarrhythmic drugs may be effective. If antiarrhythmics are administered, we recommend amiodarone (Class IIa). Give 150 mg IV over 10 minutes; repeat as needed to a maximum dose of 2.2 g IV per 24 hours. Alternative drugs for wide-complex regular tachycardias are procainamide and sotalol (see below).

Evidence in support of amiodarone comes from 3 observational studies (LOE 5)[28–30] that indicate that amiodarone is effective for the termination of shock-resistant or drug-refractory VT. One randomized parallel study (LOE 2)[31] indicated that aqueous amiodarone is more effective than lidocaine in the treatment of shock-resistant VT. Amiodarone administration is also supported by extrapolated evidence (LOE 7) from studies of out-of-hospital cardiac arrest with shock-refractory VF/VT, which showed that amiodarone improved survival to hospital admission (but not discharge) compared with placebo[32] or lidocaine.[33]

Irregular Tachycardias

Atrial Fibrillation and Flutter

Evaluation

An irregular narrow-complex or wide-complex tachycardia is most likely atrial fibrillation with an uncontrolled ventricular response. Other diagnostic possibilities include MAT. We recommend a 12-lead ECG and expert consultation if the patient is stable.

Therapy

Management (Box 11) should focus on control of the rapid ventricular rate (rate control) and conversion of hemodynamically unstable atrial fibrillation to sinus rhythm (rhythm control). Patients with atrial fibrillation for >48 hours are at increased risk for cardioembolic events and must first undergo anticoagulation before rhythm control. Electric or pharmacologic cardioversion (conversion to normal sinus rhythm) should *not be attempted* in these patients unless the patient is unstable or the absence of a left atrial thrombus is documented by transesophageal echocardiography.

Magnesium (LOE 3),[34] diltiazem (LOE 2),[35] and β-blockers (LOE 2)[36,37] have been shown to be effective for rate control in the treatment of atrial fibrillation with a rapid ventricular response in both the prehospital (LOE 3)[38] and hospital settings.

Ibutilide and amiodarone (LOE 2)[39–41] have been shown to be effective for rhythm control in the treatment of atrial fibrillation in the hospital setting.

In summary, we recommend expert consultation and initial *rate* control with diltiazem, β-blockers, or magnesium for patients with atrial fibrillation and a rapid ventricular response. Amiodarone, ibutilide, propafenone, flecainide, digoxin, clonidine, or magnesium can be considered for *rhythm* control in patients with atrial fibrillation of ≤48 hours duration.

If a pre-excitation syndrome was identified before the onset of atrial fibrillation (ie, a delta wave, characteristic of WPW, was visible during normal sinus rhythm), expert consultation is advised. Do not administer AV nodal blocking agents such as adenosine, calcium channel blockers, digoxin, and possibly β-blockers to patients with pre-excitation atrial fibrillation or atrial flutter (Box 14) because these drugs can cause a paradoxical increase in the ventricular response to the rapid atrial impulses of atrial fibrillation.

Polymorphic (Irregular) VT (Box 14)

Polymorphic (irregular) VT requires immediate treatment because it is likely to deteriorate to pulseless arrest. Providers should consider consultation with an expert in arrhythmia management.

Pharmacologic treatment of recurrent polymorphic VT is determined by the presence or absence of a long QT during sinus rhythm. If a long QT interval is observed during sinus rhythm (ie, the VT is torsades de pointes), the first step is to stop medications known to prolong the QT interval. Correct electrolyte imbalance and other acute precipitants (eg, drug overdose or poisoning—see Part 10.2: "Toxicology in ECC").

Although magnesium is commonly used to treat torsades de pointes VT (polymorphic VT associated with long QT interval), it is supported by only 2 observational studies (LOE 5)[42,43] showing effectiveness in patients with prolonged QT interval. One adult case series (LOE 5)[44] showed that isoproterenol or ventricular pacing can be effective in terminating torsades de pointes associated with bradycardia and drug-induced QT prolongation. Magnesium is unlikely to be effective in terminating polymorphic VT in patients with a normal QT interval (LOE 5),[43] but amiodarone may be effective (LOE 4).[45]

If the patient with polymorphic VT is or becomes unstable (ie, demonstrates altered level of consciousness, hypotension, or other signs of shock, such as severe pulmonary edema), provide high-energy (ie, defibrillation dose) *unsynchronized* shocks. Although synchronized cardioversion is always preferred for an organized ventricular rhythm, synchronization is not possible for some arrhythmias. The many QRS configurations and irregular rates present in polymorphic VT make it difficult or impossible to reliably synchronize to a QRS complex. A good rule of thumb is that if your eye cannot synchronize to each QRS complex, neither can the defibrillator/cardioverter.

If there is any doubt whether monomorphic or polymorphic VT is present in the *unstable* patient, do not delay shock delivery for detailed rhythm analysis—provide high-energy unsynchronized shocks (ie, defibrillation doses). Current research confirms that it is reasonable to use selected energies of 150 J to 200 J with a biphasic truncated exponential waveform or 120 J with a rectilinear biphasic waveform for the initial shock. For second and subsequent biphasic shocks use the same or higher energy (Class IIa). Providers should use the biphasic device-specific dose; the default dose is 200 J. If a monophasic defibrillator is used, use a dose of 360 J for all unsynchronized shocks (for further information see Part 5: "Electrical Therapies: Automated External Defibrillators, Defibrillation, Cardioversion, and Pacing"). Lower energy levels should not be used for these unsynchronized shocks because low-energy shocks have a high likelihood of provoking VF when they are given in an unsynchronized mode.

After shock delivery the healthcare provider should be prepared to provide immediate CPR (beginning with chest compressions) and follow the ACLS Pulseless Arrest Algorithm if pulseless arrest develops. For further information see Part 7.2: "Management of Cardiac Arrest."

Antiarrhythmic Drugs

Adenosine

Adenosine is an endogenous purine nucleoside that briefly depresses AV node and sinus node activity. Adenosine is recommended for the following indications:

- For defined, stable, narrow-complex AV nodal or sinus nodal reentry tachycardias.[16–21] The most frequent example of these is reentry SVT (Class I). Adenosine will not terminate arrhythmias such as atrial flutter, atrial fibrillation, or atrial or ventricular tachycardias, because these arrhythmias are not due to reentry involving the AV or sinus node. Adenosine will not terminate the arrhythmia but may produce transient AV or retrograde (ventriculoatrial) block clarifying the underlying rhythm.
- For unstable reentry SVT while preparations are made for cardioversion (Class IIb).
- For undefined, stable, narrow-complex SVT as a combination therapeutic and diagnostic maneuver.
- For stable, wide-complex tachycardias in patients with a recurrence of a known reentry pathway that has been previously defined.

Amiodarone IV

IV amiodarone is a complex drug with effects on sodium, potassium, and calcium channels as well as α- and β-adrenergic blocking properties. Amiodarone is recommended for tachyarrhythmias, with the following indications:

- For narrow-complex tachycardias that originated from a reentry mechanism (reentry SVT) if the rhythm remains uncontrolled by adenosine, vagal maneuvers, and AV nodal blockade in patients with preserved or impaired ventricular function (Class IIb)[22]
- Control of hemodynamically stable VT, polymorphic VT with a normal QT interval, and wide-complex tachycardia of uncertain origin (Class IIb)[28–31]
- To control rapid ventricular rate due to accessory pathway conduction in pre-excited atrial arrhythmias (Class IIb)[22]

Administer 150 mg of IV amiodarone over 10 minutes, followed by a 1 mg/min infusion for 6 hours and then a 0.5 mg/min maintenance infusion over 18 hours. Supplementary infusions of 150 mg can be repeated every 10 minutes as necessary for recurrent or resistant arrhythmias to a maximum manufacturer-recommended total daily IV dose of 2.2 g. One study found amiodarone to be effective in patients with atrial fibrillation when administered at relatively high doses of 125 mg/h for 24 hours (total dose 3 g).[41] In patients known to have severely impaired heart function, IV amiodarone is preferable to other antiarrhythmic agents for atrial and ventricular arrhythmias.

The major adverse effects of amiodarone are hypotension and bradycardia, which can be prevented by slowing the rate of drug infusion.

Calcium Channel Blockers: Verapamil and Diltiazem

Verapamil and diltiazem are nondihydropyridine calcium channel blocking agents that slow conduction and increase refractoriness in the AV node. These actions may terminate reentrant arrhythmias and control ventricular response rate in patients with a variety of atrial tachycardias. These medications are indicated in the following circumstances:

- For stable, narrow-complex, reentry mechanism tachycardias (reentry SVT) if rhythm remains uncontrolled or unconverted by adenosine or vagal maneuvers (Class IIa)[25–27]
- For stable, narrow-complex, automaticity mechanism tachycardias (junctional, ectopic, multifocal) if the rhythm is not controlled or converted by adenosine or vagal maneuvers
- To control rate of ventricular response in patients with atrial fibrillation or atrial flutter (Class IIa)[35,38]

IV verapamil is effective for terminating narrow-complex reentry SVT, and it may also be used for rate control in atrial fibrillation. The initial dose of verapamil is 2.5 to 5 mg IV given over 2 minutes. In the absence of a therapeutic response or a drug-induced adverse event, repeat doses of 5 to 10 mg may be administered every 15 to 30 minutes to a total dose of 20 mg. An alternative dosing regimen is to give a 5-mg bolus every 15 minutes to a total dose of 30 mg. Verapamil should be given *only* to patients with narrow-complex reentry SVT or arrhythmias known with certainty to be of supraventricular origin. It should not be given to patients with impaired ventricular function or heart failure.

Diltiazem at a dose of 0.25 mg/kg, followed by a second dose of 0.35 mg/kg, seems to be equivalent in efficacy to verapamil.[25–27] Verapamil and, to a lesser extent, diltiazem may decrease myocardial contractility and critically reduce cardiac output in patients with severe left ventricular dysfunction. Calcium channel blockers that affect the AV node (eg, verapamil and diltiazem) are considered harmful when given to patients with atrial fibrillation or atrial flutter associated with known pre-excitation (WPW) syndrome.

β-Adrenergic Blockers

β-Blocking agents (atenolol, metoprolol, labetalol, propranolol, esmolol) reduce the effects of circulating catecholamines and decrease heart rate and blood pressure. They also have various cardioprotective effects for patients with acute coronary syndromes. For acute tachyarrhythmias, these agents are indicated for rate control in the following situations:

- For narrow-complex tachycardias that originate from either a *reentry mechanism* (reentry SVT) or an *automatic focus* (junctional, ectopic, or multifocal tachycardia) uncontrolled by vagal maneuvers and adenosine in the patient with preserved ventricular function (Class IIa)
- To control rate in atrial fibrillation and atrial flutter in the patient with preserved ventricular function[36,37]

The recommended dose of atenolol (β_1) is 5 mg *slow* IV (over 5 minutes). If the arrhythmia persists 10 minutes after that dose and the first dose was well tolerated, give a second dose of 5 mg slow IV (over 5 minutes).

Metoprolol (β_1) is given in doses of 5 mg by slow IV/IO push at 5-minute intervals to a total of 15 mg.

An alternative agent is propranolol (β_1 and β_2 effects) 0.1 mg/kg by slow IV push divided into 3 equal doses at 2- to 3-minute intervals. The rate of administration should not exceed 1 mg/min. May repeat total dose in 2 minutes if necessary.

IV esmolol is a short-acting (half-life 2 to 9 minutes) β_1-selective β-blocker that is administered in an IV loading dose of 500 μg/kg (0.5 mg/kg) over 1 minute, followed by a 4-minute infusion of 50 μg/kg per minute (0.05 mg/kg per minute) for a total of 200 μg/kg. If the response is inadequate, a second bolus of 0.5 mg/kg is infused over 1 minute, with an increase of the maintenance infusion to 100 μg/kg (0.1 mg/kg) per minute (maximum infusion rate: 300 μg/kg [0.3 mg/kg] per minute).

Side effects related to β-blockade include bradycardias, AV conduction delays, and hypotension. Cardiovascular decompensation and cardiogenic shock after β-adrenergic blocker therapy are infrequent complications. Contraindications to the use of β-adrenergic blocking agents include second-degree or third-degree heart block, hypotension, severe congestive heart failure, and lung disease associated with bronchospasm. These agents may be harmful for patients with atrial fibrillation or atrial flutter associated with known pre-excitation (WPW) syndrome.

Ibutilide

Ibutilide is a short-acting antiarrhythmic that acts by prolonging the action potential duration and increasing the refractory period of cardiac tissue. This agent may be used in the following circumstances:

- For acute pharmacologic rhythm conversion of atrial fibrillation or atrial flutter in patients with normal cardiac function when duration of the arrhythmia is ≤48 hours (Class IIb).[39]
- To control rate in atrial fibrillation or atrial flutter in patients with preserved ventricular function when calcium channel blockers or β-blockers are ineffective.
- For acute pharmacologic rhythm conversion of atrial fibrillation or atrial flutter in patients with WPW syndrome and preserved ventricular function when the duration of the arrhythmia is ≤48 hours. But the intervention of choice for this indication is DC cardioversion.

Ibutilide seems most effective for the pharmacologic conversion of atrial fibrillation or atrial flutter of relatively brief duration. For adults weighing ≥60 kg, ibutilide is administered intravenously, diluted or undiluted, as 1 mg (10 mL) over 10 minutes. If the first dose is unsuccessful in terminating the arrhythmia, a second 1-mg dose can be administered at the same rate 10 minutes after the first. In patients weighing <60 kg, an initial dose of 0.01 mg/kg is recommended.

Ibutilide has minimal effects on blood pressure and heart rate. Its major limitation is a relatively high incidence of ventricular arrhythmias (polymorphic VT, including torsades de pointes). Correct hyperkalemia or low magnesium before administration. Monitor patients receiving ibutilide *continuously* for arrhythmias at the time of its administration and for *at least 4 to 6 hours* thereafter. Ibutilide is contraindicated in baseline QT_C (QT interval corrected for heart rate) of >440 msec.

Lidocaine

Lidocaine is one of a number of antiarrhythmic drugs available for treatment of ventricular ectopy, VT, and VF. At this time there is good evidence that alternative agents are superior to lidocaine in terminating VT.[46] Lidocaine may be considered in the following conditions (although it is not considered the drug of choice):

- For *stable monomorphic VT* in patients with preserved ventricular function (Class Indeterminate). Alternative agents are preferred.
- For *polymorphic VT* with *normal baseline QT interval* when ischemia is treated and electrolyte imbalance is corrected.
- If ventricular function is preserved: lidocaine may be administered.
- If ventricular function is impaired: use amiodarone as an antiarrhythmic agent. If unsuccessful, perform DC cardioversion.
- Lidocaine can be used for polymorphic VT with a prolonged baseline QT interval that suggests torsades de pointes.

Initial doses ranging from 0.5 to 0.75 mg/kg and up to 1 to 1.5 mg/kg may be used. Repeat 0.5 to 0.75 mg/kg every 5 to 10 minutes to a maximum total dose of 3 mg/kg. A maintenance infusion of 1 to 4 mg/min (30 to 50 μg/kg per minute) is acceptable.

Toxic reactions and side effects include slurred speech, altered consciousness, muscle twitching, seizures, and bradycardia.

Magnesium

Magnesium is recommended for the treatment of torsades de pointes VT with or without cardiac arrest, but it has not been shown to be helpful for treatment of non-torsades pulseless arrest. Low-level evidence suggests that magnesium is effective for rate control (LOE 3)[34] in patients with atrial fibrillation with a rapid ventricular response (LOE 2),[40] so it may be considered for this arrhythmia.

Give magnesium sulfate in a dose of 1 to 2 g diluted in D_5W over 5 to 60 minutes. Slower rates are preferable in the stable patient. A more rapid infusion may be used for the unstable patient.

Procainamide

Procainamide hydrochloride suppresses both atrial and ventricular arrhythmias by slowing conduction in myocardial tissue. One randomized trial (LOE 2)[47] indicated that procainamide is superior to lidocaine in terminating spontaneously occurring VT. Procainamide may be considered in the following situations:

- As one of several drugs that may be used for treatment of stable monomorphic VT in patients with preserved ventricular function (Class IIa)[46]
- One of several equivalent drugs that can be used for control of heart rate in atrial fibrillation or atrial flutter in patients with preserved ventricular function
- One of several drugs that can be used for acute control of heart rhythm in atrial fibrillation or atrial flutter in patients

with known pre-excitation (WPW) syndrome and preserved ventricular function
- One of several drugs that can be used for AV reentrant, narrow-complex tachycardias such as reentry SVT if rhythm is uncontrolled by adenosine and vagal maneuvers in patients with preserved ventricular function

Procainamide hydrochloride for non-VF/VT arrest may be given in an infusion of 20 mg/min until the arrhythmia is suppressed, hypotension ensues, the QRS complex is prolonged by 50% from its original duration, or a total of 17 mg/kg (1.2 g for a 70-kg patient) of the drug has been given. Bolus administration of the drug can result in toxic concentrations and significant hypotension. The maintenance infusion rate of procainamide hydrochloride is 1 to 4 mg/min, diluted in D_5W or normal saline. This should be reduced in the presence of renal failure.

Procainamide should be used cautiously in patients with preexisting QT prolongation. In general it should be used with caution if at all in combination with other drugs that prolong the QT interval (consider obtaining expert consultation). Monitor the ECG and blood pressure continuously during administration of procainamide.

Sotalol

Sotalol is not a first-line antiarrhythmic. Sotalol hydrochloride is an antiarrhythmic agent that, like amiodarone, prolongs action potential duration and increases cardiac tissue refractoriness. It also has nonselective β-blocking properties. One randomized controlled trial (LOE 1)[48] indicated that sotalol is significantly more effective than lidocaine for terminating acute sustained VT. This agent may be used in the following circumstances with expert consultation:

- To control rhythm in atrial fibrillation or atrial flutter in patients with pre-excitation (WPW) syndrome and preserved ventricular function when the duration of the arrhythmia is ≤48 hours. But the intervention of choice for this indication is DC cardioversion.
- For monomorphic VT.

IV sotalol is usually administered at a dose of 1 to 1.5 mg/kg body weight, then infused at a rate of 10 mg/min. Side effects include bradycardia, hypotension, and arrhythmia. The incidence of torsades de pointes following a single dose of sotalol for treatment of VT is reportedly 0.1%.[45] Use of IV sotalol is limited by the need to infuse it relatively slowly.

Summary

The goal of therapy for bradycardia or tachycardia is to rapidly identify and treat patients who are hemodynamically unstable. Pacing or drugs, or both, may be used to control symptomatic bradycardia. Cardioversion or drugs, or both, may be used to control symptomatic tachycardia. ALS providers should closely monitor stable patients pending expert consultation and should be prepared to aggressively treat those who develop decompensation.

References

1. Chiriboga D, Yarzebski J, Goldberg RJ, Gore JM, Alpert JS. Temporal trends (1975 through 1990) in the incidence and case-fatality rates of primary ventricular fibrillation complicating acute myocardial infarction: a communitywide perspective. *Circulation.* 1994;89:998–1003.
2. American Heart Association in collaboration with International Liaison Committee on Resuscitation. Guidelines 2000 for Cardiopulmonary Resuscitation and Emergency Cardiovascular Care. *Circulation.* 2000; 102(suppl):I1–I384.
3. Blomstrom-Lundqvist C, Scheinman MM, Aliot EM, Alpert JS, Calkins H, Camm AJ, Campbell WB, Haines DE, Kuck KH, Lerman BB, Miller DD, Shaeffer CW Jr, Stevenson WG, Tomaselli GF, Antman EM, Smith SC Jr, Alpert JS, Faxon DP, Fuster V, Gibbons RJ, Gregoratos G, Hiratzka LF, Hunt SA, Jacobs AK, Russell RO Jr, Priori SG, Blanc JJ, Budaj A, Burgos EF, Cowie M, Deckers JW, Garcia MA, Klein WW, Lekakis J, Lindahl B, Mazzotta G, Morais JC, Oto A, Smiseth O, Trappe HJ; American College of Cardiology; American Heart Association Task Force on Practice Guidelines; European Society of Cardiology Committee for Practice Guidelines, Writing Committee to Develop Guidelines for the Management of Patients With Supraventricular Arrhythmias. ACC/AHA/ESC guidelines for the management of patients with supraventricular tachycardias—executive summary: a report of the American College of Cardiology/American Heart Association Task Force on Practice Guidelines and the European Society of Cardiology Committee for Practice Guidelines (Writing Committee to Develop Guidelines for the Management of Patients With Supraventricular Arrhythmias). *Circulation.* 2003;108:1871–1909.
4. Cummins RO, Field JM, Hazinski MF, eds. *ACLS: Principles and Practice.* Dallas, Tex: American Heart Association; 2003:239–375.
5. Smith I, Monk TG, White PF. Comparison of transesophageal atrial pacing with anticholinergic drugs for the treatment of intraoperative bradycardia. *Anesth Analg.* 1994;78:245–252.
6. Brady WJ, Swart G, DeBehnke DJ, Ma OJ, Aufderheide TP. The efficacy of atropine in the treatment of hemodynamically unstable bradycardia and atrioventricular block: prehospital and emergency department considerations. *Resuscitation.* 1999;41:47–55.
7. Chadda KD, Lichstein E, Gupta PK, Kourtesis P. Effects of atropine in patients with bradyarrhythmia complicating myocardial infarction: usefulness of an optimum dose for overdrive. *Am J Med.* 1977;63:503–510.
8. Dauchot P, Gravenstein JS. Effects of atropine on the ECG in different age groups. *Clin Pharmacol Ther.* 1971;12:272–280.
9. Bernheim A, Fatio R, Kiowski W, Weilenmann D, Rickli H, Rocca HP. Atropine often results in complete atrioventricular block or sinus arrest after cardiac transplantation: an unpredictable and dose-independent phenomenon. *Transplantation.* 2004;77:1181–1185.
10. Love JN, Sachdeva DK, Bessman ES, Curtis LA, Howell JM. A potential role for glucagon in the treatment of drug-induced symptomatic bradycardia. *Chest.* 1998;114:323–326.
11. Lown B. Electrical reversion of cardiac arrhythmias. *Br Heart J.* 1967; 29:469–489.
12. Kerber RE, Martins JB, Kienzle MG, Constantin L, Olshansky B, Hopson R, Charbonnier F. Energy, current, and success in defibrillation and cardioversion: clinical studies using an automated impedance-based method of energy adjustment. *Circulation.* 1988;77:1038–1046.
13. Kerber RE, Kienzle MG, Olshansky B, Waldo AL, Wilber D, Carlson MD, Aschoff AM, Birger S, Fugatt L, Walsh S, et al. Ventricular tachycardia rate and morphology determine energy and current requirements for transthoracic cardioversion. *Circulation.* 1992;85: 158–163.
14. Lim SH, Anantharaman V, Teo WS, Goh PP, Tan AT. Comparison of treatment of supraventricular tachycardia by Valsalva maneuver and carotid sinus massage. *Ann Emerg Med.* 1998;31:30–35.
15. Ornato JP, Hallagan LF, Reese WA, Clark RF, Tayal VS, Garnett AR, Gonzalez ER. Treatment of paroxysmal supraventricular tachycardia in the emergency department by clinical decision analysis [published correction appears in *Am J Emerg Med.* 1990;8:85]. *Am J Emerg Med.* 1988;6:555–560.
16. DiMarco JP, Miles W, Akhtar M, Milstein S, Sharma AD, Platia E, McGovern B, Scheinman MM, Govier WC. Adenosine for paroxysmal supraventricular tachycardia: dose ranging and comparison with verapamil: assessment in placebo-controlled, multicenter trials. The Adenosine for PSVT Study Group [published correction appears in *Ann Intern Med.* 1990;113:996]. *Ann Intern Med.* 1990;113:104–110.
17. Brady WJ Jr, DeBehnke DJ, Wickman LL, Lindbeck G. Treatment of out-of-hospital supraventricular tachycardia: adenosine vs verapamil. *Acad Emerg Med.* 1996;3:574–585.
18. Furlong R, Gerhardt RT, Farber P, Schrank K, Willig R, Pittaluga J. Intravenous adenosine as first-line prehospital management of narrow-

complex tachycardias by EMS personnel without direct physician control. *Am J Emerg Med.* 1995;13:383–388.

19. Madsen CD, Pointer JE, Lynch TG. A comparison of adenosine and verapamil for the treatment of supraventricular tachycardia in the prehospital setting. *Ann Emerg Med.* 1995;25:649–655.
20. Morrison LJ, Allan R, Vermeulen M, Dong SL, McCallum AL. Conversion rates for prehospital paroxysmal supraventricular tachycardia (PSVT) with the addition of adenosine: a before-and-after trial. *Prehosp Emerg Care.* 2001;5:353–359.
21. Cheng KA. [A randomized, multicenter trial to compare the safety and efficacy of adenosine versus verapamil for termination of paroxysmal supraventricular tachycardia.] *Zhonghua Nei Ke Za Zhi.* 2003;42:773–776.
22. Cybulski J, Kulakowski P, Makowska E, Czepiel A, Sikora-Frac M, Ceremuzynski L. Intravenous amiodarone is safe and seems to be effective in termination of paroxysmal supraventricular tachyarrhythmias. *Clin Cardiol.* 1996;19:563–566.
23. Gowda RM, Khan IA, Mehta NJ, Vasavada BC, Sacchi TJ. Cardiac arrhythmias in pregnancy: clinical and therapeutic considerations. *Int J Cardiol.* 2003;88:129–133.
24. Camm AJ, Garratt CJ. Adenosine and supraventricular tachycardia. *N Engl J Med.* 1991;325:1621–1629.
25. Gupta A, Naik A, Vora A, Lokhandwala Y. Comparison of efficacy of intravenous diltiazem and esmolol in terminating supraventricular tachycardia. *J Assoc Physicians India.* 1999;47:969–972.
26. Lim SH, Anantharaman V, et al. Slow infusion of calcium channel blockers are more effective in the emergency management of supraventricular tachycardia. *Circulation.* 1999;100:722.
27. Lim SH, Anantharaman V, Teo WS. Slow-infusion of calcium channel blockers in the emergency management of supraventricular tachycardia. *Resuscitation.* 2002;52:167–174.
28. Schutzenberer W, Leisch F, Kerschner K, Harringer W, Herbinger W. Clinical efficacy of intravenous amiodarone in the short term treatment of recurrent sustained ventricular tachycardia and ventricular fibrillation. *Br Heart J.* 1989;62:367–371.
29. Credner SC, Klingenheben T, Maus O, Sticherling C, Hohnloser SH. Electrical storm in patients with transvenous implantable cardioverter-defibrillators: incidence, management and prognostic implications. *J Am Coll Cardiol.* 1998;32:1909–1915.
30. Helmy I, Herre JM, Gee G, Sharkey H, Malone P, Sauve MJ, Griffin JC, Scheinman MM. Use of intravenous amiodarone for emergency treatment of life-threatening ventricular arrhythmias. *J Am Coll Cardiol.*1989;12:1015–1022.
31. Somberg JC, Bailin SJ, Haffajee CI, Paladino WP, Kerin NZ, Bridges D, Timar S, Molnar J. Intravenous lidocaine versus intravenous amiodarone (in a new aqueous formulation) for incessant ventricular tachycardia. *Am J Cardiol.* 2002;90:853–859.
32. Kudenchuk PJ, Cobb LA, Copass MK, Cummins RO, Doherty AM, Fahrenbruch CE, Hallstrom AP, Murray WA, Olsufka M, Walsh T. Amiodarone for resuscitation after out-of-hospital cardiac arrest due to ventricular fibrillation. *N Engl J Med.* 1999;341:871–878.
33. Dorian P, Cass D, Schwartz B, Cooper R, Gelaznikas R, Barr A. Amiodarone as compared with lidocaine for shock-resistant ventricular fibrillation. *N Engl J Med.* 2002;346:884–890.
34. Chiladakis JA, Stathopoulos C, Davlouros P, Manolis AS. Intravenous magnesium sulfate versus diltiazem in paroxysmal atrial fibrillation. *Int J Cardiol.* 2001;79:287–291.
35. Wattanasuwan N, Khan IA, Mehta NJ, Arora P, Singh N, Vasavada BC, Sacchi TJ. Acute ventricular rate control in atrial fibrillation: IV combination of diltiazem and digoxin vs. IV diltiazem alone. *Chest.* 2001;119:502–506.
36. Sticherling C, Tada H, Hsu W, Bares AC, Oral H, Pelosi F, Knight BP, Strickberger SA, Morady F. Effects of diltiazem and esmolol on cycle length and spontaneous conversion of atrial fibrillation. *J Cardiovasc Pharmacol Ther.* 2002;7:81–88.
37. Shettigar UR, Toole JG, Appunn DO. Combined use of esmolol and digoxin in the acute treatment of atrial fibrillation or flutter. *Am Heart J.* 1993;126:368–374.
38. Wang HE, O'Connor RE, Megargel RE, Schnyder ME, Morrison DM, Barnes TA, Fitzkee A. The use of diltiazem for treating rapid atrial fibrillation in the out-of-hospital setting. *Ann Emerg Med.* 2001;37:38–45.
39. Martinez-Marcos FJ, Garcia-Garmendia JL, Ortega-Carpio A, Fernandez-Gomez JM, Santos JM, Camacho C. Comparison of intravenous flecainide, propafenone, and amiodarone for conversion of acute atrial fibrillation to sinus rhythm. *Am J Cardiol.* 2000;86:950–953.
40. Kalus JS, Spencer AP, Tsikouris JP, Chung JO, Kenyon KW, Ziska M, Kluger J, White CM. Impact of prophylactic i.v. magnesium on the efficacy of ibutilide for conversion of atrial fibrillation or flutter. *Am J Health Syst Pharm.* 2003;60:2308–2312.
41. Cotter G, Blatt A, Kaluski E, Metzkor-Cotter E, Koren M, Litinski I, Simantov R, Moshkovitz Y, Zaidenstein R, Peleg E, Vered Z, Golik A. Conversion of recent onset paroxysmal atrial fibrillation to normal sinus rhythm: the effect of no treatment and high-dose amiodarone: a randomized, placebo-controlled study. *Eur Heart J.* 1999;20:1833–1842.
42. Manz M, Pfeiffer D, Jung W, Lueritz B. Intravenous treatment with magnesium in recurrent persistent ventricular tachycardia. *New Trends in Arrhythmias.* 1991;7:437–442.
43. Tzivoni D, Banai S, Schuger C, Benhorin J, Keren A, Gottlieb S, Stern S. Treatment of torsade de pointes with magnesium sulfate. *Circulation.* 1988;77:392–397.
44. Keren A, Tzivoni D, Gavish D, Levi J, Gottlieb S, Benhorin J, Stern S. Etiology, warning signs and therapy of torsade de pointes: a study of 10 patients. *Circulation.* 1981;64:1167–1174.
45. Nguyen PT, Scheinman MM, Seger J. Polymorphous ventricular tachycardia: clinical characterization, therapy, and the QT interval. *Circulation.* 1986;74:340–349.
46. Marill KA, Greenbeg GM, Kay D, Nelson BK. Analysis of the treatment of spontaneous sustained stable ventricular tachycardia. *Acad Emerg Med.* 1997;12:1122–1128.
47. Gorgels AR, van den Dool A, Hofs A, Mulleneers R, Smees JL, Vos MA, Wellens HJ. Comparison of procainamide and lidocaine in terminating sustained monomorphic ventricular tachycardia. *Am J Cardiol.* 1996;78:43–46.
48. Ho DS, Zecchin RP, Richards DA, Uther JB, Ross DL. Double-blind trial of lignocaine versus sotalol for acute termination of spontaneous sustained ventricular tachycardia. *Lancet.* 1994;344:18–23.

Part 7.4: Monitoring and Medications

This section provides an overview of monitoring techniques and medications that may be useful during CPR and in the immediate prearrest and postarrest settings.

Monitoring Immediately Before, During, and After Arrest

Assessment During CPR

At present there are no reliable clinical criteria that clinicians can use to assess the efficacy of CPR. Although end-tidal CO_2 serves as an indicator of cardiac output produced by chest compressions and may indicate return of spontaneous circulation (ROSC),[1,2] there is little other technology available to provide real-time feedback on the effectiveness of CPR.

Assessment of Hemodynamics

Coronary Perfusion Pressure

Coronary perfusion pressure (CPP = aortic relaxation [diastolic] pressure minus right atrial relaxation phase blood pressure) during CPR correlates with both myocardial blood flow and ROSC (LOE 3).[3,4] A CPP of ≥15 mm Hg is predictive of ROSC. Increased CPP correlates with improved 24-hour survival rates in animal studies (LOE 6)[5] and is associated with improved myocardial blood flow and ROSC in animal studies of epinephrine, vasopressin, and angiotensin II (LOE 6).[5–7]

When intra-arterial monitoring is in place during the resuscitative effort (eg, in an intensive care setting), the clinician should try to maximize arterial diastolic pressures to achieve an optimal CPP. Assuming a right atrial diastolic pressure of 10 mm Hg means that the aortic diastolic pressure should ideally be at least 30 mm Hg to maintain a CPP of ≥20 mm Hg during CPR. Unfortunately such monitoring is rarely available outside the intensive care environment.

Pulses

Clinicians frequently try to palpate arterial pulses during chest compressions to assess the effectiveness of compressions. No studies have shown the validity or clinical utility of checking pulses during ongoing CPR. Because there are no valves in the inferior vena cava, retrograde blood flow into the venous system may produce femoral vein pulsations.[8] Thus palpation of a pulse in the femoral triangle may indicate venous rather than arterial blood flow. Carotid pulsations during CPR do not indicate the efficacy of coronary blood flow or myocardial or cerebral perfusion during CPR.

Assessment of Respiratory Gases

Arterial Blood Gases

Arterial blood gas monitoring during cardiac arrest is not a reliable indicator of the severity of tissue hypoxemia, hypercarbia (and therefore the adequacy of ventilation during CPR), or tissue acidosis. This conclusion is supported by 1 case series (LOE 5)[9] and 10 case reports[10–19] that showed that arterial blood gas values are an inaccurate indicator of the magnitude of tissue acidosis during cardiac arrest and CPR both in and out of hospital.

Oximetry

During cardiac arrest, pulse oximetry will not function because pulsatile blood flow is inadequate in peripheral tissue beds. But pulse oximetry is commonly used in emergency departments and critical care units for monitoring patients who are not in arrest because it provides a simple, continuous method of tracking oxyhemoglobin saturation. Normal pulse oximetry saturation, however, does not ensure adequate systemic oxygen delivery because it does not calculate the total oxygen content (O_2 bound to hemoglobin + dissolved O_2) and adequacy of blood flow (cardiac output).

Tissue oxygen tension is not commonly evaluated during CPR, but it may provide a mechanism to assess tissue perfusion because transconjunctival oxygen tension falls rapidly with cardiac arrest and returns to baseline when spontaneous circulation is restored.[20,21]

End-Tidal CO_2 Monitoring

End-tidal CO_2 monitoring is a safe and effective noninvasive indicator of cardiac output during CPR and may be an early indicator of ROSC in intubated patients. During cardiac arrest CO_2 continues to be generated throughout the body. The major determinant of CO_2 excretion is its rate of delivery from the peripheral production sites to the lungs. In the low-flow state during CPR, ventilation is relatively high compared with blood flow, so that the end-tidal CO_2 concentration is low. If ventilation is reasonably constant, then changes in end-tidal CO_2 concentration reflect changes in cardiac output.

Eight case series have shown that patients who were successfully resuscitated from cardiac arrest had significantly higher end-tidal CO_2 levels than patients who could not be resuscitated (LOE 5).[2,22–28] Capnometry can also be used as an early indicator of ROSC (LOE 5[29,30]; LOE 6[31]).

In case series totaling 744 intubated adults in cardiac arrest receiving CPR who had a *maximum* end-tidal CO_2 of <10 mm Hg, the prognosis was poor even if CPR was optimized (LOE 5).[1,2,24,25,32,33] But this prognostic indicator was unreliable immediately after starting CPR in 4 studies (LOE 5)[1,2,32,33] that showed no difference in rates of ROSC and survival in those with an *initial* end-tidal CO_2 of <10 mm Hg compared with higher end-tidal CO_2. Five patients achieved ROSC (one survived to discharge) despite an initial end-tidal CO_2 of <10 mm Hg.

In summary, end-tidal CO_2 monitoring during cardiac arrest can be useful as a noninvasive indicator of cardiac output generated during CPR (Class IIa). Further research is needed to define the capability of end-tidal CO_2 monitoring to

(*Circulation*. 2005;112:IV-78-IV-83.)

This special supplement to *Circulation* is freely available at http://www.circulationaha.org

DOI: 10.1161/CIRCULATIONAHA.105.166559

guide more aggressive interventions or a decision to abandon resuscitative efforts.

In the patient with ROSC, continuous or intermittent monitoring of end-tidal CO_2 provides assurance that the endotracheal tube is maintained in the trachea. End-tidal CO_2 can guide ventilation, especially when correlated with the Pa_{CO_2} from an arterial blood gas measurement.

Medications for Cardiovascular Support

Vasoactive drugs may be administered immediately before, during, and after an arrest to support cardiac output, especially blood flow to the heart and brain. Drugs may be selected to improve heart rate (chronotropic effects), myocardial contractility (inotropic effects), or arterial pressure (vasoconstrictive effects), or to reduce afterload (vasodilator effects). Unfortunately many adrenergic drugs are not selective and may increase or decrease heart rate and afterload, increase cardiac arrhythmias, and increase myocardial ischemia by creating a mismatch between myocardial oxygen demand and delivery. Myocardial ischemia, in turn, may decrease heart function. Moreover, some agents may also have metabolic effects that increase blood glucose, lactate, and metabolic rate.

Specific drug infusion rates cannot be recommended because of variations in pharmacokinetics (relation between drug dose and concentration) and pharmacodynamics (relation between drug concentration and effect) in critically ill patients,[34,35] so initial dose ranges are listed below. Vasoactive drugs must be titrated at the bedside to secure the intended effect while limiting side effects. Providers must also be aware of the concentrations delivered and compatibilities with previously and concurrently administered drugs.

In general, adrenergic drugs should not be mixed with sodium bicarbonate or other alkaline solutions in the intravenous (IV) line because there is evidence that adrenergic agents are inactivated in alkaline solutions.[36,37] Norepinephrine (levarterenol) and other catecholamines that activate α-adrenergic receptors may produce tissue necrosis if extravasation occurs. If extravasation develops, infiltrate 5 to 10 mg of phentolamine diluted in 10 to 15 mL of saline into the site of extravasation as soon as possible to prevent tissue death and sloughing.

Epinephrine

The use of epinephrine in cardiac arrest is discussed in Part 7.2: "Management of Cardiac Arrest." Epinephrine can also be used in patients who are not in cardiac arrest but who require inotropic or vasopressor support. For example, epinephrine is considered Class IIb for symptomatic bradycardia if atropine and transcutaneous pacing fail or pacing is not available (eg, in the out-of-hospital setting). It may also be used in cases of anaphylaxis associated with hemodynamic instability or respiratory distress.[38]

To create a continuous infusion of epinephrine hydrochloride for treatment of bradycardia or hypotension, add 1 mg (1 mL of a 1:1000 solution) to 500 mL of normal saline or D_5W. The initial dose for adults is 1 μg/min titrated to the desired hemodynamic response, which is typically achieved in doses of 2 to 10 μg/min. Note that this is the nonarrest infusion preparation and dose (ie, for bradycardia or hypotension).

Vasopressin

The use of vasopressin in cardiac arrest is discussed in Part 7.2. Like epinephrine, vasopressin may be used in prearrest and postarrest conditions. Vasopressin has been used for management of vasodilatory shock, such as septic shock and sepsis syndrome.[39,40] Standard therapy for vasodilatory septic shock includes antimicrobial agents, intravascular volume expansion, vasopressors, and inotropic agents that increase myocardial contractility. Inotropic agents and vasoconstrictor drugs that are commonly used in this setting, however, may have a diminished vasopressor action.[41] If conventional adrenergic vasopressor drugs are ineffective, a continuous infusion of vasopressin may be beneficial (Class IIb).[42]

Norepinephrine

Norepinephrine (levarterenol) is a naturally occurring potent vasoconstrictor and inotropic agent. Cardiac output may increase or decrease in response to norepinephrine, depending on vascular resistance, the functional state of the left ventricle, and reflex responses (eg, those mediated by carotid and aortic baroreceptors). Norepinephrine usually induces renal and mesenteric vasoconstriction; in sepsis, however, norepinephrine improves renal blood flow and urine output.[43,44] It may be effective for management of patients with severe hypotension (eg, systolic blood pressure <70 mm Hg) and a low total peripheral resistance who fail to respond to less potent adrenergic drugs such as dopamine, phenylephrine, or methoxamine.

Norepinephrine is relatively contraindicated in patients with hypovolemia. It may increase myocardial oxygen requirements, mandating cautious use in patients with ischemic heart disease. As noted above, extravasation may cause ischemic necrosis and sloughing of superficial tissues and must be treated promptly.

Norepinephrine is administered by adding 4 mg of norepinephrine or 8 mg of norepinephrine bitartrate (1 mg of norepinephrine is equivalent to 2 mg of norepinephrine bitartrate) to 250 mL of D_5W or 5% dextrose in normal saline (but not in normal saline alone), resulting in a concentration of 16 μg/mL of norepinephrine or 32 μg/mL of norepinephrine bitartrate. The initial dose of norepinephrine is 0.5 to 1 μg/min titrated to effect. It should not be administered in the same IV line as alkaline solutions, which may inactivate it.

Dopamine

Dopamine hydrochloride is a catecholamine-like agent and a chemical precursor of norepinephrine that stimulates both α- and β-adrenergic receptors. In addition, there are receptors specific for this compound (DA_1, DA_2 dopaminergic receptors). Physiologically dopamine stimulates the heart through both α- and β-receptors. Pharmacologically dopamine is both a potent adrenergic receptor agonist and a strong peripheral dopamine receptor agonist. These effects are dose dependent.

During resuscitation dopamine is often used to treat hypotension, especially if it is associated with symptomatic bradycardia or after ROSC. Dopamine in combination with other agents, including dobutamine, remains an option for management of postresuscitation hypotension. If hypotension persists after filling pressure (ie, intravascular volume) is optimized, drugs with combined inotropic and vasopressor actions like epinephrine or norepinephrine may be used. Positive effects include increases in both cardiac output and arterial perfusion pressure. Although low-dose dopamine infusion has been frequently recommended to maintain renal blood flow or improve renal function, more recent data has failed to show a beneficial effect from such therapy.[45,46]

The usual dose of dopamine ranges from 2 to 20 μg/kg per minute. Doses >10 to 20 μg/kg per minute may be associated with systemic and splanchnic vasoconstriction. Higher doses of dopamine, like all adrenergic vasoconstrictor drugs, can be associated with adverse effects on splanchnic perfusion in some patients.

Dobutamine

Dobutamine hydrochloride is a synthetic catecholamine and potent inotropic agent useful for treatment of severe systolic heart failure. Dobutamine has complex pharmacology because of the effects of the different racemic components. The (+) isomer is a potent β-adrenergic agonist, whereas the (−) isomer is a potent α_1-agonist.[47] The vasodilating β_2-adrenergic effects of the (+) isomer counterbalance the vasoconstricting α-adrenergic effects, often leading to little change or a reduction in systemic vascular resistance. The beneficial effects of dobutamine may be associated with decreased left ventricular filling pressure. In addition to its direct inotropic effects, dobutamine may further increase stroke volume through reflex peripheral vasodilation (baroreceptor mediated), reducing ventricular afterload, so that arterial pressure is unchanged or may fall even though cardiac output increases. Hemodynamic end points rather than a specific dose should be used to optimize treatment with dobutamine.

The usual dose of dobutamine ranges from 2 to 20 μg/kg per minute; however, there is a wide variation in individual response to the drug in critically ill patients. Elderly patients may have a significantly decreased response to dobutamine. At doses >20 μg/kg per minute, increases in heart rate of >10% may induce or exacerbate myocardial ischemia. Doses of dobutamine as high as 40 μg/kg per minute have been used, but such doses may greatly increase adverse effects, especially tachycardia and hypotension.

Inodilators (Inamrinone and Milrinone)

Inamrinone (formerly amrinone) and milrinone are phosphodiesterase III inhibitors that have inotropic and vasodilatory properties. Phosphodiesterase inhibitors are often used in conjunction with catecholamines for severe heart failure, cardiogenic shock, and other forms of shock unresponsive to catecholamine therapy alone. Optimal use requires hemodynamic monitoring. These drugs are contraindicated in patients with heart valve stenosis that limits cardiac output.

Inamrinone is administered as a loading dose of 0.75 mg/kg over 10 to 15 minutes (may give over 2 to 3 minutes if no left ventricular dysfunction) followed by an infusion of 5 to 15 μg/kg per minute, titrated to clinical effect. An additional bolus may be given in 30 minutes.

Milrinone is more often used today because it has a shorter half-life than inamrinone and is less likely to cause thrombocytopenia.[48,49] Milrinone is renally excreted with a half-life of around 1½ to 2 hours, so it requires 4½ to 6 hours to achieve near–steady state concentrations if given without a loading dose. A slow milrinone IV loading dose (50 μg/kg over 10 minutes) is followed by an IV infusion at a rate of 0.375 to 0.75 μg/kg per minute (375 to 750 ng/kg per minute) for 2 to 3 days. In renal failure the dose should be reduced. Adverse effects include nausea, vomiting, and hypotension.

Calcium

Although calcium ions play a critical role in myocardial contractile performance and impulse formation, retrospective and prospective studies in the cardiac arrest setting have shown no benefit from calcium administration.[50,51] Furthermore, high serum calcium levels induced by calcium administration may be detrimental. For this reason, calcium should not be used routinely to support circulation in the setting of cardiac arrest. When hyperkalemia, ionized hypocalcemia (eg, after multiple blood transfusions), or calcium channel blocker toxicity is present, use of calcium is probably helpful.[52] Ideally, ionized calcium concentration should be measured because total calcium concentration does not correlate well with ionized concentration in critically ill patients.[53,54]

When necessary, a 10% solution (100 mg/mL) of calcium chloride can be given in a dose of 8 to 16 mg/kg of the salt (usually 5 to 10 mL) and repeated as necessary. (The 10% solution contains 1.36 mEq of calcium or 27.2 mg elemental calcium per milliliter.)

Digitalis

Digitalis preparations have limited use as inotropic agents in emergency cardiovascular care. Digitalis decreases the ventricular rate in some patients with atrial flutter or fibrillation by slowing atrioventricular nodal conduction. The toxic to therapeutic ratio is narrow, especially when potassium depletion is present. Digitalis toxicity may cause serious ventricular arrhythmias and precipitate cardiac arrest. Digoxin-specific antibody is available for the treatment of serious toxicity (Digibind, Digitalis Antidote BM).

Nitroglycerin

Nitrates are used for their ability to relax vascular smooth muscle. Nitroglycerin is the initial treatment of choice for suspected ischemic-type pain or discomfort (see Part 8: "Stabilization of the Patient With Acute Coronary Syndromes").

IV nitroglycerin is also an effective adjunct in the treatment of congestive heart failure from any cause,[55] and it may be useful in hypertensive emergencies, particularly if related to volume overload. The action of nitroglycerin is mediated through local endothelial production of nitric oxide, particularly in the venous capacitance system. Nitroglycerin is most effective in patients with increased intravascular volume. Hypovolemia blunts the beneficial hemodynamic effects of nitroglycerin and increases the risk of hypotension; nitrate-induced hypotension typically responds well to fluid replacement therapy. Other potential complications of use of IV nitroglycerin are tachycardia, paradoxical bradycardia, hypoxemia caused by increased pulmonary ventilation-perfusion mismatch, and headache. Nitroglycerin should be avoided with bradycardia and extreme tachycardia or within 24 to 48 hours of the use of phosphodiesterase inhibitors to treat erectile dysfunction.

Nitroglycerin is administered by continuous infusion (nitroglycerin 50 or 100 mg in 250 mL of D_5W or 0.9% sodium chloride) at 10 to 20 μg/min and increased by 5 to 10 μg/min every 5 to 10 minutes until the desired hemodynamic or clinical response occurs. Low doses (30 to 40 μg/min) predominantly produce venodilatation; high doses (≥150 μg/min) provide arteriolar dilatation. Uninterrupted administration of nitroglycerin (>24 hours) produces tolerance.[56]

Sodium Nitroprusside

Sodium nitroprusside is a potent, rapid-acting, direct peripheral vasodilator useful in the treatment of severe heart failure and hypertensive emergencies.[57] Its direct venodilatory effects decrease right and left ventricular filling pressure by increasing venous compliance. The net effect on venous return (preload) depends on the intravascular volume. In many patients cardiac output improves secondary to the afterload-reducing effects of nitroprusside, meaning that venous return must also increase, but the latter occurs at a lower end-diastolic pressure, resulting in relief of pulmonary congestion and reduced left ventricular volume and pressure. Arteriolar relaxation causes decreases in peripheral arterial resistance (afterload), resulting in enhanced systolic emptying with reduced left ventricular volume and wall stress and reduced myocardial oxygen consumption. In the presence of hypovolemia, nitroprusside can cause hypotension with reflex tachycardia. Invasive hemodynamic monitoring is useful during nitroprusside therapy.

Although nitroprusside may be useful for the treatment of pulmonary artery hypertension, it reverses hypoxic pulmonary vasoconstriction in patients with pulmonary disease (eg, pneumonia, adult respiratory distress syndrome). The latter effect may exacerbate intrapulmonary shunting, resulting in worse hypoxemia. The major complication of nitroprusside is hypotension. Patients may also complain of headaches, nausea, vomiting, and abdominal cramps.

Nitroprusside is rapidly metabolized by nonenzymatic means to cyanide, which is then detoxified in the liver and kidney to thiocyanate. Cyanide is also metabolized by forming a complex with vitamin B_{12}.[58] Thiocyanate undergoes renal elimination. Patients with hepatic or renal insufficiency and patients requiring >3 μg/kg per minute for more than 72 hours may accumulate cyanide or thiocyanate, and they should be monitored for signs of cyanide or thiocyanate intoxication, such as metabolic acidosis.[59] When thiocyanate concentrations exceed 12 mg/dL, toxicity is manifested as confusion, hyperreflexia, and ultimately convulsions. Treatment of elevated cyanide or thiocyanate levels includes immediate discontinuation of the infusion. If the patient is experiencing signs and symptoms of cyanide toxicity, sodium nitrite and sodium thiosulfate should be administered.

Sodium nitroprusside is prepared by adding 50 or 100 mg to 250 mL of D_5W. The solution and tubing should be wrapped in opaque material because nitroprusside deteriorates when exposed to light. The recommended dosing range for sodium nitroprusside is 0.1 to 5 μg/kg per minute, but higher doses (up to 10 μg/kg per minute) may be needed.

IV Fluid Administration

Limited evidence is available to guide therapy. Volume loading during cardiac arrest causes an increase in right atrial pressure relative to aortic pressure,[60] which can have the detrimental effect of decreasing CPP. The increase in CPP produced by epinephrine during CPR is not augmented by either an IV or intra-aortic fluid bolus in experimental CPR in dogs.[61]

If cardiac arrest is associated with extreme volume losses, hypovolemic arrest should be suspected. These patients present with signs of circulatory shock advancing to pulseless electrical activity (PEA). In these settings intravascular volume should be promptly restored. In the absence of human studies the treatment of PEA arrest with volume repletion is based on evidence from animal studies.[60–63] Current evidence in patients presenting with ventricular fibrillation (VF) neither supports nor refutes the use of routine IV fluids (Class Indeterminate).

Animal studies suggest that hypertonic saline may improve survival from VF when compared with normal saline.[64,65] Human studies are needed, however, before the use of hypertonic saline can be recommended. If fluids are administered during an arrest, solutions containing dextrose should be avoided unless there is evidence of hypoglycemia.

Sodium Bicarbonate

Tissue acidosis and resulting acidemia during cardiac arrest and resuscitation are dynamic processes resulting from no blood flow during arrest and low blood flow during CPR. These processes are affected by the duration of cardiac arrest, the level of blood flow, and the arterial oxygen content during CPR. Restoration of oxygen content with appropriate ventilation with oxygen, support of some tissue perfusion and some cardiac output with good chest compressions, then rapid ROSC are the mainstays of restoring acid-base balance during cardiac arrest.

Little data supports therapy with buffers during cardiac arrest. There is no evidence that bicarbonate improves likelihood of defibrillation or survival rates in animals with VF cardiac arrest. A wide variety of adverse effects have been linked to bicarbonate administration during cardiac arrest. Bicarbonate compromises CPP by reducing systemic vascular resistance.[66] It can create extracellular alkalosis that will shift the oxyhemoglobin saturation curve and inhibits oxygen release. It can produce hypernatremia and therefore hyperosmolarity. It produces excess carbon dioxide, which freely diffuses into myocardial and cerebral cells and may paradoxically contribute to intracellular acidosis.[67] It can exacerbate central venous acidosis and may inactivate simultaneously administered catecholamines.

In some special resuscitation situations, such as preexisting metabolic acidosis, hyperkalemia, or tricyclic antidepressant overdose, bicarbonate can be beneficial (see Part 10: "Special Resuscitation Situations").

Sodium bicarbonate is not considered a first-line agent for the patient in cardiac arrest. When bicarbonate is used for special situations, an initial dose of 1 mEq/kg is typical. Whenever possible, bicarbonate therapy should be guided by the bicarbonate concentration or calculated base deficit obtained from blood gas analysis or laboratory measurement. To minimize the risk of iatrogenically induced alkalosis, providers should not attempt complete correction of the calculated base deficit. Other non–CO_2-generating buffers such as Carbicarb, Tham, or Tribonat have shown potential for minimizing some adverse effects of sodium bicarbonate, including CO_2 generation, hyperosmolarity, hypernatremia, hypoglycemia, intracellular acidosis, myocardial acidosis, and "overshoot" alkalosis.[68–70] But clinical experience is greatly limited and outcome studies are lacking.

Diuretics

Furosemide is a potent diuretic agent that inhibits reabsorption of sodium in the proximal and distal renal tubule and the loop of Henle. Furosemide has little or no direct vascular effect, but it reduces venous and pulmonary vascular resistance through stimulation of local prostaglandin production[71] and therefore may be very useful in the treatment of pulmonary edema. The vascular effects occur within 5 minutes, whereas diuresis is delayed. Although often used in acute renal failure to stimulate increased urine output, there is no data to support this indication, and some data suggests an association with increased mortality.[72] The initial dose of furosemide is 0.5 to 1 mg/kg IV injected slowly.

Newer "loop" diuretics that have an action similar to that of furosemide and a similar profile of side effects include torsemide and bumetanide. In patients who do not respond to high doses of loop diuretics alone, a combination of such agents together with the administration of "proximal tubule"–acting thiazide diuretics (such as chlorothiazide or metolazone) may be effective. Such combinations require close observation with serial measurement of serum electrolytes to avoid profound potassium depletion from their use.

Summary

Maintenance of adequate CPP is linked with survival following CPR. Rescuers can support adequate CPP by providing compressions of adequate rate and depth, allowing full chest recoil after each compression, avoiding overventilation, and minimizing interruptions in chest compressions (see Part 4: "Adult Basic Life Support"). Exhaled CO_2 can be a useful indicator of cardiac output produced by chest compressions. Pulse oximetry is not helpful during arrest, but it should be monitored in high-risk patients to ensure adequate oxygenation. No medications have been shown to improve neurologically intact survival from cardiac arrest. Better tools are needed to monitor effectiveness of CPR.

References

1. Levine RL, Wayne MA, Miller CC. End-tidal carbon dioxide and outcome of out-of-hospital cardiac arrest. *N Engl J Med.* 1997;337:301–306.
2. Wayne MA, Levine RL, Miller CC. Use of end-tidal carbon dioxide to predict outcome in prehospital cardiac arrest. *Ann Emerg Med.* 1995;25:762–767.
3. Paradis NA, Martin GB, Rivers EP, Goetting MG, Appleton TJ, Feingold M, Nowak RM. Coronary perfusion pressure and the return of spontaneous circulation in human cardiopulmonary resuscitation. *JAMA.* 1990;263:1106–1113.
4. Halperin HR, Tsitlik JE, Gelfand M, Weisfeldt ML, Gruben KG, Levin HR, Rayburn BK, Chandra NC, Scott CJ, Kreps BJ, et al. A preliminary study of cardiopulmonary resuscitation by circumferential compression of the chest with use of a pneumatic vest. *N Engl J Med.* 1993;329:762–768.
5. Kern KB, Ewy GA, Voorhees WD, Babbs CF, Tacker WA. Myocardial perfusion pressure: a predictor of 24-hour survival during prolonged cardiac arrest in dogs. *Resuscitation.* 1988;16:241–250.
6. Lindner KH, Prengel AW, Pfenninger EG, Lindner IM, Strohmenger HU, Georgieff M, Lurie KG. Vasopressin improves vital organ blood flow during closed-chest cardiopulmonary resuscitation in pigs. *Circulation.* 1995;91:215–221.
7. Little CM, Angelos MG, Paradis NA. Compared to angiotensin II, epinephrine is associated with high myocardial blood flow following return of spontaneous circulation after cardiac arrest. *Resuscitation.* 2003;59:353–359.
8. Connick M, Berg RA. Femoral venous pulsations during open-chest cardiac massage. *Ann Emerg Med.* 1994;24:1176–1179.
9. Weil MH, Rackow EC, Trevino R, Grundler W, Falk JL, Griffel MI. Difference in acid-base state between venous and arterial blood during cardiopulmonary resuscitation. *N Engl J Med.* 1986;315:153–156.
10. Kette F, Weil MH, Gazmuri RJ, Bisera J, Rackow EC. Intramyocardial hypercarbic acidosis during cardiac arrest and resuscitation. *Crit Care Med.* 1993;21:901–906.
11. Adrogue HJ, Rashad MN, Gorin AB, Yacoub J, Madias NE. Arteriovenous acid-base disparity in circulatory failure: studies on mechanism. *Am J Physiol.* 1989;257:F1087–F1093.
12. Tucker KJ, Idris AH, Wenzel V, Orban DJ. Changes in arterial and mixed venous blood gases during untreated ventricular fibrillation and cardiopulmonary resuscitation. *Resuscitation.* 1994;28:137–141.
13. Tang W, Weil MH, Sun S, Kette D, Gazmuri RJ, O'Connell F, Bisera J. Cardiopulmonary resuscitation by precordial compression but without mechanical ventilation. *Am J Respir Crit Care Med.* 1994;150:1709–1713.
14. Gudipati CV, Weil MH, Gazmuri RJ, Deshmukh HG, Bisera J, Rackow EC. Increases in coronary vein CO2 during cardiac resuscitation. *J Appl Physiol.* 1990;68:1405–1408.
15. Capparelli EV, Chow MS, Kluger J, Fieldman A. Differences in systemic and myocardial blood acid-base status during cardiopulmonary resuscitation. *Crit Care Med.* 1989;17:442–446.
16. von Planta M, Weil MH, Gazmuri RJ, Bisera J, Rackow EC. Myocardial acidosis associated with CO2 production during cardiac arrest and resuscitation. *Circulation.* 1989;80:684–692.
17. Grundler W, Weil MH, Rackow EC. Arteriovenous carbon dioxide and pH gradients during cardiac arrest. *Circulation.* 1986;74:1071–1074.
18. Sanders AB, Ewy GA, Taft TV. Resuscitation and arterial blood gas abnormalities during prolonged cardiopulmonary resuscitation. *Ann Emerg Med.* 1984;13:676–679.
19. Nowak RM, Martin GB, Carden DL, Tomlanovich MC. Selective venous hypercarbia during human CPR: implications regarding blood flow. *Ann Emerg Med.* 1987;16:527–530.
20. American Heart Association in collaboration with International Liaison Committee on Resuscitation. Guidelines 2000 for Cardiopulmonary Resuscitation and Emergency Cardiovascular Care: International Consensus on Science, Part 6: Advanced Cardiovascular Life Support: Section 4: Devices to Assist Circulation. *Circulation.* 2000;102(suppl I):I105–I111.
21. Abraham E, Fink S. Conjunctival oxygen tension monitoring in emergency department patients. *Am J Emerg Med.* 1988;6:549–554.
22. Bhende MS, Thompson AE. Evaluation of an end-tidal CO2 detector during pediatric cardiopulmonary resuscitation. *Pediatrics.* 1995;95:395–399.
23. Callaham M, Barton C. Prediction of outcome of cardiopulmonary resuscitation from end-tidal carbon dioxide concentration. *Crit Care Med.* 1990;18:358–362.
24. Grmec S, Klemen P. Does the end-tidal carbon dioxide (EtCO2) concentration have prognostic value during out-of-hospital cardiac arrest? *Eur J Emerg Med.* 2001;8:263–269.
25. Grmec S, Kupnik D. Does the Mainz Emergency Evaluation Scoring (MEES) in combination with capnometry (MEESc) help in the prognosis of outcome from cardiopulmonary resuscitation in a prehospital setting? *Resuscitation.* 2003;58:89–96.

26. Grmec S, Lah K, Tusek-Bunc K. Difference in end-tidal CO2 between asphyxia cardiac arrest and ventricular fibrillation/pulseless ventricular tachycardia cardiac arrest in the prehospital setting. *Crit Care.* 2003;7: R139–R144.
27. Mauer D, Schneider T, Elich D, Dick W. Carbon dioxide levels during pre-hospital active compression–decompression versus standard cardiopulmonary resuscitation. *Resuscitation.* 1998;39:67–74.
28. Sanders AB, Kern KB, Otto CW, Milander MM, Ewy GA. End-tidal carbon dioxide monitoring during cardiopulmonary resuscitation: a prognostic indicator for survival. *JAMA.* 1989;262:1347–1351.
29. Entholzner E, Felber A, Mielke L, Hargasser S, Breinbauer B, Hundelshausen VB, Hipp R. Assessment of end-tidal CO2 measurement in reanimation. *Anasthesiol Intensivmed Notfallmed Schmerzther.* 1992;27: 473–476.
30. Garnett AR, Ornato JP, Gonzalez ER, Johnson EB. End-tidal carbon dioxide monitoring during cardiopulmonary resuscitation. *JAMA.* 1987; 257:512–515.
31. Bhende MS, Karasic DG, Karasic RB. End-tidal carbon dioxide changes during cardiopulmonary resuscitation after experimental asphyxial cardiac arrest. *Am J Emerg Med.* 1996;14:349–350.
32. Ahrens T, Schallom L, Bettorf K, Ellner S, Hurt G, O'Mara V, Ludwig J, George W, Marino T, Shannon W. End-tidal carbon dioxide measurements as a prognostic indicator of outcome in cardiac arrest. *Am J Crit Care.* 2001;10:391–398.
33. Cantineau JP, Lambert Y, Merckx P, Reynaud P, Porte F, Bertrand C, Duvaldestin P. End-tidal carbon dioxide during cardiopulmonary resuscitation in humans presenting mostly with asystole: a predictor of outcome. *Crit Care Med.* 1996;24:791–796.
34. Kellum JA, Pinsky MR. Use of vasopressor agents in critically ill patients. *Curr Opin Crit Care.* 2002;8:236–241.
35. Zaritsky AL. Catecholamines, inotropic medications, and vasopressor agents. In: Chernow B, ed. *The Pharmacologic Approach to the Critically Ill Patient.* 3rd ed. Baltimore, Md: Williams & Wilkins; 1994:387–404.
36. Grillo JA, Gonzalez ER, Ramaiya A, Karnes HT, Wells B. Chemical compatibility of inotropic and vasoactive agents delivered via a multiple line infusion system. *Crit Care Med.* 1995;23:1061–1066.
37. Bonhomme L, Benhamou D, Comoy E, Preaux N. Stability of epinephrine in alkalinized solutions. *Ann Emerg Med.* 1990;19:1242–1244.
38. Ellis AK, Day JH. Diagnosis and management of anaphylaxis. *CMAJ.* 2003;169:307–311.
39. Dunser MW, Mayr AJ, Ulmer H, Knotzer H, Sumann G, Pajk W, Friesenecker B, Hasibeder WR. Arginine vasopressin in advanced vasodilatory shock: a prospective, randomized, controlled study. *Circulation.* 2003;107:2313–2319.
40. Mutlu GM, Factor P. Role of vasopressin in the management of septic shock. *Intensive Care Med.* 2004;30:1276–1291.
41. American Heart Association in collaboration with International Liaison Committee on Resuscitation. Guidelines 2000 for Cardiopulmonary Resuscitation and Emergency Cardiovascular Care: International Consensus on Science, Part 6: advanced cardiovascular life support: Section 6: pharmacology II. Agents to optimize cardiac output and blood pressure. *Circulation.* 2000;102(suppl I):I129–I135.
42. Delmas A, Leone M, Rousseau S, Albanese J, Martin C. Clinical review: vasopressin and terlipressin in septic shock patients. *Crit Care.* 2005;9: 212–222.
43. Marin C, Eon B, Saux P, Aknin P, Gouin F. Renal effects of norepinephrine used to treat septic shock patients. *Crit Care Med.* 1990;18:282–285.
44. Bellomo R, Giantomasso DD. Noradrenaline and the kidney: friends or foes? *Crit Care.* 2001;5:294–298.
45. Bellomo R, Chapman M, Finfer S, Hickling K, Myburgh J. Low-dose dopamine in patients with early renal dysfunction: a placebo-controlled randomised trial. Australian and New Zealand Intensive Care Society (ANZICS) Clinical Trials Group. *Lancet.* 2000;356:2139–2143.
46. Holmes CL, Walley KR. Bad medicine: low-dose dopamine in the ICU. *Chest.* 2003;123:1266–1275.
47. Ruffolo RR Jr. The pharmacology of dobutamine. *Am J Med Sci.* 1987; 294:244–248.
48. Alousi AA, Johnson DC. Pharmacology of the bipyridines: amrinone and milrinone. *Circulation.* 1986;73(suppl III):III10–III24.
49. Edelson J, Stroshane R, Benziger DP, Cody R, Benotti J, Hood WB Jr, Chatterjee K, Luczkowec C, Krebs C, Schwartz R. Pharmacokinetics of the bipyridines amrinone and milrinone. *Circulation.* 1986;73(suppl III): III145–III152.
50. Stueven HA, Thompson B, Aprahamian C, Tonsfeldt DJ, Kastenson EH. The effectiveness of calcium chloride in refractory electromechanical dissociation. *Ann Emerg Med.* 1985;14:626–629.
51. Stueven H, Thompson BM, Aprahamian C, Darin JC. Use of calcium in prehospital cardiac arrest. *Ann Emerg Med.* 1983;12:136–139.
52. Ramoska EA, Spiller HA, Winter M, Borys D. A one-year evaluation of calcium channel blocker overdoses: toxicity and treatment. *Ann Emerg Med.* 1993;22:196–200.
53. Urban P, Scheidegger D, Buchmann B, Barth D. Cardiac arrest and blood ionized calcium levels. *Ann Intern Med.* 1988;109:110–113.
54. Cardenas-Rivero N, Chernow B, Stoiko MA, Nussbaum SR, Todres ID. Hypocalcemia in critically ill children. *J Pediatr.* 1989;114:946–951.
55. DiDomenico RJ, Park HY, Southworth MR, Eyrich HM, Lewis RK, Finley JM, Schumock GT. Guidelines for acute decompensated heart failure treatment. *Ann Pharmacother.* 2004;38:649–660.
56. Kirsten R, Nelson K, Kirsten D, Heintz B. Clinical pharmacokinetics of vasodilators. Part II. *Clin Pharmacokinet.* 1998;35:9–36.
57. Vaughan CJ, Delanty N. Hypertensive emergencies. *Lancet.* 2000;356: 411–417.
58. Zerbe NF, Wagner BK. Use of vitamin B12 in the treatment and prevention of nitroprusside-induced cyanide toxicity. *Crit Care Med.* 1993; 21:465-467.
59. Rindone JP, Sloane EP. Cyanide toxicity from sodium nitroprusside: risks and management [published correction appears in *Ann Pharmacother.* 1992;26:1160]. *Ann Pharmacother.* 1992;26:515–519.
60. Ditchey RV, Lindenfeld J. Potential adverse effects of volume loading on perfusion of vital organs during closed-chest resuscitation. *Circulation.* 1984;69:181–189.
61. Gentile NT, Martin GB, Appleton TJ, Moeggenberg J, Paradis NA, Nowak RM. Effects of arterial and venous volume infusion on coronary perfusion pressures during canine CPR. *Resuscitation.* 1991;22:55–63.
62. Jameson SJ, Mateer JR, DeBehnke DJ. Early volume expansion during cardiopulmonary resuscitation. *Resuscitation.* 1993;26:243–250.
63. Voorhees WD, Ralston SH, Kougias C, Schmitz PM. Fluid loading with whole blood or Ringer's lactate solution during CPR in dogs. *Resuscitation.* 1987;15:113–123.
64. Fischer M, Dahmen A, Standop J, Hagendorff A, Hoeft A, Krep H. Effects of hypertonic saline on myocardial blood flow in a porcine model of prolonged cardiac arrest. *Resuscitation.* 2002;54:269–280.
65. Breil M, Krep H, Sinn D, Hagendorff A, Dahmen A, Eichelkraut W, Hoeft A, Fischer M. Hypertonic saline improves myocardial blood flow during CPR, but is not enhanced further by the addition of hydroxy ethyl starch. *Resuscitation.* 2003;56:307–317.
66. Kette F, Weil MH, Gazmuri RJ. Buffer solutions may compromise cardiac resuscitation by reducing coronary perfusion pressure. *JAMA.* 1991;266:2121–2126.
67. Graf H, Leach W, Arieff AI. Evidence for a detrimental effect of bicarbonate therapy in hypoxic lactic acidosis. *Science.* 1985;227:754–756.
68. Katz LM, Wang Y, Rockoff S, Bouldin TW. Low-dose Carbicarb improves cerebral outcome after asphyxial cardiac arrest in rats. *Ann Emerg Med.* 2002;39:359–365.
69. Sun S, Weil MH, Tang W, Fukui M. Effects of buffer agents on postresuscitation myocardial dysfunction. *Crit Care Med.* 1996;24: 2035–2041.
70. Blecic S, De Backer D, Deleuze M, Vachiery JL, Vincent JL. Correction of metabolic acidosis in experimental CPR: a comparative study of sodium bicarbonate, carbicarb, and dextrose. *Ann Emerg Med.* 1991;20: 235-238.
71. Pickkers P, Dormans TP, Russel FG, Hughes AD, Thien T, Schaper N, Smits P. Direct vascular effects of furosemide in humans. *Circulation.* 1997;96:1847–1852.
72. Mehta RL, Pascual MT, Soroko S, Chertow GM. Diuretics, mortality, and nonrecovery of renal function in acute renal failure. *JAMA.* 2002;288: 2547–2553.

Part 7.5: Postresuscitation Support

Few randomized controlled clinical trials deal specifically with supportive care following cardio-pulmonary-cerebral resuscitation (CPCR) from cardiac arrest. Nevertheless, postresuscitation care has significant potential to improve early mortality caused by hemodynamic instability and multi-organ failure and later mortality/morbidity resulting from brain injury.[1] This section summarizes our evolving understanding of the hemodynamic, neurologic, and metabolic abnormalities encountered in patients who are resuscitated from cardiac arrest.

Initial objectives of postresuscitation care are to

- Optimize cardiopulmonary function and systemic perfusion, especially perfusion to the brain
- Transport the victim of out-of-hospital cardiac arrest to the hospital emergency department (ED) and continue care in an appropriately equipped critical care unit
- Try to identify the precipitating causes of the arrest
- Institute measures to prevent recurrence
- Institute measures that may improve long-term, neurologically intact survival

Improving Postresuscitation Outcomes

Postresuscitation care is a critical component of advanced life support. Patient mortality remains high after return of spontaneous circulation (ROSC) and initial stabilization. Ultimate prognosis in the first 72 hours may be difficult to determine,[2] yet survivors of cardiac arrest have the potential to lead normal lives.[3–5] During postresuscitation care providers should (1) optimize hemodynamic, respiratory, and neurologic support; (2) identify and treat reversible causes of arrest; and (3) monitor temperature and consider treatment for disturbances of temperature regulation and metabolism. The first sections below discuss initial stabilization and temperature/metabolic factors that may be relevant to improving postresuscitation outcome, particularly in the critically ill survivor. Subsequent sections highlight organ-specific evaluation and support.

Return of Spontaneous Circulation

The principal objective of postresuscitation care is the re-establishment of effective perfusion of organs and tissue. After ROSC in the out-of-hospital or in-hospital setting, the provider must consider and treat the cause of the arrest and the consequences of any hypoxemic/ischemic/reperfusion injury. In most cases the acidemia associated with cardiac arrest improves spontaneously when adequate ventilation and perfusion are restored. But restoration of blood pressure and improvement in gas exchange do not ensure survival and functional recovery. Significant myocardial stunning and hemodynamic instability can develop, requiring vasopressor support. Most postresuscitation deaths occur during the first 24 hours.[6,7]

Ideally the patient will be awake, responsive, and breathing spontaneously. Alternatively the patient may initially be comatose but have the potential for full recovery after postresuscitation care.[3] Indeed, up to 20% of initially comatose survivors of cardiac arrest have been reported to have good 1-year neurologic outcome.[8] The pathway to the best hospital postresuscitation care of all initial survivors is not completely known, but there is increasing interest in identifying and optimizing practices that can improve outcome.[9] Regardless of the patient's initial status, the provider should support adequate airway and breathing, administer supplementary oxygen, monitor the patient's vital signs, establish or verify existing intravenous access, and verify the function of any catheters in place.

The clinician should assess the patient frequently and treat abnormalities of vital signs or cardiac arrhythmias and request studies that will further aid in the evaluation of the patient. It is important to identify and treat any cardiac, electrolyte, toxicologic, pulmonary, and neurologic precipitants of arrest. The clinician may find it helpful to review the H's and T's mnemonic to recall factors that may contribute to cardiac arrest or complicate resuscitation or postresuscitation care: hypovolemia, hypoxia, hydrogen ion (acidosis), hyper-/hypokalemia, hypoglycemia, hypothermia; toxins, tamponade (cardiac), tension pneumothorax, thrombosis of the coronary or pulmonary vasculature, and trauma. For further information see Part 10: "Special Resuscitation Situations."

After initial assessment and stabilization of airway, ventilation, and circulation, transfer the patient to a special care unit for observation, continuous monitoring, and further therapy. Personnel with appropriate training and resuscitation equipment must accompany the patient during transport to the special care unit.

Temperature Regulation

Induced Hypothermia

Both permissive hypothermia (allowing a mild degree of hypothermia >33°C [91.5°F] that often develops spontaneously after arrest) and active induction of hypothermia may play a role in postresuscitation care. In 2 randomized clinical trials (LOE 1[3]; LOE 2[4]) induced hypothermia (cooling within minutes to hours after ROSC) resulted in improved outcome in adults who remained comatose after initial resuscitation from out-of-hospital ventricular fibrillation (VF) cardiac arrest. Patients in the study were cooled to 33°C (91.5°F)[3] or to the range of 32°C to 34°C (89.6°F to 93.2°F)[4] for 12 to 24 hours. The Hypothermia After Cardiac Arrest (HACA) study[3] included a small subset of patients with in-hospital cardiac arrest.

(*Circulation.* 2005;000:IV-84-IV-88.)

DOI: 10.1161/CIRCULATIONAHA.105.166560

A third study (LOE 2)[10] documented improvement in metabolic end points (lactate and O_2 extraction) when comatose adult patients were cooled after ROSC from out-of-hospital cardiac arrest in which the initial rhythm was pulseless electrical activity (PEA)/asystole.

In the HACA[3] and Bernard[4] studies, only about 8% of patients with cardiac arrest were selected for induced hypothermia (ie, patients were hemodynamically stable but comatose after a witnessed arrest of presumed cardiac etiology). This highlights the importance of identifying the subset of patients who may most benefit. Although the number of patients who may benefit from hypothermia induction is limited at present, it is possible that with more rapid and controlled cooling and better insights into optimal target temperature, timing, duration, and mechanism of action, such cooling may prove more widely beneficial in the future.[11] A recent multicenter study in asphyxiated neonates showed that hypothermia can be beneficial in another select population.[12]

Complications associated with cooling can include coagulopathy and arrhythmias, particularly with an unintentional drop below target temperature. Although not significantly higher, cases of pneumonia and sepsis increased in the hypothermia-induction group.[3,4] Cooling may also increase hyperglycemia.[4]

Most clinical studies of cooling have used external cooling techniques (eg, cooling blankets and frequent applications of ice bags) that may require a number of hours to attain target temperature. More recent studies[13] suggest that internal cooling techniques (eg, cold saline, endovascular cooling catheter) can also be used to induce hypothermia. Providers should continuously monitor the patient's temperature during cooling.[3,4]

In summary, providers should not actively rewarm hemodynamically stable patients who spontaneously develop a mild degree of hypothermia (>33°C [91.5°F]) after resuscitation from cardiac arrest. Mild hypothermia may be beneficial to neurologic outcome and is likely to be well tolerated without significant risk of complications. In a select subset of patients who were initially comatose but hemodynamically stable after a witnessed VF arrest of presumed cardiac etiology, active induction of hypothermia was beneficial.[3,4,13] Thus, unconscious adult patients with ROSC after out-of-hospital cardiac arrest should be cooled to 32°C to 34°C (89.6°F to 93.2°F) for 12 to 24 hours when the initial rhythm was VF (Class IIa). Similar therapy may be beneficial for patients with non-VF arrest out of hospital or for in-hospital arrest (Class IIb).

Hyperthermia

After resuscitation, temperature elevation above normal can create a significant imbalance between oxygen supply and demand that can impair brain recovery. Few studies (with either frequent use of antipyretics or "controlled normothermia" with cooling techniques) have directly examined the effect of temperature control immediately after resuscitation. Because fever may be a symptom of brain injury, it may be difficult to control it with conventional antipyretics. Many studies of brain injury in animal models, however, show exacerbation of injury if body/brain temperature is increased during or after resuscitation from cardiac arrest.[14–17] Moreover, several studies have documented worse neurologic outcome in humans with fever after cardiac arrest (LOE 3)[18] and ischemic brain injury (LOE 7 extrapolated from stroke victims[18]). Thus, the provider should monitor the patient's temperature after resuscitation and avoid hyperthermia.

Glucose Control

The postresuscitation patient is likely to develop electrolyte abnormalities that may be detrimental to recovery. Although many studies have documented a strong association between high blood glucose after resuscitation from cardiac arrest and poor neurologic outcomes (LOE 4[21,22]; LOE 5[9,22–26]; LOE 6[27]), they did not show that control of serum glucose level alters outcome.

A prospective randomized study by van den Berghe (LOE 1)[28] did show that tight control of blood glucose using insulin reduced hospital mortality rates in critically ill patients who required mechanical ventilation. The study did not specifically focus on postresuscitation patients, but the effect of blood glucose control on outcome is compelling. The study documented not only improved survival but decreased mortality from infectious complications, a common problem in the postresuscitation setting.

In comatose patients, signs of hypoglycemia are less apparent, so clinicians must monitor serum glucose closely to avoid hypoglycemia when treating hyperglycemia. On the basis of findings of improved outcomes in critically ill patients when glucose levels are maintained in the normal range, it is reasonable for providers to maintain strict glucose control during the postresuscitation period. Additional study is needed, however, to identify the precise blood glucose concentration that requires insulin therapy, the target range of blood glucose concentration, and the effect of tight glucose control on outcomes of patients after cardiac arrest.

Organ-Specific Evaluation and Support

After ROSC patients may remain comatose or have decreased responsiveness for a variable period of time. If spontaneous breathing is absent or inadequate, mechanical ventilation via an endotracheal tube or other advanced airway device may be required. Hemodynamic status may be unstable with abnormalities of cardiac rate, rhythm, systemic blood pressure, and organ perfusion.

Clinicians must prevent, detect, and treat hypoxemia and hypotension because these conditions can exacerbate brain injury. Clinicians should determine the baseline postarrest status of each organ system and support organ function as needed.

The remainder of this chapter focuses on organ-specific measures that should be provided in the immediate postresuscitation period.

Respiratory System

After ROSC patients may exhibit respiratory dysfunction. Some patients will remain dependent on mechanical ventilation and will need an increased inspired concentration of oxygen. Providers should perform a full physical examination and evaluate the chest radiograph to verify appropriate endotracheal tube depth of insertion and identify cardiopulmonary complications of resuscitation. Providers should adjust mechanical ventilatory support based on the patient's blood gas values, respiratory rate, and work of breathing. As the patient's spontaneous ventilation becomes more efficient, the level of respiratory support may be decreased until spontaneous respiration returns. If the patient continues to require high inspired oxygen concentrations, providers should determine if the cause is pulmonary or cardiac and direct care accordingly.

Debate exists as to the length of time patients who require ventilatory support should remain sedated. To date there is little evidence to guide therapy. One observational study (LOE 3)[29] found an association between use of sedation and development of pneumonia in intubated patients during the first 48 hours of therapy. The study, however, was not designed to investigate sedation as a risk factor for either pneumonia or death in patients with cardiac arrest. At this time there is inadequate data to recommend for or against the use of a defined period of sedation or neuromuscular blockade after cardiac arrest (Class Indeterminate). Use of neuromuscular blocking agents should be kept to a minimum because these agents preclude thorough neurologic assessments during the first 12 to 72 hours after ROSC.[2]

Sedation may be necessary to control shivering during hypothermia. If shivering continues despite optimal sedation, neuromuscular blockade may be required in addition to deep sedation.

Ventilatory Parameters

Sustained hypocapnea (low P_{CO_2}) may reduce cerebral blood flow.[30–31] After cardiac arrest, restoration of blood flow results in an initial hyperemic blood flow response that lasts 10 to 30 minutes, followed by a more prolonged period of low blood flow.[32,33] During this latter period of late hypoperfusion, a mismatch between blood flow (oxygen delivery) and oxygen requirement may occur. If the patient is hyperventilated at this stage, cerebral vasoconstriction may further decrease cerebral blood flow and increase cerebral ischemia and ischemic injury.

There is no evidence that hyperventilation protects the brain or other vital organs from further ischemic damage after cardiac arrest. In fact, Safar et al[34] provided evidence that hyperventilation may worsen neurologic outcome. Hyperventilation may also generate increased airway pressures and augment intrinsic positive end-expiratory pressure (so-called "auto PEEP"), leading to an increase in cerebral venous and intracranial pressures.[35,36] Increases in cerebral venous pressure can decrease cerebral blood flow and increase brain ischemia.

In summary, no data supports targeting a specific arterial Pa_{CO_2} level after resuscitation from cardiac arrest. But data extrapolated from patients with brain injury supports ventilation to normocarbic levels as appropriate. Routine hyperventilation is detrimental (Class III).

Cardiovascular System

Both the ischemia/reperfusion of cardiac arrest and electrical defibrillation can cause transient myocardial stunning and dysfunction[37] that can last many hours but may improve with vasopressors.[38] Cardiac biomarker levels may be increased in association with global ischemia caused by absent or decreased coronary blood flow during cardiac arrest and CPR. Increased cardiac biomarkers may also indicate acute myocardial infarction as the cause of cardiac arrest.

Hemodynamic instability is common after cardiac arrest, and early death due to multi-organ failure is associated with a persistently low cardiac index during the first 24 hours after resuscitation (LOE 5).[6,39] Thus, after resuscitation clinicians should evaluate the patient's electrocardiogram, radiographs, and laboratory analyses of serum electrolytes and cardiac biomarkers. Echocardiographic evaluation within the first 24 hours after arrest is useful to guide ongoing management.[5,40]

One large case series (LOE 5)[6] of patients resuscitated following out-of-hospital cardiac arrest documented significant early but reversible myocardial dysfunction and low cardiac output, followed by later vasodilation. The hemodynamic instability responded to fluid administration and vasoactive support.[6] Invasive monitoring may be necessary to measure blood pressure accurately and to determine the most appropriate combination of medications to optimize blood flow and distribution. The provider should titrate volume administration and vasoactive (eg, norepinephrine), inotropic (eg, dobutamine), and inodilator (eg, milrinone) drugs as needed to support blood pressure, cardiac index, and systemic perfusion. The ideal target blood pressure or hemodynamic parameters associated with optimal survival have not been established.

Both cardiac arrest and sepsis are thought to involve multi-organ ischemic injury and microcirculatory dysfunction. Goal-directed therapy with volume and vasoactive drug administration has been effective in improving survival from sepsis.[41] The greatest survival benefit is due to a decreased incidence of acute hemodynamic collapse, a challenge also seen in the postresuscitation setting. Data extrapolated from a study of goal-directed therapy for sepsis (LOE 1[41] for sepsis; LOE 7 [extrapolated] for cardiac arrest) suggests that providers should try to normalize oxygen content and oxygen transport.

Relative adrenal insufficiency may develop following the stress of cardiac arrest, but the use of early corticosteroid supplementation in such patients to improve either hemodynamics or outcome is unproven and requires further evaluation.[42]

Although sudden cardiac arrest may be precipitated by cardiac arrhythmia, it is unclear if antiarrhythmics are beneficial or detrimental in the postresuscitation period. Thus, there is insufficient evidence to recommend for or against prophylactic administration of antiarrhythmic drugs to patients who have survived cardiac arrest from any cause. It may be reasonable, however, to continue an infusion of an antiarrhythmic drug that was associated with ROSC (Class Indeterminate). Also, given the cardioprotective effects of β-blockers in the context of ischemic heart disease, the use of β-blockers in the postresuscitation setting seems prudent if there are no contraindications.[9]

Central Nervous System

A healthy brain and a functional patient are the primary goals of cardio-pulmonary-cerebral resuscitation. Following ROSC, after a brief initial period of hyperemia cerebral blood flow is reduced (the "no-reflow phenomenon") as a result of microvascular dysfunction. This reduction occurs even when cerebral perfusion pressure is normal.[43,44]

Neurologic support for the unresponsive patient should include measures to optimize cerebral perfusion pressure by maintaining a normal or slightly elevated mean arterial pressure and reducing intracranial pressure if it is elevated. Because hyperthermia and seizures increase the oxygen requirements of the brain, providers should treat hyperthermia and consider therapeutic hypothermia. Witnessed seizures should be promptly controlled and maintenance anticonvulsant therapy initiated (Class IIa). Because of a paucity of data, routine seizure prophylaxis is a Class Indeterminate recommendation at present.

Prognostic Factors

The period after resuscitation is often stressful to medical staff and family members as questions arise about the patient's ultimate prognosis. Ideally a clinical assessment, laboratory test, or biochemical marker would reliably predict outcome during or immediately after cardiac arrest. Unfortunately no such predictors are available. Determination of prognosis based on initial physical examination findings can be difficult, and coma scores may be less predictive than individual motor and brainstem reflexes found in the first 12 to 72 hours after arrest.[2]

In a meta-analysis (LOE 1)[44] bilateral absence of cortical response to median nerve somatosensory-evoked potentials predicted poor outcome in normothermic patients who were comatose for at least 72 hours after hypoxic-ischemic insult. A case report[46] also documents the usefulness of this evaluation. Therefore, median nerve somatosensory-evoked potentials measured 72 hours after cardiac arrest can be used to predict neurologic outcome in patients with hypoxic-anoxic coma.

A recent meta-analysis (LOE 1) of 11 studies involving 1914 patients[2] documented 5 clinical signs that were found to strongly predict death or poor neurologic outcome, with 4 of the 5 predictors detectable at 24 hours after resuscitation:

- Absent corneal reflex at 24 hours
- Absent pupillary response at 24 hours
- Absent withdrawal response to pain at 24 hours
- No motor response at 24 hours
- No motor response at 72 hours

An electroencephalogram performed >24 to 48 hours after resuscitation has also been shown to provide useful predictive information (LOE 5[47–50]) and can help define prognosis.

Other Complications

Sepsis is a potentially fatal postresuscitation complication.[51] Patients with sepsis will benefit from goal-directed therapy. Renal failure[52] and pancreatitis, while often transient, should be diagnosed and evaluated.[3,53]

Summary

The postresuscitation period is often marked by hemodynamic instability as well as laboratory abnormalities. This is also a period for which promising technological interventions such as controlled therapeutic hypothermia are being evaluated. Every organ system is at risk during this time, and patients may ultimately develop multi-organ dysfunction. A complete discussion of this topic is beyond the scope of this chapter. The goal of the postresuscitation period is to manage the patient's vital signs and laboratory abnormalities and support organ system function to increase the likelihood of intact neurologic survival.

References

1. Safar P. Resuscitation from clinical death: pathophysiologic limits and therapeutic potentials. *Crit Care Med.* 1988;16:923–941.
2. Booth CM, Boone RH, Tomlinson G, Detsky AS. Is this patient dead, vegetative, or severely neurologically impaired? Assessing outcome for comatose survivors of cardiac arrest. *JAMA.* 2004;291:870–879.
3. Hypothermia After Cardiac Arrest Study Group. Mild therapeutic hypothermia to improve the neurologic outcome after cardiac arrest. *N Engl J Med.* 2002;346:549–556.
4. Bernard SA, Gray TW, Buist MD, Jones BM, Silvester W, Gutteridge G, Smith K. Treatment of comatose survivors of out-of-hospital cardiac arrest with induced hypothermia. *N Engl J Med.* 2002;346:557–563.
5. Bunch TJ, White RD, Gersh BJ, Meverden RA, Hodge DO, Ballman KV, Hammill SC, Shen WK, Packer DL. Long-term outcomes of out-of-hospital cardiac arrest after successful early defibrillation. *N Engl J Med.* 2003;348:2626–2633.
6. Laurent I, Monchi M, Chiche JD, Joly LM, Spaulding C, Bourgeois B, Cariou A, Rozenberg A, Carli P, Weber S, Dhainaut JF. Reversible myocardial dysfunction in survivors of out-of-hospital cardiac arrest. *J Am Coll Cardiol.* 2002;40:2110–2116.
7. Negovsky VA. The second step in resuscitation—the treatment of the 'post-resuscitation disease.' *Resuscitation.* 1972;1:1–7.
8. A randomized clinical study of cardiopulmonary-cerebral resuscitation: design, methods, and patient characteristics. Brain Resuscitation Clinical Trial I Study Group. *Am J Emerg Med.* 1986;4:72–86.
9. Skrifvars MB, Pettila V, Rosenberg PH, Castren M. A multiple logistic regression analysis of in-hospital factors related to survival at six months in patients resuscitated from out-of-hospital ventricular fibrillation. *Resuscitation.* 2003;59:319–328.
10. Hachimi-Idrissi S, Corne L, Ebinger G, Michotte Y, Huyghens L. Mild hypothermia induced by a helmet device: a clinical feasibility study. *Resuscitation.* 2001;51:275–281.
11. Nolan JP, Morley PT, Hoek TL, Hickey RW. Therapeutic hypothermia after cardiac arrest: an advisory statement by the Advancement Life Support Task Force of the International Liaison Committee on Resuscitation. *Resuscitation.* 2003;57:231–235.
12. Shankaran S, Laptook AR, Ehrenkranz RA, Tyson JE, McDonald SA, Donovan EF, Fanaroff AA, Poole WK, Wright LL, Higgins RD, Finer NN, Carlo WA, Duara S, Oh W, Cotten CM, Stevenson DK, Stoll BJ, Lemons JA, Guillet R, Jobe AH. Whole-body hypothermia for neonates with hypoxic-ischemic encephalopathy. *N Engl J Med.* 2005;353: 1574–1584.
13. Bernard S, Buist M, Monteiro O, Smith K. Induced hypothermia using large volume, ice-cold intravenous fluid in comatose survivors of out-of-hospital cardiac arrest: a preliminary report. *Resuscitation.* 2003;56:9–13.
14. Hickey RW, Kochanek PM, Ferimer H, Alexander HL, Garman RH, Graham SH. Induced hyperthermia exacerbates neurologic neuronal histologic damage after asphyxial cardiac arrest in rats. *Crit Care Med.* 2003;31:531–535.
15. Dietrich WD, Busto R, Halley M, Valdes I. The importance of brain temperature in alterations of the blood-brain barrier following cerebral ischemia. *J Neuropathol Exp Neurol.* 1990;49:486–497.
16. Dietrich WD, Busto R, Valdes I, Loor Y. Effects of normothermic versus mild hyperthermic forebrain ischemia in rats. *Stroke.* 1990;21: 1318–1325.
17. Kim Y, Busto R, Dietrich WD, Kraydieh S, Ginsberg MD. Delayed postischemic hyperthermia in awake rats worsens the histopathological

outcome of transient focal cerebral ischemia. *Stroke.* 1996;27: 2274–2280; discussion 2281.
18. Zeiner A, Holzer M, Sterz F, Schorkhuber W, Eisenburger P, Havel C, Kliegel A, Laggner AN. Hyperthermia after cardiac arrest is associated with an unfavorable neurologic outcome. *Arch Intern Med.* 2001;161: 2007–2012.
19. Hajat C, Hajat S, Sharma P. Effects of poststroke pyrexia on stroke outcome: a meta-analysis of studies in patients. *Stroke.* 2000;31: 410–414.
20. Mullner M, Sterz F, Binder M, Schreiber W, Deimel A, Laggner AN. Blood glucose concentration after cardiopulmonary resuscitation influences functional neurological recovery in human cardiac arrest survivors. *J Cereb Blood Flow Metab.* 1997;17:430–436.
21. Langhelle A, Tyvold SS, Lexow K, Hapnes SA, Sunde K, Steen PA. In-hospital factors associated with improved outcome after out-of-hospital cardiac arrest: a comparison between four regions in Norway. *Resuscitation.* 2003;56:247–263.
22. Calle PA, Buylaert WA, Vanhaute OA. Glycemia in the post-resuscitation period. The Cerebral Resuscitation Study Group. *Resuscitation.* 1989; 17(suppl):S181–S188; discussion S199–S206.
23. Mackenzie CF. A review of 100 cases of cardiac arrest and the relation of potassium, glucose, and haemoglobin levels to survival. *West Indian Med J.* 1975;24:39–45.
24. Longstreth WT Jr, Diehr P, Inui TS. Prediction of awakening after out-of-hospital cardiac arrest. *N Engl J Med.* 1983;308:1378–1382.
25. Longstreth WT Jr, Inui TS. High blood glucose level on hospital admission and poor neurological recovery after cardiac arrest. *Ann Neurol.* 1984;15:59–63.
26. Longstreth WT Jr, Copass MK, Dennis LK, Rauch-Matthews ME, Stark MS, Cobb LA. Intravenous glucose after out-of-hospital cardiopulmonary arrest: a community-based randomized trial. *Neurology.* 1993;43: 2534–2541.
27. Sheldon RA, Partridge JC, Ferriero DM. Postischemic hyperglycemia is not protective to the neonatal rat brain. *Pediatr Res.* 1992;32:489–493.
28. van den Berghe G, Wouters P, Weekers F, Verwaest C, Bruyninckx F, Schetz M, Vlasselaers D, Ferdinande P, Lauwers P, Bouillon R. Intensive insulin therapy in the critically ill patients. *N Engl J Med.* 2001;345: 1359–1367.
29. Rello J, Diaz E, Roque M, Valles J. Risk factors for developing pneumonia within 48 hours of intubation. *Am J Respir Crit Care Med.* 1999;159:1742–1746.
30. Ausina A, Baguena M, Nadal M, Manrique S, Ferrer A, Sahuquillo J, Garnacho A. Cerebral hemodynamic changes during sustained hypocapnia in severe head injury: can hyperventilation cause cerebral ischemia? *Acta Neurochir Suppl.* 1998;71:1–4.
31. Yundt KD, Diringer MN. The use of hyperventilation and its impact on cerebral ischemia in the treatment of traumatic brain injury. *Crit Care Clin.* 1997;13:163–184.
32. Wolfson SK Jr, Safar P, Reich H, Clark JM, Gur D, Stezoski W, Cook EE, Krupper MA. Dynamic heterogeneity of cerebral hypoperfusion after prolonged cardiac arrest in dogs measured by the stable xenon/CT technique: a preliminary study. *Resuscitation.* 1992;23:1–20.
33. Fischer M, Hossmann KA. No-reflow after cardiac arrest. *Intensive Care Med.* 1995;21:132–141.
34. Safar P, Xiao F, Radovsky A, Tanigawa K, Ebmeyer U, Bircher N, Alexander H, Stezoski SW. Improved cerebral resuscitation from cardiac arrest in dogs with mild hypothermia plus blood flow promotion. *Stroke.* 1996;27:105–113.
35. Gottfried SB, Rossi A, Milic-Emili J. Dynamic hyperinflation, intrinsic PEEP, and the mechanically ventilated patient. *Crit Care Digest.* 1986; 5:30–33.
36. Ligas JR, Mosiehi F, Epstein MAF. Occult positive end-expiratory pressure with different types of mechanical ventilators. *J Crit Care.* 1990;52:95–100.
37. Weaver WD, Cobb LA, Copass MK, Hallstrom AP. Ventricular defibrillation: a comparative trial using 175-J and 320-J shocks. *N Engl J Med.* 1982;307:1101–1106.
38. Vasquez A, Kern KB, Hilwig RW, Heidenreich J, Berg RA, Ewy GA. Optimal dosing of dobutamine for treating post-resuscitation left ventricular dysfunction. *Resuscitation.* 2004;61:199–207.
39. Mullner M, Domanovits H, Sterz F, Herkner H, Gamper G, Kurkciyan I, Laggner AN. Measurement of myocardial contractility following successful resuscitation: quantitated left ventricular systolic function utilising non-invasive wall stress analysis. *Resuscitation.* 1998;39:51–59.
40. Spaulding CM, Joly LM, Rosenberg A, Monchi M, Weber SN, Dhainaut JF, Carli P. Immediate coronary angiography in survivors of out-of-hospital cardiac arrest. *N Engl J Med.* 1997;336:1629–1633.
41. Rivers E, Nguyen B, Havstad S, Ressler J, Muzzin A, Knoblich B, Peterson E, Tomlanovich M. Early goal-directed therapy in the treatment of severe sepsis and septic shock. *N Engl J Med.* 2001;345:1368–1377.
42. Ito T, Saitoh D, Takasu A, Kiyozumi T, Sakamoto T, Okada Y. Serum cortisol as a predictive marker of the outcome in patients resuscitated after cardiopulmonary arrest. *Resuscitation.* 2004;62:55–60.
43. Gisvold SE, Sterz F, Abramson NS, Bar-Joseph G, Ebmeyer U, Gervais H, Ginsberg M, Katz LM, Kochanek PM, Kuboyama K, Miller B, Obrist W, Roine RO, Safar P, Sim KM, Vandevelde K, White RJ, Xiao F. Cerebral resuscitation from cardiac arrest: treatment potentials. *Crit Care Med.* 1996;24(2 suppl):S69–S80.
44. del Zoppo GJ, Mabuchi T. Cerebral microvessel responses to focal ischemia. *J Cereb Blood Flow Metab.* 2003;23:879–894.
45. Zandbergen EG, de Haan RJ, Stoutenbeek CP, Koelman JH, Hijdra A. Systematic review of early prediction of poor outcome in anoxic-ischaemic coma. *Lancet.* 1998;352:1808–1812.
46. Rothstein TL. Recovery from near death following cerebral anoxia: a case report demonstrating superiority of median somatosensory evoked potentials over EEG in predicting a favorable outcome after cardiopulmonary resuscitation. *Resuscitation.* 2004;60:335–341.
47. Kaplan PW, Genoud D, Ho TW, Jallon P. Etiology, neurologic correlations, and prognosis in alpha coma. *Clin Neurophysiol.* 1999;110: 205–213.
48. Ajisaka H. Early electroencephalographic findings in patients with anoxic encephalopathy after cardiopulmonary arrest and successful resuscitation. *J Clin Neurosci.* 2004;11:616–618.
49. Bassetti C, Bomio F, Mathis J, Hess CW. Early prognosis in coma after cardiac arrest: a prospective clinical, electrophysiological, and biochemical study of 60 patients. *J Neurol Neurosurg Psychiatry.* 1996;61: 610–615.
50. Berkhoff M, Donati F, Bassetti C. Postanoxic alpha (theta) coma: a reappraisal of its prognostic significance. *Clin Neurophysiol.* 2000;111: 297–304.
51. Dellinger RP, Carlet JM, Masur H, Gerlach H, Calandra T, Cohen J, Gea-Banacloche J, Keh D, Marshall JC, Parker MM, Ramsay G, Zimmerman JL, Vincent JL, Levy MM. Surviving Sepsis Campaign guidelines for management of severe sepsis and septic shock. *Crit Care Med.* 2004;32:858–873.
52. Zeiner A, Sunder-Plassmann G, Sterz F, Holzer M, Losert H, Laggner AN, Mullner M. The effect of mild therapeutic hypothermia on renal function after cardiopulmonary resuscitation in men. *Resuscitation.* 2004; 60:253–261.
53. Mattana J, Singhal PC. Prevalence and determinants of acute renal failure following cardiopulmonary resuscitation. *Arch Intern Med.* 1993;153: 235–239.

Part 8: Stabilization of the Patient With Acute Coronary Syndromes

Acute myocardial infarction (AMI) and unstable angina (UA) are part of a spectrum of clinical disease collectively identified as *acute coronary syndromes* (ACS). The pathophysiology common to this spectrum of disease is a ruptured or eroded atheromatous plaque.[1–5] The electrocardiographic (ECG) presentation of these syndromes encompasses ST-segment elevation myocardial infarction (STEMI), ST-segment depression, and nondiagnostic ST-segment and T-wave abnormalities. A non–ST-elevation myocardial infarction (NSTEMI) is diagnosed if cardiac markers are positive with ST-segment depression or with nonspecific or normal ECGs. Sudden cardiac death may occur with any of these conditions. ACS is the most common proximate cause of sudden cardiac death.[6–10]

Effective interventions for patients with ACS, particularly STEMI, are extremely time-sensitive. The first healthcare providers to encounter the ACS patient can have a big impact on patient outcome if they provide efficient risk stratification, initial stabilization, and referral for cardiology care. It is critical that basic life support (BLS) and advanced cardiovascular life support (ACLS) healthcare providers who care for ACS patients in the out-of-hospital, emergency department (ED), and hospital environments be aware of the principles and priorities of assessment and stabilization of these patients.

These guidelines target BLS and ACLS healthcare providers who treat patients with ACS within the first hours after onset of symptoms, summarizing key out-of-hospital, ED, and some initial critical-care topics that are relevant to stabilization. They also continue to build on recommendations from the ACC/AHA Guidelines,[11,12] which are used throughout the United States and Canada.[13] As with any medical guidelines, these general recommendations must be considered within the context of local resources and application to individual patients by knowledgeable healthcare providers.

The primary goals of therapy for patients with ACS are to

- Reduce the amount of myocardial necrosis that occurs in patients with MI, preserving left ventricular (LV) function and preventing heart failure
- Prevent major adverse cardiac events (MACE): death, nonfatal MI, and need for urgent revascularization
- Treat acute, life-threatening complications of ACS, such as ventricular fibrillation (VF)/pulseless ventricular tachycardia (VT), symptomatic bradycardias, and unstable tachycardias (see Part 7.2: "Management of Cardiac Arrest" and Part 7.3: "Management of Symptomatic Bradycardia and Tachycardia")

(*Circulation*. 2005;112:IV-89-IV-110.)

This special supplement to *Circulation* is freely available at http://www.circulationaha.org

DOI: 10.1161/CIRCULATIONAHA.105.166561

An overview of recommended care for the ACS patient is illustrated in Figure 1, the Acute Coronary Syndromes Algorithm. Part 8 provides details of the care highlighted in the numbered algorithm boxes. Box numbers in the text correspond to the numbered boxes in the algorithm.

In this part the abbreviation AMI refers to acute myocardial infarction, whether associated with STEMI or NSTEMI. The diagnosis and treatment of AMI, however, will often differ for patients with STEMI versus NSTEMI. Note carefully which is being discussed.

Out-of-Hospital Management

Recognition (Figure 1, Box 1)

Treatment offers the greatest potential benefit for myocardial salvage in the first hours of STEMI. Thus, it is imperative that healthcare providers evaluate, triage, and treat patients with ACS as quickly as possible. Delays to therapy occur during 3 intervals: from onset of symptoms to patient recognition, during out-of-hospital transport, and during in-hospital evaluation. Patient delay to symptom recognition often constitutes the longest period of delay to treatment.[14]

The classic symptom associated with ACS is chest discomfort, but symptoms may also include discomfort in other areas of the upper body, shortness of breath, sweating, nausea, and lightheadedness. The symptoms of AMI are characteristically more intense than angina and last >15 minutes. Atypical symptoms or unusual presentations of ACS are more common in elderly, female, and diabetic patients.[15–19]

Public education campaigns increase public awareness and knowledge of the symptoms of heart attack but have only transient effects.[20] For patients at risk for ACS (and for their families), physicians should discuss the appropriate use of nitroglycerin and aspirin, activation of the emergency medical services (EMS) system, and location of the nearest hospital that offers 24-hour emergency cardiovascular care. Recent ACC/AHA guidelines recommend that the patient or family members activate the EMS system rather than call their physician or drive to the hospital if chest discomfort is unimproved or worsening 5 minutes after taking 1 nitroglycerin tablet or using nitroglycerin spray.[12]

Initial EMS Care (Figure 1, Box 2)

Half of the patients who die of AMI do so before reaching the hospital. VF or pulseless VT is the precipitating rhythm in most of these deaths,[21–23] and it is most likely to develop during the first 4 hours after onset of symptoms.[24–27] Communities should develop programs to respond to out-of-hospital cardiac arrest that include prompt recognition of symptoms of ACS, early activation of the EMS system, and

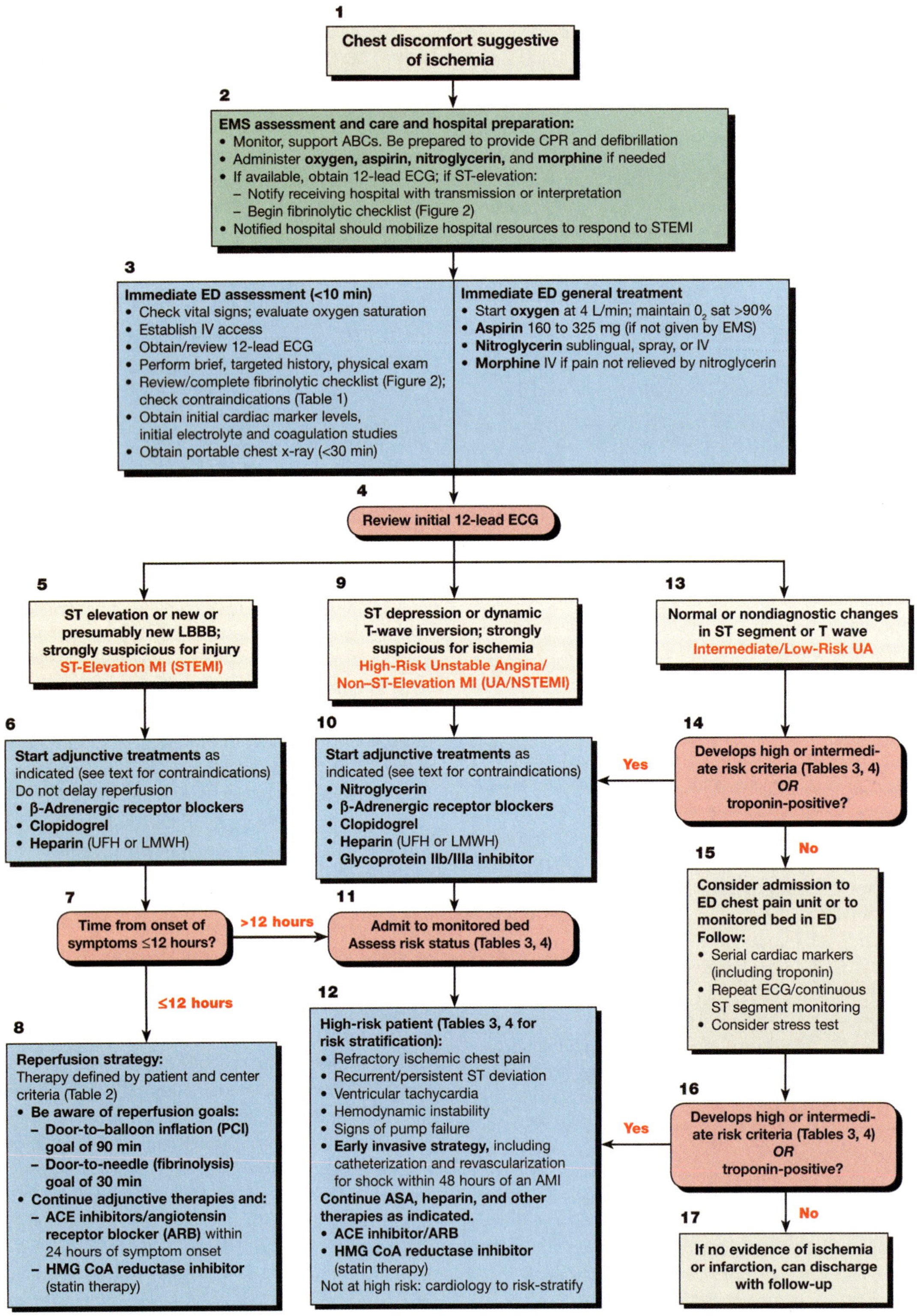

Figure 1. Acute Coronary Syndromes Algorithm.

if needed, early CPR (see Part 4: "Adult Basic Life Support") and early access to an automated external defibrillator (AED) through community AED programs (see Part 5: "Electrical Therapies").[28] EMS and dispatch system personnel should be trained to respond to cardiovascular emergencies.

Dispatchers and EMS providers must be trained to recognize symptoms of ACS. Dispatchers should advise patients with no history of aspirin allergy or signs of active or recent gastrointestinal bleeding to chew an aspirin (160 to 325 mg) while awaiting the arrival of EMS providers (Class IIa).[29]

EMS providers should be trained to determine the time of onset of symptoms and to stabilize, triage, and transport the patient to an appropriate facility and to provide prearrival notification. EMS providers should monitor vital signs and cardiac rhythm and be prepared to provide CPR and defibrillation if needed.

EMS providers may administer oxygen to all patients. If the patient is hypoxemic, providers should titrate therapy based on monitoring of oxyhemoglobin saturation (Class I).[30–44] If the patient has not taken aspirin and has no history of aspirin allergy and no evidence of recent gastrointestinal bleeding, EMS providers should give the patient nonenteric aspirin (160 to 325 mg) to chew (Class I).[45–48]

EMS providers should administer up to 3 nitroglycerin tablets (or spray) for ongoing symptoms at intervals of 3 to 5 minutes if permitted by medical control and if the patient remains hemodynamically stable (systolic blood pressure [SBP] >90 mm Hg [or no more than 30 mm Hg below baseline], heart rate between 50 and 100 beats per minute [bpm]).[49,50] EMS providers can administer morphine for chest pain unresponsive to nitroglycerin if authorized by protocol or medical control. Additional information about out-of-hospital stabilization and care is included in the following sections.

Out-of-Hospital ECGs

Out-of-hospital 12-lead ECGs and advance notification to the receiving facility speed the diagnosis, shorten the time to fibrinolysis, and may be associated with decreased mortality rates.[51–64] The reduction in door-to–reperfusion therapy interval in most studies ranges from 10 to 60 minutes. EMS providers can efficiently acquire and transmit diagnostic-quality ECGs to the ED[53,58,65,66] with a minimal increase (0.2 to 5.6 minutes) in the on-scene time interval.[52,56,65–68]

Qualified and specially trained paramedics and prehospital nurses can accurately identify typical ST-segment elevation (>1 mm in 2 or more contiguous leads) in the 12-lead ECG with specificity ranging from 91% to 100% and sensitivity ranging from 71% to 97% when compared with emergency medicine physicians or cardiologists.[69,70] Using radio or cell phone, they can also provide advance notification to the receiving hospital of the arrival of a patient with ACS.[56,61–64]

We recommend implementation of out-of-hospital 12-lead ECG diagnostic programs in urban and suburban EMS systems (Class I). Routine use of 12-lead out-of-hospital ECG and advance notification is recommended for patients with signs and symptoms of ACS (Class IIa). A 12-lead out-of-hospital ECG with advance notification to the ED may be beneficial for STEMI patients by reducing time to reperfusion therapy. We recommend that out-of-hospital paramedics acquire and transmit either diagnostic-quality ECGs or their interpretation of them to the receiving hospital with advance notification of the arrival of a patient with ACS (Class IIa). If EMS providers identify STEMI on the ECG, it is reasonable for them to begin to complete a fibrinolytic checklist (Figure 2).

Out-of-Hospital Fibrinolysis

Clinical trials have shown the benefit of initiating fibrinolysis as soon as possible after onset of ischemic-type chest pain in patients with STEMI or new or presumably new left bundle branch block (LBBB).[67,71] Several prospective studies (LOE 1)[72–74] have documented reduced time to administration of fibrinolytics and decreased mortality rates when out-of-hospital fibrinolytics were administered to patients with STEMI and no contraindications to fibrinolytics.

Physicians in the Grampian Region Early Anistreplase Trial (GREAT)[73] administered fibrinolytic therapy to patients at home 130 minutes earlier than to patients at the hospital and noted a 50% reduction in hospital mortality rates and greater 1-year and 5-year survival rates in those treated earlier.[75,76] Delaying fibrinolytic treatment by 1 hour increased the hazard ratio of death by 20%, which is equivalent to the loss of 43 lives per 1000 patients over 5 years.

A meta-analysis of out-of-hospital fibrinolytic trials found a relative improvement of 17% in outcome associated with out-of-hospital fibrinolytic therapy, particularly when therapy was initiated 60 to 90 minutes earlier than in the hospital.[71] A meta-analysis of 6 trials involving 6434 patients (LOE 1)[72] documented decreased all-cause hospital mortality rates among patients treated with out-of-hospital fibrinolysis compared with in-hospital fibrinolysis (odds ratio [OR]: 0.83; 95% confidence interval [CI]: 0.70 to 0.98) with a number needed to treat of 62 to save 1 extra life with out-of-hospital fibrinolysis. Results were similar regardless of the training and experience of the provider.

The *ECC Guidelines 2000*[77] recommended consideration of out-of-hospital fibrinolysis for patients with a transport time >1 hour. But in a recent Swiss study (LOE 1),[74] prehospital administration of fibrinolytics significantly decreased the time to drug administration even in an urban setting with relatively short transport intervals (<15 minutes).[74]

In summary, out-of-hospital administration of fibrinolytics to patients with STEMI with no contraindications is safe, feasible, and reasonable (Class IIa). This intervention may be performed by trained paramedics, nurses, and physicians for patients with symptom duration of 30 minutes to 6 hours. System requirements include protocols with fibrinolytic checklists, ECG acquisition and interpretation, experience in ACLS, the ability to communicate with the receiving institution, and a medical director with training/experience in management of STEMI. A process of continuous quality improvement is required. Given the operational challenges required to provide out-of-hospital fibrinolytics, most EMS systems should focus on early diagnosis with 12-lead ECG, rapid transport, and advance notification of the ED (verbal

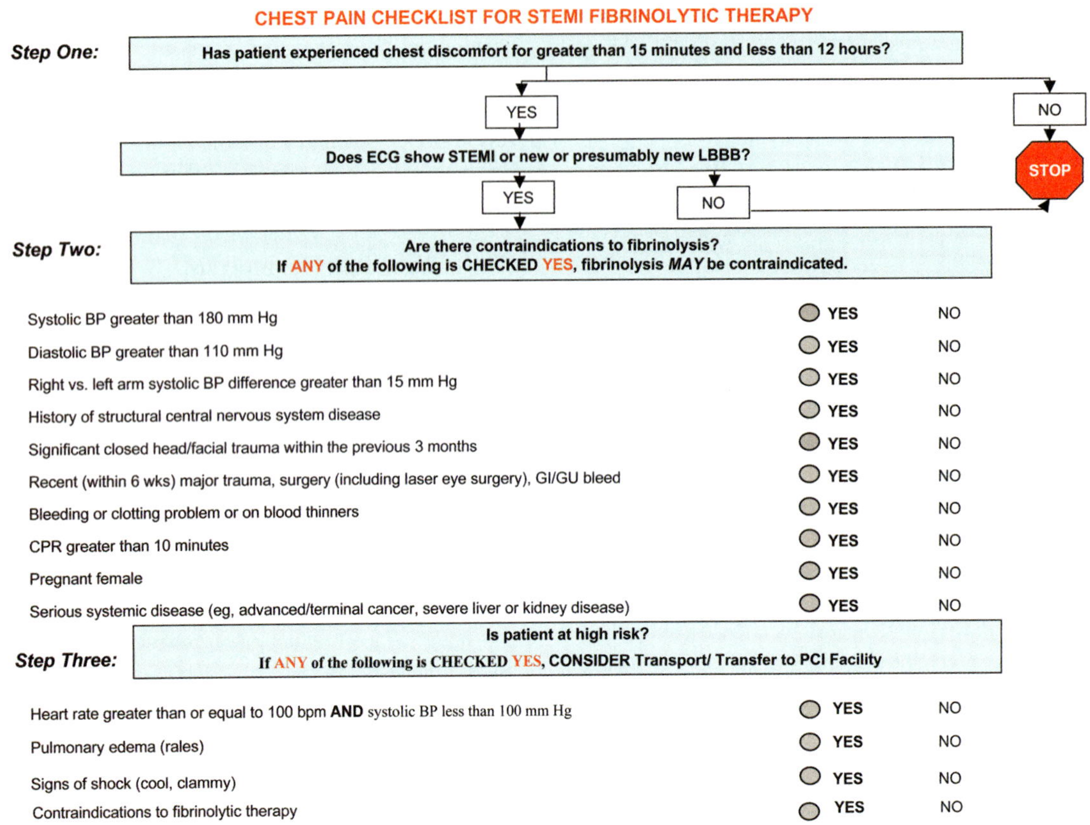

Figure 2. Fibrinolytic Checklist.

interpretation or direct transmission of ECG) instead of out-of-hospital delivery of fibrinolysis.

Triage and Transfer

Out-of-Hospital Triage

Hospital and EMS protocols should clearly identify criteria for transfer of patients to specialty centers and conditions under which fibrinolytics should be initiated before transfer. When transfer is indicated, the ACC/AHA guidelines recommend a door-to-departure time ≤30 minutes.[12] It may be appropriate for the EMS medical director to institute a policy of out-of-hospital bypass of hospitals that provide medical therapy only, particularly for patients who require interventional therapy. Patients who require interventional therapy may include those with cardiogenic shock, pulmonary edema, large infarctions, and contraindications to fibrinolytic therapy.

At present no randomized studies have directly compared triage with an experienced percutaneous coronary intervention (PCI) center with medical management at the local hospital. Extrapolation from several randomized trials on interfacility transfer[78–80] suggests that STEMI patients triaged directly to a primary PCI facility may have better outcomes related to the potential for earlier treatment. A cost-efficacy substudy of the Comparison of Angioplasty and Prehospital Thrombolysis in Acute Myocardial Infarction (CAPTIM) trial[81] suggests that direct transport to a primary PCI facility may be more cost-effective than out-of-hospital fibrinolysis when transport can be completed in ≤60 minutes with a physician in a mobile intensive care unit. There is no direct evidence, however, to suggest that these strategies are safe or effective. Patients judged to be at highest risk for a complicated transfer were excluded from some of these studies.

In summary, at this time there is inadequate evidence to recommend out-of-hospital triage to bypass non–PCI-capable hospitals to bring patients to a PCI center (Class Indeterminate). Local protocols for EMS providers are appropriate to guide the destination of patients with suspected or confirmed STEMI.

Interfacility Transfer

All patients with STEMI and symptom duration of ≤12 hours are candidates for reperfusion therapy with either fibrinolysis or PCI (Class I). When patients present directly to a facility capable of providing only fibrinolysis, 3 treatment options are available: administering fibrinolytics with admission to that hospital, transferring the patient for primary PCI, or giving fibrinolytics and then transferring the patient to a specialized center. The decision is guided by a risk-benefit assessment that includes evaluation of duration of symptoms, complications, contraindications, and the time delay from patient contact to fibrinolysis versus potential delay to PCI balloon inflation.

In 2 prospective studies (LOE 2)[78–80] and a meta-analysis,[82] patients with STEMI who presented 3 to 12 hours after onset of symptoms to a hospital without capability for primary PCI had better outcome (improved 30-day combined incidence of death, reinfarction, or stroke) when they were transferred to a skilled PCI center (interventionalist performing >75 procedures per year) rather than receiving fibrinolytics at the presenting hospital. In these studies balloon inflation occurred ≤93 minutes after decision to treat.[80,83–85] Thus, interfacility transfer is indicated for patients with STEMI presenting >3 hours from onset of symptoms from hospitals that lack primary PCI capability to centers capable of providing primary PCI when the transfer can be accomplished as soon as possible. The ACC/AHA guidelines recommend a treatment delay of no more than 90 minutes.[12] In patients with STEMI presenting <3 hours from onset of symptoms, the superiority of immediate administration of fibrinolytics in the hospital or transfer for primary PCI is not established (Class Indeterminate).

In-Hospital Fibrinolytics and Interfacility Transfer for PCI

Data from the 1980s to 1990s did not support a strategy of fibrinolytic therapy combined with transfer for facilitated PCI (LOE 1[86–88] and meta-analyses[89–91]). But all of the studies involved in-hospital administration of fibrinolytics, and most were completed before the era of coronary stenting and without use of contemporary pharmacologic therapies or PCI techniques. Three small randomized trials (LOE 1)[92–94] supported the strategy of fibrinolytics plus transfer for PCI; however, the timing of PCI after administration of fibrinolytics, the inclusion of patients who required transfer for PCI, the use of coronary stents, and the control group interventions differ considerably among these trials. The most recent study[79] was fairly small and showed a benefit of early PCI with 1-year follow-up.[94]

At present there is inadequate evidence to recommend the routine transfer of patients for early PCI (ie, within 24 hours) after successful administration of fibrinolytics in a community hospital. The use of out-of-hospital administration of fibrinolytics followed by early PCI has not been specifically studied.

Special Transfer Considerations

Special transfer considerations are appropriate for patients with signs of shock (pulmonary congestion, heart rate >100 bpm, *and* SBP <100 mm Hg). The Second National Registry of Myocardial Infarction found that the mortality rate in patients with AMI and shock was lower in those treated with PCI as a primary strategy than in those treated with fibrinolysis.[95] In the SHOCK (Should We Emergently Revascularize Occluded Coronaries for Cardiogenic Shock) trial, 152 patients with cardiogenic shock were randomly assigned to an early revascularization (ERV) strategy, 150 patients were assigned to a strategy of initial medical stabilization that included fibrinolytics, and 25% had delayed revascularization.[96] Although there was no difference in the 30-day mortality rate, the mortality rate at 6 months was significantly lower in the ERV group (50.3% versus 63.1%). In a prespecified subgroup analysis for patients <75 years of age, early revascularization was associated with a 15.4% reduction in 30-day mortality and improvement in 1-year survival rates.[97] A direct comparison of the outcome of primary or early PCI patients with patients who received fibrinolytic therapy only was not reported.

There is inadequate evidence to recommend routine transfer of stable patients for early PCI after successful administration of fibrinolytics in community hospitals or the out-of-hospital setting. Patients <75 years of age and selected patients >75 years of age who develop cardiogenic shock or persistent ischemic symptoms within 36 hours of STEMI should be transferred to experienced facilities capable of ERV if ERV can be performed within 18 hours of onset of shock.[12]

ED Evaluation and Risk Stratification (Figure 1, Boxes 3 and 4)

Focused Assessment and ECG Risk Stratification

ED providers should quickly assess patients with possible ACS. Ideally within 10 minutes of ED arrival, providers should obtain a targeted history while a monitor is attached to the patient and a 12-lead ECG is obtained (if not done in the prehospital setting).[98] The evaluation should focus on chest discomfort, associated signs and symptoms, prior cardiac history, risk factors for ACS, and historical features that may preclude the use of fibrinolytics or other therapies. This initial evaluation must be efficient because if the patient has STEMI, the goals of reperfusion are to administer fibrinolytics within 30 minutes of arrival (30-minute interval "door-to-drug") or to provide PCI within 90 minutes of arrival (90-minute interval "door-to–balloon inflation" in the catheterization suite).

Potential delay during the in-hospital evaluation period may occur from **d**oor to **d**ata, from data (ECG) to **d**ecision, and from decision to **d**rug (or PCI). These 4 major points of in-hospital therapy are commonly referred to as the "4 D's."[99] All providers must focus on minimizing delays at each of these points. Out-of-hospital transport time constitutes only 5% of delay to treatment time; in-hospital evaluation constitutes 25% to 33% of this delay.[100,101]

The physical examination is performed to aid diagnosis, rule out other causes of the patient's symptoms, and evaluate the patient for complications related to ACS. Although the use of clinical signs and symptoms may increase suspicion of ACS, evidence does not support the use of any single sign or combination of clinical signs and symptoms alone to confirm the diagnosis.[102–105]

When the patient presents with signs of ACS, the clinician uses ECG findings (Figure 1, Box 4) to classify the patient into 1 of 3 groups:

1. ST-segment elevation or presumed new LBBB (Box 5) is characterized by ST-segment elevation >1 mm (0.1 mV) in 2 or more contiguous precordial leads or 2 or more adjacent limb leads and is classified as *ST-elevation MI (STEMI)*.
2. Ischemic ST-segment depression ≥0.5 mm (0.05 mV) or dynamic T-wave inversion with pain or discomfort (Box 9) is classified as *high-risk UA/non–ST-elevation MI (NSTEMI)*. Nonpersistent or transient ST-segment elevation ≥0.5 mm for <20 minutes is also included in this category.

3. Normal or nondiagnostic changes in ST segment or T waves (Box 13) are inconclusive and require further risk stratification. This classification includes patients with normal ECGs and those with ST-segment deviation of <0.5 mm (0.05 mV) or T-wave inversion of ≤0.2 mV. Serial cardiac studies (and functional testing) are appropriate.

Cardiac Biomarkers

New cardiac biomarkers, which are more sensitive than the myocardial muscle creatine kinase isoenzyme (CK-MB), are useful in diagnosis, risk stratification, and determination of prognosis. An elevated level of *troponin* correlates with an increased risk of death, and greater elevations predict greater risk of adverse outcome.[106] Patients with increased troponin levels have increased thrombus burden and microvascular embolization.

Cardiac biomarkers should be obtained during the initial evaluation of the patient, but therapeutic decisions and reperfusion therapy for patients with STEMI should not be delayed pending the results of these tests. Important limitations to these tests exist because they are insensitive during the first 4 to 6 hours of presentation unless continuous persistent pain has been present for 6 to 8 hours. For this reason cardiac biomarkers are not useful in the prehospital setting.[107–112]

Serial marker testing (CK-MB and cardiac troponin) over time improves sensitivity for detection of myocardial infarction but remains insensitive in the first 4 to 6 hours.[113,114]

ST-Segment Elevation MI (Figure 1, Boxes 5 Through 8)

Patients with STEMI usually have complete occlusion of an epicardial coronary vessel. The mainstay of treatment is reperfusion therapy through administration of fibrinolytics (pharmacologic reperfusion) or primary PCI (mechanical reperfusion). Providers should rapidly identify patients with STEMI and quickly screen them for indications and contraindications to fibrinolytic therapy and PCI.

The first physician who encounters a patient with AMI should be able to determine the need for reperfusion therapy and direct its administration (see Tables 1 and 2). If the patient meets the criteria for fibrinolytic therapy, a door-to-needle time (needle time is the beginning of infusion of a fibrinolytic agent) ≤30 minutes is desired. Results of cardiac biomarkers do not delay the administration of fibrinolytic therapy or referral for PCI. They are normal in a significant percentage of patients who present early with STEMI. Consultation with a cardiologist or the patient's personal physician delays therapy, is associated with increased hospital mortality rates, and is recommended only in equivocal or uncertain cases.[115] Hospitals with capabilities for angiography and PCI should have a clear protocol directing ED triage and initial management. Confusion about the method of reperfusion, eg, fibrinolysis or PCI, delays definitive therapy.

UA and NSTEMI (Figure 1, Boxes 9 Through 17)

In the absence of ST-segment elevation, patients with ischemic-type chest pain can present with ST-segment depression or nondiagnostic or normal ECGs. ST-segment depression identifies a population at increased risk for MACE. Patients with ischemic-type pain and ECGs consistent with NSTEMI or normal or nondiagnostic ECGs do not benefit from fibrinolytic therapy, and fibrinolysis may be harmful.[116]

Although many patients will not have ACS (ie, the ECG change is due to an alternative diagnosis, such as LV hypertrophy), initial triage and therapy appropriately includes antiplatelet, antithrombin, and antianginal therapy. These patients usually have a partially or intermittently occluding thrombus. Clinical features can correlate with the dynamic nature of clot formation and degradation, eg, waxing and waning clinical symptoms.

Serial cardiac markers are often obtained during evaluation, including CK-MB and cardiac troponins. At any point during evaluation, elevation of cardiac troponin places a patient at increased risk for MACE. Studies have shown that patients with increased troponin are best managed with a strategy of small-molecule glycoprotein (GP) IIb/IIIa inhibitor therapy and an early invasive strategy (cardiac catheterization with possible revascularization). Troponin serves as an additional and incremental adjunct to the ECG. Physicians

TABLE 1. Fibrinolytic Therapy: Contraindications and Cautions for Fibrinolytic Use in STEMI From ACC/AHA 2004 Guideline Update*

Absolute Contraindications

- Any prior intracranial hemorrhage
- Known structural cerebral vascular lesion (eg, AVM)
- Known malignant intracranial neoplasm (primary or metastatic)
- Ischemic stroke within 3 months EXCEPT acute ischemic stroke within 3 hours
- Suspected aortic dissection
- Active bleeding or bleeding diathesis (excluding menses)
- Significant closed head trauma or facial trauma within 3 months

Relative Contraindications

- History of chronic, severe, poorly controlled hypertension
- Severe uncontrolled hypertension on presentation (SBP >180 mm Hg or DBP >110 mm Hg)†
- History of prior ischemic stroke >3 months, dementia, or known intracranial pathology not covered in contraindications
- Traumatic or prolonged (>10 minutes) CPR or major surgery (<3 weeks)
- Recent (within 2 to 4 weeks) internal bleeding
- Noncompressible vascular punctures
- For streptokinase/anistreplase: prior exposure (>5 days ago) or prior allergic reaction to these agents
- Pregnancy
- Active peptic ulcer
- Current use of anticoagulants: the higher the INR, the higher the risk of bleeding

AVM indicates arteriovenous malformation; SBP, systolic blood pressure; DBP, diastolic blood pressure; and INR, International Normalized Ratio.

*Viewed as advisory for clinical decision making and may not be all-inclusive or definitive.

†Could be an absolute contraindication in low-risk patients with myocardial infarction.

TABLE 2. ST-Segment Elevation or New or Presumably New LBBB: Evaluation for Reperfusion

Step 1: Assess time and risk	
Time since onset of symptoms	
Risk of STEMI	
Risk of fibrinolysis	
Time required to transport to skilled PCI catheterization suite	
Step 2: Select reperfusion (fibrinolysis or invasive) strategy	
Note: If presentation <3 hours and no delay for PCI, then no preference for either strategy.	
Fibrinolysis is generally preferred if:	**An invasive strategy is generally preferred if:**
• Early presentation (≤3 hours from symptom onset)	• Late presentation (symptom onset >3 hours ago)
• Invasive strategy is not an option (eg, lack of access to skilled PCI facility or difficult vascular access) or would be delayed	• Skilled PCI facility available with surgical backup
—Medical contact-to-balloon or door-balloon >90 min	• Medical contact-to-balloon or door-balloon <90 min
—(Door-to-balloon) minus (door-to-needle) is >1 hour	• (Door-to-balloon) minus (door-to-needle) is <1 hour
• No contraindications to fibrinolysis	• Contraindications to fibrinolysis, including increased risk of bleeding and ICH
	• High risk from STEMI (CHF, Killip class is ≥3)
	• Diagnosis of STEMI is in doubt

Modified from ACC/AHA 2004 Update Recommendations.[112]

need to appreciate that other disorders can increase cardiac troponin, eg, myocarditis, congestive heart failure, and pulmonary embolism.

Risk Stratification

Braunwald Stratification

There are many ways to risk-stratify patients with chest pain. A well-recognized approach is the one initially proposed and later refined by Braunwald and colleagues on the ACC/AHA Task Force on the Management of Patients With Unstable Angina.[11,117–120] This approach is based on a combination of historical, clinical, laboratory, and ECG variables.

Table 3 is a modified version of what has been a work in progress by Braunwald and colleagues over several publications.[118,120,121] Patients are initially risk-stratified according to the likelihood that symptoms are due to unstable coronary artery disease (CAD). Patients at intermediate or high risk for CAD are further classified by their risk of MACE. This second classification is useful for prospectively identifying patients at intermediate or high risk who can benefit from an invasive strategy and more aggressive pharmacology with antiplatelet and antithrombin agents.

TIMI Risk Score

The risk of MACE has been further studied and refined. Researchers who derived the important Thrombolysis in Myocardial Ischemia (TIMI) risk score used data from the TIMI-11B and ESSENCE (Efficacy and Safety of Subcutaneous Enoxaparin in Non–Q-Wave Coronary Events) trials for UA/NSTEMI[122,123] and from the In-TIME trial for STEMI.[124] The TIMI risk score comprises 7 independent prognostic variables (Table 4). These 7 variables were significantly associated with the occurrence within 14 days of at least one of the primary end points: death, new or recurrent MI, or need for urgent revascularization. The score is derived from complex multivariate logistic regression and includes variables that seem counterintuitive. It is useful to note that traditional cardiac risk factors are only weakly associated with MACE. Use of aspirin within the previous 7 days, for example, would not seem to be an indicator of a bad outcome. But aspirin use was in fact found to be one of the most powerful predictors.[122] It is possible that aspirin use identified a subgroup of patients at higher risk or on active but failed therapy for CAD.

The creators of the TIMI risk score validated it with 3 groups of patients, and 4 clinical trials showed a significant interaction between the TIMI risk score and outcome.[124–128] These findings confirm the value of the TIMI risk score as a guide to therapeutic decisions. A PDA download of this risk assessment is available at *www.TIMI.org*.

By classifying patients into 1 of 3 risk strata, the Braunwald (Table 3) and TIMI (Table 4) risk scores serve as the dominant clinical guides for predicting the risk of MACE in patients with ACS. Risk stratification is applicable to patients at intermediate or high risk of symptoms due to CAD and not the larger general population of patients presenting with chest pain or symptoms possibly due to anginal equivalents. Risk stratification enables clinicians to direct therapy to those patients at intermediate or high risk of MACE and avoids unnecessary therapy and the potential for adverse consequences in patients who are at lower risk.

The TIMI risk score has become the primary tool for evaluating therapeutic recommendations. Incrementally greater benefit from some of the newer therapies may be gained for patients with higher risk scores.

One additional product of the TIMI trials is the TIMI grading system of coronary artery blood flow. Investigators from the TIMI study developed and validated a coronary artery perfusion scoring system, characterizing the degree of reperfusion of a coronary artery on a scale of 0 (no flow) to 3 (normal, brisk flow). This TIMI grading system is now used as an outcome measure in many studies of ACS interventions.

Indicators for Early Invasive Strategies

Risk stratification (Figure 1, Box 12) helps the clinician identify patients with NSTEMI and UA who should be

TABLE 3. Likelihood of Ischemic Etiology and Short-Term Risk

Part I. Chest Pain Patients Without ST-Segment Elevation: Likelihood of Ischemic Etiology

	A. High likelihood High likelihood that chest pain is of ischemic etiology if patient has *any* of the findings in the column below:	**B. Intermediate likelihood** Intermediate likelihood that chest pain is of ischemic etiology if patient has NO findings in column A and *any* of the findings in the column below:	**C. Low likelihood** Low likelihood that chest pain is of ischemic etiology if patient has NO findings in column A or B. Patients may have any of the findings in the column below:
History	• Chief symptom is chest or left arm pain or discomfort *plus* Current pain reproduces pain of prior documented angina *and* Known CAD, including MI	• Chief symptom is chest or left arm pain or discomfort • Age >70 years • Male sex • Diabetes mellitus	• Probable ischemic symptoms • Recent cocaine use
Physical exam	• Transient mitral regurgitation • Hypotension • Diaphoresis • Pulmonary edema or rales	• Extracardiac vascular disease	• Chest discomfort reproduced by palpation
ECG	• New (or presumed new) transient ST deviation (≥0.5 mm) *or* T-wave inversion (≥2 mm) with symptoms	• Fixed Q waves • Abnormal ST segments *or* T waves that are not new	• Normal ECG *or* T-wave flattening *or* T-wave inversion in leads with dominant R waves
Cardiac markers	• Elevated troponin I or T • Elevated CK-MB	*Any finding in column B above PLUS* • Normal	• Normal

[High (A) or Intermediate (B) Likelihood of Ischemia]

Part II. Risk of Death or Nonfatal MI Over the Short Term in Patients With Chest Pain With High or Intermediate Likelihood of Ischemia (Columns A and B in Part I)

	High risk: Risk is high if patient has *any* of the following findings:	**Intermediate risk:** Risk is intermediate if patient has *any* of the following findings:	**Low risk:** Risk is low if patient has NO high- or intermediate-risk features; may have any of the following:
History	• Accelerating tempo of ischemic symptoms over prior 48 hours	• Prior MI *or* • Peripheral-artery disease *or* • Cerebrovascular disease *or* • CABG, prior aspirin use	
Character of pain	• Prolonged, continuing (>20 min) rest pain	• Prolonged (>20 min) rest angina is now resolved (moderate to high likelihood of CAD) • Rest angina (<20 min) or relieved by rest or sublingual nitrates	• New-onset functional angina (Class III or IV) in past 2 weeks without prolonged rest pain (but with moderate or high likelihood of CAD)
Physical exam	• Pulmonary edema secondary to ischemia • New or worse mitral regurgitation murmur • Hypotension, bradycardia, tachycardia • S_3 gallop or new or worsening rales • Age >75 years	• Age >70 years	
ECG	• Transient ST-segment deviation (≥0.5 mm) with rest angina • New or presumably new bundle branch block • Sustained VT	• T-wave inversion ≥2 mm • Pathologic Q waves or T waves that are not new	• Normal or unchanged ECG during an episode of chest discomfort
Cardiac markers	• Elevated cardiac troponin I or T • Elevated CK-MB	*Any of the above findings PLUS* • Normal	• Normal

Modified from Braunwald et al. *Circulation*. 2002;106:1893–1900.

TABLE 4. TIMI Risk Score for Patients With Unstable Angina and Non–ST-Segment Elevation MI: Predictor Variables

Predictor Variable	Point Value of Variable	Definition
Age ≥65 years	1	
≥3 risk factors for CAD	1	Risk factors • Family history of CAD • Hypertension • Hypercholesterolemia • Diabetes • Current smoker
Aspirin use in last 7 days	1	
Recent, severe symptoms of angina	1	≥2 anginal events in last 24 hours
Elevated cardiac markers	1	CK-MB or cardiac-specific troponin level
ST deviation ≥0.5 mm	1	ST depression ≥0.5 mm is significant; transient ST elevation >0.5 mm for <20 minutes is treated as ST-segment depression and is high risk; ST elevation ≥1 mm for more than 20 minutes places these patients in the STEMI treatment category
Prior coronary artery stenosis ≥50%	1	Risk predictor remains valid even if this information is unknown

Calculated TIMI Risk Score	Risk of ≥1 Primary End Point* in ≤14 Days	Risk Status
0 or 1	5%	Low
2	8%	
3	13%	Intermediate
4	20%	
5	26%	High
6 or 7	41%	

*Primary end points: death, new or recurrent MI, or need for urgent revascularization.

managed with an invasive strategy. Coronary angiography then allows the clinician to determine whether patients are appropriate candidates for revascularization with PCI or coronary artery bypass grafting (CABG).

The *2005 AHA Guidelines for CPR and ECC* define high-risk patients with indicators that overlap to a considerable degree with the more rigorously validated TIMI risk score[122]:

- New ST-segment depression and positive troponins
- Persistent or recurrent symptoms
- Hemodynamic instability or VT
- Depressed LV function (ejection fraction <40%)
- ECG or functional study that suggests multivessel CAD

Normal or Nondiagnostic ECG Changes (Boxes 13 to 17)

The majority of patients with normal or nondiagnostic ECGs do not have ACS. Patients in this category with ACS are most often at low or intermediate risk. The physician's goal involves risk stratification (see above) to provide appropriate diagnostic or treatment strategies for an individual patient. These strategies then target patients at increased risk for benefit while avoiding risk (eg, anticoagulation therapy and invasive cardiac catheterization) in patients with low or minimal risk.

Initial General Therapy for ACS

Several initial measures are appropriate for all patients with suspected ACS in both the out-of-hospital and ED setting. These include immediate oxygen therapy, continuous cardiac monitoring, establishment of intravenous (IV) access, and several medications discussed below.

Oxygen

Administer oxygen to all patients with overt pulmonary congestion or arterial oxygen saturation <90% (Class I). It is also reasonable to administer supplementary oxygen to all patients with ACS for the first 6 hours of therapy (Class IIa). Supplementary oxygen limited ischemic myocardial injury in animals,[31] and oxygen therapy in patients with STEMI reduced the amount of ST-segment elevation.[35] Although a human trial of supplementary oxygen versus room air failed to show a long-term benefit of supplementary oxygen therapy for patients with MI,[30] short-term oxygen administration is beneficial for the patient with unrecognized hypoxemia or unstable pulmonary function. In patients with severe chronic obstructive pulmonary disease, as with any other patient, monitor for hypoventilation.

Aspirin

Early administration of aspirin (acetylsalicylic acid [ASA]), including administration in the out-of-hospital setting,[47] has been associated with decreased mortality rates in several clinical trials.[47,129–131] Multiple studies support the safety of aspirin administration. Therefore, unless the patient has a known aspirin allergy, nonenteric aspirin should be given as soon as possible to all patients with suspected ACS.

Aspirin produces a rapid clinical antiplatelet effect with near-total inhibition of thromboxane A_2 production. It reduces coronary reocclusion and recurrent ischemic events after fibrinolytic therapy. Aspirin alone reduced death from AMI in the Second International Study of Infarct Survival (ISIS-2), and its effect was additive to that of streptokinase.[129] In a review of 145 trials, aspirin was found to substantially reduce vascular events in all patients with AMI, and in high-risk patients it reduced nonfatal AMI and vascular death.[132] Aspirin is also effective in patients with UA. The standard dose (160 to 325 mg) is recommended, although higher doses may be used. Chewable or soluble aspirin is absorbed more quickly than swallowed tablets.[133,134]

The early administration of a single chewed dose of aspirin (160 to 325 mg) is recommended in either the out-of-hospital or ED setting for patients with suspected ACS (Class I). Other formulations of ASA (soluble, IV) may be as effective as chewed tablets. Aspirin suppositories (300 mg) are safe and can be considered for patients with severe nausea, vomiting, or disorders of the upper gastrointestinal tract.

Nitroglycerin (or Glyceryl Trinitrate)

Nitroglycerin is an effective analgesic for ischemic chest discomfort. It also has beneficial hemodynamic effects, including dilation of the coronary arteries (particularly in the region of plaque disruption), the peripheral arterial bed, and venous capacitance vessels. The treatment benefits of nitroglycerin are limited, however, and no conclusive evidence has been shown to support *routine* use of IV, oral, or topical nitrate therapy in patients with AMI.[135] With this in mind, these agents should be carefully considered, especially when low blood pressure precludes the use of other agents shown to be effective in reducing morbidity and mortality (eg, β-blockers and angiotensin-converting enzyme [ACE] inhibitors).

IV nitroglycerin is indicated in the following clinical situations (Class I):

- Ongoing ischemic chest discomfort
- Management of hypertension
- Management of pulmonary congestion

Patients with ischemic discomfort may receive up to 3 doses of sublingual or aerosol nitroglycerin at 3- to 5-minute intervals until pain is relieved or low blood pressure limits its use (Class I). IV nitroglycerin is indicated for ongoing chest discomfort, control of hypertension, or management of pulmonary congestion in patients with STEMI associated with LV failure (Class I). In patients with recurrent ischemia, nitrates are indicated in the first 24 to 48 hours. IV rather than long-acting preparations should be used acutely to enable titration.

Do not use nitrates (Class III) in patients with hypotension (SBP <90 mm Hg or >30 mm Hg below baseline), extreme bradycardia (<50 bpm), or tachycardia (>100 bpm). Administer nitrates with extreme caution if at all to patients with suspected inferior wall MI with possible right ventricular (RV) involvement because these patients require adequate RV preload. Do not administer nitrates (Class III) to patients who have received a phosphodiesterase inhibitor for erectile dysfunction within the last 24 hours (longer for some preparations).

Morphine Sulfate

Morphine sulfate is the analgesic of choice for continuing pain unresponsive to nitrates, and it is also effective in patients with pulmonary vascular congestion complicating ACS. Morphine is a venodilator that reduces ventricular preload and oxygen requirements. For this reason it should not be used in patients who may have hypovolemia. If hypotension develops, elevate the patient's legs, administer volume, and monitor for signs of worsening pulmonary vascular congestion. Start with a 2 to 4 mg IV dose, and give additional doses of 2 to 8 mg IV at 5- to 15-minute intervals.

Reperfusion Therapies (Figure 1, Box 8)

Perhaps the most significant advance in the treatment of cardiovascular disease in the last decade is reperfusion therapy for AMI. Many clinical trials have established early fibrinolytic therapy as a standard of care for patients with AMI who present within 12 hours of the onset of symptoms with no contraindications.[136–140] Reperfusion reduces mortality, and the shorter the time to reperfusion, the greater the benefit: a 47% reduction in mortality was noted when fibrinolytic therapy was provided within the first hour after onset of symptoms.[139,140]

The major determinants of myocardial salvage and long-term prognosis are

- Short time to reperfusion[136,140]
- Complete and sustained patency of the infarct-related artery with normal (TIMI grade 3) flow[141,142]
- Normal microvascular perfusion[116,143–145]

Fibrinolytics

In the absence of contraindications and the presence of a favorable risk-benefit stratification, fibrinolytic therapy is one option for reperfusion in those STEMI patients with onset of symptoms of ≤12 hours and ECG findings of STEMI (elevation >1 mm in 2 or more contiguous precordial or adjacent limb leads or new or presumably new LBBB) (Class I). In the absence of contraindications, it is also reasonable to administer fibrinolytics to patients with onset of symptoms within the prior 12 hours and ECG findings consistent with true posterior MI (Class IIa).

The ED physician should administer fibrinolytics to eligible patients as early as possible according to a predetermined process of care developed by the ED and cardiology staff. The goal is a door-to-needle time of ≤30 minutes. Every effort must be made to minimize the time to therapy. Patients treated within the first 70 minutes of onset of symptoms have >50% reduction in infarct size and 75% reduction in mortality rates.[146] Pooled data from 22 randomized controlled trials of fibrinolytic therapy documents 65 lives saved per 1000 patients treated if fibrinolytics are provided in the first hour and pooled total of 131 lives saved per 1000 patients treated if fibrinolytics are provided within the first 3 hours of onset of symptoms.[147] Fibrinolytics may be beneficial ≤12 hours after onset of symptoms.[148,149]

Fibrinolytic therapy is generally not recommended for patients presenting >12 hours after onset of symptoms, although it may be considered if continuing ischemic pain is present with ST elevation >1 mm in 2 or more contiguous precordial or adjacent limb leads (Class IIa).

Fibrinolytic therapy should not be administered (Class III) to patients who present >24 hours after the onset of symptoms or to patients who show ST-segment depression (unless a true posterior MI is suspected).

Risks of Fibrinolytic Therapy

Physicians who administer fibrinolytic agents should be aware of the indications, contraindications, benefits, and major risks of administration so that they may be able to weigh the net clinical benefit for each patient (see Table 1).[150,151] This net clinical benefit requires integration of relative and absolute contraindications versus overall potential clinical gain.

Patients who present with extensive ECG changes (consistent with a large AMI) and a low risk of intracranial bleeding receive the greatest benefit from fibrinolytic therapy.[136] Patients with symptoms highly suggestive of ACS and ECG findings consistent with LBBB are also appropriate candidates for intervention because they have the highest mortality rate when LBBB is due to extensive AMI. Fibrinolytics have been shown to be beneficial across a spectrum of patient subgroups with comorbidities such as previous MI, diabetes, cardiogenic shock, tachycardia, and hypotension.[136] The benefits of fibrinolytic therapy are less impressive in inferior wall infarction except when it is associated with RV infarction (ST-segment elevation in lead V_4R or anterior ST-segment depression).

Although older patients (>75 years) have a higher absolute risk of death, their absolute benefit appears to be similar to that of younger patients. There is only a small trend for benefit of fibrinolytic therapy administered 12 to 24 hours following the onset of symptoms. The incidence of stroke does increase with advancing age,[152,153] reducing the relative benefit of fibrinolytic therapy. Older age is the most important baseline variable predicting nonhemorrhagic stroke.[152] Although 1 large trial reported lower early and 1-year mortality rates with accelerated administration of tissue plasminogen activator (tPA) in patients <85 years of age,[154] a recent retrospective analysis found no specific survival advantage and possible risk for patients >75 years of age.[155] Additional studies are needed to clarify risk-benefit parameters in the elderly.

The presence of high blood pressure (SBP >175 mm Hg) on presentation to the ED increases the risk of stroke after fibrinolytic therapy.[156] Current clinical practice is directed at lowering blood pressure before administration of fibrinolytic agents, although this has not been shown to reduce the risk of stroke.[156] Fibrinolytic treatment of ACS patients who present with an SBP >180 mm Hg or a diastolic blood pressure >110 mm Hg is relatively contraindicated. Note that this SBP limit is slightly lower than the upper limit of 185 mm Hg used in eligibility criteria for fibrinolytic therapy for acute ischemic stroke; the diastolic limit of 110 mm Hg is consistent with the diastolic limit for tPA administration for stroke (see Part 9: "Adult Stroke").

Several fibrinolytics are available for clinical use, including streptokinase,[129,140,157] anistreplase,[158,159] various regimens of alteplase,[147,160,161] reteplase,[162,163] and tenecteplase.[138,164] Choice of agent is typically based on ease of administration, cost, and preferences of each institution.

Intracranial Hemorrhage

Fibrinolytic therapy is associated with a small but definite increase in the risk of hemorrhagic stroke, which contributes to increased mortality.[136] More intensive fibrinolytic regimens using tPA (alteplase) and heparin pose a greater risk than streptokinase and aspirin.[147,165] Clinical factors that may help risk-stratify patients at the time of presentation are age (≥65 years), low body weight (<70 kg), initial hypertension (≥180/110 mm Hg), and use of tPA. The number of risk factors can be used to estimate the frequency of stroke, which ranges from 0.25% with no risk factors to 2.5% with 3 risk factors.[151] Several risk factor estimates are available for use by clinicians, including Simoons,[151] the Co-Operative Cardiovascular Project,[166] and the In-Time 2 trial.[167]

Percutaneous Coronary Intervention

Coronary angioplasty with or without stent placement is the most common form of PCI. PCI has been shown to be superior to fibrinolysis in combined end points of death, stroke, and reinfarction in many studies.[78,80,82,96,168–173] These results, however, have been achieved in experienced medical environments with skilled providers (performing >75 PCIs per year) at a skilled PCI facility (performing >200 PCIs annually for STEMI, with cardiac surgery capabilities).

At this time primary PCI is preferred in patients with STEMI and symptom duration of >3 and ≤12 hours if skilled personnel can ensure that door-to-balloon time is ≤90 minutes or the difference in time between administration of fibrinolysis versus inflation of the PCI balloon is ≤60 minutes (Class I). PCI is also preferred in patients with contraindications to fibrinolysis and is reasonable in patients with cardiogenic shock or heart failure complicating MI.

In patients with STEMI presenting ≤3 hours from onset of symptoms, treatment is more time-sensitive, and there is inadequate research to recommend one treatment over the other (Class Indeterminate). In these "early presenters," any possible benefit from primary PCI will be lost in prolonged transfers.

Complicated AMI

Cardiogenic Shock, LV Failure, and Congestive Heart Failure

Infarction of ≥40% of the LV myocardium usually results in cardiogenic shock and carries a high mortality rate. Of those who developed shock,[174] patients with ST-segment elevation developed shock significantly earlier than patients without ST-segment elevation.

Cardiogenic shock and congestive heart failure are not contraindications to fibrinolysis, but PCI is preferred if the patient is at a facility with PCI capabilities. The ACC/AHA guidelines note that primary PCI is reasonable in those who develop shock within 36 hours of MI and are suitable candidates for revascularization that can be performed within 18 hours of the onset of shock.[12] In hospitals without PCI facilities, rapidly administer a fibrinolytic agent and transfer the patient to a tertiary care facility where adjunct PCI can be performed if low-output syndromes or ischemia continues.[175] The ACC/AHA STEMI guidelines recommend a door-to-departure time of ≤30 minutes for transfer.[12]

RV Infarction

RV infarction or ischemia may occur in up to 50% of patients with inferior wall MI. The clinician should suspect RV infarction in patients with inferior wall infarction, hypotension, and clear lung fields. In patients with inferior wall infarction, obtain a right-sided or 15-lead ECG; ST-segment elevation (>1 mm) in lead V_4R is sensitive (sensitivity, 88%; specificity, 78%; diagnostic accuracy, 83%) for RV infarction and a strong predictor of increased in-hospital complications and mortality.[176] The in-hospital mortality rate of patients with RV dysfunction is 25% to 30%, and these patients should be routinely considered for reperfusion therapy. Fibrinolytic therapy reduces the incidence of RV dysfunction.[177] Similarly PCI is an alternative for patients with RV infarction and is preferred for patients in shock. Patients with shock caused by RV failure have a mortality rate similar to that for patients with shock due to LV failure.

Patients with RV dysfunction and acute infarction are dependent on maintenance of RV "filling" pressure (RV end-diastolic pressure) to maintain cardiac output.[178] Thus, nitrates, diuretics, and other vasodilators (ACE inhibitors) should be avoided because severe hypotension may result. This hypotension is often easily treated with an IV fluid bolus.

Adjunctive Therapies for ACS and AMI

Clopidogrel

Clopidogrel irreversibly inhibits the platelet adenosine diphosphate receptor, resulting in a reduction in platelet aggregation through a different mechanism than aspirin. Since the publication of the *ECC Guidelines 2000*, several important clopidogrel studies have been published that document its efficacy for patients with both UA/NSTEMI and STEMI.

Clopidogrel was shown to be effective in 2 in-hospital randomized controlled trials (LOE 1)[179,180] and 4 post-hoc analyses (LOE 7).[181–184] In these studies patients with ACS and a rise in cardiac biomarkers or ECG changes consistent with ischemia had reduced stroke and MACE if clopidogrel was added to aspirin and heparin within 4 hours of hospital presentation. One study confirmed that clopidogrel did not increase risk of bleeding in comparison with aspirin.[185] Clopidogrel given 6 hours or more before elective PCI for patients with ACS without ST elevation reduced adverse ischemic events at 28 days (LOE 1).[186]

In patients up to 75 years of age with STEMI who are treated with fibrinolysis, aspirin, and heparin (low-molecular-weight heparin [LMWH] or unfractionated heparin [UFH]), a 300-mg oral loading dose of clopidogrel given at the time of initial management (followed by a 75-mg daily dose for up to 8 days in hospital) improved coronary artery patency and reduced MACE.[187]

The Clopidogrel in Unstable angina to prevent Recurrent ischemic Events (CURE) trial documented an increased rate of bleeding (but not intracranial hemorrhage) in the 2072 patients undergoing CABG within 5 to 7 days of administration of this agent.[184] In addition, a post-hoc analysis of this trial reported a trend toward life-threatening bleeding. A subsequent risk-to-benefit ratio analysis concluded that the bleeding risk with clopidogrel in patients undergoing CABG was modest.[184] One recent large prospective trial (LOE 1)[187] failed to show any increase in bleeding in 136 patients undergoing CABG within 5 to 7 days of administration of clopidogrel. In patients with ACS, the risk of bleeding must be weighed against the risk of perioperative ACS events recurring if these agents are withheld. Current ACC/AHA guidelines, published soon after the large CURE trial, recommend withholding clopidogrel for 5 to 7 days in patients for whom CABG is anticipated.[12] Ongoing studies are evaluating the efficacy and risk-benefit issues.

On the basis of these findings, providers should administer a 300-mg loading dose of clopidogrel in addition to standard care (aspirin, UFH, or LMWH and GP IIb/IIIa inhibitors if indicated) to ED patients with ACS with elevated cardiac markers or new ECG changes consistent with ischemia (excluding STEMI)[184] in whom a medical approach or PCI is planned (Class I). It is reasonable to administer a 300-mg oral dose of clopidogrel to ED patients with suspected ACS (without ECG or cardiac marker changes) who are unable to take aspirin because of hypersensitivity or major gastrointestinal intolerance (Class IIa). Providers should administer a 300-mg oral dose of clopidogrel to ED patients up to 75 years of age with STEMI who receive aspirin, heparin, and fibrinolysis.

β-Adrenergic Receptor Blockers

In-hospital administration of β-blockers reduces the size of the infarct, incidence of cardiac rupture, and mortality in patients who do not receive fibrinolytic therapy.[188–190] They also reduce the incidence of ventricular ectopy and fibrillation.[191,192] In patients who do receive fibrinolytic agents, IV β-blockers decrease postinfarction ischemia and nonfatal AMI. A small but significant decrease in death and nonfatal infarction has been observed in patients treated with β-blockers soon after infarction.[193] IV β-blockers may also be beneficial for NSTEMI ACS.

Oral β-blockers should be administered in the ED for ACS of all types unless contraindications are present. They should be given irrespective of the need for revascularization therapies (Class I). Use IV β-blockers for the treatment of tachyarrhythmias or hypertension (Class IIa).

Contraindications to β-blockers are moderate to severe LV failure and pulmonary edema, bradycardia (<60 bpm), hypotension (SBP <100 mm Hg), signs of poor peripheral perfusion, second-degree or third-degree heart block, or reactive airway disease. In the presence of moderate or severe heart failure, oral β-blockers are preferred. They may need to be given in low and titrated doses after the patient is stabilized. This permits earlier administration of ACE inhibitors that are documented to be efficacious in reducing 30-day mortality rates (see below).

Heparins

Heparin is an indirect inhibitor of thrombin that has been widely used in ACS as adjunctive therapy for fibrinolysis and in combination with aspirin and other platelet inhibitors for the treatment of UA and NSTEMI. UFH is a heterogeneous mixture of sulfated glycosaminoglycans with varying chain lengths. UFH has several disadvantages, including an unpredictable anticoagulant response in individual patients, the need for IV administration, and the requirement for frequent monitoring of the activated partial thromboplastin time (aPTT). Heparin can also stimulate platelet activation, causing thrombocytopenia.[194]

When UFH is used as adjunctive therapy with fibrin-specific lytics in STEMI, the current recommendations call for a bolus dose of 60 U/kg followed by infusion at a rate of 12 U/kg per hour (a maximum bolus of 4000 U and infusion of 1000 U/h for patients weighing >70 kg).[195] An aPTT of 50 to 70 seconds is considered optimal. Because of the limitations of heparin, newer preparations of LMWH have been developed.

Unfractionated Heparin Versus Low-Molecular-Weight Heparin in UA/NSTEMI

Six in-hospital randomized controlled trials (LOE 1[196,197] and LOE 2[130,198,199] <24 hours; LOE 1[200] <36 hours) and additional studies (including 7 meta-analyses [LOE 1[201–207]]) document similar or improved composite outcomes (death, MI and/or recurrent angina, or recurrent ischemia or revascularization) when LMWH is given instead of UFH to patients with UA/NSTEMI within the first 24 to 36 hours after onset of symptoms.

Although major bleeding events are not significantly different with LMWH compared with UFH, there is a consistent increase in minor and postoperative bleeding with the use of LMWH.[208] Omission of LMWH (enoxaparin) on the morning of angiography resulted in vascular complication rates comparable to that of UFH.[209]

Four trials have compared UFH and LMWH in patients with NSTEMI who were treated with a GP IIb/IIIa inhibitor.[210–213] In terms of efficacy, LMWH compared favorably with UFH, and in terms of safety there were similar or less frequent major bleeding events with LMWH but again an increased frequency of minor bleeding complications.

In summary, ED administration of LMWH (specifically enoxaparin) is beneficial compared with UFH when given in addition to antiplatelet therapy such as aspirin for patients with UA/NSTEMI (Class IIb). UFH should be considered if reperfusion is planned in the first 24 to 36 hours after onset of symptoms. Changing from one form of heparin to another (crossover of antithrombin therapy) during an acute event is not recommended because it may lead to an increase in bleeding complications.[214]

Unfractionated Heparin Versus Low-Molecular-Weight Heparin in STEMI

LMWHs have been found to be superior to UFH in patients with STEMI in terms of overall TIMI flow[215,216] and reducing the frequency of ischemic complications,[217] with a trend to a 14% reduction in mortality rates in a meta-analysis.[218] No superiority was found in studies in which an invasive strategy (PCI) was used.

Two randomized controlled trials compared UFH with LMWH as ancillary treatment with fibrinolysis in the out-of-hospital setting.[219,220] Administration of LMWH for patients with STEMI showed superiority in composite end points compared with UFH. This must be balanced against an increase in intracranial hemorrhage in patients >75 years of age who received LMWH (enoxaparin) documented in one of these randomized controlled trials (LOE 2).[220]

LMWH (enoxaparin) is an acceptable alternative to UFH in the ED as ancillary therapy for patients <75 years of age who are receiving fibrinolytic therapy, provided that significant renal dysfunction (serum creatinine >2.5 mg/dL in men or 2 mg/dL in women) is not present (Class IIb). UFH is recommended for patients ≥75 years of age as ancillary therapy to fibrinolysis (Class IIa) and for any STEMI patient who is undergoing revascularization. In patients with STEMI who are not receiving fibrinolysis or revascularization, LMWH (specifically enoxaparin) may be considered an acceptable alternative to UFH in the ED setting (Class IIb).

Glycoprotein IIb/IIIa Inhibitors

After plaque rupture in the coronary artery, tissue factor in the lipid-rich core is exposed and forms complexes with factor VIIa, setting in motion the coagulation cascade resulting in platelet activation. The integrin GP IIb/IIIa receptor is considered the final common pathway to platelet aggregation. GP IIb/IIIa inhibitors modulate this receptor activity. Three agents are available for use: abciximab, eptifibatide, and tirofiban.

GP IIb/IIIa Inhibitors in UA/NSTEMI

Several large studies of GP IIb/IIIa inhibitors in UA/NSTEMI have shown a clear benefit when combined with standard aspirin and heparin and a strategy of mechanical reperfusion (LOE 1[221]; LOE 2[222]; and 3 meta-analyses[221,223,224]). Severe bleeding complications (and no increase in intracranial hemorrhage) in the GP IIb/IIIa group were offset by the large benefit of these agents. The benefit of GP IIb/IIIa inhibitors extends to high-risk patients with UA/NSTEMI treated with PCI.[223]

In UA/NSTEMI patients not treated with PCI, the effect of GP IIb/IIIa inhibitors has been mixed. In 2 studies (LOE 1)[212,221] and 3 meta-analyses (LOE 1),[223–225] GP IIb/IIIa inhibitors produced no mortality advantage and only a slight reduction in recurrent ischemic events in one large meta-analysis[224] but did show a reduction in 30-day mortality in a later, equally large meta-analysis.[225] Of note, the benefit of GP IIb/IIIa inhibitors was dependent on coadministration of UFH or LMWH. Interestingly abciximab appears to behave differently from the other 2 GP IIb/IIIa inhibitors. In the Global Utilization of Streptokinase and Tissue Plasminogen Activator for Occluded Coronary Arteries (GUSTO) IV-ACS trial and 1-year follow-up involving 7800 patients,[226,227] abciximab showed a lack of treatment effect compared with placebo in patients treated medically only.

On the basis of these findings, GP IIb/IIIa inhibitors should be used in patients with high-risk stratification UA/NSTEMI as soon as possible in conjunction with aspirin, heparin, and clopidogrel and a strategy of early PCI (Class I). High-risk features include persistent pain, hemodynamic or rhythm instability, diabetes, acute or dynamic ECG changes, and any elevation in cardiac troponins attributed to cardiac injury. Extrapolation from efficacy studies suggests that this therapy may be administered in the ED once a decision has been made to proceed to PCI (Class IIa).

GP IIb/IIIa inhibitors tirofiban and eptifibatide may be used in patients with high-risk stratification UA/NSTEMI in conjunction with standard therapy if PCI is not planned (Class IIb), although studies are not conclusive at this time. As a result of the lack of benefit demonstrated in the GUSTO IV ACS trial, abciximab should not be given unless PCI is planned (Class III).

GP IIa/IIIb Inhibitors in STEMI

There is insufficient evidence to recommend for or against GP IIb/IIIa inhibitor therapy in STEMI; studies are ongoing. These agents have been used to facilitate antiplatelet therapy in patients undergoing direct PCI, but relatively few patients have been evaluated. GP IIb/IIIa inhibitors are now being evaluated early in STEMI to "facilitate" fibrinolytic therapy and serve as "upstream" adjuncts to planned direct PCI for STEMI, for example, achieving some degree of infarct artery patency during preparation or transfer. One study using abciximab (Facilitated Intervention with Enhanced Reperfusion Speed to Stop Events [*FINESSE*]) is ongoing. Use of these agents in STEMI requires institutional-individualized protocols developed in conjunction with interventional cardiologists.

Calcium Channel Blockers

Calcium channel blocking agents may be added as an alternative or additional therapy if β-blockers are contraindicated or the maximum dose has been achieved.

The 1996 ACC/AHA guidelines for the management of patients with AMI[228] make the following comment about calcium channel blockers:

> Calcium channel blocking agents have not been shown to reduce mortality after acute MI, and in certain patients with cardiovascular disease there is data to suggest that they are harmful. There is concern that these agents are still used too frequently in patients with acute MI and that β-adrenergic receptor blocking agents are a more appropriate choice across a broad spectrum of patients with MI. In general, give calcium antagonists only when β-blockers are contraindicated or have been given at maximum clinical doses without effect (Class Indeterminate).

ACE Inhibitor Therapy

ACE inhibitor therapy has improved survival rates in patients with AMI, particularly when started early.[229–233] Evidence from 7 large clinical trials,[135,232–237] 2 meta-analyses,[238,239] and 10 minor trials[237,240–249] documents consistent improvement in mortality when oral ACE inhibitors are administered in the hospital setting to patients with AMI with or without early reperfusion therapy. In these studies ACE inhibitors were not administered in the presence of hypotension (SBP <100 mm Hg or more than 30 mm Hg below baseline). The beneficial effects are most pronounced in patients with anterior infarction, pulmonary congestion, or LV ejection fraction <40%.

Administration of an oral ACE inhibitor is recommended within the first 24 hours after onset of symptoms in STEMI patients with pulmonary congestion or LV ejection fraction <40%, in the absence of hypotension (SBP <100 mm Hg or more than 30 mm Hg below baseline) (Class I). Oral ACE inhibitor therapy can also be recommended for all other patients with AMI with or without early reperfusion therapy (Class IIa). IV administration of ACE inhibitors is contraindicated in the first 24 hours because of risk of hypotension (Class III).

HMG Coenzyme A Reductase Inhibitors (Statins)

A variety of studies documented consistent reduction in indicators of inflammation and complications such as reinfarction, recurrent angina, and arrhythmias when statin treatment is administered within a few days after onset of an ACS.[250–253] There is little data to suggest that this therapy should be initiated within the ED; however, early initiation (within 24 hours of presentation) of statin therapy is safe and feasible in patients with an ACS or AMI (Class I). If patients are already on statin therapy, continue the therapy (Class IIb).

Glucose-Insulin-Potassium

Although glucose-insulin-potassium (GIK) therapy was formerly thought to reduce the chance of mortality during AMI by several mechanisms, recent clinical trials found that GIK did not show any benefit in STEMI.[254,255] At this time there is little evidence to suggest that this intervention is helpful.

Management of Arrhythmias

This section discusses management of arrhythmias during acute ischemia and infarction.

Ventricular Rhythm Disturbances

Treatment of ventricular arrhythmias during and after AMI has been a controversial topic for 2 decades. Primary VF accounts for the majority of early deaths during AMI.[21–23] The incidence of primary VF is highest during the first 4 hours after onset of symptoms[24–27] but remains an important contributor to mortality during the first 24 hours. Secondary VF occurring in the setting of CHF or cardiogenic shock can also contribute to death from AMI. VF is a less common cause of death in the hospital setting with the early use of fibrinolytics in conjunction with β-blockers.

Although prophylaxis with lidocaine reduces the incidence of VF, an analysis of data from ISIS-3 and a meta-analysis suggest that lidocaine increased all-cause mortality rates.[256] Thus, the practice of prophylactic administration of lidocaine has been largely abandoned.

Routine IV administration of β-blockers to patients without hemodynamic or electrical contraindications is associated with a reduced incidence of primary VF. Low serum potassium but not magnesium has been associated with ventricular arrhythmias. It is prudent clinical practice to maintain serum potassium >4 mEq/L and magnesium >2 mEq/L.

Routine administration of magnesium to patients with MI has no significant clinical mortality benefit, particularly in patients receiving fibrinolytic therapy. The definitive study on the subject is the ISIS-4 study (LOE 1).[135] ISIS-4 enrolled >58 000 patients and showed a trend toward increased mortality rates when magnesium was given in-hospital for primary prophylaxis to patients within the first 4 hours of known or suspected AMI.

Following an episode of VF, there is no conclusive data to support the use of lidocaine or any particular strategy for preventing VF recurrence. β-Blockers are the preferred treatment if not initiated before the episode of VF. If lidocaine is used, continue it for a short time after MI but no more than 24 hours unless symptomatic VT persists. Exacerbating or modulating factors should be identified and corrected. Further management of ventricular rhythm disturbances is discussed in Part 7.2: "Management of Cardiac Arrest" and Part 7.3: "Management of Symptomatic Bradycardia and Tachycardia."

Summary

There has been tremendous progress in reducing disability and death from ACS. But many patients still die before reaching the hospital because patients and family members fail to recognize the signs of ACS and fail to activate the EMS system. Once the patient with ACS contacts the healthcare system, providers must focus on support of cardiorespiratory function, rapid transport, and early classification of the patient based on ECG characteristics. Patients with STEMI require prompt reperfusion; the shorter the interval from symptom onset to reperfusion, the greater the benefit. Patients with UA/NSTEMI or nonspecific or normal ECGs require risk stratification and appropriate monitoring and therapy. Healthcare providers can improve survival rates and myocardial function of patients with ACS by providing skilled, efficient, and coordinated out-of-hospital and in-hospital care.

References

1. Chesebro JH, Rauch U, Fuster V, Badimon JJ. Pathogenesis of thrombosis in coronary artery disease. *Haemostasis*. 1997;27(suppl 1):12–18.
2. Fuster V. Elucidation of the role of plaque instability and rupture in acute coronary events. *Am J Cardiol*. 1995;76:24C–33C.
3. Fuster V, Badimon L, Badimon JJ, Chesebro JH. The pathogenesis of coronary artery disease and the acute coronary syndromes (1). *N Engl J Med*. 1992;326:242–250.
4. Fuster V, Badimon L, Badimon JJ, Chesebro JH. The pathogenesis of coronary artery disease and the acute coronary syndromes (2). *N Engl J Med*. 1992;326:310–318.
5. Fuster V, Fallon JT, Badimon JJ, Nemerson Y. The unstable atherosclerotic plaque: clinical significance and therapeutic intervention. *Thromb Haemost*. 1997;78:247–255.
6. Davies MJ. Anatomic features in victims of sudden coronary death: coronary artery pathology. *Circulation*. 1992;85(suppl I):I-19–I-24.
7. Burke AP, Farb A, Malcom GT, Liang Y, Smialek JE, Virmani R. Plaque rupture and sudden death related to exertion in men with coronary artery disease. *JAMA*. 1999;281:921–926.
8. Farb A, Tang AL, Burke AP, Sessums L, Liang Y, Virmani R. Sudden coronary death: frequency of active coronary lesions, inactive coronary lesions, and myocardial infarction. *Circulation*. 1995;92:1701–1709.
9. Virmani R, Burke AP, Farb A. Plaque morphology in sudden coronary death. *Cardiologia*. 1998;43:267–271.
10. Falk E. Unstable angina with fatal outcome: dynamic coronary thrombosis leading to infarction and/or sudden death: autopsy evidence of recurrent mural thrombosis with peripheral embolization culminating in total vascular occlusion. *Circulation*. 1985;71:699–708.
11. Braunwald E, Antman EM, Beasley JW, Califf RM, Cheitlin MD, Hochman JS, Jones RH, Kereiakes D, Kupersmith J, Levin TN, Pepine CJ, Schaeffer JW, Smith EE III, Steward DE, Theroux P, Gibbons RJ, Alpert JS, Faxon DP, Fuster V, Gregoratos G, Hiratzka LF, Jacobs AK, Smith SC Jr. ACC/AHA 2002 guideline update for the management of patients with unstable angina and non-ST-segment elevation myocardial infarction—summary article: a report of the American College of Cardiology/American Heart Association task force on practice guidelines (Committee on the Management of Patients With Unstable Angina). *J Am Coll Cardiol*. 2002;40:1366–1374.
12. Antman EM, Anbe DT, Armstrong PW, Bates ER, Green LA, Hand M, Hochman JS, Krumholz HM, Kushner FG, Lamas GA, Mullany CJ, Ornato JP, Pearle DL, Sloan MA, Smith SC Jr, Alpert JS, Anderson JL, Faxon DP, Fuster V, Gibbons RJ, Gregoratos G, Halperin JL, Hiratzka LF, Hunt SA, Jacobs AK. ACC/AHA guidelines for the management of patients with ST-elevation myocardial infarction—executive summary: a report of the American College of Cardiology/American Heart Association Task Force on Practice Guidelines (Writing Committee to Revise the 1999 Guidelines for the Management of Patients With Acute Myocardial Infarction). *Circulation*. 2004;110:588–636.
13. Armstrong PW, Bogaty P, Buller CE, Dorian P, O'Neill BJ. The 2004 ACC/AHA Guidelines: a perspective and adaptation for Canada by the Canadian Cardiovascular Society Working Group. *Can J Cardiol*. 2004; 20:1075–1079.
14. Nallamothu BK, Bates ER, Herrin J, Wang Y, Bradley EH, Krumholz HM; NRMI Investigators. Times to treatment in transfer patients undergoing primary percutaneous coronary intervention in the United States: National Registry of Myocardial Infarction (NRMI)-3/4 analysis. *Circulation*. 2005;111:761–767.
15. Douglas PS, Ginsburg GS. The evaluation of chest pain in women. *N Engl J Med*. 1996;334:1311–1315.
16. Solomon CG, Lee TH, Cook EF, Weisberg MC, Brand DA, Rouan GW, Goldman L. Comparison of clinical presentation of acute myocardial infarction in patients older than 65 years of age to younger patients: the Multicenter Chest Pain Study experience. *Am J Cardiol*. 1989;63: 772–776.
17. Peberdy MA, Ornato JP. Coronary artery disease in women. *Heart Dis Stroke*. 1992;1:315–319.
18. Sullivan AK, Holdright DR, Wright CA, Sparrow JL, Cunningham D, Fox KM. Chest pain in women: clinical, investigative, and prognostic features. *BMJ*. 1994;308:883–886.
19. Dempsey SJ, Dracup K, Moser DK. Women's decision to seek care for symptoms of acute myocardial infarction. *Heart Lung*. 1995;24: 444–456.
20. Blohm M, Herlitz J, Schroder U, Hartford M, Karlson BW, Risenfors M, Larsson E, Luepker R, Wennerblom B, Holmberg S. Reaction to a media campaign focusing on delay in acute myocardial infarction. *Heart Lung*. 1991;20:661–666.
21. Pantridge JF, Geddes JS. A mobile intensive-care unit in the management of myocardial infarction. *Lancet*. 1967;2:271–273.
22. Cohen MC, Rohtla KM, Lavery CE, Muller JE, Mittleman MA. Meta-analysis of the morning excess of acute myocardial infarction and sudden cardiac death [published correction appears in *Am J Cardiol*. 1998;81:260]. *Am J Cardiol*. 1997;79:1512–1516.
23. Colquhoun MC, Julien DG. Sudden death in the community: the arrhythmia causing cardiac arrest and results of immediate resuscitation. *Resuscitation*. 1992;24:177A.
24. Campbell RW, Murray A, Julian DG. Ventricular arrhythmias in first 12 hours of acute myocardial infarction: natural history study. *Br Heart J*. 1981;46:351–357.
25. O'Doherty M, Tayler DI, Quinn E, Vincent R, Chamberlain DA. Five hundred patients with myocardial infarction monitored within one hour of symptoms. *BMJ*. 1983;286:1405–1408.
26. Lie KI, Wellens HJ, Downar E, Durrer D. Observations on patients with primary ventricular fibrillation complicating acute myocardial infarction. *Circulation*. 1975;52:755–759.
27. Chiriboga D, Yarzebski J, Goldberg RJ, Gore JM, Alpert JS. Temporal trends (1975 through 1990) in the incidence and case-fatality rates of primary ventricular fibrillation complicating acute myocardial infarction: a communitywide perspective. *Circulation*. 1994;89: 998–1003.

28. The Public Access Defibrillation Trial Investigators. Public-access defibrillation and survival after out-of-hospital cardiac arrest. *N Engl J Med.* 2004;351:637–646.
29. Eisenberg MJ, Topol EJ. Prehospital administration of aspirin in patients with unstable angina and acute myocardial infarction. *Arch Intern Med.* 1996;156:1506–1510.
30. Rawles JM, Kenmure AC. Controlled trial of oxygen in uncomplicated myocardial infarction. *BMJ.* 1976;1:1121–1123.
31. Maroko PR, Radvany P, Braunwald E, Hale SL. Reduction of infarct size by oxygen inhalation following acute coronary occlusion. *Circulation.* 1975;52:360–368.
32. Kelly RF, Hursey TL, Parrillo JE, Schaer GL. Effect of 100% oxygen administration on infarct size and left ventricular function in a canine model of myocardial infarction and reperfusion. *Am Heart J.* 1995;130: 957–965.
33. Radvany P, Maroko PR, Braunwald E. Effects of hypoxemia on the extent of myocardial necrosis after experimental coronary occlusion. *Am J Cardiol.* 1975;35:795–800.
34. Shnier CB, Cason BA, Horton AF, Hickey RF. Hyperoxemic reperfusion does not increase myocardial infarct size. *Am J Physiol.* 1991; 260:H1307–H1312.
35. Madias JE, Madias NE, Hood WB Jr. Precordial ST-segment mapping: 2: effects of oxygen inhalation on ischemic injury in patients with acute myocardial infarction. *Circulation.* 1976;53:411–417.
36. Horvat M, Yoshida S, Prakash R, Marcus HS, Swan HJ, Ganz W. Effect of oxygen breathing on pacing-induced angina pectoris and other manifestations of coronary insufficiency. *Circulation.* 1972;45:837–844.
37. Kenmure AC, Murdoch WR, Beattie AD, Marshall JC, Cameron AJ. Circulatory and metabolic effects of oxygen in myocardial infarction. *BMJ.* 1968;4:360–364.
38. Fillmore SJ, Shapiro M, Killip T. Arterial oxygen tension in acute myocardial infarction: serial analysis of clinical state and blood gas changes. *Am Heart J.* 1970;79:620–629.
39. Bourassa MG, Campeau L, Bois MA, Rico O. The effects of inhalation of 100 percent oxygen on myocardial lactate metabolism in coronary heart disease. *Am J Cardiol.* 1969;24:172–177.
40. Malm A, Arborelius MJ, Bornmyr S, Lilja B, Gill RL. Effects of oxygen on acute myocardial infarction: a thermographic study in the dog. *Cardiovasc Res.* 1977;11:512–518.
41. Sayen JJ, Sheldon WF, Horwitz O, Kuo PT, Peirce G, Zinsser HF, Mead J Jr. Studies of coronary disease in the experimental animal, II: polarographic determinations of local oxygen availability in the dog's left ventricle during coronary occlusion and pure oxygen breathing. *J Clin Invest.* 1951;30:932–940.
42. Sayen JJ, Sheldon WF, Peirce G, Kuo PT. Polarographic oxygen, the epicardial electrocardiogram and muscle contraction in experimental acute regional ischemia of the left ventricle. *Circ Res.* 1958;6:779–798.
43. Rivas F, Rembert JC, Bache RJ, Cobb FR, Greenfield JC Jr. Effect of hyperoxia on regional blood flow after coronary occlusion in awake dogs. *Am J Physiol.* 1980;238:H244–H248.
44. Baron JF, Vicaut E, Hou X, Duvelleroy M. Independent role of arterial O2 tension in local control of coronary blood flow. *Am J Physiol.* 1990;258:H1388–H1394.
45. Haynes BE, Pritting J. A rural emergency medical technician with selected advanced skills. *Prehosp Emerg Care.* 1999;3:343–346.
46. Funk D, Groat C, Verdile VP. Education of paramedics regarding aspirin use. *Prehosp Emerg Care.* 2000;4:62–64.
47. Freimark D, Matetzky S, Leor J, Boyko V, Barbash IM, Behar S, Hod H. Timing of aspirin administration as a determinant of survival of patients with acute myocardial infarction treated with thrombolysis. *Am J Cardiol.* 2002;89:381–385.
48. Verheugt FW, van der Laarse A, Funke-Kupper AJ, Sterkman LG, Galema TW, Roos JP. Effects of early intervention with low-dose aspirin (100 mg) on infarct size, reinfarction and mortality in anterior wall acute myocardial infarction. *Am J Cardiol.* 1990;66:267–270.
49. Held P. Effects of nitrates on mortality in acute myocardial infarction and in heart failure. *Br J Clin Pharmacol.* 1992;34(suppl 1):25S–28S.
50. Tan WA, Moliterno DJ. Aspirin, ticlopidine, and clopidogrel in acute coronary syndromes: underused treatments could save thousands of lives. *Cleve Clin J Med.* 1999;66:615–618, 621–624, 627–628.
51. Access to timely and optimal care of patients with acute coronary syndromes: community planning considerations. A report by the National Heart Attack Alert Program. *J Thromb Thrombolysis.* 1998;6: 19–46.
52. Karagounis L, Ipsen SK, Jessop MR, Gilmore KM, Valenti DA, Clawson JJ, Teichman S, Anderson JL. Impact of field-transmitted electrocardiography on time to in-hospital thrombolytic therapy in acute myocardial infarction. *Am J Cardiol.* 1990;66:786–791.
53. Grim P, Feldman T, Martin M, Donovan R, Nevins V, Childers RW. Cellular telephone transmission of 12-lead electrocardiograms from ambulance to hospital. *Am J Cardiol.* 1987;60:715–720.
54. Kudenchuk PJ, Ho MT, Weaver WD, Litwin PE, Martin JS, Eisenberg MS, Hallstrom AP, Cobb LA, Kennedy JW. Accuracy of computer-interpreted electrocardiography in selecting patients for thrombolytic therapy. MITI Project Investigators. *J Am Coll Cardiol.* 1991;17: 1486–1491.
55. Kereiakes DJ, Gibler WB, Martin LH, Pieper KS, Anderson LC. Relative importance of emergency medical system transport and the prehospital electrocardiogram on reducing hospital time delay to therapy for acute myocardial infarction: a preliminary report from the Cincinnati Heart Project. *Am Heart J.* 1992;123(pt 1):835–840.
56. Foster DB, Dufendach JH, Barkdoll CM, Mitchell BK. Prehospital recognition of AMI using independent nurse/paramedic 12-lead ECG evaluation: impact on in-hospital times to thrombolysis in a rural community hospital. *Am J Emerg Med.* 1994;12:25–31.
57. Aufderheide TP, Kereiakes DJ, Weaver WD, Gibler WB, Simoons ML. Planning, implementation, and process monitoring for prehospital 12-lead ECG diagnostic programs. *Prehospital Disaster Med.* 1996;11: 162–171.
58. Aufderheide TP, Hendley GE, Woo J, Lawrence S, Valley V, Teichman SL. A prospective evaluation of prehospital 12-lead ECG application in chest pain patients. *J Electrocardiol.* 1992;24(suppl):8–13.
59. Weaver W, Cerqueira M, Hallstrom A, Litwin P, Martin J, Kudenchuk P, Eisenberg M. Prehospital-initiated vs hospital-initiated thrombolytic therapy: the Myocardial Infarction Triage and Intervention Trial (MITI). *JAMA.* 1993;270:1203–1210.
60. Canto JG, Rogers WJ, Bowlby LJ, French WJ, Pearce DJ, Weaver WD. The prehospital electrocardiogram in acute myocardial infarction: is its full potential being realized? National Registry of Myocardial Infarction 2 Investigators. *J Am Coll Cardiol.* 1997;29:498–505.
61. Banerjee S, Rhoden WE. Fast-tracking of myocardial infarction by paramedics. *J R Coll Physicians Lond.* 1998;32:36–38.
62. Melville MR, Gray D, et al. The potential impact of prehospital electrocardiography and telemetry on time to thrombolysis in a United Kingdom center. *Ann Noninvasive Electrocardiol.* 1998;3:327–333.
63. Millar-Craig MW, Joy AV, Adamowicz M, Furber R, Thomas B. Reduction in treatment delay by paramedic ECG diagnosis of myocardial infarction with direct CCU admission. *Heart.* 1997;78:456–461.
64. Wall T, Albright J, Livingston B, Isley L, Young D, Nanny M, Jacobowitz S, Maynard C, Mayer N, Pierce K, Rathbone C, Stuckey T, Savona M, Leibrandt P, Brodie B, Wagner G. Prehospital ECG transmission speeds reperfusion for patients with acute myocardial infarction. *N C Med J.* 2000;61:104–108.
65. Aufderheide TP, Hendley GE, Thakur RK, Mateer JR, Stueven HA, Olson DW, Hargarten KM, Laitinen F, Robinson N, Preuss KC, et al. The diagnostic impact of prehospital 12-lead electrocardiography. *Ann Emerg Med.* 1990;19:1280–1287.
66. Grim PS, Feldman T, Childers RW. Evaluation of patients for the need of thrombolytic therapy in the prehospital setting. *Ann Emerg Med.* 1989;18:483–488.
67. Weaver WD, Cerqueira M, Hallstrom AP, Litwin PE, Martin JS, Kudenchuk PJ, Eisenberg M. Prehospital-initiated vs hospital-initiated thrombolytic therapy. The Myocardial Infarction Triage and Intervention Trial. *JAMA.* 1993;270:1211–1216.
68. Aufderheide TP, Haselow WC, Hendley GE, Robinson NA, Armaganian L, Hargarten KM, Olson DW, Valley VT, Stueven HA. Feasibility of prehospital r-TPA therapy in chest pain patients. *Ann Emerg Med.* 1992;21:379–383.
69. Brinfield K. Identification of ST elevation AMI on prehospital 12 lead ECG: accuracy of unaided paramedic interpretation. *J Emerg Med.* 1998;16:22S.
70. Ioannidis JP, Salem D, Chew PW, Lau J. Accuracy and clinical effect of out-of-hospital electrocardiography in the diagnosis of acute cardiac ischemia: a meta-analysis. *Ann Emerg Med.* 2001;37:461–470.
71. Prehospital thrombolytic therapy in patients with suspected acute myocardial infarction. The European Myocardial Infarction Project Group. *N Engl J Med.* 1993;329:383–389.

72. Morrison LJ, Verbeek PR, McDonald AC, Sawadsky BV, Cook DJ. Mortality and prehospital thrombolysis for acute myocardial infarction: a meta-analysis. *JAMA*. 2000;283:2686–2692.
73. GREAT. Feasibility, safety, and efficacy of domiciliary thrombolysis by general practitioners: Grampian region early anistreplase trial. GREAT Group. *BMJ*. 1992;305:548–553.
74. Dussoix P, Reuille O, Verin V, Gaspoz JM, Unger PF. Time savings with prehospital thrombolysis in an urban area. *Eur J Emerg Med*. 2003;10:2–5.
75. Rawles J. Halving of mortality at 1 year by domiciliary thrombolysis in the Grampian Region Early Anistreplase Trial (GREAT). *J Am Coll Cardiol*. 1994;23:1–5.
76. Rawles JM. Quantification of the benefit of earlier thrombolytic therapy: five-year results of the Grampian Region Early Anistreplase Trial (GREAT). *J Am Coll Cardiol*. 1997;30:1181–1186.
77. American Heart Association in collaboration with International Liaison Committee on Resuscitation. Guidelines 2000 for Cardiopulmonary Resuscitation and Emergency Cardiovascular Care: International Consensus on Science, Part 7: the Era of Reperfusion: Section 1: Acute Coronary Syndromes (Acute Myocardial Infarction). *Circulation*. 2000; 102(suppl I):I-172–I-203.
78. Andersen HR, Nielsen TT, Rasmussen K, Thuesen L, Kelbaek H, Thayssen P, Abildgaard U, Pedersen F, Madsen JK, Grande P, Villadsen AB, Krusell LR, Haghfelt T, Lomholt P, Husted SE, Vigholt E, Kjaergard HK, Mortensen LS. A comparison of coronary angioplasty with fibrinolytic therapy in acute myocardial infarction. *N Engl J Med*. 2003;349:733–742.
79. Widimsky P, Groch L, Zelizko M, Aschermann M, Bednar F, Suryapranata H. Multicentre randomized trial comparing transport to primary angioplasty vs immediate thrombolysis vs combined strategy for patients with acute myocardial infarction presenting to a community hospital without a catheterization laboratory. The PRAGUE Study. *Eur Heart J*. 2000;21:823–831.
80. Widimsky P, Budesinsky T, Vorac D, Groch L, Zelizko M, Aschermann M, Branny M, St'asek J, Formanek P. Long distance transport for primary angioplasty vs immediate thrombolysis in acute myocardial infarction: final results of the randomized national multicentre trial–PRAGUE-2. *Eur Heart J*. 2003;24:94–104.
81. Bonnefoy E, Lapostolle F, Leizorovicz A, Steg G, McFadden EP, Dubien PY, Cattan S, Boullenger E, Machecourt J, Lacroute JM, Cassagnes J, Dissait F, Touboul P, Comparison of Angioplasty and Prehospital Thrombolysis in Acute Myocardial Infarction Study Group. Primary angioplasty versus prehospital fibrinolysis in acute myocardial infarction: a randomised study. *Lancet*. 2002;360:825–829.
82. Dalby M, Bouzamondo A, Lechat P, Montalescot G. Transfer for primary angioplasty versus immediate thrombolysis in acute myocardial infarction: a meta-analysis. *Circulation*. 2003;108:1809–1814.
83. Steg PG, Bonnefoy E, Chabaud S, Lapostolle F, Dubien PY, Cristofini P, Leizorovicz A, Touboul P, Comparison of Angioplasty and Prehospital Thrombolysis in Acute Myocardial Infarction Study Group. Impact of time to treatment on mortality after prehospital fibrinolysis or primary angioplasty: data from the CAPTIM randomized clinical trial. *Circulation*. 2003;108:2851–2856.
84. Berger PB, Ellis SG, Holmes DR Jr, Granger CB, Criger DA, Betriu A, Topol EJ, Califf RM. Relationship between delay in performing direct coronary angioplasty and early clinical outcome in patients with acute myocardial infarction: results from the global use of strategies to open occluded arteries in Acute Coronary Syndromes (GUSTO-IIb) trial. *Circulation*. 1999;100:14–20.
85. Canto JG, Every NR, Magid DJ, Rogers WJ, Malmgren JA, Frederick PD, French WJ, Tiefenbrunn AJ, Misra VK, Kiefe CI, Barron HV. The volume of primary angioplasty procedures and survival after acute myocardial infarction. *N Engl J Med*. 2000;342:1573–1580.
86. Immediate vs delayed catheterization and angioplasty following thrombolytic therapy for acute myocardial infarction. TIMI II A results. The TIMI Research Group. *JAMA*. 1988;260:2849–2858.
87. Simoons ML, Arnold AE, Betriu A, de Bono DP, Col J, Dougherty FC, von Essen R, Lambertz H, Lubsen J, Meier B, et al. Thrombolysis with tissue plasminogen activator in acute myocardial infarction: no additional benefit from immediate percutaneous coronary angioplasty. *Lancet*. 1988;1:197–203.
88. Topol EJ, Califf RM, George BS, Kereiakes DJ, Abbottsmith CW, Candela RJ, Lee KL, Pitt B, Stack RS, O'Neill WW. A randomized trial of immediate versus delayed elective angioplasty after intravenous tissue plasminogen activator in acute myocardial infarction. *N Engl J Med*. 1987;317:581–588.
89. Michels KB, Yusuf S. Does PTCA in acute myocardial infarction affect mortality and reinfarction rates? A quantitative overview (meta-analysis) of the randomized clinical trials. *Circulation*. 1995;91:476–485.
90. Topol EJ. Thrombolytic or angioplasty therapy of evolving myocardial infarction? *J Thromb Thrombolysis*. 1998;5:S125–S131.
91. Jovell AJ, Lau J, Berkey C, Kupelnick B, Chalmers TC. Early angiography and angioplasty following thrombolytic therapy of acute myocardial infarction: metaanalysis of the randomized control trials. *Online J Curr Clin Trials*. 1993; Document No 67.
92. Califf RM, Topol EJ, Stack RS, Ellis SG, George BS, Kereiakes DJ, Samaha JK, Worley SJ, Anderson JL, Harrelson-Woodlief L, Wall TC, Phillips HR III, Abbottsmith CW, Candela RJ, Flanagan WH, Sasahara AA, Mantell SJ, Lee KL. Evaluation of combination thrombolytic therapy and timing of cardiac catheterization in acute myocardial infarction: results of thrombolysis and angioplasty in myocardial infarction—Phase 5 randomized trial. *Circulation*. 1991;83:1543–1556.
93. Fernandez-Aviles F, Alonso JJ, Castro-Beiras A, Vazquez N, Blanco J, Alonso-Briales J, Lopez-Mesa J, Fernandez-Vazquez F, Calvo I, Martinez-Elbal L, San Roman JA, Ramos B. Routine invasive strategy within 24 hours of thrombolysis versus ischaemia-guided conservative approach for acute myocardial infarction with ST-segment elevation (GRACIA-1): a randomised controlled trial. *Lancet*. 2004;364: 1045–1053.
94. Bednar F, Widimsky P, Krupicka J, Groch L, Aschermann M, Zelizko M. Interhospital transport for primary angioplasty improves the long-term outcome of acute myocardial infarction compared with immediate thrombolysis in the nearest hospital (one-year follow-up of the PRAGUE-1 study). *Can J Cardiol*. 2003;19:1133–1137.
95. Tiefenbrunn AJ, Chandra NC, French WJ, Gore JM, Rogers WJ. Clinical experience with primary percutaneous transluminal coronary angioplasty compared with alteplase (recombinant tissue-type plasminogen activator) in patients with acute myocardial infarction: a report from the Second National Registry of Myocardial Infarction (NRMI- 2). *J Am Coll Cardiol*. 1998;31:1240–1245.
96. Hochman JS, Sleeper LA, Webb JG, Sanborn TA, White HD, Talley JD, Buller CE, Jacobs AK, Slater JN, Col J, McKinlay SM, LeJemtel TH. Early revascularization in acute myocardial infarction complicated by cardiogenic shock. SHOCK Investigators. Should We Emergently Revascularize Occluded Coronaries for Cardiogenic Shock. *N Engl J Med*. 1999;341:625–634.
97. Hochman JS, Sleeper LA, White HD, Dzavik V, Wong SC, Menon V, Webb JG, Steingart R, Picard MH, Menegus MA, Boland J, Sanborn T, Buller CE, Modur S, Forman R, Desvigne-Nickens P, Jacobs AK, Slater JN, LeJemtel TH. One-year survival following early revascularization for cardiogenic shock. *JAMA*. 2001;285:190–192.
98. Emergency department: rapid identification and treatment of patients with acute myocardial infarction. National Heart Attack Alert Program Coordinating Committee, 60 Minutes to Treatment Working Group. *Ann Emerg Med*. 1994;23:311–329.
99. Lambrew CT, Bowlby LJ, Rogers WJ, Chandra NC, Weaver WD. Factors influencing the time to thrombolysis in acute myocardial infarction. Time to Thrombolysis Substudy of the National Registry of Myocardial Infarction-1. *Arch Intern Med*. 1997;157:2577–2582.
100. Bleeker JK, Simoons ML, Erdman RA, Leenders CM, Kruyssen HA, Lamers LM, van der Does E. Patient and doctor delay in acute myocardial infarction: a study in Rotterdam, The Netherlands. *Br J Gen Pract*. 1995;45:181–184.
101. Goldberg RJ, McGovern PG, Guggina T, Savageau J, Rosamond WD, Luepker RV. Prehospital delay in patients with acute coronary heart disease: concordance between patient interviews and medical records. *Am Heart J*. 1998;135(pt 1):293–299.
102. Goodacre SW, Angelini K, Arnold J, Revill S, Morris F. Clinical predictors of acute coronary syndromes in patients with undifferentiated chest pain. *QJM*. 2003;96:893–898.
103. Goodacre S, Locker T, Morris F, Campbell S. How useful are clinical features in the diagnosis of acute, undifferentiated chest pain? *Acad Emerg Med*. 2002;9:203–208.
104. Everts B, Karlson BW, Wahrborg P, Hedner T, Herlitz J. Localization of pain in suspected acute myocardial infarction in relation to final diagnosis, age and sex, and site and type of infarction. *Heart Lung*. 1996;25:430–437.

105. McSweeney JC, Cody M, O'Sullivan P, Elberson K, Moser DK, Garvin BJ. Women's early warning symptoms of acute myocardial infarction. *Circulation.* 2003;108:2619–2623.
106. Antman EM, Tanasijevic MJ, Thompson B, Schactman M, McCabe CH, Cannon CP, Fischer GA, Fung AY, Thompson C, Wybenga D, Braunwald E. Cardiac-specific troponin I levels to predict the risk of mortality in patients with acute coronary syndromes. *N Engl J Med.* 1996;335:1342–1349.
107. Svensson L, Axelsson C, Nordlander R, Herlitz J. Elevation of biochemical markers for myocardial damage prior to hospital admission in patients with acute chest pain or other symptoms raising suspicion of acute coronary syndrome. *J Intern Med.* 2003;253:311–319.
108. Gust R, Gust A, Bottiger BW, Bohrer H, Martin E. Bedside troponin T testing is not useful for early out-of-hospital diagnosis of myocardial infarction. *Acta Anaesthesiol Scand.* 1998;42:414–417.
109. Newman J, Aulick N, Cheng T, Faynor S, Curtis R, Mercer D, Williams J, Hobbs G. Prehospital identification of acute coronary ischemia using a troponin T rapid assay. *Prehosp Emerg Care.* 1999;3:97–101.
110. Svensson L, Axelsson C, Nordlander R, Herlitz J. Prognostic value of biochemical markers, 12-lead ECG and patient characteristics amongst patients calling for an ambulance due to a suspected acute coronary syndrome. *J Intern Med.* 2004;255:469–477.
111. Schuchert A, Hamm C, Scholz J, Klimmeck S, Goldmann B, Meinertz T. Prehospital testing for troponin T in patients with suspected acute myocardial infarction. *Am Heart J.* 1999;138:45–48.
112. Tanaka K, Seino Y, Ohbayashi K, Takano T. Cardiac emergency triage and therapeutic decisions using whole blood rapid troponin T test for patients with suspicious acute coronary syndrome. *Jpn Circ J.* 2001;65: 424–428.
113. Ng SM, Krishnaswamy P, Morrissey R, Clopton P, Fitzgerald R, Maisel AS. Ninety-minute accelerated critical pathway for chest pain evaluation. *Am J Cardiol.* 2001;88:611–617.
114. Ng SM, Krishnaswamy P, Morrisey R, Clopton P, Fitzgerald R, Maisel AS. Mitigation of the clinical significance of spurious elevations of cardiac troponin I in settings of coronary ischemia using serial testing of multiple cardiac markers. *Am J Cardiol.* 2001;87:994–999.
115. al-Mubarak N, Rogers WJ, Lambrew CT, Bowlby LJ, French WJ. Consultation before thrombolytic therapy in acute myocardial infarction. Second National Registry of Myocardial Infarction (NRMI 2) Investigators. *Am J Cardiol.* 1999;83:89–93.
116. Topol EJ. Inflammation and embolization in ischemic heart disease. *J Invasive Cardiol.* 2000;12(suppl B):2B–7B.
117. Braunwald E, Antman EM, Beasley JW, Califf RM, Cheitlin MD, Hochman JS, Jones RH, Kereiakes D, Kupersmith J, Levin TN, Pepine CJ, Schaeffer JW, Smith EE III, Steward DE, Theroux P, Gibbons RJ, Alpert JS, Faxon DP, Fuster V, Gregoratos G, Hiratzka LF, Jacobs AK, Smith SC Jr. ACC/AHA guideline update for the management of patients with unstable angina and non-ST-segment elevation myocardial infarction—2002: summary article: a report of the American College of Cardiology/American Heart Association Task Force on Practice Guidelines (Committee on the Management of Patients With Unstable Angina). *Circulation.* 2002;106:1893–1900.
118. Braunwald E, Antman EM, Beasley JW, Califf RM, Cheitlin MD, Hochman JS, Jones RH, Kereiakes D, Kupersmith J, Levin TN, Pepine CJ, Schaeffer JW, Smith EE III, Steward DE, Theroux P, Alpert JS, Eagle KA, Faxon DP, Fuster V, Gardner TJ, Gregoratos G, Russell RO, Smith SC Jr. ACC/AHA guidelines for the management of patients with unstable angina and non-ST-segment elevation myocardial infarction: a report of the American College of Cardiology/American Heart Association Task Force on Practice Guidelines (Committee on the Management of Patients With Unstable Angina). *J Am Coll Cardiol.* 2000; 36:970–1062.
119. Effects of tissue plasminogen activator and a comparison of early invasive and conservative strategies in unstable angina and non-Q-wave myocardial infarction: results of the TIMI IIIB Trial. Thrombolysis in Myocardial Ischemia. *Circulation.* 1994;89:1545–1556.
120. Scanlon PJ, Faxon DP, Audet AM, Carabello B, Dehmer GJ, Eagle KA, Legako RD, Leon DF, Murray JA, Nissen SE, Pepine CJ, Watson RM, Ritchie JL, Gibbons RJ, Cheitlin MD, Gardner TJ, Garson A Jr, Russell RO Jr, Ryan TJ, Smith SC Jr. ACC/AHA guidelines for coronary angiography: executive summary and recommendations: a report of the American College of Cardiology/American Heart Association Task Force on Practice Guidelines (Committee on Coronary Angiography) developed in collaboration with the Society for Cardiac Angiography and Interventions. *Circulation.* 1999;99:2345–2357.
121. Alpert JS, Thygesen K, Antman E, Bassand JP. Myocardial infarction redefined—a consensus document of the Joint European Society of Cardiology/American College of Cardiology Committee for the redefinition of myocardial infarction. *J Am Coll Cardiol.* 2000;36:959–969.
122. Guideline for the management of patients with acute coronary syndromes without persistent ECG ST segment elevation. British Cardiac Society Guidelines and Medical Practice Committee and Royal College of Physicians Clinical Effectiveness and Evaluation Unit. *Heart.* 2001; 85:133–142.
123. Clinical policy: critical issues in the evaluation and management of adult patients presenting with suspected acute myocardial infarction or unstable angina. American College of Emergency Physicians. *Ann Emerg Med.* 2000;35:521–525.
124. Doukky R, Calvin JE. Risk stratification in patients with unstable angina and non-ST segment elevation myocardial infarction: evidence-based review. *J Invasive Cardiol.* 2002;14:215–220.
125. Doukky R, Calvin JE. Part II: risk stratification in patients with unstable angina and non-ST segment elevation myocardial infarction: evidence-based review. *J Invasive Cardiol.* 2002;14:254–262.
126. Braunwald E, Jones RH, Mark DB, Brown J, Brown L, Cheitlin MD, Concannon CA, Cowan M, Edwards C, Fuster V, et al. Diagnosing and managing unstable angina. Agency for Health Care Policy and Research. *Circulation.* 1994;90:613–622.
127. Antman EM, Cohen M, Bernink PJ, McCabe CH, Horacek T, Papuchis G, Mautner B, Corbalan R, Radley D, Braunwald E. The TIMI risk score for unstable angina/non-ST elevation MI: a method for prognostication and therapeutic decision making. *JAMA.* 2000;284:835–842.
128. Smith SC Jr, Dove JT, Jacobs AK, Kennedy JW, Kereiakes D, Kern MJ, Kuntz RE, Popma JJ, Schaff HV, Williams DO, Gibbons RJ, Alpert JP, Eagle KA, Faxon DP, Fuster V, Gardner TJ, Gregoratos G, Russell RO. ACC/AHA guidelines for percutaneous coronary intervention (revision of the 1993 PTCA guidelines) executive summary: a report of the American College of Cardiology/American Heart Association task force on practice guidelines (Committee to revise the 1993 guidelines for percutaneous transluminal coronary angioplasty) endorsed by the Society for Cardiac Angiography and Interventions. *Circulation.* 2001; 103:3019–3041.
129. Randomised trial of intravenous streptokinase, oral aspirin, both, or neither among 17,187 cases of suspected acute myocardial infarction: ISIS-2. ISIS-2 (Second International Study of Infarct Survival) Collaborative Group. *Lancet.* 1988;2:349–360.
130. Gurfinkel EP, Manos EJ, Mejail RI, Cerda MA, Duronto EA, Garcia CN, Daroca AM, Mautner B. Low molecular weight heparin versus regular heparin or aspirin in the treatment of unstable angina and silent ischemia. *J Am Coll Cardiol.* 1995;26:313–318.
131. Collaborative meta-analysis of randomised trials of antiplatelet therapy for prevention of death, myocardial infarction, and stroke in high risk patients. *BMJ.* 2002;324:71–86.
132. Collaborative overview of randomised trials of antiplatelet therapy–I: prevention of death, myocardial infarction, and stroke by prolonged antiplatelet therapy in various categories of patients. Antiplatelet Trialists' Collaboration [published correction appears in *BMJ.* 1994;308: 1540]. *BMJ.* 1994;308:81–106.
133. Feldman M, Cryer B. Aspirin absorption rates and platelet inhibition times with 325-mg buffered aspirin tablets (chewed or swallowed intact) and with buffered aspirin solution. *Am J Cardiol.* 1999;84:404–409.
134. Sagar KA, Smyth MR. A comparative bioavailability study of different aspirin formulations using on-line multidimensional chromatography. *J Pharm Biomed Anal.* 1999;21:383–392.
135. ISIS-4: a randomised factorial trial assessing early oral captopril, oral mononitrate, and intravenous magnesium sulphate in 58,050 patients with suspected acute myocardial infarction. ISIS-4 (Fourth International Study of Infarct Survival) Collaborative Group. *Lancet.* 1995;345: 669–685.
136. Indications for fibrinolytic therapy in suspected acute myocardial infarction: collaborative overview of early mortality and major morbidity results from all randomised trials of more than 1000 patients. Fibrinolytic Therapy Trialists' (FTT) Collaborative Group. *Lancet.* 1994;343:311–322.
137. A comparison of reteplase with alteplase for acute myocardial infarction. The Global Use of Strategies to Open Occluded Coronary Arteries (GUSTO III) Investigators. *N Engl J Med.* 1997;337:1118–1123.
138. Single-bolus tenecteplase compared with front-loaded alteplase in acute myocardial infarction: the ASSENT-2 double-blind randomised trial.

Assessment of the Safety and Efficacy of a New Thrombolytic Investigators. *Lancet.* 1999;354:716–722.

139. Franzosi MG, Santoro E, De Vita C, Geraci E, Lotto A, Maggioni AP, Mauri F, Rovelli F, Santoro L, Tavazzi L, Tognoni G. Ten-year follow-up of the first megatrial testing thrombolytic therapy in patients with acute myocardial infarction: results of the Gruppo Italiano per lo Studio della Sopravvivenza nell'Infarto-1 study. The GISSI Investigators. *Circulation.* 1998;98:2659–2665.

140. Effectiveness of intravenous thrombolytic treatment in acute myocardial infarction. Gruppo Italiano per lo Studio della Streptochinasi nell'Infarto Miocardico (GISSI). *Lancet.* 1986;1:397–402.

141. Brodie BR, Stuckey TD, Kissling G, Hansen CJ, Weintraub RA, Kelly TA. Importance of infarct-related artery patency for recovery of left ventricular function and late survival after primary angioplasty for acute myocardial infarction. *J Am Coll Cardiol.* 1996;28:319–325.

142. Puma JA, Sketch MHJ, Thompson TD, Simes RJ, Morris DC, White HD, Topol EJ, Califf RM. Support for the open-artery hypothesis in survivors of acute myocardial infarction: analysis of 11,228 patients treated with thrombolytic therapy. *Am J Cardiol.* 1999;83:482–487.

143. de Lemos JA, Antman EM, Gibson CM, McCabe CH, Giugliano RP, Murphy SA, Coulter SA, Anderson K, Scherer J, Frey MJ, Van Der Wieken R, Van De Werf F, Braunwald E. Abciximab improves both epicardial flow and myocardial reperfusion in ST-elevation myocardial infarction: observations from the TIMI 14 trial. *Circulation.* 2000;101: 239–243.

144. Claeys MJ, Bosmans J, Veenstra L, Jorens P, De R, Vrints CJ. Determinants and prognostic implications of persistent ST-segment elevation after primary angioplasty for acute myocardial infarction: importance of microvascular reperfusion injury on clinical outcome. *Circulation.* 1999; 99:1972–1977.

145. Gibson CM, Murphy SA, Rizzo MJ, Ryan KA, Marble SJ, McCabe CH, Cannon CP, Van de Werf F, Braunwald E. Relationship between TIMI frame count and clinical outcomes after thrombolytic administration. Thrombolysis In Myocardial Infarction (TIMI) Study Group. *Circulation.* 1999;99:1945–1950.

146. Brouwer MA, Martin JS, Maynard C, Wirkus M, Litwin PE, Verheugt FW, Weaver WD. Influence of early prehospital thrombolysis on mortality and event-free survival (the Myocardial Infarction Triage and Intervention [MITI] Randomized Trial). MITI Project Investigators. *Am J Cardiol.* 1996;78:497–502.

147. An international randomized trial comparing four thrombolytic strategies for acute myocardial infarction. The GUSTO investigators. *N Engl J Med.* 1993;329:673–682.

148. Randomised trial of late thrombolysis in patients with suspected acute myocardial infarction. EMERAS (Estudio Multicentrico Estreptoquinasa Republicas de America del Sur) Collaborative Group. *Lancet.* 1993;342:767–772.

149. Late Assessment of Thrombolytic Efficacy (LATE) study with alteplase 6–24 hours after onset of acute myocardial infarction. *Lancet.* 1993; 342:759–766.

150. Hillis LD, Forman S, Braunwald E. Risk stratification before thrombolytic therapy in patients with acute myocardial infarction. The Thrombolysis in Myocardial Infarction (TIMI) Phase II Co-Investigators. *J Am Coll Cardiol.* 1990;16:313–315.

151. Simoons ML, Maggioni AP, Knatterud G, Leimberger JD, de Jaegere P, van Domburg R, Boersma E, Franzosi MG, Califf R, Schroder R, et al. Individual risk assessment for intracranial haemorrhage during thrombolytic therapy. *Lancet.* 1993;342:1523–1528.

152. Mahaffey KW, Granger CB, Sloan MA, Thompson TD, Gore JM, Weaver WD, White HD, Simoons ML, Barbash GI, Topol EJ, Califf RM. Risk factors for in-hospital nonhemorrhagic stroke in patients with acute myocardial infarction treated with thrombolysis: results from GUSTO-I. *Circulation.* 1998;97:757–764.

153. Gore JM, Granger CB, Simoons ML, Sloan MA, Weaver WD, White HD, Barbash GI, Van de Werf F, Aylward PE, Topol EJ, et al. Stroke after thrombolysis: mortality and functional outcomes in the GUSTO-I trial. Global Use of Strategies to Open Occluded Coronary Arteries. *Circulation.* 1995;92:2811–2818.

154. White HD, Barbash GI, Califf RM, Simes RJ, Granger CB, Weaver WD, Kleiman NS, Aylward PE, Gore JM, Vahanian A, Lee KL, Ross AM, Topol EJ. Age and outcome with contemporary thrombolytic therapy: results from the GUSTO-I trial. Global Utilization of Streptokinase and TPA for Occluded coronary arteries trial. *Circulation.* 1996;94: 1826–1833.

155. Thiemann DR, Coresh J, Schulman SP, Gerstenblith G, Oetgen WJ, Powe NR. Lack of benefit for intravenous thrombolysis in patients with myocardial infarction who are older than 75 years. *Circulation.* 2000; 101:2239–2246.

156. Aylward PE, Wilcox RG, Horgan JH, White HD, Granger CB, Califf RM, Topol EJ. Relation of increased arterial blood pressure to mortality and stroke in the context of contemporary thrombolytic therapy for acute myocardial infarction: a randomized trial. GUSTO-I Investigators. *Ann Intern Med.* 1996;125:891–900.

157. Kennedy JW, Martin GV, Davis KB, Maynard C, Stadius M, Sheehan FH, Ritchie JL. The Western Washington Intravenous Streptokinase in Acute Myocardial Infarction Randomized Trial. *Circulation.* 1988;77: 345–352.

158. Effect of intravenous APSAC on mortality after acute myocardial infarction: preliminary report of a placebo-controlled clinical trial. AIMS Trial Study Group. *Lancet.* 1988;1:545–549.

159. Timmis AD, Griffin B, Crick JC, Sowton E. Anisoylated plasminogen streptokinase activator complex in acute myocardial infarction: a placebo-controlled arteriographic coronary recanalization study. *J Am Coll Cardiol.* 1987;10:205–210.

160. Verstraete M, Bernard R, Bory M, Brower RW, Collen D, de Bono DP, Erbel R, Huhmann W, Lennane RJ, Lubsen J, et al. Randomised trial of intravenous recombinant tissue-type plasminogen activator versus intravenous streptokinase in acute myocardial infarction: report from the European Cooperative Study Group for Recombinant Tissue-type Plasminogen Activator. *Lancet.* 1985;1:842–847.

161. Wilcox RG, von der Lippe G, Olsson CG, Jensen G, Skene AM, Hampton JR. Trial of tissue plasminogen activator for mortality reduction in acute myocardial infarction. Anglo-Scandinavian Study of Early Thrombolysis (ASSET). *Lancet.* 1988;2:525–530.

162. Bode C, Smalling RW, Berg G, Burnett C, Lorch G, Kalbfleisch JM, Chernoff R, Christie LG, Feldman RL, Seals AA, Weaver WD. Randomized comparison of coronary thrombolysis achieved with double-bolus reteplase (recombinant plasminogen activator) and front-loaded, accelerated alteplase (recombinant tissue plasminogen activator) in patients with acute myocardial infarction. The RAPID II Investigators. *Circulation.* 1996;94:891–898.

163. Randomised, double-blind comparison of reteplase double-bolus administration with streptokinase in acute myocardial infarction (INJECT): trial to investigate equivalence. International Joint Efficacy Comparison of Thrombolytics. *Lancet.* 1995;346:329–336.

164. Van de Werf F, Cannon CP, Luyten A, Houbracken K, McCabe CH, Berioli S, Bluhmki E, Sarelin H, Wang-Clow F, Fox NL, Braunwald E. Safety assessment of single-bolus administration of TNK tissue-plasminogen activator in acute myocardial infarction: the ASSENT-1 trial. The ASSENT-1 Investigators. *Am Heart J.* 1999;137:786–791.

165. Collins R, Peto R, Parish S, Sleight P. ISIS-3 and GISSI-2: no survival advantage with tissue plasminogen activator over streptokinase, but a significant excess of strokes with tissue plasminogen activator in both trials [letter]. *Am J Cardiol.* 1993;71:1127–1130.

166. The EPISTENT Investigators (Evaluation of Platelet IIb/IIIa Inhibitor for Stenting). Randomised placebo-controlled and balloon-angioplasty-controlled trial to assess safety of coronary stenting with use of platelet glycoprotein-IIb/IIIa blockade. *Lancet.* 1998;352:87–92.

167. Selker HP, Griffith JL, D'Agostino RB. A tool for judging coronary care unit admission appropriateness, valid for both real-time and retrospective use: a time-insensitive predictive instrument (TIPI) for acute cardiac ischemia: a multicenter study. *Med Care.* 1991;29:610–627.

168. A clinical trial comparing primary coronary angioplasty with tissue plasminogen activator for acute myocardial infarction. The Global Use of Strategies to Open Occluded Coronary Arteries in Acute Coronary Syndromes (GUSTO IIb) Angioplasty Substudy Investigators. *N Engl J Med.* 1997;336:1621–1628.

169. Weaver WD, Simes RJ, Betriu A, Grines CL, Zijlstra F, Garcia E, Grinfeld L, Gibbons RJ, Ribeiro EE, DeWood MA, Ribichini F. Comparison of primary coronary angioplasty and intravenous thrombolytic therapy for acute myocardial infarction: a quantitative review [published correction appears in *JAMA.* 1998;279:1876]. *JAMA.* 1997;278: 2093–2098.

170. Berger AK, Schulman KA, Gersh BJ, Pirzada S, Breall JA, Johnson AE, Every NR. Primary coronary angioplasty vs thrombolysis for the management of acute myocardial infarction in elderly patients. *JAMA.* 1999; 282:341–348.

171. Keeley EC, Boura JA, Grines CL. Primary angioplasty versus intravenous thrombolytic therapy for acute myocardial infarction: a quantitative review of 23 randomised trials. *Lancet*. 2003;361:13–20.
172. Nallamothu BK, Bates ER. Percutaneous coronary intervention versus fibrinolytic therapy in acute myocardial infarction: is timing (almost) everything? *Am J Cardiol*. 2003;92:824–826.
173. Zijlstra F, Patel A, Jones M, Grines CL, Ellis S, Garcia E, Grinfeld L, Gibbons RJ, Ribeiro EE, Ribichini F, Granger C, Akhras F, Weaver WD, Simes RJ. Clinical characteristics and outcome of patients with early (<2 h), intermediate (2–4 h) and late (>4 h) presentation treated by primary coronary angioplasty or thrombolytic therapy for acute myocardial infarction. *Eur Heart J*. 2002;23:550–557.
174. Holmes DR Jr, Bates ER, Kleiman NS, Sadowski Z, Horgan JH, Morris DC, Califf RM, Berger PB, Topol EJ. Contemporary reperfusion therapy for cardiogenic shock: the GUSTO-I trial experience. The GUSTO-I Investigators. Global Utilization of Streptokinase and Tissue Plasminogen Activator for Occluded Coronary Arteries. *J Am Coll Cardiol*. 1995;26:668–674.
175. Califf RM, Bengtson JR. Cardiogenic shock. *N Engl J Med*. 1994;330: 1724–1730.
176. Zehender M, Kasper W, Kauder E, Schonthaler M, Geibel A, Olschewski M, Just H. Right ventricular infarction as an independent predictor of prognosis after acute inferior myocardial infarction. *N Engl J Med*. 1993;328:981–988.
177. Berger PB, Ruocco NA Jr, Ryan TJ, Jacobs AK, Zaret BL, Wackers FJ, Frederick MM, Faxon DP. Frequency and significance of right ventricular dysfunction during inferior wall left ventricular myocardial infarction treated with thrombolytic therapy (results from the thrombolysis in myocardial infarction [TIMI] II trial). The TIMI Research Group. *Am J Cardiol*. 1993;71:1148–1152.
178. Goldstein JA, Barzilai B, Rosamond TL, Eisenberg PR, Jaffe AS. Determinants of hemodynamic compromise with severe right ventricular infarction. *Circulation*. 1990;82:359–368.
179. Yusuf S, Zhao F, Mehta SR, Chrolavicius S, Tognoni G, Fox KK. Effects of clopidogrel in addition to aspirin in patients with acute coronary syndromes without ST-segment elevation. *N Engl J Med*. 2001;345:494–502.
180. Mehta SR, Yusuf S, Peters RJ, Bertrand ME, Lewis BS, Natarajan MK, Malmberg K, Rupprecht H, Zhao F, Chrolavicius S, Copland I, Fox KA. Effects of pretreatment with clopidogrel and aspirin followed by long-term therapy in patients undergoing percutaneous coronary intervention: the PCI-CURE study. *Lancet*. 2001;358:527–533.
181. Yusuf S, Mehta SR, Zhao F, Gersh BJ, Commerford PJ, Blumenthal M, Budaj A, Wittlinger T, Fox KA. Early and late effects of clopidogrel in patients with acute coronary syndromes. *Circulation*. 2003;107: 966–972.
182. Budaj A, Yusuf S, Mehta SR, Fox KA, Tognoni G, Zhao F, Chrolavicius S, Hunt D, Keltai M, Franzosi MG. Benefit of clopidogrel in patients with acute coronary syndromes without ST-segment elevation in various risk groups. *Circulation*. 2002;106:1622–1626.
183. Peters RJ, Mehta SR, Fox KA, Zhao F, Lewis BS, Kopecky SL, Diaz R, Commerford PJ, Valentin V, Yusuf S. Effects of aspirin dose when used alone or in combination with clopidogrel in patients with acute coronary syndromes: observations from the Clopidogrel in Unstable angina to prevent Recurrent Events (CURE) study. *Circulation*. 2003;108: 1682–1687.
184. Fox KA, Mehta SR, Peters R, Zhao F, Lakkis N, Gersh BJ, Yusuf S. Benefits and risks of the combination of clopidogrel and aspirin in patients undergoing surgical revascularization for non-ST-elevation acute coronary syndrome: the Clopidogrel in Unstable angina to prevent Recurrent ischemic Events (CURE) Trial. *Circulation*. 2004;110: 1202–1208.
185. CAPRIE Steering Committee. A randomised, blinded, trial of clopidogrel versus aspirin in patients at risk of ischaemic events (CAPRIE). *Lancet*. 1996;348:1329–1339.
186. Steinhubl SR, Berger PB, Mann JT III, Fry ET, DeLago A, Wilmer C, Topol EJ. Early and sustained dual oral antiplatelet therapy following percutaneous coronary intervention: a randomized controlled trial. *JAMA*. 2002;288:2411–2420.
187. Sabatine MS, Cannon CP, Gibson CM, Lopez-Sendon JL, Montalescot G, Theroux P, Claeys MJ, Cools F, Hill KA, Skene AM, McCabe CH, Braunwald E. Addition of clopidogrel to aspirin and fibrinolytic therapy for myocardial infarction with ST-segment elevation. *N Engl J Med*. 2005;352:1179–1189.
188. Hjalmarson A, Herlitz J, Holmberg S, Ryden L, Swedberg K, Vedin A, Waagstein F, Waldenstrom A, Waldenstrom J, Wedel H, Wilhelmsen L, Wilhelmsson C. The Goteborg metoprolol trial: effects on mortality and morbidity in acute myocardial infarction: limitation of infarct size by beta blockers and its potential role for prognosis. *Circulation*. 1983; 67(suppl I):I26–I32.
189. Metoprolol in acute myocardial infarction (MIAMI). A randomised placebo-controlled international trial. The MIAMI Trial Research Group. *Eur Heart J*. 1985;6:199–226.
190. Randomised trial of intravenous atenolol among 16 027 cases of suspected acute myocardial infarction: ISIS-1. First International Study of Infarct Survival Collaborative Group. *Lancet*. 1986;2:57–66.
191. Rehnqvist N, Olsson G, Erhardt L, Ekman AM. Metoprolol in acute myocardial infarction reduces ventricular arrhythmias both in the early stage and after the acute event. *Int J Cardiol*. 1987;15:301–308.
192. Herlitz J, Edvardsson N, Holmberg S, Ryden L, Waagstein F, Waldenstrom A, Swedberg K, Hjalmarson A. Goteborg Metoprolol Trial: effects on arrhythmias. *Am J Cardiol*. 1984;53:27D–31D.
193. Roberts R, Rogers WJ, Mueller HS, Lambrew CT, Diver DJ, Smith HC, Willerson JT, Knatterud GL, Forman S, Passamani E, et al. Immediate versus deferred beta-blockade following thrombolytic therapy in patients with acute myocardial infarction: results of the Thrombolysis in Myocardial Infarction (TIMI) II-B Study. *Circulation*. 1991;83: 422–437.
194. Brieger DB, Mak KH, Kottke-Marchant K, Topol EJ. Heparin-induced thrombocytopenia. *J Am Coll Cardiol*. 1998;31:1449–1459.
195. Ryan TJ, Antman EM, Brooks NH, Califf RM, Hillis LD, Hiratzka LF, Rapaport E, Riegel B, Russell RO, Smith EE III, Weaver WD, Gibbons RJ, Alpert JS, Eagle KA, Gardner TJ, Garson A Jr, Gregoratos G, Smith SC Jr. 1999 update: ACC/AHA guidelines for the management of patients with acute myocardial infarction: a report of the American College of Cardiology/American Heart Association Task Force on Practice Guidelines (Committee on Management of Acute Myocardial Infarction). *J Am Coll Cardiol*. 1999;34:890–911.
196. Antman EM, McCabe CH, Gurfinkel EP, Turpie AG, Bernink PJ, Salein D, Bayes De Luna A, Fox K, Lablanche JM, Radley D, Premmereur J, Braunwald E. Enoxaparin prevents death and cardiac ischemic events in unstable angina/non-Q-wave myocardial infarction: results of the thrombolysis in myocardial infarction (TIMI) 11B trial. *Circulation*. 1999;100:1593–1601.
197. Comparison of two treatment durations (6 days and 14 days) of a low molecular weight heparin with a 6-day treatment of unfractionated heparin in the initial management of unstable angina or non-Q wave myocardial infarction: FRAX.I.S. (FRAxiparine in Ischaemic Syndrome). *Eur Heart J*. 1999;20:1553–1562.
198. Suvarna TT, Parikh JA, Keshav R, Pillai MG, Pahlajani DB, Gandhi MJ. Comparison of clinical outcome of fixed-dose subcutaneous low molecular weight heparin (tinzaparin) with conventional heparin in unstable angina: a pilot study. *Indian Heart J*. 1997;49:159–162.
199. Ferguson JJ, Califf RM, Antman EM, Cohen M, Grines CL, Goodman S, Kereiakes DJ, Langer A, Mahaffey KW, Nessel CC, Armstrong PW, Avezum A, Aylward P, Becker RC, Biasucci L, Borzak S, Col J, Frey MJ, Fry E, Gulba DC, Guneri S, Gurfinkel E, Harrington R, Hochman JS, Kleiman NS, Leon MB, Lopez-Sendon JL, Pepine CJ, Ruzyllo W, Steinhubl SR, Teirstein PS, Toro-Figueroa L, White H. Enoxaparin vs unfractionated heparin in high-risk patients with non-ST-segment elevation acute coronary syndromes managed with an intended early invasive strategy: primary results of the SYNERGY randomized trial. *JAMA*. 2004;292:45–54.
200. Cohen M, Demers C, Gurfinkel EP, Turpie AG, Fromell GJ, Goodman S, Langer A, Califf RM, Fox KA, Premmereur J, Bigonzi F. A comparison of low-molecular-weight heparin with unfractionated heparin for unstable coronary artery disease. Efficacy and Safety of Subcutaneous Enoxaparin in Non-Q-Wave Coronary Events Study Group. *N Engl J Med*. 1997;337:447–452.
201. Petersen JL, Mahaffey KW, Hasselblad V, Antman EM, Cohen M, Goodman SG, Langer A, Blazing MA, Le-Moigne-Amrani A, de Lemos JA, Nessel CC, Harrington RA, Ferguson JJ, Braunwald E, Califf RM. Efficacy and bleeding complications among patients randomized to enoxaparin or unfractionated heparin for antithrombin therapy in non-ST-segment elevation acute coronary syndromes: a systematic overview. *JAMA*. 2004;292:89–96.
202. Magee KD, Sevcik W, Moher D, Rowe BH. Low molecular weight heparins versus unfractionated heparin for acute coronary syndromes. *Cochrane Database Syst Rev*. 2004;2:2.

203. Antman EM, Cohen M, Radley D, McCabe C, Rush J, Premmereur J, Braunwald E. Assessment of the treatment effect of enoxaparin for unstable angina/non-Q-wave myocardial infarction: TIMI 11B-ESSENCE meta-analysis. *Circulation*. 1999;100:1602–1608.
204. Antman EM, Cohen M, McCabe C, Goodman SG, Murphy SA, Braunwald E. Enoxaparin is superior to unfractionated heparin for preventing clinical events at 1-year follow-up of TIMI 11B and ESSENCE. *Eur Heart J*. 2002;23:308–314.
205. Le Nguyen MT, Spencer FA. Low molecular weight heparin and unfractionated heparin in the early pharmacologic management of acute coronary syndromes: a meta-analysis of randomized clinical trials. *J Thromb Thrombolysis*. 2001;12:289–295.
206. Malhotra S, Bhargava VK, Grover A, Pandhi P, Sharma YP. A randomized trial to compare the efficacy, safety, cost and platelet aggregation effects of enoxaparin and unfractionated heparin (the ESCAPEU trial). *Int J Clin Pharmacol Ther*. 2001;39:110–115.
207. Eikelboom JW, Anand SS, Malmberg K, Weitz JI, Ginsberg JS, Yusuf S. Unfractionated heparin and low-molecular-weight heparin in acute coronary syndrome without ST elevation: a meta-analysis [published correction appears in *Lancet*. 2000;356:600]. *Lancet*. 2000;355: 1936–1942.
208. Clark SC, Vitale N, Zacharias J, Forty J. Effect of low molecular weight heparin (Fragmin) on bleeding after cardiac surgery. *Ann Thorac Surg*. 2000;69:762–764.
209. Brieger D, Solanki V, Gaynor M, Booth V, MacDonald R, Freedman SB. Optimal strategy for administering enoxaparin to patients undergoing coronary angiography without angioplasty for acute coronary syndromes. *Am J Cardiol*. 2002;89:1167–1170.
210. Goodman SG, Fitchett D, Armstrong PW, Tan M, Langer A. Randomized evaluation of the safety and efficacy of enoxaparin versus unfractionated heparin in high-risk patients with non-ST-segment elevation acute coronary syndromes receiving the glycoprotein IIb/IIIa inhibitor eptifibatide. *Circulation*. 2003;107:238–244.
211. Kovar D, Canto JG, Rogers WJ. Safety and effectiveness of combined low molecular weight heparin and glycoprotein IIb/IIIa inhibitors. *Am J Cardiol*. 2002;90:911–915.
212. Cohen M, Theroux P, Borzak S, Frey MJ, White HD, Van Mieghem W, Senatore F, Lis J, Mukherjee R, Harris K, Bigonzi F. Randomized double-blind safety study of enoxaparin versus unfractionated heparin in patients with non-ST-segment elevation acute coronary syndromes treated with tirofiban and aspirin: the ACUTE II study. The Antithrombotic Combination Using Tirofiban and Enoxaparin. *Am Heart J*. 2002;144:470–477.
213. Cohen M, Theroux P, Weber S, Laramee P, Huynh T, Borzak S, Diodati JG, Squire IB, Deckelbaum LI, Thornton AR, Harris KE, Sax FL, Lo MW, White HD. Combination therapy with tirofiban and enoxaparin in acute coronary syndromes. *Int J Cardiol*. 1999;71:273–281.
214. Ferguson J. Low-molecular-weight heparins and glycoprotein IIb/IIIa antagonists in acute coronary syndromes. *J Invasive Cardiol*. 2004;16: 136–144.
215. Wallentin L, Bergstrand L, Dellborg M, Fellenius C, Granger CB, Lindahl B, Lins LE, Nilsson T, Pehrsson K, Siegbahn A, Swahn E. Low molecular weight heparin (dalteparin) compared to unfractionated heparin as an adjunct to rt-PA (alteplase) for improvement of coronary artery patency in acute myocardial infarction—the ASSENT Plus study. *Eur Heart J*. 2003;24:897–908.
216. Ross AM, Molhoek P, Lundergan C, Knudtson M, Draoui Y, Regalado L, Le Louer V, Bigonzi F, Schwartz W, De Jong E, Coyne K. Randomized comparison of enoxaparin, a low-molecular-weight heparin, with unfractionated heparin adjunctive to recombinant tissue plasminogen activator thrombolysis and aspirin: second trial of Heparin and Aspirin Reperfusion Therapy (HART II). *Circulation*. 2001;104: 648–652.
217. Van de Werf FJ, Armstrong PW, Granger C, Wallentin L. Efficacy and safety of tenecteplase in combination with enoxaparin, abciximab, or unfractionated heparin: the ASSENT-3 randomised trial in acute myocardial infarction. *Lancet*. 2001;358:605–613.
218. Theroux P, Welsh RC. Meta-analysis of randomized trials comparing enoxaparin versus unfractionated heparin as adjunctive therapy to fibrinolysis in ST-elevation acute myocardial infarction. *Am J Cardiol*. 2003;91:860–864.
219. Baird SH, Menown IB, McBride SJ, Trouton TG, Wilson C. Randomized comparison of enoxaparin with unfractionated heparin following fibrinolytic therapy for acute myocardial infarction. *Eur Heart J*. 2002;23:627–632.
220. Wallentin L, Goldstein P, Armstrong PW, Granger CB, Adgey AA, Arntz HR, Bogaerts K, Danays T, Lindahl B, Makijarvi M, Verheugt F, Van de Werf F. Efficacy and safety of tenecteplase in combination with the low-molecular-weight heparin enoxaparin or unfractionated heparin in the prehospital setting: the Assessment of the Safety and Efficacy of a New Thrombolytic Regimen (ASSENT)-3 PLUS randomized trial in acute myocardial infarction. *Circulation*. 2003;108:135–142.
221. PURSUIT Trial Investigators. Inhibition of platelet glycoprotein IIb/IIIa with eptifibatide in patients with acute coronary syndromes. The PURSUIT Trial Investigators. Platelet Glycoprotein IIb/IIIa in Unstable Angina: Receptor Suppression Using Integrilin Therapy. *N Engl J Med*. 1998;339:436–443.
222. Cannon CP, Weintraub WS, Demopoulos LA, Vicari R, Frey MJ, Lakkis N, Neumann FJ, Robertson DH, DeLucca PT, DiBattiste PM, Gibson CM, Braunwald E. Comparison of early invasive and conservative strategies in patients with unstable coronary syndromes treated with the glycoprotein IIb/IIIa inhibitor tirofiban. *N Engl J Med*. 2001;344: 1879–1887.
223. Roffi M, Chew DP, Mukherjee D, Bhatt DL, White JA, Heeschen C, Hamm CW, Moliterno DJ, Califf RM, White HD, Kleiman NS, Theroux P, Topol EJ. Platelet glycoprotein IIb/IIIa inhibitors reduce mortality in diabetic patients with non-ST-segment-elevation acute coronary syndromes. *Circulation*. 2001;104:2767–2771.
224. Bosch X, Marrugat J. Platelet glycoprotein IIb/IIIa blockers for percutaneous coronary revascularization, and unstable angina and non-ST-segment elevation myocardial infarction. *Cochrane Database Syst Rev*. 2001;CD002130.
225. Boersma E, Harrington RA, Moliterno DJ, White H, Theroux P, Van de Werf F, de Torbal A, Armstrong PW, Wallentin LC, Wilcox RG, Simes J, Califf RM, Topol EJ, Simoons ML. Platelet glycoprotein IIb/IIIa inhibitors in acute coronary syndromes: a meta-analysis of all major randomised clinical trials [published correction appears in *Lancet*. 2002; 359:2120]. *Lancet*. 2002;359:189–198.
226. Simoons ML. Effect of glycoprotein IIb/IIIa receptor blocker abciximab on outcome in patients with acute coronary syndromes without early coronary revascularisation: the GUSTO IV-ACS randomised trial. *Lancet*. 2001;357:1915–1924.
227. Ottervanger JP, Armstrong P, Barnathan ES, Boersma E, Cooper JS, Ohman EM, James S, Topol E, Wallentin L, Simoons ML. Long-term results after the glycoprotein IIb/IIIa inhibitor abciximab in unstable angina: one-year survival in the GUSTO IV-ACS (Global Use of Strategies To Open Occluded Coronary Arteries IV—Acute Coronary Syndrome) Trial. *Circulation*. 2003;107:437–442.
228. Ryan T, Anderson J, Antman E, Braniff B, Brooks N, Califf R, Hillis L, Hiratzka L, Rapaport E, Riegel B, Russell R, Smith E Jr, Weaver W. ACC/AHA guidelines for the management of patients with acute myocardial infarction: a report of the American College of Cardiology/ American Heart Association Task Force on Practice Guidelines (Committee on Management of Acute Myocardial Infarction). *J Am Coll Cardiol*. 1996;28:1328–1428.
229. ISIS-4 (Fourth International Study of Infarct Survival) Collaborative Group. ISIS-4: a randomised factorial trial assessing early oral captopril, oral mononitrate, and intravenous magnesium sulphate in 58,050 patients with suspected acute myocardial infarction. *Lancet*. 1995;345: 669–685.
230. Gruppo Italiano per lo Studio della Sopravvivenza nell'infarto Miocardico. GISSI-3: effects of lisinopril and transdermal glyceryl trinitrate singly and together on 6-week mortality and ventricular function after acute myocardial infarction. *Lancet*. 1994;343:1115–1122.
231. Chinese Cardiac Study (CCS-1) Collaborative Group. Oral captopril versus placebo among 14,962 patients with suspected acute myocardial infarction: a multicenter, randomized, double-blind, placebo controlled clinical trial. *Chin Med J*. 1997;110:834–838.
232. Ambrosioni E, Borghi C, Magnani B. The effect of the angiotensin-converting-enzyme inhibitor zofenopril on mortality and morbidity after anterior myocardial infarction: the Survival of Myocardial Infarction Long-Term Evaluation (SMILE) Study Investigators. *N Engl J Med*. 1995;332:80–85.
233. Borghi C, Marino P, Zardini P, Magnani B, Collatina S, Ambrosioni E. Short- and long-term effects of early fosinopril administration in patients with acute anterior myocardial infarction undergoing intravenous thrombolysis: results from the Fosinopril in Acute Myocardial Infarction Study. FAMIS Working Party. *Am Heart J*. 1998;136:213–225.

234. Oral captopril versus placebo among 13,634 patients with suspected acute myocardial infarction: interim report from the Chinese Cardiac Study (CCS-1). *Lancet.* 1995;345:686–687.

235. Oral captopril versus placebo among 14,962 patients with suspected acute myocardial infarction: a multicenter, randomized, double-blind, placebo controlled clinical trial. Chinese Cardiac Study (CCS-1) Collaborative Group. *Chin Med J (Engl).* 1997;110:834–838.

236. GISSI-3: effects of lisinopril and transdermal glyceryl trinitrate singly and together on 6-week mortality and ventricular function after acute myocardial infarction. Gruppo Italiano per lo Studio della Sopravvivenza nell'infarto Miocardico. *Lancet.* 1994;343:1115–1122.

237. Pfeffer MA, Greaves SC, Arnold JM, Glynn RJ, LaMotte FS, Lee RT, Menapace FJ Jr, Rapaport E, Ridker PM, Rouleau JL, Solomon SD, Hennekens CH. Early versus delayed angiotensin-converting enzyme inhibition therapy in acute myocardial infarction. The Healing and Early Afterload Reducing Therapy Trial. *Circulation.* 1997;95:2643–2651.

238. Indications for ACE inhibitors in the early treatment of acute myocardial infarction: systematic overview of individual data from 100,000 patients in randomized trials. ACE Inhibitor Myocardial Infarction Collaborative Group. *Circulation.* 1998;97:2202–2651.

239. Teo KK, Yusuf S, Pfeffer M, Torp-Pedersen C, Kober L, Hall A, Pogue J, Latini R, Collins R. Effects of long-term treatment with angiotensin-converting-enzyme inhibitors in the presence or absence of aspirin: a systematic review. *Lancet.* 2002;360:1037–1043.

240. Borghi C, Ambrosioni E. Double-blind comparison between zofenopril and lisinopril in patients with acute myocardial infarction: results of the Survival of Myocardial Infarction Long-term Evaluation-2 (SMILE-2) study. *Am Heart J.* 2003;145:80–87.

241. Latini R, Maggioni AP, Flather M, Sleight P, Tognoni G. ACE inhibitor use in patients with myocardial infarction: summary of evidence from clinical trials. *Circulation.* 1995;92:3132–3137.

242. Latini R, Tognoni G, Maggioni AP, Baigent C, Braunwald E, Chen ZM, Collins R, Flather M, Franzosi MG, Kjekshus J, Kober L, Liu LS, Peto R, Pfeffer M, Pizzetti F, Santoro E, Sleight P, Swedberg K, Tavazzi L, Wang W, Yusuf S. Clinical effects of early angiotensin-converting enzyme inhibitor treatment for acute myocardial infarction are similar in the presence and absence of aspirin: systematic overview of individual data from 96,712 randomized patients. Angiotensin-converting Enzyme Inhibitor Myocardial Infarction Collaborative Group. *J Am Coll Cardiol.* 2000;35:1801–1807.

243. Lu CY. [Treatment of acute myocardial infarction with oral captopril. A randomized, double blind and placebo controlled pilot study.] *Zhonghua Xin Xue Guan Bing Za Zhi.* 1993;21:74–76, 121–122.

244. Ray SG, Pye M, Oldroyd KG, Christie J, Connelly DT, Northridge DB, Ford I, Morton JJ, Dargie HJ, Cobbe SM. Early treatment with captopril after acute myocardial infarction. *Br Heart J.* 1993;69:215–222.

245. Di Pasquale P, Paterna S, Cannizzaro S, Bucca V. Does captopril treatment before thrombolysis in acute myocardial infarction attenuate reperfusion damage? Short-term and long-term effects. *Int J Cardiol.* 1994;43:43–50.

246. Spinar J, Vitovec J, Pluhacek L, Spinarova L, Fischerova B, Toman J. First dose hypotension after angiotensin converting enzyme inhibitor captopril and angiotensin II blocker losartan in patients with acute myocardial infarction. *Int J Cardiol.* 2000;75:197–204.

247. Wagner A, Herkner H, Schreiber W, Bur A, Woisetschlager C, Stix G, Laggner AN, Hirschl MM. Ramipril prior to thrombolysis attenuates the early increase of PAI-1 in patients with acute myocardial infarction. *Thromb Haemost.* 2002;88:180–185.

248. Mehta PM, Przyklenk K, Kloner RA. Cardioprotective effects of captopril in myocardial ischaemia, ischaemia/reperfusion and infarction. *Eur Heart J.* 1990;(suppl B):94–99.

249. Pfeffer MA, McMurray JJ, Velazquez EJ, Rouleau JL, Kober L, Maggioni AP, Solomon SD, Swedberg K, Van de Werf F, White H, Leimberger JD, Henis M, Edwards S, Zelenkofske S, Sellers MA, Califf RM. Valsartan, captopril, or both in myocardial infarction complicated by heart failure, left ventricular dysfunction, or both. *N Engl J Med.* 2003;349:1893–1906.

250. Kayikcioglu M, Can L, Kultursay H, Payzin S, Turkoglu C. Early use of pravastatin in patients with acute myocardial infarction undergoing coronary angioplasty. *Acta Cardiol.* 2002;57:295–302.

251. Kayikcioglu M, Can L, Evrengul H, Payzin S, Kultursay H. The effect of statin therapy on ventricular late potentials in acute myocardial infarction. *Int J Cardiol.* 2003;90:63–72.

252. Kinlay S, Schwartz GG, Olsson AG, Rifai N, Leslie SJ, Sasiela WJ, Szarek M, Libby P, Ganz P. High-dose atorvastatin enhances the decline in inflammatory markers in patients with acute coronary syndromes in the MIRACL study. *Circulation.* 2003;108:1560–1566.

253. Correia LC, Sposito AC, Lima JC, Magalhaes LP, Passos LC, Rocha MS, D'Oliveira A, Esteves JP. Anti-inflammatory effect of atorvastatin (80 mg) in unstable angina pectoris and non-Q-wave acute myocardial infarction. *Am J Cardiol.* 2003;92:298–301.

254. Mehta SR, Yusuf S, Diaz R, Zhu J, Pais P, Xavier D, Paolasso E, Ahmed R, Xie C, Kazmi K, Tai J, Orlandini A, Pogue J, Liu L. Effect of glucose-insulin-potassium infusion on mortality in patients with acute ST-segment elevation myocardial infarction: the CREATE-ECLA randomized controlled trial. *JAMA.* 2005;293:437–446.

255. Timmer J. Glucose-insulin-potassium study in patients with ST-elevation myocardial infarction without signs of heart failure: the Gips-II Trial. Paper presented at: Late-Breaking Clinical Trials III, American College of Cardiology Scientific Sessions; March 9, 2005; Orlando, Fla.

256. MacMahon S, Collins R, Peto R, Koster RW, Yusuf S. Effects of prophylactic lidocaine in suspected acute myocardial infarction: an overview of results from the randomized, controlled trials. *JAMA.* 1988;260:1910–1916.

Part 9: Adult Stroke

Each year in the United States about 700 000 people of all ages suffer a new or repeat stroke. Approximately 158 000 of these people will die, making stroke the third leading cause of death in the United States.[1,2] Many advances have been made in stroke prevention, treatment, and rehabilitation.[3,4] For example, fibrinolytic therapy can limit the extent of neurologic damage from stroke and improve outcome, but the time available for treatment is limited.[5,6] Healthcare providers, hospitals, and communities must develop systems to increase the efficiency and effectiveness of stroke care.[3] The "7 D's of Stroke Care"—detection, dispatch, delivery, door (arrival and urgent triage in the emergency department [ED]), data, decision, and drug administration—highlight the major steps in diagnosis and treatment and the key points at which delays can occur.[7,8]

This chapter summarizes the management of acute stroke in the adult patient. It summarizes out-of-hospital care through the first hours of therapy. For additional information about the management of acute ischemic stroke, see the AHA/American Stroke Association (ASA) guidelines for the management of acute ischemic stroke.[9,10]

Management Goals

The goal of stroke care is to minimize brain injury and maximize patient recovery. The AHA and ASA developed a community-oriented "Stroke Chain of Survival" that links actions to be taken by patients, family members, and healthcare providers to maximize stroke recovery. These links are

- Rapid recognition and reaction to stroke warning signs
- Rapid emergency medical services (EMS) dispatch
- Rapid EMS system transport and hospital prenotification
- Rapid diagnosis and treatment in the hospital

The AHA ECC stroke guidelines focus on the initial out-of-hospital and ED assessment and management of the patient with acute stroke as depicted in the algorithm Goals for Management of Patients With Suspected Stroke (Figure). The time goals of the National Institute of Neurological Disorders and Stroke (NINDS)[11] are illustrated along the left side of the algorithm as clocks with a sweep hand depicting the goal in minutes from ED arrival to task completion to remind the clinician of the time-sensitive nature of management of acute ischemic stroke.

The sections below summarize the principles and goals of stroke assessment and management, highlighting key controversies, new recommendations, and training issues. The text refers to the numbered boxes in the algorithm.

(*Circulation.* **2005;112:IV-111-IV-120.**)

This special supplement to *Circulation* is freely available at http://www.circulationaha.org

DOI: 10.1161/CIRCULATIONAHA.105.166562

Stroke Recognition and EMS Care

Stroke Warning Signs

Identifying clinical signs of possible stroke (Box 1) is important because fibrinolytic treatment must be provided within a few hours of onset of symptoms.[5,12] Most strokes occur at home, and only half of all victims of acute stroke use EMS for transport to the hospital.[13–15] In addition, stroke victims often deny or rationalize[16] their symptoms. This can delay EMS access and treatment and result in increased morbidity and mortality. Even high-risk patients fail to recognize the signs of a stroke.[16] Community and professional education is essential,[17] and it has successfully increased the proportion of stroke victims treated with fibrinolytic therapy.[18,19]

The signs and symptoms of a stroke may be subtle. They include sudden weakness or numbness of the face, arm, or leg, especially on one side of the body; sudden confusion, trouble speaking or understanding; sudden trouble seeing in one or both eyes; sudden trouble walking, dizziness, loss of balance or coordination; or sudden severe headache with no known cause.

EMS Dispatch

Currently $<10\%$ of patients with acute ischemic stroke are ultimately eligible for fibrinolytic therapy because they fail to arrive at the receiving hospital within 3 hours of onset of symptoms.[20–24]

EMS systems must provide education and training to minimize delays in prehospital dispatch, assessment, and transport. Emergency medical dispatchers must identify potential stroke victims and provide high-priority dispatch to patients with possible stroke. EMS providers must be able to support cardiopulmonary function, perform rapid stroke assessment, establish time of onset of symptoms (or last time the patient was known to be normal), triage and transport the patient, and provide prearrival notification to the receiving hospital (Box 2).[25–28]

Stroke Assessment Tools

EMS providers can identify stroke patients with reasonable sensitivity and specificity, using abbreviated out-of-hospital tools such as the Cincinnati Prehospital Stroke Scale (CPSS)[27,29–31] (Table 1) or the Los Angeles Prehospital Stroke Screen (LAPSS) (Table 2).[32,33] The CPSS is based on physical examination only. The EMS provider checks for 3 physical findings: facial droop, arm weakness, and speech abnormalities. The presence of a single abnormality on the CPSS has a sensitivity of 59% and a specificity of 89% when scored by prehospital providers.[30] The LAPSS requires the examiner to rule out other causes of altered level of consciousness (eg, history of seizures, hypoglycemia) and then identify asymmetry in any of 3 examination categories: facial smile or grimace, grip, and arm strength. The LAPSS has a specificity of 97% and a sensitivity of 93%.[32,33]

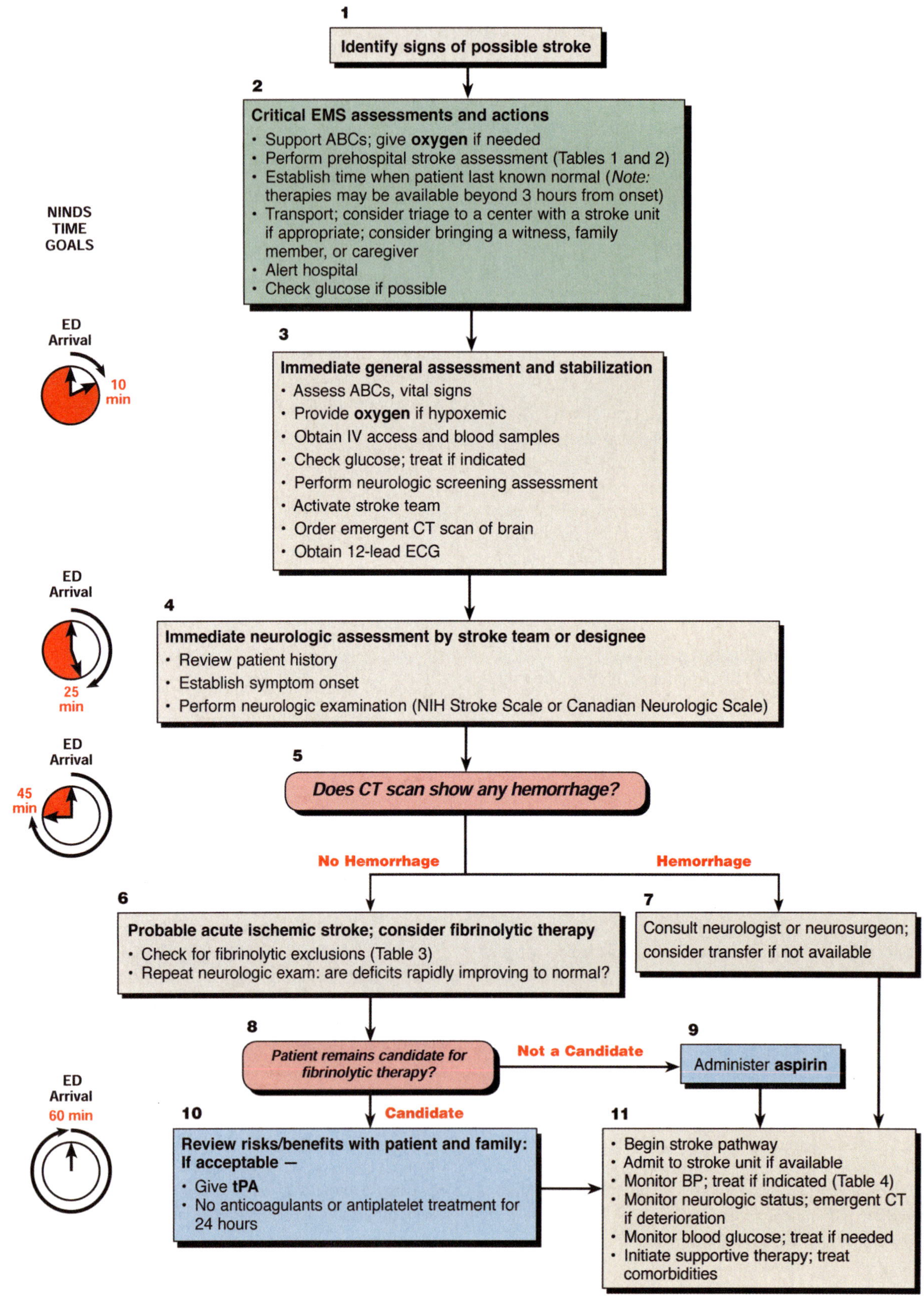

Goals for Management of Patients With Suspected Stroke Algorithm.

TABLE 1. The Cincinnati Prehospital Stroke Scale

Facial Droop (have patient show teeth or smile):

- Normal—both sides of face move equally
- Abnormal—one side of face does not move as well as the other side

Left: normal. Right: stroke patient with facial droop (right side of face). Kothari R, et al. *Acad Emerg Med.* 1997;4:986–990.

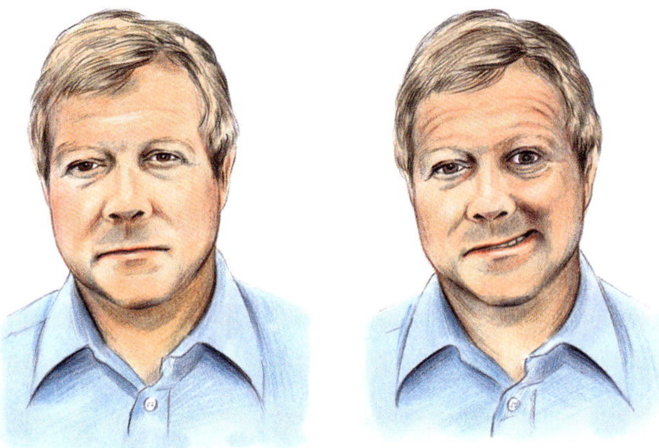

Arm Drift (patient closes eyes and holds both arms straight out for 10 seconds):

- Normal—both arms move the same or both arms do not move at all (other findings, such as pronator drift, may be helpful)
- Abnormal—one arm does not move or one arm drifts down compared with the other

Abnormal Speech (have the patient say "you can't teach an old dog new tricks"):

- Normal—patient uses correct words with no slurring
- Abnormal—patient slurs words, uses the wrong words, or is unable to speak

Interpretation: If any 1 of these 3 signs is abnormal, the probability of a stroke is 72%.

With standard training in stroke recognition, paramedics have demonstrated a sensitivity of 61% to 66% for identifying patients with stroke.[31,34,35] After training in using a stroke assessment tool, paramedic sensitivity for identifying patients with stroke increased to 86% to 97% (LOE 3 to 5).[33,36,37] Therefore, all paramedics and emergency medical technicians-basic (EMT-basic) should be trained in the recognition of stroke using a validated, abbreviated out-of-hospital screening tool, such as the CPSS or the LAPSS (Class IIa).

Transport and Care

Once EMS providers suspect the diagnosis of stroke, they should establish the time of onset of symptoms. This time represents time zero for the patient. If the patient wakes from sleep or is found with symptoms of a stroke, time zero is the last time the patient was observed to be normal. EMS providers must rapidly deliver the patient to a medical facility capable of providing acute stroke care and provide prearrival notification to the receiving facility.[25]

EMS providers should consider transporting a witness, family member, or caregiver with the patient to verify the time of onset of stroke symptoms. En route to the facility providers should support cardiopulmonary function, monitor neurologic status, and if authorized by medical control, check blood glucose.

Patients with acute stroke are at risk for respiratory compromise from aspiration, upper airway obstruction, hypoventilation, and (rarely) neurogenic pulmonary edema. The combination of poor perfusion and hypoxemia will exacerbate and extend ischemic brain injury, and it has been associated with worse outcome from stroke.[38] Although one small randomized clinical trial (LOE 2)[39] of selected stroke patients suggested a transient improvement in clinical deficit and MRI abnormalities following 8 hours of high-flow supplementary oxygen (by face mask), a larger quasi-randomized trial (LOE 3)[40] did not show any clinical benefit from routine administration of low-flow (3 L/min) oxygen for 24 hours to all patients with ischemic stroke. In contrast, the administration of supplementary oxygen to the subset of stroke patients who are hypoxemic is indirectly supported by several studies showing improved functional outcomes and survival of stroke patients treated in dedicated stroke units in which higher supplementary oxygen concentrations were used (LOE 7).[38,39,41,42]

Both out-of-hospital and in-hospital medical personnel should administer supplementary oxygen to hypoxemic (ie, oxygen saturation <92%) stroke patients (Class I) or those with unknown oxygen saturation. Clinicians may consider giving oxygen to patients who are not hypoxemic (Class IIb).

The role of stroke centers and stroke units continues to be debated.[43] Initial evidence[44–50] indicated a favorable benefit from triage of stroke patients directly to designated stroke centers (Class IIb), but the concept of routine out-of-hospital triage of stroke patients requires more rigorous evaluation.

Each receiving hospital should define its capability for treating patients with acute stroke and should communicate this information to the EMS system and the community. Although not every hospital is capable of organizing the necessary resources to safely administer fibrinolytic therapy, every hospital with an ED should have a written plan describing how patients with acute stroke are to be managed in that institution. The plan should detail the roles of healthcare professionals in the care of patients with acute stroke and define which patients will be treated with fibrinolytic therapy at that facility and when transfer to another hospital with a dedicated stroke unit is appropriate (Class IIa).

Multiple randomized clinical trials and meta-analyses in adults (LOE 1)[51–54] document consistent improvement in 1-year survival rate, functional outcomes, and quality of life when patients hospitalized with acute stroke are cared for in a dedicated stroke unit by a multidisciplinary team experienced in managing stroke. Although the studies reported were conducted outside the United States in in-hospital units that provided both acute care and rehabilitation, the improved outcomes were apparent very early in the stroke care. These results should be relevant to the outcome of dedicated stroke units staffed with experienced multidisciplinary teams in the United States. When such a facility is available within a reasonable transport interval, stroke patients who require hospitalization should be admitted there (Class I).

TABLE 2. Los Angeles Prehospital Stroke Screen (LAPSS)

For evaluation of acute, noncomatose, nontraumatic neurologic complaint. If items 1 through 6 are all checked "Yes" (or "Unknown"), provide prearrival notification to hospital of potential stroke patient. If any item is checked "No," return to appropriate treatment protocol. Interpretation: 93% of patients with stroke will have a positive LAPSS score (sensitivity=93%), and 97% of those with a positive LAPSS score will have a stroke (specificity=97%). Note that the patient may still be experiencing a stroke if LAPSS criteria are not met.

Criteria	Yes	Unknown	No
1. Age >45 years	☐	☐	☐
2. History of seizures or epilepsy absent	☐	☐	☐
3. Symptom duration <24 hours	☐	☐	☐
4. At baseline, patient is not wheelchair bound or bedridden	☐	☐	☐
5. Blood glucose between 60 and 400	☐	☐	☐
6. Obvious asymmetry (right vs left) in any of the following 3 exam categories (must be unilateral):	☐	☐	☐
	Equal	**R Weak**	**L Weak**
Facial smile/grimace	☐	☐ Droop	☐ Droop
Grip	☐	☐ Weak grip ☐ No grip	☐ Weak grip ☐ No grip
Arm strength	☐	☐ Drifts down ☐ Falls rapidly	☐ Drifts down ☐ Falls rapidly

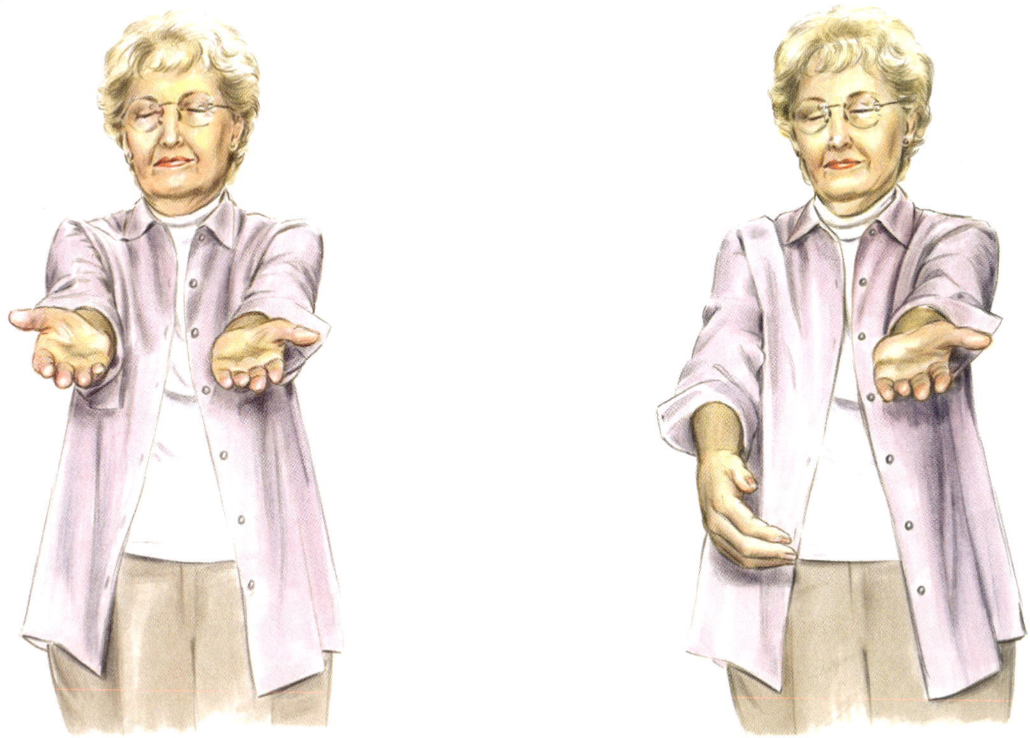

One-sided motor weakness (right arm).

Kidwell CS, Saver JL, Schubert GB, Eckstein M, Starkman S. Design and retrospective analysis of the Los Angeles prehospital stroke screen (LAPSS). *Prehosp Emerg Care.* 1998;2:267–273.

Kidwell CS, Starkman S, Eckstein M, Weems K, Saver JL. Identifying stroke in the field: prospective validation of the Los Angeles Prehospital Stroke Screen (LAPSS). *Stroke.* 2000;31:71–76.

In-Hospital Care

Initial ED Assessment and Stabilization

Protocols should be used in the ED to minimize delay to definitive diagnosis and therapy.[28] As a goal, ED personnel should assess the patient with suspected stroke within 10 minutes of arrival in the ED (Box 3). General care includes assessment and support of airway, breathing, and circulation and evaluation of baseline vital signs. We recommend that providers administer oxygen to hypoxemic patients in the ED (Class I) and consider oxygen administration for patients without hypoxemia (Class IIb).

Establish or confirm intravenous (IV) access and obtain blood samples for baseline studies (blood count, coagulation studies, blood glucose, etc). Promptly treat hypoglycemia. The ED physician should perform a neurologic screening assessment, order an emergent computerized tomography (CT) scan of the brain, and activate the stroke team or arrange consultation with a stroke expert.

A 12-lead ECG does not take priority over the CT scan, but it may identify a recent acute myocardial infarction or arrhythmias (eg, atrial fibrillation) as the cause of an embolic stroke. If the patient is hemodynamically stable, treatment of other arrhythmias, including bradycardia, premature atrial or ventricular contractions, or defects or blocks in atrioventricular conduction, may not be necessary.[55] There is general agreement to recommend cardiac monitoring during the initial evaluation of patients with acute ischemic stroke to detect atrial fibrillation and potentially life-threatening arrhythmias.[10]

Assessment

The stroke team, another expert, or an emergency physician with access to remote stroke expert support will review the patient history and verify time of onset of symptoms (Box 4).[56–58] This may require interviewing out-of-hospital providers, witnesses, and family members to establish the time that the patient was last known to be normal. Neurologic assessment is performed incorporating either the National Institutes of Health (NIH) Stroke Scale or Canadian Neurologic Scale (see the ASA website: *www.strokeassociation.org*).

Management of hypertension in the stroke patient is controversial. For patients eligible for fibrinolytic therapy, however, control of blood pressure is required to reduce the potential risk of bleeding. If a patient who is otherwise eligible for treatment with tissue plasminogen activator (tPA) has elevated blood pressure, providers can try to lower it to a systolic pressure of <185 mm Hg and a diastolic blood pressure of <110 mm Hg. Because the maximum interval from onset of stroke until effective treatment of stroke with tPA is limited, most patients with sustained hypertension above these levels (ie, systolic blood pressure >185 mm Hg or diastolic blood pressure >110 mm Hg) cannot be treated with IV tPA (Table 4).[9,10]

Ideally the CT scan should be completed within 25 minutes of the patient's arrival in the ED and should be read within 45 minutes of ED arrival (Box 5). Emergent CT or magnetic resonance imaging (MRI) scans of patients with suspected stroke should be promptly evaluated by a physician with expertise in interpretation of these studies.[59,60] During the first few hours of an ischemic stroke, the noncontrast CT scan may not indicate signs of brain ischemia. If the CT scan shows no evidence of hemorrhage, the patient may be a candidate for fibrinolytic therapy (Boxes 6 and 8).

If hemorrhage is noted on the CT scan, the patient is not a candidate for fibrinolytic therapy. Consult a neurologist or neurosurgeon and consider transfer as needed for appropriate care (Box 7).

If hemorrhage is not present on the initial CT scan and the patient is not a candidate for fibrinolytic therapy for other reasons, consider administration of aspirin (Box 9) either rectally or orally after the patient is screened for dysphagia (see below). Admit the patient to a stroke unit (if available) for careful monitoring (Box 11). Although the aspirin is not a time-critical intervention, it is appropriate to administer aspirin in the ED if the patient is not a candidate for fibrinolysis.

Fibrinolytic Therapy (Boxes 6, 8, and 10)

If the CT scan shows no hemorrhage, the probability of acute ischemic stroke remains. The physician should review the inclusion and exclusion criteria for IV fibrinolytic therapy (Table 3) and perform a repeat neurologic examination (incorporating the NIH Stroke Scale or Canadian Neurologic Scale). If the patient's neurologic signs are spontaneously clearing (ie, function is rapidly improving toward normal) and is near baseline, fibrinolytic administration is not recommended (Box 6).[10]

As with all medications, fibrinolytics have potential adverse effects. The physician must verify that there are no exclusion criteria, consider the risks and benefits to the patient, and be prepared to monitor and treat any potential complications. The major complication of IV tPA for stroke is symptomatic intracranial hemorrhage. This complication occurred in 6.4% of the 312 patients treated in the NINDS trials[5] and 4.6% of the 1135 patients treated in 60 Canadian centers.[61] A meta-analysis of 15 published case series on the open-label use of tPA for acute ischemic stroke in general clinical practice shows a symptomatic hemorrhage rate of 5.2% of 2639 patients treated.[62] Other complications include orolingual angioedema (occurs in about 1.5% of patients), acute hypotension, and systemic bleeding. In one large prospective registry, major systemic bleeding was uncommon (0.4%) and usually occurred at the site of femoral groin puncture for acute angiography.[61,63]

If the patient remains a candidate for fibrinolytic therapy (Box 8), the physician should discuss the risks and potential benefits of the therapy with the patient or family if available (Box 10). After this discussion, if the patient/family elects to proceed with fibrinolytic therapy, give the patient tPA and begin the stroke pathway of care (see below). Neither anticoagulants nor antiplatelet treatment is administered for 24 hours after administration of tPA, typically until a follow-up CT scan at 24 hours shows no hemorrhage.

Several studies (LOE 1)[5,12,61] have documented a higher likelihood of good to excellent functional outcome when tPA is administered to adult patients with acute ischemic stroke within 3 hours of onset of symptoms. These results are obtained when tPA is administered by physicians in hospitals with a stroke protocol that rigorously adheres to the eligibility criteria and therapeutic regimen of the NINDS protocol. These results have been supported by subsequent 1-year follow-up,[64] reanalysis of the NINDS data,[65] and a meta-analysis (LOE 1).[66] Evidence from prospective, randomized (LOE 1)[5,12,65,67] studies in adults also documents a greater likelihood of benefit the earlier treatment is begun. Many physicians have emphasized the flaws in the NINDS trials.[68,69] But additional analyses of the original NINDS data by an independent group of investigators confirmed the validity of the results,[65] veri-

TABLE 3. Fibrinolytic Checklist

Use of tPA in Patients With Acute Ischemic Stroke

All boxes must be checked before tPA can be given.

Note: The following checklist includes FDA-approved indications and contraindications for tPA administration for acute ischemic stroke. A physician with expertise in acute stroke care may modify this list.

Inclusion Criteria (all Yes boxes in this section must be checked):

Yes

☐ Age 18 years or older?

☐ Clinical diagnosis of ischemic stroke with a measurable neurologic deficit?

☐ Time of symptom onset (when patient was last seen normal) well established as <180 minutes (3 hours) before treatment would begin?

Exclusion Criteria (all No boxes in "Contraindications" section must be checked):

Contraindications:

No

☐ Evidence of intracranial hemorrhage on pretreatment noncontrast head CT?

☐ Clinical presentation suggestive of subarachnoid hemorrhage even with normal CT?

☐ CT shows multilobar infarction (hypodensity greater than one third cerebral hemisphere)?

☐ History of intracranial hemorrhage?

☐ Uncontrolled hypertension: At the time treatment should begin, systolic pressure remains >185 mm Hg or diastolic pressure remains >110 mm Hg despite repeated measurements?

☐ Known arteriovenous malformation, neoplasm, or aneurysm?

☐ Witnessed seizure at stroke onset?

☐ Active internal bleeding or acute trauma (fracture)?

☐ Acute bleeding diathesis, including but not limited to

—Platelet count <100 000/mm^3?

—Heparin received within 48 hours, resulting in an activated partial thromboplastin time (aPTT) that is greater than upper limit of normal for laboratory?

—Current use of anticoagulant (eg, warfarin sodium) that has produced an elevated international normalized ratio (INR) >1.7 or prothrombin time (PT) >15 seconds?*

☐ Within 3 months of intracranial or intraspinal surgery, serious head trauma, or previous stroke?

☐ Arterial puncture at a noncompressible site within past 7 days?

Relative Contraindications/Precautions:

Recent experience suggests that under some circumstances—with careful consideration and weighing of risk-to-benefit ratio—patients may receive fibrinolytic therapy despite one or more relative contraindications. Consider the pros and cons of tPA administration carefully if any of these relative contraindications is present:

- Only minor or rapidly improving stroke symptoms (clearing spontaneously)
- Within 14 days of major surgery or serious trauma
- Recent gastrointestinal or urinary tract hemorrhage (within previous 21 days)
- Recent acute myocardial infarction (within previous 3 months)
- Postmyocardial infarction pericarditis
- Abnormal blood glucose level (<50 or >400 mg/dL [<2.8 or >22.2 mmol/L])

*In patients without recent use of oral anticoagulants or heparin, treatment with tPA can be initiated before availability of coagulation study results but should be discontinued if the INR is >1.7 or the partial thromboplastin time is elevated by local laboratory standards.

fying that improved outcomes in the tPA treatment arm persist even when imbalances in the baseline stroke severity among treatment groups is corrected.[70]

Administration of IV tPA to patients with acute ischemic stroke who meet the NINDS eligibility criteria is recommended if tPA is administered by physicians in the setting of a clearly defined protocol, a knowledgeable team, and institutional commitment (Class I). It is important to note that the superior outcomes reported in both community and tertiary care hospitals in the NINDS trials have been difficult to replicate in hospitals with less experience in, and institutional commitment to, acute stroke care.[71,72] There is strong evidence to avoid all delays and treat patients as soon as possible. Failure to adhere to protocol is associated with an increased rate of complications, particularly the risk of symptomatic intracranial hemorrhage.[71,73]

Community hospitals have reported outcomes comparable to the results of the NINDS trials after implementing a stroke program with a focus on quality improvement.[61,74,75] The experience of the Cleveland Clinic system is instructive.[71,75] A quality improvement program increased compliance with the tPA treatment protocol in 9 community hospitals, and the rate of symptomatic intracerebral hemorrhage fell from 13.4% to 6.4%.[75]

TABLE 4. Approach to Elevated Blood Pressure in Acute Ischemic Stroke[9]

Blood Pressure Level, mm Hg	Treatment
A. Not eligible for fibrinolytic therapy	
Systolic ≤220 OR diastolic ≤120	Observe unless other end-organ involvement (eg, aortic dissection, acute myocardial infarction, pulmonary edema, hypertensive encephalopathy) Treat other symptoms of stroke (eg, headache, pain, agitation, nausea, vomiting) Treat other acute complications of stroke, including hypoxia, increased intracranial pressure, seizures, or hypoglycemia
Systolic >220 OR diastolic 121 to 140	Labetalol 10 to 20 mg IV for 1 to 2 min May repeat or double every 10 min (max dose 300 mg) OR Nicardipine 5 mg/h IV infusion as initial dose; titrate to desired effect by increasing 2.5 mg/h every 5 min to max of 15 mg/h Aim for a 10% to 15% reduction in blood pressure
Diastolic >140	Nitroprusside 0.5 μg/kg per minute IV infusion as initial dose with continuous blood pressure monitoring Aim for a 10% to 15% reduction in blood pressure
B. Eligible for fibrinolytic therapy	
Pretreatment	
Systolic >185 OR diastolic >110	Labetalol 10 to 20 mg IV for 1 to 2 min May repeat 1 time or nitropaste 1 to 2 in
During/after treatment	
1. Monitor blood pressure	Check blood pressure every 15 min for 2 h, then every 30 min for 6 h, and finally every hour for 16 h
2. Diastolic >140	Sodium nitroprusside 0.5 μg/kg per minute IV infusion as initial dose and titrate to desired blood pressure
3. Systolic >230 OR diastolic 121 to 140	Labetalol 10 mg IV for 1 to 2 min May repeat or double labetalol every 10 min to maximum dose of 300 mg, or give initial labetalol dose, then start labetalol drip at 2 to 8 mg/min OR Nicarpidine 5 mg/h IV infusion as initial dose and titrate to desired effect by increasing 2.5 mg/h every 5 min to maximum of 15 mg/h; if blood pressure is not controlled by labetalol, consider sodium nitroprusside
4. Systolic 180 to 230 OR diastolic 105 to 120	Labetalol 10 mg IV for 1 to 2 min May repeat or double labetalol every 10 to 20 min to maximum dose of 300 mg, or give initial labetalol dose, then start labetalol drip at 2 to 8 mg/min

There is a relationship between violations of the NINDS treatment protocol and increased risk of symptomatic intracerebral hemorrhage and death.[62] In Germany there was an increased risk of death after administration of tPA for acute ischemic stroke in hospitals that treated ≤5 patients per year, which suggests that clinical experience is an important factor in ensuring adherence to protocol.[63] Adding a dedicated stroke team to a community hospital can increase the number of patients with acute stroke treated with fibrinolytic therapy and produce excellent clinical outcomes.[76] These findings show that it is important to have an institutional commitment to ensure optimal patient outcomes.

Evidence from 2 prospective randomized studies in adults and a meta-analysis[77,78] and additional case series[79–86] documented improved outcome from therapies such as intra-arterial tPA. Thus, for patients with acute ischemic stroke who are not candidates for standard IV fibrinolysis, administration of intra-arterial fibrinolysis in centers that have the resources and expertise available may be considered within the first few hours after the onset of symptoms (Class IIb). Intra-arterial administration of tPA has not yet been approved by the US Food and Drug Administration (FDA).

General Stroke Care

Admit the patient to a stroke unit (if available) for careful observation (Box 11), including monitoring of blood pressure and neurologic status and treatment of hypertension if indicated (Table 4). If the patient's neurologic status deteriorates, order an emergent CT scan to determine if cerebral edema or hemorrhage is responsible for the deterioration and treat if possible.

Hyperglycemia is associated with worse clinical outcome in patients with acute ischemic stroke than is normoglycemia,[87–94] but there is no direct evidence that active glucose control improves clinical outcome.[95,96] There is evidence that insulin treatment of hyperglycemia in other critically ill patients improves survival rates (LOE 7 for stroke).[97] For this reason administration of IV or subcutaneous insulin may be considered (Class IIb) to lower blood glucose in patients with acute ischemic stroke when the serum glucose level is >10 mmol/L (>about 200 mg/dL).

Additional stroke care includes support of the airway, oxygenation and ventilation, and nutritional support. Administer approximately 75 to 100 mL/h of normal saline to maintain euvolemia if needed. Seizure prophylaxis is not recommended, but we recommend treatment of acute seizures followed by administration of anticonvulsants to prevent further seizures.[98] Monitor the patient for signs of increased intracranial pressure. Continued control of blood pressure is required to reduce the potential risk of bleeding (see Table 4).

All patients with stroke should be screened for dysphagia before anything is given by mouth. A simple bedside screening evaluation involves asking the patient to sip water from a cup. If the patient can sip and swallow without difficulty, the patient is asked to take a large gulp of water and swallow. If there are no signs of coughing or aspiration after 30 seconds, then it is safe for the patient to have a thickened diet until formally assessed by a speech pathologist. Medications may be given in applesauce or jam. Any patient who fails a swallow test may be given medications such as aspirin rectally or if appropriate via the IV, intramuscular, or subcutaneous route.

Temperature Control

Treat fever >37.5°C (99.5°F). Hyperthermia in the setting of acute cerebral ischemia is associated with increased morbidity and mortality.[99–102]

Induced hypothermia can exert neuroprotective effects following stroke.[103–111] Hypothermia has been shown to improve survival and functional outcome in patients following resuscitation from ventricular fibrillation (VF) sudden cardiac arrest (LOE 1[112]; LOE 2[113]), but it has not been shown to be effective for acute ischemic stroke in controlled human trials. In some small human pilot studies and in animal models, hypothermia (33°C to 36°C) for acute ischemic stroke has been shown to be relatively safe and feasible (LOE 3 to 5).[106,109,110] Although effects of hypothermia on both global and focal cerebral ischemia in animals have been promising,[111] cooling to ≤33°C appears to be associated with increased complications, including hypotension, cardiac arrhythmias, cardiac failure, pneumonia, thrombocytopenia, and a rebound increase in intracranial pressure during rewarming.[104,105,107,108,111]

Ongoing larger clinical trials of induced hypothermia will likely increase our understanding of the role of hypothermia in acute cerebral ischemia. There is insufficient scientific evidence to recommend for or against the use of hypothermia in the treatment of acute ischemic stroke (Class Indeterminate).

Summary

Advances in stroke care will have the greatest effect on stroke outcome if care is delivered within a system designed to improve both efficiency and effectiveness. The ultimate goal of stroke therapy is to maximize functional recovery.

References

1. *Know the Facts, Get the Stats: Our Guide to Heart Disease, Stroke and Risks*. Dallas, Tex: American Heart Association; 2002. Publication No. 55-0576 2002-04.
2. American Heart Association. *Heart Disease and Stroke Statistics—2006 Update*. Dallas, Tex: American Heart Association. In press.
3. Schwamm LH, Pancioli A, Acker JE III, Goldstein LB, Zorowitz RD, Shephard TJ, Moyer P, Gorman M, Johnston SC, Duncan PW, Gorelick P, Frank J, Stranne SK, Smith R, Federspiel W, Horton KB, Magnis E, Adams RJ. Recommendations for the establishment of stroke systems of care: recommendations from the American Stroke Association's Task Force on the Development of Stroke Systems. *Circulation*. 2005;111:1078–1091.
4. Dobkin BH. Clinical practice: rehabilitation after stroke. *N Engl J Med*. 2005;352:1677–1684.
5. Tissue plasminogen activator for acute ischemic stroke. The National Institute of Neurological Disorders and Stroke rt-PA Stroke Study Group. *N Engl J Med*. 1995;333:1581–1587.
6. Albers GW, Bates VE, Clark WM, Bell R, Verro P, Hamilton SA. Intravenous tissue-type plasminogen activator for treatment of acute stroke: the Standard Treatment with Alteplase to Reverse Stroke (STARS) study. *JAMA*. 2000;283:1145–1150.
7. Hazinski M. D-mystifying recognition and management of stroke. *Curr Emerg Cardiac Care*. 1996;7:8.
8. Acute stroke: current treatment and paradigms. In: Cummins RO, Field JM, Hazinski MF, eds. *ACLS: Principles and Practice*. Dallas, Tex: American Heart Association; 2003:437–482.
9. Adams H, Adams R, Del Zoppo G, Goldstein LB. Guidelines for the early management of patients with ischemic stroke: 2005 guidelines update: a scientific statement from the Stroke Council of the American Heart Association/American Stroke Association. *Stroke*. 2005;36:916–923.
10. Adams HP Jr, Adams RJ, Brott T, del Zoppo GJ, Furlan A, Goldstein LB, Grubb RL, Higashida R, Kidwell C, Kwiatkowski TG, Marler JR, Hademenos GJ. Guidelines for the early management of patients with ischemic stroke: a scientific statement from the Stroke Council of the American Stroke Association. *Stroke*. 2003;34:1056–1083.
11. Marler JR, Jones PW, Emr M, eds. *Setting New Directions for Stroke Care: Proceedings of a National Symposium on Rapid Identification and Treatment of Acute Stroke*. Bethesda, Md: National Institute of Neurological Disorders and Stroke; 1997.
12. Hacke W, Donnan G, Fieschi C, Kaste M, von Kummer R, Broderick JP, Brott T, Frankel M, Grotta JC, Haley EC Jr, Kwiatkowski T, Levine SR, Lewandowski C, Lu M, Lyden P, Marler JR, Patel S, Tilley BC, Albers G, Bluhmki E, Wilhelm M, Hamilton S. Association of outcome with early stroke treatment: pooled analysis of ATLANTIS, ECASS, and NINDS rt-PA stroke trials. *Lancet*. 2004;363:768–774.
13. Barsan WG, Brott TG, Olinger CP, Adams HP Jr, Haley EC Jr, Levy DE. Identification and entry of the patient with acute cerebral infarction. *Ann Emerg Med*. 1988;17:1192–1195.
14. Barsan WG, Brott TG, Broderick JP, Haley EC, Levy DE, Marler JR. Time of hospital presentation in patients with acute stroke. *Arch Intern Med*. 1993;153:2558–2561.
15. Pepe PE, Zachariah BS, Sayre MR, Floccare D. Ensuring the chain of recovery for stroke in your community. Chain of Recovery Writing Group. *Prehosp Emerg Care*. 1998;2:89–95.
16. Feldmann E, Gordon N, Brooks JM, Brass LM, Fayad PB, Sawaya KL, Nazareno F, Levine SR. Factors associated with early presentation of acute stroke. *Stroke*. 1993;24:1805–1810.
17. Lyden P, Rapp K, Babcock T, et al. Ultra-rapid identification, triage, and enrollment of stroke patients into clinical trials. *J Stroke Cerebrovasc Dis*. 1994;2:106–113.
18. Morgenstern LB, Staub L, Chan W, Wein TH, Bartholomew LK, King M, Felberg RA, Burgin WS, Groff J, Hickenbottom SL, Saldin K, Demchuk AM, Kalra A, Dhingra A, Grotta JC. Improving delivery of acute stroke therapy: the TLL Temple Foundation Stroke Project. *Stroke*. 2002;33:160–166.
19. Morgenstern LB, Bartholomew LK, Grotta JC, Staub L, King M, Chan W. Sustained benefit of a community and professional intervention to increase acute stroke therapy. *Arch Intern Med*. 2003;163:2198–2202.
20. Cocho D, Belvis R, Marti-Fabregas J, Molina-Porcel L, Diaz-Manera J, Aleu A, Pagonabarraga J, Garcia-Bargo D, Mauri A, Marti-Vilalta JL. Reasons for exclusion from thrombolytic therapy following acute ischemic stroke. *Neurology*. 2005;64:719–720.
21. Prioritizing interventions to improve rates of thrombolysis for ischemic stroke. *Neurology*. 2005;64:654–659.
22. Katzan IL, Hammer MD, Hixson ED, Furlan AJ, Abou-Chebl A, Nadzam DM. Utilization of intravenous tissue plasminogen activator for acute ischemic stroke. *Arch Neurol*. 2004;61:346–350.
23. Kleindorfer D, Kissela B, Schneider A, Woo D, Khoury J, Miller R, Alwell K, Gebel J, Szaflarski J, Pancioli A, Jauch E, Moomaw C, Shukla R, Broderick JP. Eligibility for recombinant tissue plasminogen activator in acute ischemic stroke: a population-based study. *Stroke*. 2004;35:e27–e29.
24. O'Connor R, McGraw P, Edelsohn L. Thrombolytic therapy for acute ischemic stroke: why the majority of patients remain ineligible for treatment. *Ann Emerg Med*. 1999;33:9–14.
25. Sayre MR, Swor RA, Honeykutt LK. Prehospital identification and treatment. In: Marler JR, Jones PW, Emr M, eds. *Setting New Directions for Stroke Care: Proceedings of a National Symposium on Rapid Identification and Treatment of Acute Stroke*. Bethesda, Md: National Institute of Neurological Disorders and Stroke; 1997:35–44.

26. Zachariah B, Dunford J, Van Cott CC. Dispatch life support and the acute stroke patient: making the right call. In: *Proceedings of the National Institute of Neurological Disorders and Stroke*. Bethesda, Md: National Institute of Neurological Disorders and Stroke; 1991:29–33.
27. Kothari R, Barsan W, Brott T, Broderick J, Ashbrock S. Frequency and accuracy of prehospital diagnosis of acute stroke. *Stroke*. 1995;26:937–941.
28. A systems approach to immediate evaluation and management of hyperacute stroke: experience at eight centers and implications for community practice and patient care. The National Institute of Neurological Disorders and Stroke (NINDS) rt-PA Stroke Study Group. *Stroke*. 1997;28: 1530–1540.
29. Kothari R, Hall K, Brott T, Broderick J. Early stroke recognition: developing an out-of-hospital NIH Stroke Scale. *Acad Emerg Med*. 1997; 4:986–990.
30. Kothari RU, Pancioli A, Liu T, Brott T, Broderick J. Cincinnati Prehospital Stroke Scale: reproducibility and validity. *Ann Emerg Med*. 1999;33: 373–378.
31. Smith WS, Isaacs M, Corry MD. Accuracy of paramedic identification of stroke and transient ischemic attack in the field. *Prehosp Emerg Care*. 1998;2:170–175.
32. Kidwell CS, Saver JL, Schubert GB, Eckstein M, Starkman S. Design and retrospective analysis of the Los Angeles Prehospital Stroke Screen (LAPSS). *Prehosp Emerg Care*. 1998;2:267–273.
33. Kidwell CS, Starkman S, Eckstein M, Weems K, Saver JL. Identifying stroke in the field: prospective validation of the Los Angeles prehospital stroke screen (LAPSS). *Stroke*. 2000;31:71–76.
34. Ellison SR, Gratton MC, Schwab RA, Ma OJ. Prehospital dispatch assessment of stroke. *Mo Med*. 2004;101:64–66.
35. Wojner AW, Morgenstern L, Alexandrov AV, Rodriguez D, Persse D, Grotta JC. Paramedic and emergency department care of stroke: baseline data from a citywide performance improvement study. *Am J Crit Care*. 2003;12:411–417.
36. Smith WS, Corry MD, Fazackerley J, Isaacs SM. Improved paramedic sensitivity in identifying stroke victims in the prehospital setting. *Prehosp Emerg Care*. 1999;3:207–210.
37. Zweifler RM, York D, et al. Accuracy of paramedic diagnosis of stroke. *J Stroke Cerebrovasc Dis*. 1998;7:446–448.
38. Langhorne P, Tong BL, Stott DJ. Association between physiological homeostasis and early recovery after stroke. *Stroke*. 2000;31:2518–2519.
39. Singhal AB, Benner T, Roccatagliata L, Koroshetz WJ, Schaefer PW, Lo EH, Buonanno FS, Gonzalez RG, Sorensen AG. A pilot study of normobaric oxygen therapy in acute ischemic stroke. *Stroke*. 2005;36:797–802.
40. Ronning OM, Guldvog B. Should stroke victims routinely receive supplemental oxygen? A quasi-randomized controlled trial. *Stroke*. 1999;30: 2033–2037.
41. Evans A, Perez I, Harraf F, Melbourn A, Steadman J, Donaldson N, Kalra L. Can differences in management processes explain different outcomes between stroke unit and stroke-team care? *Lancet*. 2001;358:1586–1592.
42. Indredavik B, Bakke F, Slordahl SA, Rokseth R, Haheim LL. Treatment in a combined acute and rehabilitation stroke unit: which aspects are most important? *Stroke*. 1999;30:917–923.
43. International Liaison Committee on Resuscitation. 2005 International Consensus on Cardiopulmonary Resuscitation and Emergency Cardiovascular Care Science With Treatment Recommendations. *Circulation*. 2005;112: III-1–III-136.
44. Chapman KM, Woolfenden AR, Graeb D, Johnston DC, Beckman J, Schulzer M, Teal PA. Intravenous tissue plasminogen activator for acute ischemic stroke: a Canadian hospital's experience. *Stroke*. 2000;31: 2920–2924.
45. Merino JG, Silver B, Wong E, Foell B, Demaerschalk B, Tamayo A, Poncha F, Hachinski V. Extending tissue plasminogen activator use to community and rural stroke patients. *Stroke*. 2002;33:141–146.
46. Riopelle RJ, Howse DC, Bolton C, Elson S, Groll DL, Holtom D, Brunet DG, Jackson AC, Melanson M, Weaver DF. Regional access to acute ischemic stroke intervention. *Stroke*. 2001;32:652–655.
47. Cross DT III, Tirschwell DL, Clark MA, Tuden D, Derdeyn CP, Moran CJ, Dacey RG Jr. Mortality rates after subarachnoid hemorrhage: variations according to hospital case volume in 18 states. *J Neurosurg*. 2003;99: 810–817.
48. Domeier R, Scott P, Wagner C. From research to the road: the development of EMS specialty triage. *Air Med J*. 2004;23:28–31.
49. Pepe PE, Zachariah BS, Sayre MR, Floccare D. Ensuring the chain of recovery for stroke in your community. *Acad Emerg Med*. 1998;5:352–358.
50. Wojner AW, Alexandrov AV, Rodriguez D, Persse D, Grotta JC. The Houston Paramedic and Emergency Stroke Treatment and Outcomes Study (HoPSTO). *Stroke*. In press.
51. Collaborative systematic review of the randomised trials of organised inpatient (stroke unit) care after stroke. Stroke Unit Trialists' Collaboration. *BMJ*. 1997;314:1151–1159.
52. How do stroke units improve patient outcomes? A collaborative systematic review of the randomized trials. Stroke Unit Trialists Collaboration. *Stroke*. 1997;28:2139–2144.
53. Organised inpatient (stroke unit) care for stroke. *Cochrane Database Syst Rev*. 2002:CD000197.
54. Ma RH, Wang YJ, Zhao XQ, Wang CX, Yang ZH, Qu H. [The impact of stroke unit on early outcome of cerebral infarction patients]. *Zhonghua Nei Ke Za Zhi*. 2004;43:183–185.
55. Oppenheimer SM, Cechetto DF, Hachinski VC. Cerebrogenic cardiac arrhythmias: cerebral electrocardiographic influences and their role in sudden death. *Arch Neurol*. 1990;47:513–519.
56. LaMonte MP, Bahouth MN, Hu P, Pathan MY, Yarbrough KL, Gunawardane R, Crarey P, Page W. Telemedicine for acute stroke: triumphs and pitfalls. *Stroke*. 2003;34:725–728.
57. Rymer MM, Thurtchley D, Summers D. Expanded modes of tissue plasminogen activator delivery in a comprehensive stroke center increases regional acute stroke interventions. *Stroke*. 2003;34:e58–e60.
58. Audebert HJ, Kukla C, Clarmann von Claranau S, Kuhn J, Vatankhah B, Schenkel J, Ickenstein GW, Haberl RL, Horn M. Telemedicine for safe and extended use of thrombolysis in stroke: the Telemedic Pilot Project for Integrative Stroke Care (TEMPiS) in Bavaria. *Stroke*. 2005;36:287–291.
59. Connors JJ III, Sacks D, Furlan AJ, Selman WR, Russell EJ, Stieg PE, Hadley MN. Training, competency, and credentialing standards for diagnostic cervicocerebral angiography, carotid stenting, and cerebrovascular intervention: a joint statement from the American Academy of Neurology, American Association of Neurological Surgeons, American Society of Interventional and Therapeutic Radiology, American Society of Neuroradiology, Congress of Neurological Surgeons, AANS/CNS Cerebrovascular Section, and Society of Interventional Radiology. *Radiology*. 2005;234: 26–34.
60. Schriger DL, Kalafut M, Starkman S, Krueger M, Saver JL. Cranial computed tomography interpretation in acute stroke: physician accuracy in determining eligibility for thrombolytic therapy. *JAMA*. 1998;279: 1293–1297.
61. Hill MD, Buchan AM. Thrombolysis for acute ischemic stroke: results of the Canadian Alteplase for Stroke Effectiveness Study. Canadian Alteplase for Stroke Effectiveness Study (CASES) Investigators. *CMAJ*. 2005;172: 1307–1312.
62. Graham GD. Tissue plasminogen activator for acute ischemic stroke in clinical practice: a meta-analysis of safety data. *Stroke*. 2003;34:2847–2850.
63. Heuschmann PU, Berger K, Misselwitz B, Hermanek P, Leffmann C, Adelmann M, Buecker-Nott HJ, Rother J, Neundoerfer B, Kolominsky-Rabas PL. Frequency of thrombolytic therapy in patients with acute ischemic stroke and the risk of in-hospital mortality: the German Stroke Registers Study Group. *Stroke*. 2003;34:1106–1113.
64. Kwiatkowski TG, Libman RB, Frankel M, Tilley BC, Morgenstern LB, Lu M, Broderick JP, Lewandowski CA, Marler JR, Levine SR, Brott T. Effects of tissue plasminogen activator for acute ischemic stroke at one year. National Institute of Neurological Disorders and Stroke Recombinant Tissue Plasminogen Activator Stroke Study Group. *N Engl J Med*. 1999; 340:1781–1787.
65. Ingall TJ, O'Fallon WM, Asplund K, Goldfrank LR, Hertzberg VS, Louis TA, Christianson TJ. Findings from the reanalysis of the NINDS tissue plasminogen activator for acute ischemic stroke treatment trial. *Stroke*. 2004;35:2418–2424.
66. Wardlaw JM, Zoppo G, Yamaguchi T, Berge E. Thrombolysis for acute ischaemic stroke. *Cochrane Database Syst Rev*. 2003:CD000213.
67. Marler JR, Tilley BC, Lu M, Brott TG, Lyden PC, Grotta JC, Broderick JP, Levine SR, Frankel MP, Horowitz SH, Haley EC Jr, Lewandowski CA, Kwiatkowski TP. Early stroke treatment associated with better outcome: the NINDS rt-PA stroke study. *Neurology*. 2000;55:1649–1655.
68. Mann J. Truths about the NINDS study: setting the record straight. *West J Med*. 2002;176:192–194.
69. Lindley RI. Further randomized controlled trials of tissue plasminogen activator within 3 hours are required. *Stroke*. 2001;32:2708–2709.
70. Kwiatkowski T, Libman R, Tilley BC, Lewandowski C, Grotta JC, Lyden P, Levine SR, Brott T. The impact of imbalances in baseline stroke severity on outcome in the National Institute of Neurological Disorders and Stroke

Recombinant Tissue Plasminogen Activator Stroke Study. *Ann Emerg Med.* 2005;45:377–384.

71. Katzan IL, Furlan AJ, Lloyd LE, Frank JI, Harper DL, Hinchey JA, Hammel JP, Qu A, Sila CA. Use of tissue-type plasminogen activator for acute ischemic stroke: the Cleveland area experience. *JAMA.* 2000;283: 1151–1158.
72. Bravata DM, Kim N, Concato J, Krumholz HM, Brass LM. Thrombolysis for acute stroke in routine clinical practice. *Arch Intern Med.* 2002;162: 1994–2001.
73. Lopez-Yunez AM, Bruno A, Williams LS, Yilmaz E, Zurru C, Biller J. Protocol violations in community-based rTPA stroke treatment are associated with symptomatic intracerebral hemorrhage. *Stroke.* 2001;32:12–16.
74. Asimos AW, Norton HJ, Price MF, Cheek WM. Therapeutic yield and outcomes of a community teaching hospital code stroke protocol. *Acad Emerg Med.* 2004;11:361–370.
75. Katzan IL, Hammer MD, Furlan AJ, Hixson ED, Nadzam DM. Quality improvement and tissue-type plasminogen activator for acute ischemic stroke: a Cleveland update. *Stroke.* 2003;34:799–800.
76. Lattimore SU, Chalela J, Davis L, DeGraba T, Ezzeddine M, Haymore J, Nyquist P, Baird AE, Hallenbeck J, Warach S. Impact of establishing a primary stroke center at a community hospital on the use of thrombolytic therapy: the NINDS Suburban Hospital Stroke Center experience. *Stroke.* 2003;34:e55–e57.
77. Furlan A, Higashida R, Wechsler L, Gent M, Rowley H, Kase C, Pessin M, Ahuja A, Callahan F, Clark WM, Silver F, Rivera F. Intra-arterial prourokinase for acute ischemic stroke: the PROACT II study: a randomized controlled trial. Prolyse in Acute Cerebral Thromboembolism. *JAMA.* 1999;282:2003–2011.
78. Combined intravenous and intra-arterial recanalization for acute ischemic stroke: the Interventional Management of Stroke Study. *Stroke.* 2004;35: 904–911.
79. Suarez JI, Sunshine JL, Tarr R, Zaidat O, Selman WR, Kernich C, Landis DM. Predictors of clinical improvement, angiographic recanalization, and intracranial hemorrhage after intra-arterial thrombolysis for acute ischemic stroke. *Stroke.* 1999;30:2094–2100.
80. Gonner F, Remonda L, Mattle H, Sturzenegger M, Ozdoba C, Lovblad KO, Baumgartner R, Bassetti C, Schroth G. Local intra-arterial thrombolysis in acute ischemic stroke. *Stroke.* 1998;29:1894–1900.
81. Suarez JI, Zaidat OO, Sunshine JL, Tarr R, Selman WR, Landis DM. Endovascular administration after intravenous infusion of thrombolytic agents for the treatment of patients with acute ischemic strokes. *Neurosurgery.* 2002;50:251–259; discussion 259–260.
82. Ernst R, Pancioli A, Tomsick T, Kissela B, Woo D, Kanter D, Jauch E, Carrozzella J, Spilker J, Broderick J. Combined intravenous and intra-arterial recombinant tissue plasminogen activator in acute ischemic stroke. *Stroke.* 2000;31:2552–2557.
83. Bourekas EC, Slivka AP, Shah R, Sunshine J, Suarez JI. Intra-arterial thrombolytic therapy within 3 hours of the onset of stroke. *Neurosurgery.* 2004;54:39–44; discussion 44–46.
84. Keris V, Rudnicka S, Vorona V, Enina G, Tilgale B, Fricbergs J. Combined intra-arterial/intravenous thrombolysis for acute ischemic stroke. *AJNR Am J Neuroradiol.* 2001;22:352–358.
85. Ueda T, Sakaki S, Kumon Y, Ohta S. Multivariable analysis of predictive factors related to outcome at 6 months after intra-arterial thrombolysis for acute ischemic stroke. *Stroke.* 1999;30:2360–2365.
86. Jahan R, Duckwiler GR, Kidwell CS, Sayre JW, Gobin YP, Villablanca JP, Saver J, Starkman S, Martin N, Vinuela F. Intra-arterial thrombolysis for treatment of acute stroke: experience in 26 patients with long-term follow-up. *AJNR Am J Neuroradiol.* 1999;20:1291–1299.
87. Alvarez-Sabin J, Molina CA, Montaner J, Arenillas JF, Huertas R, Ribo M, Codina A, Quintana M. Effects of admission hyperglycemia on stroke outcome in reperfused tissue plasminogen activator–treated patients. *Stroke.* 2003;34:1235–1241.
88. Baird TA, Parsons MW, Phanh T, Butcher KS, Desmond PM, Tress BM, Colman PG, Chambers BR, Davis SM. Persistent poststroke hyperglycemia is independently associated with infarct expansion and worse clinical outcome. *Stroke.* 2003;34:2208–2214.
89. Parsons MW, Barber PA, Desmond PM, Baird TA, Darby DG, Byrnes G, Tress BM, Davis SM. Acute hyperglycemia adversely affects stroke outcome: a magnetic resonance imaging and spectroscopy study. *Ann Neurol.* 2002;52:20–28.
90. Capes SE, Hunt D, Malmberg K, Pathak P, Gerstein HC. Stress hyperglycemia and prognosis of stroke in nondiabetic and diabetic patients: a systematic overview. *Stroke.* 2001;32:2426–2432.
91. Bhalla A, Sankaralingam S, Tilling K, Swaminathan R, Wolfe C, Rudd A. Effect of acute glycaemic index on clinical outcome after acute stroke. *Cerebrovasc Dis.* 2002;13:95–101.
92. Bruno A, Biller J, Adams HP Jr, Clarke WR, Woolson RF, Williams LS, Hansen MD. Acute blood glucose level and outcome from ischemic stroke. Trial of ORG 10172 in Acute Stroke Treatment (TOAST) Investigators. *Neurology.* 1999;52:280–284.
93. Celik Y, Utku U, Asil T, Balci K. Factors affecting haemorrhagic transformation in middle cerebral artery infarctions. *J Clin Neurosci.* 2004;11: 656–658.
94. Williams LS, Rotich J, Qi R, Fineberg N, Espay A, Bruno A, Fineberg SE, Tierney WR. Effects of admission hyperglycemia on mortality and costs in acute ischemic stroke. *Neurology.* 2002;59:67–71.
95. Scott JF, Robinson GM, French JM, O'Connell JE, Alberti KG, Gray CS. Glucose potassium insulin infusions in the treatment of acute stroke patients with mild to moderate hyperglycemia: the Glucose Insulin in Stroke Trial (GIST). *Stroke.* 1999;30:793–799.
96. Gray CS, Hildreth AJ, Alberti GK, O'Connell JE. Poststroke hyperglycemia: natural history and immediate management. *Stroke.* 2004;35: 122–126.
97. van den Berghe G, Wouters P, Weekers F, Verwaest C, Bruyninckx F, Schetz M, Vlasselaers D, Ferdinande P, Lauwers P, Bouillon R. Intensive insulin therapy in the critically ill patients. *N Engl J Med.* 2001;345: 1359–1367.
98. Adams HJ, Brott T, Crowell R, Furlan A, Gomez C, Grotta J, Helgason C, Marler J, Woolson R, Zivin J, Feinberg W, Mayberg M. Guidelines for the management of patients with acute ischemic stroke: a statement for healthcare professionals from a special writing group of the Stroke Council, American Heart Association. *Stroke.* 1994;25:1901–1914.
99. Hajat C, Hajat S, Sharma P. Effects of poststroke pyrexia on stroke outcome: a meta-analysis of studies in patients. *Stroke.* 2000;31:410–414.
100. Azzimondi G, Bassein L, Nonino F, Fiorani L, Vignatelli L, Re G, D'Alessandro R. Fever in acute stroke worsens prognosis: a prospective study. *Stroke.* 1995;26:2040–2043.
101. Reith J, Jorgensen HS, Pedersen PM, Nakayama H, Raaschou HO, Jeppesen LL, Olsen TS. Body temperature in acute stroke: relation to stroke severity, infarct size, mortality, and outcome. *Lancet.* 1996;347:422–425.
102. Boyson G, Christenson H. Stroke severity determines body temperature in acute stroke. *Stroke.* 2001;32:413–417.
103. De Georgia MA, Krieger DW, Abou-Chebl A, Devlin TG, Jauss M, Davis SM, Koroshetz WJ, Rordorf G, Warach S. Cooling for Acute Ischemic Brain Damage (COOL AID): a feasibility trial of endovascular cooling. *Neurology.* 2004;63:312–317.
104. Georgiadis D, Schwarz S, Aschoff A, Schwab S. Hemicraniectomy and moderate hypothermia in patients with severe ischemic stroke. *Stroke.* 2002; 33:1584–1588.
105. Georgiadis D, Schwarz S, Kollmar R, Schwab S. Endovascular cooling for moderate hypothermia in patients with acute stroke: first results of a novel approach. *Stroke.* 2001;32:2550–2553.
106. Wang H, Olivero W, Lanzino G, Elkins W, Rose J, Honings D, Rodde M, Burnham J, Wang D. Rapid and selective cerebral hypothermia achieved using a cooling helmet. *J Neurosurg.* 2004;100:272–277.
107. Schwab S, Schwarz S, Spranger M, Keller E, Bertram M, Hacke W. Moderate hypothermia in the treatment of patients with severe middle cerebral artery infarction. *Stroke.* 1998;29:2461–2466.
108. Schwab S, Georgiadis D, Berrouschot J, Schellinger PD, Graffagnino C, Mayer SA. Feasibility and safety of moderate hypothermia after massive hemispheric infarction. *Stroke.* 2001;32:2033–2035.
109. Kammersgaard LP, Rasmussen BH, Jorgensen HS, Reith J, Weber U, Olsen TS. Feasibility and safety of inducing modest hypothermia in awake patients with acute stroke through surface cooling: a case-control study: the Copenhagen Stroke Study. *Stroke.* 2000;31:2251–2556.
110. Knoll T, Wimmer ML, Gumpinger F, Haberl RL. The low normothermia concept—maintaining a core body temperature between 36 and 37 degrees C in acute stroke unit patients. *J Neurosurg Anesthesiol.* 2002;14:304–308.
111. Krieger DW, De Georgia MA, Abou-Chebl A, Andrefsky JC, Sila CA, Katzan IL, Mayberg MR, Furlan AJ. Cooling for acute ischemic brain damage (COOL AID): an open pilot study of induced hypothermia in acute ischemic stroke. *Stroke.* 2001;32:1847–1854.
112. Hypothermia After Cardiac Arrest Study Group. Mild therapeutic hypothermia to improve the neurologic outcome after cardiac arrest. *N Engl J Med.* 2002;346:549–556.
113. Bernard SA, Gray TW, Buist MD, Jones BM, Silvester W, Gutteridge G, Smith K. Treatment of comatose survivors of out-of-hospital cardiac arrest with induced hypothermia. *N Engl J Med.* 2002;346:557–563.

Part 10.1: Life-Threatening Electrolyte Abnormalities

Electrolyte abnormalities are commonly associated with cardiovascular emergencies. These abnormalities may cause or contribute to cardiac arrest and may hinder resuscitative efforts. In some cases therapy for life-threatening electrolyte disorders should be initiated before laboratory results become available.

Potassium (K^+)

The magnitude of the potassium gradient across cell membranes determines excitability of nerve and muscle cells, including the myocardium. Rapid or significant changes in the serum potassium concentration can have life-threatening consequences.

Evaluation of serum potassium must consider the effects of changes in serum pH. When serum pH falls, serum potassium rises because potassium shifts from the cellular to the vascular space. When serum pH rises, serum potassium falls because potassium shifts from the vascular space into the cells. Effects of pH changes on serum potassium should be anticipated during therapy for hyperkalemia or hypokalemia and during any therapy that may cause changes in serum pH (eg, treatment of diabetic ketoacidosis).

Hyperkalemia

Although hyperkalemia is defined as a serum potassium concentration >5 mEq/L, it is moderate (6 to 7 mEq/L) and severe (>7 mEq/L) hyperkalemia that are life-threatening and require immediate therapy. Hyperkalemia is most commonly seen in patients with end-stage renal disease. Other causes are listed in the Table. Many medications can contribute to the development of hyperkalemia. Identification of potential causes of hyperkalemia will contribute to rapid identification and treatment.[1–3]

Signs and symptoms of hyperkalemia include weakness, ascending paralysis, and respiratory failure. A variety of electrocardiographic (ECG) changes suggest hyperkalemia. Early findings include peaked T waves (tenting). As the serum potassium rises further, flattened P waves, prolonged PR interval (first-degree heart block), widened QRS complex, deepened S waves, and merging of S and T waves can be seen. If hyperkalemia is left untreated, a sine-wave pattern, idioventricular rhythms, and asystolic cardiac arrest may develop.

Treatment of Hyperkalemia

The treatment of hyperkalemia is determined by its severity and the patient's clinical condition. Stop sources of exogenous potassium administration (eg, consider supplements and maintenance IV fluids) and evaluate drugs that can increase serum potassium (eg, potassium-sparing diuretics, angiotensin-converting enzyme [ACE] inhibitors, nonsteroidal anti-inflammatory agents). Additional treatment is based on the severity of the hyperkalemia and its clinical consequences. The following sequences list the treatments for hyperkalemia in order of priority.

For *mild* elevation (5 to 6 mEq/L), remove potassium from the body with

1. Diuretics: furosemide 40 to 80 mg IV
2. Resins: Kayexalate 15 to 30 g in 50 to 100 mL of 20% sorbitol either orally or by retention enema

For *moderate* elevation (6 to 7 mEq/L), shift potassium intracellularly with

1. Glucose plus insulin: mix 25 g (50 mL of D_{50}) glucose and 10 U regular insulin and give IV over 15 to 30 minutes
2. Sodium bicarbonate: 50 mEq IV over 5 minutes (sodium bicarbonate alone is less effective than glucose plus insulin or nebulized albuterol, particularly for treatment of patients with renal failure; it is best used in conjunction with these medications[4,5])
3. Nebulized albuterol: 10 to 20 mg nebulized over 15 minutes

For *severe* elevation (>7 mEq/L with toxic ECG changes), you need to shift potassium into the cells and eliminate potassium from the body. Therapies that shift potassium will act rapidly but they are temporary; if the serum potassium rebounds you may need to repeat those therapies. In order of priority, treatment includes the following:

TABLE. Common Causes of Hyperkalemia

Endogenous Causes

- Chronic renal failure
- Metabolic acidosis (eg, diabetic ketoacidosis)
- Pseudohypoaldosteronism type II (also known as Gordon's syndrome; familial hyperkalemia and hypertension)
- Chemotherapy causing tumor lysis
- Muscle breakdown (rhabdomyolysis)
- Renal tubular acidosis
- Hemolysis
- Hypoaldosteronism (Addison's disease, hyporeninemia)
- Hyperkalemic periodic paralysis

Exogenous Causes

- Medications: K^+-sparing diuretics, ACE inhibitors, nonsteroidal anti-inflammatory drugs, potassium supplements, penicillin derivatives, succinylcholine, heparin therapy (especially in patients with other risk factors), β-blockers
- Blood administration (particularly with large transfusions of older "bank" blood)
- Diet (rarely the sole cause), salt substitutes
- Pseudohyperkalemia (due to blood sampling or hemolysis, high white blood cell count, high platelets, tumor lysis syndrome)

(*Circulation.* 2005;112:IV-121-IV-125.)

This special supplement to *Circulation* is freely available at http://www.circulationaha.org

DOI: 10.1161/CIRCULATIONAHA.105.166563

- *Shift potassium into cells:*

1. Calcium chloride (10%): 500 to 1000 mg (5 to 10 mL) IV over 2 to 5 minutes to reduce the effects of potassium at the myocardial cell membrane (lowers risk of ventricular fibrillation [VF])
2. Sodium bicarbonate: 50 mEq IV over 5 minutes (may be less effective for patients with end-stage renal disease)
3. Glucose plus insulin: mix 25 g (50 mL of D_{50}) glucose and 10 U regular insulin and give IV over 15 to 30 minutes
4. Nebulized albuterol: 10 to 20 mg nebulized over 15 minutes[5–7]

- *Promote potassium excretion:*

5. Diuresis: furosemide 40 to 80 mg IV
6. Kayexalate enema: 15 to 50 g plus sorbitol PO or per rectum
7. Dialysis

Hypokalemia

Hypokalemia is defined as a serum potassium level <3.5 mEq/L. The most common causes of low serum potassium are gastrointestinal loss (diarrhea, laxatives), renal loss (hyperaldosteronism, severe hyperglycemia, potassium-depleting diuretics, carbenicillin, sodium penicillin, amphotericin B), intracellular shift (alkalosis or a rise in pH), and malnutrition.

The major consequences of severe hypokalemia result from its effects on nerves and muscles (including the heart). The myocardium is extremely sensitive to the effects of hypokalemia, particularly if the patient has coronary artery disease or is taking a digitalis derivative. Symptoms of mild hypokalemia are weakness, fatigue, paralysis, respiratory difficulty, constipation, paralytic ileus, and leg cramps; more severe hypokalemia will alter cardiac tissue excitability and conduction. Hypokalemia can produce ECG changes such as U waves, T-wave flattening, and arrhythmias (especially if the patient is taking digoxin), particularly ventricular arrhythmias. Pulseless electrical activity or asystole may develop.

Treatment of Hypokalemia

The treatment of hypokalemia consists of minimizing further potassium loss and providing potassium replacement. IV administration of potassium is indicated when arrhythmias are present or hypokalemia is severe (potassium level of <2.5 mEq/L). Gradual correction of hypokalemia is preferable to rapid correction unless the patient is clinically unstable.

Administration of potassium may be empirical in emergent conditions. When indicated, the maximum amount of IV potassium replacement should be 10 to 20 mEq/h with continuous ECG monitoring during infusion. A more concentrated solution of potassium may be infused if a central line is used, but the tip of the catheter used for the infusion should not extend into the right atrium.

If cardiac arrest from hypokalemia is imminent (ie, malignant ventricular arrhythmias are present), rapid replacement of potassium is required. Give an initial infusion of 10 mEq IV over 5 minutes; repeat once if needed. *Document in the patient's chart that rapid infusion is intentional in response to life-threatening hypokalemia.*

Sodium (Na^+)

Sodium is the major intravascular ion that influences serum osmolality. An acute increase in serum sodium will produce an acute increase in serum osmolality; an acute decrease in serum sodium will produce an acute fall in serum osmolality.

Sodium concentration and osmolality in the intravascular and interstitial spaces equilibrate across the vascular membrane. *Acute* changes in serum sodium will produce free water shifts into and out of the vascular space until osmolality equilibrates in these compartments. An acute fall in serum sodium will produce an acute shift of free water from the vascular into the interstitial space and may cause cerebral edema.[8,9] An acute rise in serum sodium will produce an acute shift of free water from the interstitial to the vascular space. Rapid correction of hyponatremia has been associated with development of pontine myelinolysis and cerebral bleeding.[10–12] For these reasons, monitor neurologic function closely in the patient with hypernatremia or hyponatremia, particularly during correction of these conditions. Whenever possible, correct serum sodium slowly, carefully controlling the total change in serum sodium over 48 hours and avoiding overcorrection.[13,14]

Hypernatremia

Hypernatremia is defined as a serum sodium concentration >145 to 150 mEq/L. It may be caused by a primary gain in Na^+ or excess loss of water. Gains in sodium can result from hyperaldosteronism (excess mineralocorticoid), Cushing's syndrome (excess glucocorticoid), or excessive hypertonic saline or sodium bicarbonate administration. Loss of free water can result from gastrointestinal losses or renal excretion (eg, osmotic diuresis or diabetes insipidus).

Hypernatremia may cause neurologic symptoms such as altered mental status, weakness, irritability, focal neurologic deficits, and even coma or seizures. The severity of symptoms is determined by the speed and magnitude of the change in serum sodium concentration.

Treatment of Hypernatremia

Treatment of hypernatremia includes reduction of ongoing water losses (by treating the underlying cause) and correction of the water deficit. For stable, asymptomatic patients, replacement of fluid by mouth or through a nasogastric tube is effective and safe.

In hypovolemic patients the extracellular fluid (ECF) volume is typically restored with normal saline or a 5% dextrose in half-normal saline solution to prevent a rapid fall in the serum sodium concentration. Avoid D_5W because it will reduce the serum sodium too rapidly. During rehydration, monitor serum sodium closely to ensure a gradual fall (and prevent rapid fall) in serum sodium.

The quantity of water needed to correct hypernatremia can be calculated by using the following equation:

$$\text{Water deficit (in liters)} = \frac{\text{plasma Na}^+ \text{ concentration} - 140}{140} \times \text{total body water}$$

Total body water is approximately 50% of lean body weight in men and 40% of lean body weight in women. For example, if a 70-kg man had a serum Na^+ level of 160 mEq/L, the estimated free water deficit would be

$$\frac{160-140}{140}\times(0.5\times70)=5\text{ L}$$

Once the free water deficit is calculated, administer fluid to lower serum sodium at a rate of 0.5 to 1 mEq/h with a decrease of no more than approximately 12 mEq/L in the first 24 hours and the remainder over the next 48 to 72 hours.

Hyponatremia

Hyponatremia is defined as a serum sodium concentration <130 to 135 mEq/L. It is caused by an excess of water relative to sodium. Most cases of hyponatremia are caused by reduced renal excretion of water with continued water intake or by loss of sodium in the urine. Impairment of renal water excretion may be caused by

- Use of thiazide diuretics
- Renal failure
- ECF depletion (eg, vomiting with continued water intake)
- Syndrome of inappropriate antidiuretic hormone (SIADH) secretion
- Edematous states (eg, congestive heart failure, cirrhosis with ascites)
- Hypothyroidism
- Adrenal insufficiency

Most cases of hyponatremia are associated with low serum osmolality (so-called hypo-osmolar hyponatremia). The one common exception to this is in uncontrolled diabetes, in which hyperglycemia leads to a hyperosmolar state despite a serum sodium that is below normal (hyperosmolar hyponatremia).

Hyponatremia is usually asymptomatic unless it is acute or severe (<120 mEq/L). An abrupt fall in serum sodium produces a free water shift from the vascular to the interstitial space that can cause cerebral edema. In this case the patient may present with nausea, vomiting, headache, irritability, lethargy, seizures, coma, or even death.

Treatment of Hyponatremia

Treatment of hyponatremia involves administration of sodium and elimination of intravascular free water. If SIADH is present, the treatment is restriction of fluid intake to 50% to 66% of estimated maintenance fluid requirement. Correction of asymptomatic hyponatremia should be gradual: typically increase the Na^+ by 0.5 mEq/L per hour to a maximum change of about 12 mEq/L in the first 24 hours. Rapid correction of hyponatremia can cause coma, which may be associated with osmotic demyelination syndrome or central pontine myelinolysis, lethal disorders thought to be caused by rapid fluid shifts into and out of brain tissue.[10–12]

If the patient develops neurologic compromise, administer 3% saline IV immediately to correct (raise) the serum sodium at a rate of 1 mEq/L per hour until neurologic symptoms are controlled. Some experts recommend a faster rate of correction (ie, increase concentration 2 to 4 mEq/L per hour) when seizures are present. After neurologic symptoms are controlled, provide 3% saline IV to correct (raise) the serum sodium at a rate of 0.5 mEq/L per hour.

To determine the amount of sodium (eg, 3% saline) required to correct the deficit, calculate the total body sodium deficit. The following formula may be used:

Na^+ deficit=(desired $[Na^+]$−current $[Na^+]$)×0.6*×body wt (kg) (*use 0.6 for men and 0.5 for women).

Once the deficit is estimated, determine the volume of 3% saline (513 mEq/L Na^+) necessary to correct the deficit (divide the deficit by 513 mEq/L). Plan to increase the sodium by 1 mEq/L per hour over 4 hours (or until neurologic symptoms improve); then increase the sodium by 0.5 mEq/L per hour. To calculate this amount, use the amount you wish to correct the sodium in an hour (eg, 0.5 mEq/L) and multiply by 0.6 (or 0.5 in women) and then multiply by the body weight; that will calculate the amount of sodium to administer that hour. Check serum sodium frequently and monitor neurologic status.

Magnesium (Mg^{++})

Magnesium is the fourth most common mineral and the second most abundant intracellular cation (after potassium) in the human body. Because extracellular magnesium is bound to serum albumin, magnesium levels do not reliably reflect total body magnesium stores. Magnesium is necessary for the movement of sodium, potassium, and calcium into and out of cells, and magnesium plays an important role in stabilizing excitable membranes. Low potassium in combination with low magnesium is a risk factor for severe arrhythmias. Thus, magnesium balance is closely tied to sodium, calcium, and potassium balance.

Hypermagnesemia

Hypermagnesemia is defined as a serum magnesium concentration >2.2 mEq/L (normal: 1.3 to 2.2 mEq/L). The most common cause of hypermagnesemia is renal failure. Note that pre-eclampsia in pregnant women is treated with magnesium administration, often titrated to maintain the serum magnesium near the maximum normal concentration, without complications of hypermagnesemia.

Neurologic symptoms of hypermagnesemia are muscular weakness, paralysis, ataxia, drowsiness, and confusion. Moderate hypermagnesemia can produce vasodilation; severe hypermagnesemia can produce hypotension. Extremely high serum magnesium levels may produce a depressed level of consciousness, bradycardia, cardiac arrhythmias, hypoventilation, and cardiorespiratory arrest.[15]

Treatment of Hypermagnesemia

Hypermagnesemia is treated with administration of calcium, which removes magnesium from serum. It is important to eliminate sources of ongoing magnesium intake. Cardiorespiratory support may be needed until magnesium levels are reduced. Administration of 10% solution of calcium chloride (5 to 10 mL [500 to 1000 mg] IV) will often correct lethal arrhythmias. This dose may be repeated if needed.

Dialysis is the treatment of choice for severe hypermagnesemia. If renal function is normal and cardiovascular function adequate, IV saline diuresis (administration of IV normal saline and furosemide [1 mg/kg]) can be used to increase renal excretion of magnesium until dialysis can be performed. Diuresis can also increase calcium excretion; the development of hypocalcemia will make signs and symptoms of hypermagnesemia worse.

Hypomagnesemia

Hypomagnesemia, defined as a serum magnesium concentration <1.3 mEq/L, is far more common than hypermagnesemia. Hypomagnesemia usually results from decreased absorption or increased loss of magnesium from either the kidneys or intestines (diarrhea). Alterations in thyroid hormone function and certain medications (eg, pentamidine, diuretics, alcohol) can also induce hypomagnesemia.

Hypomagnesemia interferes with the effects of parathyroid hormone, resulting in hypocalcemia. It may also cause hypokalemia. Symptoms of low serum magnesium are muscular tremors and fasciculations, ocular nystagmus, tetany, altered mental state, and cardiac arrhythmias such as torsades de pointes (multifocal ventricular tachycardia). Other possible symptoms are ataxia, vertigo, seizures, and dysphagia.

Treatment of Hypomagnesemia

The treatment of hypomagnesemia is determined by its severity and the patient's clinical status. For severe or symptomatic hypomagnesemia, give 1 to 2 g of IV $MgSO_4$ over 5 to 60 minutes. For torsades de pointes with cardiac arrest, give 1 to 2 g of $MgSO_4$ IV push over 5 to 20 minutes. If torsades de pointes is intermittent and not associated with arrest, administer the magnesium over 5 to 60 minutes IV. If seizures are present, give 2 g IV $MgSO_4$ over 10 minutes. Administration of calcium is usually appropriate because most patients with hypomagnesemia are also hypocalcemic.[16]

Calcium (Ca^{++})

Calcium is the most abundant mineral in the body. Many processes depend on intracellular calcium, such as enzymatic reactions, receptor activation, muscle contraction, cardiac contractility, and platelet aggregation. Calcium is essential for bone strength and neuromuscular function. Half of all calcium in the ECF is bound to albumin; the other half is in the biologically active, ionized form. Calcium concentration is normally regulated by parathyroid hormone and vitamin D.

Total serum calcium is directly related to the serum albumin concentration. The total serum calcium will increase 0.8 mg/dL for every 1 g/dL rise in serum albumin and will fall 0.8 mg/dL for every 1 g/dL fall in serum albumin.

Although total serum albumin is directly related to total serum calcium, the ionized calcium is *inversely* related to serum albumin. The lower the serum albumin, the higher the portion of the total calcium that is present in ionized form. In the presence of hypoalbuminemia, although total calcium level may be low, the ionized calcium level may be normal.

Calcium antagonizes the effects of both potassium and magnesium at the cell membrane. For this reason it is extremely useful for treating the effects of hyperkalemia and hypermagnesemia.

Hypercalcemia

Hypercalcemia is defined as a total serum calcium concentration >10.5 mEq/L (or an elevation in ionized calcium >4.8 mg/dL). Primary hyperparathyroidism and malignancy account for >90% of reported cases.[17] In these and most forms of hypercalcemia, release of calcium from the bones and intestines is increased, and renal clearance may be compromised.

Symptoms of hypercalcemia usually develop when the total serum calcium concentration is ≥12 to 15 mg/dL. Neurologic symptoms are depression, weakness, fatigue, and confusion at lower levels. At higher levels patients may experience hallucinations, disorientation, hypotonicity, seizures, and coma. Hypercalcemia interferes with renal concentration of urine; the diuresis can cause dehydration.

Cardiovascular symptoms of hypercalcemia are variable. Myocardial contractility may initially increase until the calcium level reaches >15 mg/dL. Above this level myocardial depression occurs. Automaticity is decreased and ventricular systole is shortened. Arrhythmias occur because the refractory period is shortened. Hypercalcemia can worsen digitalis toxicity and may cause hypertension. In addition, many patients with hypercalcemia develop hypokalemia. Both of these conditions contribute to cardiac arrhythmias.[18] The QT interval typically shortens when the serum calcium is >13 mg/dL, and the PR and QRS intervals are prolonged. Atrioventricular block may develop and progress to complete heart block and even cardiac arrest when the total serum calcium is >15 to 20 mg/dL.

Gastrointestinal symptoms of hypercalcemia include dysphagia, constipation, peptic ulcers, and pancreatitis. Effects on the kidney include diminished ability to concentrate urine; diuresis, leading to loss of sodium, potassium, magnesium, and phosphate; and a vicious cycle of calcium absorption in the intestines and calcium release from the bones that worsens hypercalcemia.

Treatment of Hypercalcemia

Treatment for hypercalcemia is required if the patient is symptomatic (typically a total serum concentration of approximately >12 mg/dL) or if the calcium level is >15 mg/dL. Immediate therapy is directed at restoring intravascular volume and promoting calcium excretion in the urine. In patients with adequate cardiovascular and renal function this is accomplished with infusion of 0.9% saline at 300 to 500 mL/h (saline diuresis) until any fluid deficit is replaced and diuresis occurs (urine output ≥200 to 300 mL/h). Once adequate rehydration has occurred, the saline infusion rate is reduced to 100 to 200 mL/h. During this therapy, monitor and maintain potassium and magnesium concentrations closely because the diuresis can reduce potassium and magnesium concentrations.

Hemodialysis is the treatment of choice to rapidly decrease serum calcium in patients with heart failure or renal insufficiency.[19] Chelating agents (eg, 50 mmol PO_4 over 8 to 12 hours or EDTA 10 to 50 mg/kg over 4 hours) may be used for extreme conditions.

Use of furosemide (1 mg/kg IV) for treatment of hypercalcemia is controversial. In the presence of heart failure, administration of furosemide is required, but it can actually foster release of calcium from bone, thus worsening hypercalcemia.

Hypocalcemia

Hypocalcemia is defined as a serum calcium concentration <8.5 mg/dL (or ionized calcium <4.2 mg/dL). Hypocalcemia may develop with toxic shock syndrome, with abnormalities in serum magnesium, after thyroid surgery, with fluoride poisoning, and with tumor lysis syndrome (rapid cell turnover with resultant hyperkalemia, hyperphosphatemia, and hypocalcemia).

Symptoms of hypocalcemia usually occur when ionized levels fall to <2.5 mg/dL. Symptoms include paresthesias of the extremities and face, followed by muscle cramps, carpopedal spasm, stridor, tetany, and seizures. Hypocalcemic patients show hyperreflexia and positive Chvostek and Trousseau signs. Cardiac effects include decreased myocardial contractility and heart failure. Hypocalcemia can exacerbate digitalis toxicity.

Treatment of Hypocalcemia

Treatment of hypocalcemia requires administration of calcium. Treat acute, symptomatic hypocalcemia with 10% calcium gluconate, 93 to 186 mg of elemental calcium (10 to 20 mL) IV over 10 minutes. Follow this with an IV infusion of 540 to 720 mg of elemental calcium (58 to 77 mL of 10% calcium gluconate) in 500 to 1000 mL D_5W at 0.5 to 2 mg/kg per hour (10 to 15 mg/kg). Alternatively, administer 10% calcium chloride, giving 5 mL (136.5 mg of elemental calcium) over 10 minutes, followed by 36.6 mL (1 g) over the next 6 to 12 hours IV. Measure serum calcium every 4 to 6 hours. Aim to maintain the total serum calcium concentration at 7 to 9 mg/dL. Correct abnormalities in magnesium, potassium, and pH simultaneously. Note that untreated hypomagnesemia will often make hypocalcemia refractory to therapy. Therefore, evaluate serum magnesium when hypocalcemia is present and particularly if hypocalcemia is refractory to initial calcium therapy.

Summary

Electrolyte abnormalities are among the most common causes of cardiac arrhythmias, and they can cause or complicate attempted resuscitation and postresuscitation care. A high degree of clinical suspicion and aggressive treatment of underlying electrolyte abnormalities can prevent these abnormalities from progressing to cardiac arrest.

References

1. Jackson MA, Lodwick R, Hutchinson SG. Hyperkalaemic cardiac arrest successfully treated with peritoneal dialysis. *BMJ*. 1996;312:1289–1290.
2. Voelckel W, Kroesen G. Unexpected return of cardiac action after termination of cardiopulmonary resuscitation. *Resuscitation*. 1996;32:27–29.
3. Niemann JT, Cairns CB. Hyperkalemia and ionized hypocalcemia during cardiac arrest and resuscitation: possible culprits for postcountershock arrhythmias? *Ann Emerg Med*. 1999;34:1–7.
4. Ngugi NN, McLigeyo SO, Kayima JK. Treatment of hyperkalaemia by altering the transcellular gradient in patients with renal failure: effect of various therapeutic approaches. *East Afr Med J*. 1997;74:503–509.
5. Allon M, Shanklin N. Effect of bicarbonate administration on plasma potassium in dialysis patients: interactions with insulin and albuterol. *Am J Kidney Dis*. 1996;28:508–514.
6. Lin JL, Lim PS, Leu ML, Huang CC. Outcomes of severe hyperkalemia in cardiopulmonary resuscitation with concomitant hemodialysis. *Intensive Care Med*. 1994;20:287–290.
7. Allon M. Hyperkalemia in end-stage renal disease: mechanisms and management [editorial]. *J Am Soc Nephrol*. 1995;6:1134–1142.
8. Adrogue HJ, Madias NE. Aiding fluid prescription for the dysnatremias. *Intensive Care Med*. 1997;23:309–316.
9. Fraser CL, Arieff AI. Epidemiology, pathophysiology, and management of hyponatremic encephalopathy. *Am J Med*. 1997;102:67–77.
10. Laureno R, Karp BI. Myelinolysis after correction of hyponatremia. *Ann Intern Med*. 1997;126:57–62.
11. Gross P, Reimann D, Neidel J, Doke C, Prospert F, Decaux G, Verbalis J, Schrier RW. The treatment of severe hyponatremia. *Kidney Int Suppl*. 1998;64:S6–S11.
12. Soupart A, Decaux G. Therapeutic recommendations for management of severe hyponatremia: current concepts on pathogenesis and prevention of neurologic complications. *Clin Nephrol*. 1996;46:149–169.
13. Brunner JE, Redmond JM, Haggar AM, Kruger DF, Elias SB. Central pontine myelinolysis and pontine lesions after rapid correction of hyponatremia: a prospective magnetic resonance imaging study. *Ann Neurol*. 1990;27:61–66.
14. Ayus JC, Krothapalli RK, Arieff AI. Treatment of symptomatic hyponatremia and its relation to brain damage: a prospective study. *N Engl J Med*. 1987;317:1190–1195.
15. Higham PD, Adams PC, Murray A, Campbell RW. Plasma potassium, serum magnesium and ventricular fibrillation: a prospective study. *Q J Med*. 1993;86:609–617.
16. al-Ghamdi SM, Cameron EC, Sutton RA. Magnesium deficiency: pathophysiologic and clinical overview. *Am J Kidney Dis*. 1994;24:737–752.
17. Barri YM, Knochel JP. Hypercalcemia and electrolyte disturbances in malignancy. *Hematol Oncol Clin North Am*. 1996;10:775–790.
18. Aldinger KA, Samaan NA. Hypokalemia with hypercalcemia: prevalence and significance in treatment. *Ann Intern Med*. 1977;87:571–573.
19. Edelson GW, Kleerekoper M. Hypercalcemic crisis. *Med Clin North Am*. 1995;79:79–92.

Part 10.2: Toxicology in ECC

Poisoning is an infrequent cause of cardiac arrest in older patients, but it is a leading cause of cardiac arrest in victims <40 years of age.[1–4] When a patient with poisoning is in cardiac arrest or near-arrest, immediate support of airway, breathing, and circulation is essential. Urgent consultation with a medical toxicologist or certified regional poison center is recommended[5,6] because standard guidelines for emergency cardiovascular care may not be optimal in the management of acute poisoning and overdose.

This section presents recommendations for the care of the patient with a toxicologic problem. Some recommendations are evidence-based, but most toxicology research in this area consists primarily of small case series (LOE 5), case reports, and animal studies (LOE 6). Hence many of these recommendations are based on expert consensus, and further research is needed to validate them.

Clinicians may see a patient with a history of ingestion of an unknown substance. In such cases the clinician must be familiar with common toxidromes and their therapies. To assist during such encounters, Table 1 lists drug-induced cardiovascular emergencies or altered vital signs, potential therapies to consider, and interventions that should be used with caution.

Clinicians may also encounter patients with a history of known ingestion. Then the clinician must anticipate the complications from that substance and be prepared to treat them. Table 2 lists potentially cardiotoxic drugs, signs of toxicity, and therapy to consider.

Drug-Induced Emergencies: Prearrest

Airway and Respiratory Management

Poisoned patients may deteriorate rapidly. Providers must assess and frequently reassess airway, breathing, and circulation and support them as needed. Although consultation with a poison control center or toxicologist may be needed to identify a particular toxin or antidote, the first priority of care is support of airway, breathing, and circulation. In patients who are obtunded or comatose, perform rapid sequence intubation before gastric lavage to decrease the risk of aspiration. Gastric lavage is recommended only for patients who have ingested a potentially lethal amount of a drug or toxin and present within 1 hour of ingestion.[7]

Reversal of benzodiazepine intoxication with flumazenil is associated with significant toxicity in patients with benzodiazepine dependence[8–12] or coingestion of proconvulsant medications such as tricyclic antidepressants. But it may be useful to reverse excessive sedation when benzodiazepines are used for procedural sedation.[13] Thus, the routine use of flumazenil in "coma cocktail" protocols is not recommended.

(*Circulation*. 2005;112:IV-126-IV-132.)

DOI: 10.1161/CIRCULATIONAHA.105.166564

Opiate Poisoning

Opiate poisoning commonly causes respiratory depression followed by respiratory insufficiency or arrest. Heroin overdose may cause respiratory depression, and it frequently causes pulmonary edema. The respiratory effects of opioids are rapidly reversed by the opiate antagonist naloxone.

In the hospital setting the administration of naloxone for acute opioid exposure has been successful without prior ventilation (LOE: 4[14,15]; 5[16,17]; 7[18]) if the airway was maintained and high-flow oxygen administered and the patient was otherwise healthy with no chronic opioid addiction and no cardiovascular disease. In the out-of-hospital setting, however, the evidence indicates fewer adverse events when emergency medical services (EMS) system personnel provide ventilation (ie, provide positive-pressure ventilation with bag and mask) before administration of naloxone to all patients with opioid-induced respiratory depression (LOE 5[19–21] in adults, extrapolated from pediatric cases [LOE 7[22,23]; LOE 8]).[24] The adverse effects seen in patients receiving naloxone prior to ventilation may be due to the underlying cardiovascular disorders or chronic epileptic conditions, and thus the hazards of naloxone might be overstated in some cases.

As a general practice for the treatment of suspected opiate overdose, providers should try to support ventilation before administration of naloxone. Naloxone may be administered before intubation (ie, with bag and mask), however, because significant complications after administration of naloxone are uncommon and effective reversal of opiate-induced respiratory depression may make intubation unnecessary. Naloxone can be administered by the intravenous (IV), intramuscular (IM), intranasal, or subcutaneous (SC) routes. IV is preferred. If the patient is already intubated and vascular access is not available, naloxone may be administered by the endotracheal route, although a slightly higher dose may be needed than that administered by other routes. There is only anecdotal (case report) support for endotracheal administration of naloxone for opioid overdose; intravenous and other routes (SC, IM) are preferred to the endotracheal route.

The duration of action of naloxone is approximately 45 to 70 minutes, but respiratory depression may persist for 4 to 5 hours with opiate ingestion or overdose. Thus, the clinical effects of naloxone may not last as long as those of a significant opioid overdose, and repeat doses of naloxone may be needed. The end points of opiate reversal are adequate airway reflexes and ventilation, not complete arousal.

Acute withdrawal from opiates produces a state of sympathetic excess and severe agitation. Pulmonary edema and ventricular arrhythmias are less common complications. Naloxone reversal of opiate intoxication should be used with caution in patients who are suspected of being opiate-dependent, especially if they have cardiovascular disease.

In the emergency setting the recommended adult dose range is 0.4 mg to 2 mg IV or 0.4 mg to 0.8 mg IM or SC, repeated as needed. Some opiate overdoses may require

TABLE 1. Drug-Induced Cardiovascular Emergencies or Altered Vital Signs*: Therapies to Consider† and Contraindicated Interventions

Drug-Induced Cardiovascular Emergency or Altered Vital Signs*	Therapies to Consider†	Contraindicated Interventions (or Use With Caution)
Bradycardia	• Pacemaker (transcutaneous or transvenous) • Toxic drug—*calcium channel blocker:* epinephrine, calcium salt? glucose/insulin? glucagon? NS (if hypotensive) • Toxic drug—*β-blocker:* NS, epinephrine, calcium salt? glucose/insulin? glucagon?	• Atropine (seldom helpful except for cholinesterase inhibitor poisonings) • Isoproterenol if hypotensive • Prophylactic transvenous pacing
Tachycardia	• Toxic drug—*sympathomimetics:* benzodiazepines, lidocaine, sodium bicarbonate, nitroglycerin, nitroprusside, labetalol • Toxic drug—*tricyclic antidepressants:* sodium bicarbonate, hyperventilation, NS, magnesium sulfate, lidocaine • Toxic drug—*anticholinergics:* physostigmine	• β-Blockers (not generally useful in drug-induced tachycardia) • Do not use propranolol for cocaine intoxication • Cardioversion (rarely indicated) • Adenosine (rarely indicated) • Calcium channel blockers (rarely indicated) • Physostigmine for TCA overdose
Impaired conduction/ventricular arrhythmias	• Sodium bicarbonate • Lidocaine	• If TCA overdose: amiodarone or type I_{VW} antiarrhythmics (eg, procainamide)
Hypertensive emergencies	• Toxic drug—*sympathomimetics:* benzodiazepines, lidocaine, sodium bicarbonate, nitroglycerin, nitroprusside, phentolamine	• β-Blockers
Acute coronary syndrome	• Benzodiazepines • Lidocaine • Sodium bicarbonate • Nitroglycerin • Aspirin, heparin • Base reperfusion strategy on cardiac catheterization data	• β-Blockers
Shock	• Toxic drug—*calcium channel blocker:* NS, epinephrine, norepinephrine, dopamine, calcium salt? glucose/insulin? glucagon? • Toxic drug—*β-blocker:* NS, epinephrine, norepinephrine, dopamine, calcium salt? glucose/insulin? glucagon? • If refractory to *maximal* medical therapy: consider circulatory assist devices	• Isoproterenol • Avoid calcium salts if digoxin toxicity is suspected
Acute cholinergic syndrome	• Atropine • Pralidoxime/obidoxime	• Succinylcholine
Acute anticholinergic syndrome	• Benzodiazepine • Physostigmine (not for TCA overdose)	• Antipsychotics • Other anticholinergic agents
Opioid poisoning	• Assisted ventilation • Naloxone • Tracheal intubation	• Do not use naloxone for meperidine-induced seizures

*Unless stated otherwise, listed alterations of vital signs (bradycardia, tachycardia, tachypnea) are "hemodynamically significant."
†*Therapies to consider* should be based on specific indications. Therapies followed by "?" are *Class Indeterminate.*
NS indicates normal saline; TCA, tricyclic antidepressant; and VW, Vaughan Williams.

titration to a total naloxone dose of 6 to 10 mg over a short period. For the patient with chronic opioid addiction, use smaller dose and titrate slowly to minimize adverse cardiovascular effects and withdrawal symptoms. There is no good evidence to suggest that naloxone improves outcome in the patient with an opioid-induced cardiac arrest. Thus, once arrest has occurred, normal guidelines for advanced cardiovascular life support (ACLS) should be followed, with airway control coming before use of naloxone (Class IIa).[19–21]

Drug-Induced Hemodynamically Significant Bradycardia

Hemodynamically significant bradycardia from poisoning or drug overdose may be refractory to standard ACLS protocols because some toxins bind receptors or produce direct cellular toxicity. In these cases specific antidote therapy may be needed.

Administration of atropine may be lifesaving in organophosphate, carbamate, or nerve agent poisoning (LOE 4).[25] Atropine may be administered in an initial dose of 2 to 4 mg

TABLE 2. Potentially Cardiotoxic Drugs: Cardiopulmonary Signs* of Toxicity and Therapy to Consider†

Potentially Toxic Drugs: by Type of Agent	Cardiopulmonary Signs* of Toxicity	Therapy to Consider†
Stimulants (sympathomimetics) • Amphetamines • Methamphetamines • Cocaine • Phencyclidine (PCP) • Ephedrine	• Tachycardia • Supraventricular arrhythmias • Ventricular arrhythmias • Impaired conduction • Hypertensive crises • Acute coronary syndromes • Shock • Cardiac arrest	• Benzodiazepines • Lidocaine • Sodium bicarbonate (for cocaine-related ventricular arrhythmias) • Nitroglycerin • Nitroprusside • Reperfusion strategy based on cardiac catheterization data • Phentolamine (α_1-adrenergic blocker) • β-Blockers relatively contraindicated (do not use propranolol for cocaine intoxication)
Calcium channel blockers • Verapamil • Nifedipine (and other dihydropyridines) • Diltiazem	• Bradycardia • Impaired conduction • Shock • Cardiac arrest	• NS boluses (0.5 to 1 L) • Epinephrine IV; or other α/β-agonists • Pacemakers • Circulatory assist devices? • Calcium infusions • Glucose/insulin infusion? • Glucagon
β-Adrenergic receptor antagonists • Propranolol • Atenolol • Sotalol • Metropolol	• Bradycardia • Impaired conduction • Shock • Cardiac arrest	• NS boluses (0.5 to 1 L) • Epinephrine IV; or other α/β-agonists • Pacemakers • Circulatory assist devices? • Calcium infusions? • Glucose/insulin infusion? • Glucagon
Tricyclic antidepressants • Amitriptyline • Desipramine • Nortriptyline • Imipramine	• Tachycardia • Bradycardia • Ventricular arrhythmias • Impaired conduction • Shock • Cardiac arrest	• Sodium bicarbonate • Hyperventilation • NS boluses (0.5 to 1 L) • Magnesium sulfate • Lidocaine • Epinephrine IV; or other α/β-agonists
Cardiac glycosides • Digoxin • Digitoxin • Foxglove • Oleander	• Bradycardia • Supraventricular arrhythmias • Ventricular arrhythmias • Impaired conduction • Shock • Cardiac arrest	• Restore total body K^+, Mg^{++} • Restore intravascular volume • Digoxin-specific antibodies (Fab fragments: *Digibind* or *DigiFab*) • Atropine • Pacemakers (use caution and monitor for ventricular arrhythmias) • Lidocaine • Phenytoin?
Anticholinergics • Diphenhydramine • Doxylamine	• Tachycardia • Supraventricular arrhythmias • Ventricular arrhythmias • Impaired conduction • Shock, cardiac arrest	• Physostigmine
Cholinergics • Carbamates • Nerve agents • Organophosphates	• Bradycardia • Ventricular arrhythmias • Impaired conduction, shock • Pulmonary edema • Bronchospasm • Cardiac arrest	• Atropine • Decontamination • Pralidoxime • Obidoxime
Opioids • Heroin • Fentanyl • Methadone • Morphine	• Hypoventilation (slow and shallow respirations, apnea) • Bradycardia • Hypotension • Miosis (pupil constriction)	• Assisted ventilation • Naloxone • Tracheal intubation • Nalmefene
Isoniazid	• Lactic acidosis with/without seizures • Tachycardia or bradycardia • Shock, cardiac arrest	• Pyridoxine (vitamin B_6)—large doses may be needed (ie, 1 g pyridoxine/g of ingested isoniazid)
Sodium channel blockers (Class I_{VW} antiarrhythmics) • Procainamide • Disopyramide • Lidocaine • Propafenone • Flecainide	• Bradycardia • Ventricular arrhythmias • Impaired conduction • Seizures • Shock, cardiac arrest	• Sodium bicarbonate • Pacemakers • α- and β-agonist • Lidocaine (not for lidocaine overdose) • Hypertonic saline

*Unless stated otherwise, listed alterations of vital signs (bradycardia, tachycardia, tachypnea) are "hemodynamically significant."
†Specific *therapy to consider* should be based on specific indications. Therapies followed by "?" are *Class Indeterminate.*

for bradycardia resulting from acetylcholinesterase-inhibiting agents, and large total doses may be required. Providers should notify the pharmacy to obtain a large amount (eg, 20 to 40 mg or higher) of atropine for use if needed.

Isoproterenol is contraindicated in acetylcholinesterase-induced bradycardias, although it may be useful at high doses in refractory bradycardia induced by β-antagonist receptor blockade. Heart block and ventricular arrhythmias associated with digoxin or digitalis glycoside poisoning may be effectively treated with digoxin-specific antibody fragment therapy (LOE 5).[26] Antibody-specific therapy may also be effective in poisoning caused by plants and Chinese herbal medications containing digitalis glycosides (LOE 2, 8[27,28]; LOE 5[26]). Transcutaneous pacing may be effective in mild to moderate hemodynamically significant bradycardia associated with poisoning and overdose.

Drug-Induced Hemodynamically Significant Tachycardia

Drug-induced hemodynamically significant tachycardia may cause myocardial ischemia, myocardial infarction, or ventricular arrhythmias and may lead to high-output heart failure and shock. Adenosine and synchronized cardioversion are unlikely to be of benefit in this context given the ongoing presence of a toxin. Some drug-induced tachyarrhythmias, however, may be successfully treated with adenosine (LOE 5).[29] In patients with borderline hypotension, diltiazem and verapamil are contraindicated because they may further lower blood pressure.

Benzodiazepines such as diazepam or lorazepam are safe and effective in patients with drug-induced hemodynamically significant tachycardia resulting from sympathomimetic agents. When large quantities of benzodiazepines are used to treat poisoning or overdose, providers must closely monitor the patient's level of consciousness, ventilatory effort, and respiratory function because the sedative effects of the benzodiazepines may produce respiratory depression and loss of protective airway reflexes.

Physostigmine is a specific antidote that may be preferable for drug-induced hemodynamically significant tachycardia and central anticholinergic syndrome caused by pure anticholinergic poisoning.[30] Physostigmine must be used with caution because it can produce symptoms of cholinergic crisis such as copious tracheobronchial secretions (frequent suctioning will be required), seizures, bradycardia, and even asystole if given in excessive doses or given too rapidly. Often patients with anticholinergic intoxication can be managed with benzodiazepines alone, but at least one clinical study suggested that physostigmine used appropriately may offer superior results (LOE 4).[30] Physostigmine should not be administered for anticholinergic symptoms associated with tricyclic antidepressant overdose. Consultation with a medical toxicologist or regional poison center is recommended.

Drug-Induced Hypertensive Emergencies

Benzodiazepines are the drug class of choice for treatment of drug-induced hypertension because they decrease the effects of endogenous catecholamine release. Hypotension may follow drug-induced hypertension, and aggressive control of blood pressure may not be warranted. Thus, short-acting antihypertensive agents, such as nitroprusside, are preferred in patients who are refractory to benzodiazepine therapy. Nonselective β-antagonist receptor blocking agents, such as propranolol, are contraindicated in poisoning by sympathomimetic agents. Blockade of β-receptors with unopposed α-receptor stimulation may worsen hypertension.[31] Labetalol, a mixed α- and β-receptor antagonist, may be used with caution as third-line therapy in patients with refractory drug-induced hypertension.

Drug-Induced Acute Coronary Syndromes

Acute coronary syndromes (ACS) can develop in patients with cocaine overdose. ACS results from coronary artery vasoconstriction with resultant coronary ischemia that is exacerbated by tachycardia and hypertension associated with excess sympathetic nervous system stimulation.

Fibrinolytics are thought to have a higher risk-to-benefit ratio when used in the context of drug-induced ACS, particularly in the presence of severe hypertension, so they should be used with caution if at all.[32] Intracoronary administration of fibrinolytics or coronary vasodilators is preferred to peripheral administration.

Cardiac catheterization studies in cocaine overdose have shown that nitroglycerin and phentolamine reverse cocaine-induced vasoconstriction. Labetalol has no significant effect, and propranolol worsens it.[33–36] Therefore, nitroglycerin and benzodiazepines are first-line agents, phentolamine is a second-line agent, and propranolol is contraindicated for cocaine-induced ACS. Although labetalol has been reported to be effective in isolated cases of cocaine toxicity,[37,38] use of this agent is controversial because it blocks the peripheral signs of drug-induced sympathetic excess without affecting central nervous system effects such as seizures. Esmolol and metoprolol may induce hypotension.[39]

Drug-Induced Ventricular Tachycardia and Ventricular Fibrillation

When a patient develops sudden conversion to a wide-complex rhythm with hypotension, drug-induced ventricular tachycardia (VT) is likely and cardioversion is indicated. If the patient is unstable and polymorphic VT is present, use high-energy unsynchronized shocks (defibrillation doses).

Use of antiarrhythmics is indicated in cases of hemodynamically stable drug-induced VT. Lidocaine is the antiarrhythmic of choice in most cases of drug-induced monomorphic VT. Types I_A and I_C and other antiarrhythmics that block the fast sodium channel (eg, sotalol) are contraindicated in cases of poisoning with tricyclic antidepressants or other fast sodium channel blockers because of the risk of synergistic toxicity. The efficacy and safety of phenytoin for tricyclic antidepressant poisoning has been questioned and is no longer recommended.[40,41] Magnesium has beneficial effects in certain cases of drug-induced VT (LOE 5[42]), but it may also aggravate drug-induced hypotension.[43,44]

Torsades de pointes can occur with either therapeutic or toxic exposure to many drugs. Administration of magnesium is recommended for patients with torsades de pointes even when the serum magnesium concentration is normal (Class IIa). Summary of therapy:

- Correction of hypoxia, hypokalemia, and hypomagnesemia is critical.
- The effectiveness of lidocaine in treatment of torsades de pointes has not been demonstrated.
- Electrical overdrive pacing at rates of 100 to 120 beats per minute may terminate torsades de pointes.
- Pharmacologic overdrive pacing with isoproterenol may be effective (LOE 8).[45]
- Some toxicologists recommend potassium supplementation even when the serum potassium is normal.

High level studies have not established the safety and efficacy of any of these recommended therapies for drug-induced polymorphic VT (Class Indeterminate).

Drug-Induced Impaired Conduction

Hypertonic saline and systemic alkalinization may prevent or terminate VT secondary to poisoning from sodium channel blocking agents (eg, procainamide, flecainide) and tricyclic antidepressants (LOE 5).[46,47] Sodium bicarbonate provides hypertonic saline and induces systemic alkalinization; hypertonic saline alone may be effective in treating the impaired conduction associated with these agents.[48] When sodium bicarbonate is used to treat arrhythmias and hypotension, the goal of alkalinization is to maintain an arterial pH of 7.45 to 7.55 with repeated boluses of 1 to 2 mEq/kg of sodium bicarbonate. Although no study has investigated the optimal target pH with bicarbonate therapy, this pH range has been commonly accepted and seems reasonable. A maintenance infusion of 150 mEq/L of sodium bicarbonate plus 30 mEq KCl/L in D_5W is recommended (Class IIa). Boluses of sodium bicarbonate are used without prior determination of serum pH for acute decompensation if the QRS duration is >100 milliseconds or if hypotension develops.

There is insufficient evidence to recommend for or against the use of sodium bicarbonate in adults with calcium channel blocker overdose (Class Indeterminate). Calcium channel antagonist and β-adrenergic antagonist overdose may lead to seriously impaired conduction. These patients may require chronotropic adrenergic agents such as epinephrine, use of glucagon in high doses (although the data to support this is inadequate and primarily limited to animal studies),[49] or possibly pacing.[50]

Drug-Induced Shock

Drug-induced shock may produce a decrease in intravascular volume, a decrease in systemic vascular resistance (SVR), diminished myocardial contractility, or a combination of these factors. In addition, drugs can disable normal compensatory mechanisms. It is these combined aspects of cardiovascular dysfunction that render drug-induced shock refractory to many standard therapies.

Drug-Induced Hypovolemic Shock

Overdose of some drugs or chemicals (eg, zinc salts) can cause excessive fluid loss through the gastrointestinal tract, resulting in pure hypovolemia. Drug-induced shock, however, typically includes cardiovascular dysfunction with decreased myocardial contractility and low SVR that requires a combination of volume therapy and myocardial support. Initial treatment will require a fluid challenge to correct relative hypovolemia and optimize preload. In cardiotoxic poisoning congestive heart failure may limit tolerance of, and response to, fluid administration. Central hemodynamic monitoring with a pulmonary artery catheter may be required to titrate therapy.

Patients unresponsive to fluid loading may require inotrope or vasopressor support, or both. Dopamine is often the recommended initial agent. However, drug-induced shock following overdose of some drugs (eg, calcium channel blockers) will require administration and titration of a variety of cardiovascular medications.

Drug-Induced Distributive Shock

Distributive shock is associated with normal or even high cardiac output and low SVR. Treatment with α-adrenergic drugs such as norepinephrine or phenylephrine may be needed. Case reports suggest that vasopressin may also be useful.[51] More powerful vasoconstrictors such as endothelin are not yet available in the United States and have not been well studied. Watch for the development of ventricular arrhythmias with the use of these agents. **Caution:** Avoid dobutamine and isoproterenol, which may worsen hypotension by further decreasing SVR.

Drug-Induced Cardiogenic Shock

Drug-induced cardiogenic shock is associated with low cardiac output and high SVR. Cardiac ischemia may also be present in these patients. In addition to volume titration and use of sympathomimetic drugs such as dobutamine, inotropic support may be provided by agents such as inamrinone, calcium, glucagon, insulin, or even isoproterenol, depending on the toxic agent(s) identified.[52,53] Concurrent vasopressor therapy is often required.[54]

Drug-Induced Cardiac Arrest

Cardioversion/Defibrillation

Electric defibrillation is appropriate for pulseless patients with drug-induced VT or ventricular fibrillation (VF) and also for unstable patients with polymorphic VT. In cases of sympathomimetic poisoning with refractory VF, increase the interval between doses of epinephrine and use only standard dosing. Propranolol is contraindicated in cocaine overdose. It was thought to be contraindicated in sympathomimetic poisoning, but there are some case reports suggesting that it may be useful in the treatment of ephedrine and pseudoephedrine overdose.[55]

Prolonged CPR and Resuscitation

More prolonged CPR and resuscitation may be warranted in patients with poisoning or overdose, especially those with calcium channel blocker poisoning (LOE 5).[56] In cases of severe poisoning, recovery with good neurologic outcomes has been reported in patients who received prolonged CPR (eg, 3 to 5 hours).[52,53] Cardiopulmonary bypass (extracorporeal membrane oxygenation) has been used successfully in resuscitation of patients with severe poisoning.[57]

Summary

Use of standard ACLS protocols for all patients who are critically poisoned may not result in an optimal outcome. Care of patients with severe poisoning can be enhanced by consultation with a medical toxicologist or regional poison center. Alternative approaches that may be effective in severely poisoned patients include

- Higher doses of medication than those in standard protocols
- Nonstandard drug therapies, including inamrinone, calcium chloride, glucagon, insulin, labetalol, phenylephrine, physostigmine, and sodium bicarbonate
- Use of specific antagonists or antidotes
- Heroic measures, such as prolonged CPR and possible use of circulatory assist devices such as extracorporeal membrane oxygenation

References

1. Litovitz TL, Felberg L, White S, Klein-Schwartz W. 1995 annual report of the American Association of Poison Control Centers Toxic Exposure Surveillance System. *Am J Emerg Med.* 1996;14:487–537.
2. McCaig LF, Burt CW. Poisoning-related visits to emergency departments in the United States, 1993–1996. *J Toxicol Clin Toxicol.* 1999;37:817–826.
3. Fingerhut LA, Cox CS. Poisoning mortality, 1985–1995. *Public Health Rep.* 1998;113:218–233.
4. Watson WA, Litovitz TL, Klein-Schwartz W, Rodgers GC Jr, Youniss J, Reid N, Rouse WG, Rembert RS, Borys D. 2003 annual report of the American Association of Poison Control Centers Toxic Exposure Surveillance System. *Am J Emerg Med.* 2004;22:335–404.
5. Facility assessment guidelines for regional toxicology treatment centers. American Academy of Clinical Toxicology. *J Toxicol Clin Toxicol.* 1993;31:211–217.
6. Poison information and treatment systems. American College of Emergency Physicians. *Ann Emerg Med.* 1996;28:384.
7. Chyka PA, Seger D, Krenzelok EP, Vale JA. Position paper: single-dose activated charcoal. *Clin Toxicol (Phila).* 2005;43:61–87.
8. Amrein R, Hetzel W, Hartmann D, Lorscheid T. Clinical pharmacology of flumazenil. *Eur J Anaesth.* 1988;2:65–80.
9. Amrein R, Leishman B, Bentzinger C, et al. Flumazenil in benzodiazepine antagonism: actions and clinical use in intoxications and anaesthesiology. *Med Toxicol.* 1987;2:411–429.
10. Flückiger A, Hartmann D, Leishman B, et al. Lack of effect of the benzodiazepine antagonist flumazenil (Ro 15-1788) on the performance of healthy subjects during experimentally induced ethanol intoxication. *Eur J Clin Pharmacol.* 1988;34:273–276.
11. Lukes SE, Griffiths RR. Precipitated withdrawal by a benzodiazepine receptor antagonist (Ro-15-1788) after 7 days of diazepam. *Science.* 1982;217:1161–1163.
12. Martens F, Köppel C, Ibe K, et al. Clinical experience with the benzodiazepine antagonist flumazenil in suspected benzodiazepine or ethanol poisoning. *J Toxicol Clin Toxicol.* 1990;28:341–356.
13. Pitetti RD, Singh S, Pierce MC. Safe and efficacious use of procedural sedation and analgesia by nonanesthesiologists in a pediatric emergency department. *Arch Pediatr Adolesc Med.* 2003;157:1090–1096.
14. Gill AM, Cousins A, Nunn AJ, Choonara JA. Opiate-induced respiratory depression in pediatric patients. *Ann Pharmacother.* 1996;30:125–129.
15. Herschel M, Kloshnood B, Lass NA. Role of naloxone in newborn resuscitation. *Pediatrics.* 2000;106:831–834.
16. Lewis JM, Klein-Schwartz W, Benson BE, Oderda GM, Takai S. Continuous naloxone infusion in pediatric narcotic overdose. *Am J Dis Child.* 1984;138:944–946.
17. Romac DR. Safety of prolonged, high-dose infusion of naloxone hydrochloride for severe methadone overdose. *Clin Pharm.* 1986;5:251–254.
18. Singhal N, McMillan DD, Yee WH, Akierman AR, Yee YJ. Evaluation of the effectiveness of the standardized neonatal resuscitation program. *J Perinatol.* 2001;21:388–392.
19. Osterwalder JJ. Naloxone—for intoxications with intravenous heroin and heroin mixtures—harmless or hazardous? A prospective clinical study. *J Toxicol Clin Toxicol.* 1996;34:409–416.
20. Sporer KA, Firestone J, Isaacs SM. Out-of-hospital treatment of opioid overdoses in an urban setting. *Acad Emerg Med.* 1996;3:660–667.
21. Wanger K, Brough L, Macmillan I, Goulding J, MacPhail I, Christenson JM. Intravenous vs subcutaneous naloxone for out-of-hospital management of presumed opioid overdose. *Acad Emerg Med.* 1998;5:293–299.
22. Hasan RA, Benko AS, Nolan BM, Campe J, Duff J, Zureikat GY. Cardiorespiratory effects of naloxone in children. *Ann Pharmacother.* 2003;37:1587–1592.
23. Sporer KA. Acute heroin overdose. *Ann Intern Med.* 1999;130:584–590.
24. Schneir AB, Vadeboncoeur TF, Offerman SR, Barry JD, Ly BT, Williams SR, Clark RF. Massive OxyContin ingestion refractory to naloxone therapy. *Ann Emerg Med.* 2002;40:425–428.
25. Sungur M, Guven M. Intensive care management of organophosphate insecticide poisoning. *Crit Care.* 2001;5:211–215.
26. Bosse GM, Pope TM. Recurrent digoxin overdose and treatment with digoxin-specific Fab antibody fragments. *J Emerg Med.* 1994;12:179–185.
27. Eddleston M, Rajapakse S, Rajakanthan, Jayalath S, Sjostrom L, Santharaj W, Thenabadu PN, Sheriff MH, Warrell DA. Anti-digoxin Fab fragments in cardiotoxicity induced by ingestion of yellow oleander: a randomised controlled trial. *Lancet.* 2000;355:967–972.
28. Dasgupta A, Szelei-Stevens KA. Neutralization of free digoxin-like immunoreactive components of oriental medicines Dan Shen and Lu-Shen-Wan by the Fab fragment of antidigoxin antibody (Digibind). *Am J Clin Pathol.* 2004;121:276–281.
29. Tracey JA, Cassidy N, Casey PB, Ali I. Bupropion (Zyban) toxicity. *Ir Med J.* 2002;95:23–24.
30. Burns MJ, Linden CH, Graudins A, Brown RM, Fletcher KE. A comparison of physostigmine and benzodiazepines for the treatment of anticholinergic poisoning. *Ann Emerg Med.* 2000;35:374–381.
31. Ramoska E, Sacchetti AD. Propranolol-induced hypertension in treatment of cocaine intoxication. *Ann Emerg Med.* 1985;14:1112–1113.
32. Hollander JE, Wilson LD, Shih LP. Complications from the use of thrombolytic agents in patients with cocaine associated chest pain. *J Emerg Med.* 1996;14:731–736.
33. Brogan WCI, Lange RA, Kim AS, Moliterno DJ, Hillis LD. Alleviation of cocaine-induced coronary vasoconstriction by nitroglycerin. *J Am Coll Cardiol.* 1991;18:581–586.
34. Lange RA, Cigarroa RG, Yancy CW Jr, Willard JE, Popma JJ, Sills MN, McBride W, Kim AS, Hillis LD. Cocaine-induced coronary-artery vasoconstriction. *N Engl J Med.* 1989;321:1557–1562.
35. Lange RA, Cigarroa RG, Flores ED, McBride W, Kim AS, Wells PJ, Bedotto JB, Danziger RS, Hillis LD. Potentiation of cocaine-induced coronary vasoconstriction by beta-adrenergic blockade. *Ann Intern Med.* 1990;112:897–903.
36. Boehrer JD, Moliterno DJ, Willard JE, Hillis LD, Lange RA. Influence of labetalol on cocaine-induced coronary vasoconstriction in humans. *Am J Med.* 1993;94:608–610.
37. Gay GR, Loper KA. The use of labetalol in the management of cocaine crisis. *Ann Emerg Med.* 1988;17:282–283.
38. Dusenberry SJ, Hicks MJ, Mariani PJ. Labetalol treatment of cocaine toxicity. *Ann Emerg Med.* 1987;16:235.
39. Sand IC, Brody SL, Wrenn KD, Slovis CM. Experience with esmolol for the treatment of cocaine-associated cardiovascular complications. *Am J Emerg Med.* 1991;9:161–163.
40. Mayron R, Ruiz E. Phenytoin: does it reverse tricyclic-antidepressant-induced cardiac conduction abnormalities? *Ann Emerg Med.* 1986;15:876–880.
41. Callaham M, Schumaker H, Pentel P. Phenytoin prophylaxis of cardiotoxicity in experimental amitriptyline poisoning. *J Pharmacol Exp Ther.* 1988;245:216–220.
42. Citak A, Soysal DD, Ucsel R, Karabocuoglu M, Uzel N. Efficacy of long duration resuscitation and magnesium sulphate treatment in amitriptyline poisoning. *Eur J Emerg Med.* 2002;9:63–66.
43. Knudsen K, Abrahamsson J. Effects of magnesium sulfate and lidocaine in the treatment of ventricular arrhythmias in experimental amitriptyline poisoning in the rat. *Crit Care Med.* 1994;22:494–498.
44. Kline JA, DeStefano AA, Schroeder JD, Raymond RM. Magnesium potentiates imipramine toxicity in the isolated rat heart. *Ann Emerg Med.* 1994;24:224–232.
45. Gowda RM, Khan IA, Punukollu G, Vasavada BC, Sacchi TJ, Wilbur SL. Female preponderance in ibutilide-induced torsade de pointes. *Int J Cardiol.* 2004;95:219–222.

46. Brown TC. Sodium bicarbonate treatment for tricyclic antidepressant arrhythmias in children. *Med J Aust.* 1976;2:380–382.
47. Hoffman JR, Votey SR, Bayer M, Silver L. Effect of hypertonic sodium bicarbonate in the treatment of moderate-to-severe cyclic antidepressant overdose. *Am J Emerg Med.* 1993;11:336–341.
48. McKinney PE, Rasmussen R. Reversal of severe tricyclic antidepressant-induced cardiotoxicity with intravenous hypertonic saline solution. *Ann Emerg Med.* 2003;42:20–24.
49. Bailey PM, Little M, Jelinek GA, Wilce JA. Jellyfish envenoming syndromes: unknown toxic mechanisms and unproven therapies. *Med J Aust.* 2003;178:34–37.
50. Proano L, Chiang WK, Wang RY. Calcium channel blocker overdose. *Am J Emerg Med.* 1995;13:444–450.
51. Wenzel V, Lindner KH. Employing vasopressin during cardiopulmonary resuscitation and vasodilatory shock as a lifesaving vasopressor. *Cardiovasc Res.* 2001;51:529–541.
52. Ramsay ID. Survival after imipramine poisoning. *Lancet.* 1967;2: 1308–1309.
53. Southall DP, Kilpatrick SM. Imipramine poisoning: survival of a child after prolonged cardiac massage. *BMJ.* 1974;4:508.
54. Kollef MH. Labetalol overdose successfully treated with amrinone and alpha-adrenergic receptor agonists. *Chest.* 1994;105:626–627.
55. Burkhart KK. Intravenous propranolol reverses hypertension after sympathomimetic overdose: two case reports. *J Toxicol Clin Toxicol.* 1992; 30:109–114.
56. Durward A, Guerguerian AM, Lefebvre M, Shemie SD. Massive diltiazem overdose treated with extracorporeal membrane oxygenation. *Pediatr Crit Care Med.* 2003;4:372–376.
57. Holzer M, Sterz F, Schoerkhuber W, et al. Successful resuscitation of a verapamil-intoxicated patient with percutaneous cardiopulmonary bypass. *Crit Care Med.* 1999;27:2818–2823.

Part 10.3: Drowning

Drowning is a leading preventable cause of unintentional morbidity and mortality. Although this chapter focuses on treatment, prevention is possible, and pool fencing has been shown to reduce drowning and submersion injury (Class I).[1]

The most important and detrimental consequence of submersion is hypoxia. Therefore, oxygenation, ventilation, and perfusion should be restored as rapidly as possible. This will require immediate bystander CPR plus immediate activation of the emergency medical services (EMS) system. Victims who have spontaneous circulation and breathing when they reach the hospital usually recover with a good outcome.

Victims of drowning may develop primary or secondary hypothermia. If the drowning occurs in icy (<5°C [41°F]) water, hypothermia may develop rapidly and provide some protection against hypoxia. Such effects, however, have typically been reported only after submersion of young victims in *icy* water (see Part 10.4: "Hypothermia").[2]

All victims of drowning (see definitions below) who require any form of resuscitation (including rescue breathing alone) should be transported to the hospital for evaluation and monitoring even if they appear to be alert with effective cardiorespiratory function at the scene. The hypoxic insult can produce an increase in pulmonary capillary permeability with delayed onset of pulmonary complications.

Definitions, Classifications, and Prognostic Indicators

A number of terms are used to describe drowning. To aid in the use of consistent terminology and the uniform reporting of data from drowning, the Utstein definition and style of data reporting are recommended[3]:

Drowning. Drowning is a process resulting in primary respiratory impairment from submersion/immersion in a liquid medium. Implicit in this definition is that a liquid/air interface is present at the entrance of the victim's airway, preventing the victim from breathing air. The victim may live or die after this process, but whatever the outcome, he or she has been involved in a drowning incident.

A victim may be rescued at any time during the drowning process and may not require intervention or may receive appropriate resuscitation measures. In either case the drowning process is interrupted.

The Utstein statement recommends that the term *near-drowning* no longer be used. It also de-emphasizes classification based on type of submersion fluid (salt water versus fresh water). Although there are theoretical differences that have been reported in laboratory conditions, these have not been found to be clinically significant. The most important factors that determine outcome of drowning are the duration and severity of the hypoxia.

Although survival is uncommon in victims who have undergone prolonged submersion and require prolonged resuscitation,[4,5] successful resuscitation with full neurologic recovery has occasionally occurred with prolonged submersion in icy water.[6–8] For this reason, scene resuscitation should be initiated and the victim transported to an ED unless there is obvious physical evidence of death.

Modifications to Basic Life Support for Drowning

No modification of standard BLS sequencing is necessary. Some cautions are appropriate, however, when beginning CPR for the drowning victim.

Recovery From the Water

When attempting to rescue a drowning victim, the rescuer should get to the victim as quickly as possible, preferably by some conveyance (boat, raft, surfboard, or flotation device). The rescuer must always be aware of personal safety.

Recent evidence indicates that routine stabilization of the cervical spine is not necessary unless the circumstances leading to the submersion episode indicate that trauma is likely (Class IIa). These circumstances include a history of diving, use of a water slide, signs of injury, or signs of alcohol intoxication.[9] In the absence of such indicators, spinal injury is unlikely. Manual cervical spine stabilization and spine immobilization equipment may impede adequate opening of the airway, and they complicate and may delay the delivery of rescue breaths.

Rescue Breathing

The first and most important treatment of the drowning victim is the immediate provision of ventilation. Prompt initiation of rescue breathing increases the victim's chance of survival.[10] Rescue breathing is usually performed when the unresponsive victim is in shallow water or out of the water. If it is difficult for the rescuer to pinch the victim's nose, support the head, and open the airway in the water, mouth-to-nose ventilation may be used as an alternative to mouth-to-mouth ventilation. Untrained rescuers should not try to provide care while the victim is still in deep water.

Management of the drowning victim's airway and breathing is similar to that recommended for any victim of cardiopulmonary arrest. There is no need to clear the airway of aspirated water, because only a modest amount of water is aspirated by the majority of drowning victims and it is rapidly absorbed into the central circulation, so it does not act as an obstruction in the trachea.[5,11] Some victims aspirate nothing because they develop laryngospasm or breath-holding.[5,12] Attempts to remove water from the breathing passages by any means other than suction (eg, abdominal thrusts or the Heimlich maneuver) are unnecessary and potentially danger-

(*Circulation*. 2005;112:IV-133-IV-135.)

DOI: 10.1161/CIRCULATIONAHA.105.166565

ous.[11] The routine use of abdominal thrusts or the Heimlich maneuver for drowning victims is not recommended.

Chest Compressions

As soon as the unresponsive victim is removed from the water, the rescuer should open the airway, check for breathing, and if there is no breathing, give 2 rescue breaths that make the chest rise (if this was not done in the water). After delivery of 2 effective breaths, the lay rescuer should immediately begin chest compressions and provide cycles of compressions and ventilations. The healthcare provider should check for a central pulse. The pulse may be difficult to appreciate in a drowning victim, particularly if the victim is cold. If the healthcare provider does not definitely feel a pulse within 10 seconds, the healthcare provider should start cycles of compressions and ventilations. Only trained rescuers should try to provide chest compressions in the water.

Once the victim is out of the water, if the victim is unresponsive and not breathing (and the healthcare provider does not feel a pulse) after delivery of 2 rescue breaths, rescuers should attach an AED and attempt defibrillation if a shockable rhythm is identified. If hypothermia is present, see Part 10.4.

Vomiting by the Victim During Resuscitation

The victim may vomit when the rescuer performs chest compressions or rescue breathing. In fact, in a 10-year study in Australia, two thirds of victims who received rescue breathing and 86% of victims who required compressions and ventilations vomited.[13] If vomiting occurs, turn the victim's mouth to the side and remove the vomitus using your finger, a cloth, or suction. If spinal cord injury is possible, logroll the victim so that the head, neck, and torso are turned as a unit.

Modifications to ACLS for Drowning

The drowning victim in cardiac arrest requires ACLS, including early intubation. Every drowning victim, even one who requires only minimal resuscitation before recovery, requires monitored transport and evaluation at a medical facility.

Victims in cardiac arrest may present with asystole, pulseless electrical activity, or pulseless ventricular tachycardia/ventricular fibrillation (VF). Follow the guidelines for pediatric advanced life support and ACLS for treatment of these rhythms. Case reports document the use of surfactant for fresh water–induced respiratory distress, but further research is needed.[14–16] The use of extracorporeal membrane oxygenation in young children with severe hypothermia after submersion is documented in case reports.[8,17] There is insufficient evidence to support or refute the use of barbiturates, steroids,[18] nitric oxide,[19] therapeutic hypothermia after return of spontaneous circulation,[20] or vasopressin.[21]

Improving Neurologic Outcomes: Therapeutic Hypothermia

Recent randomized controlled trials (LOE 1)[22] and (LOE 2)[23] and subsequent consensus recommendations[24,25] support the use of therapeutic hypothermia in patients who remain in a coma after resuscitation from cardiac arrest caused by VF and note that it may be effective for other causes of cardiac arrest. However, the effectiveness of induced hypothermia for drowning victims has not been established, and evaluation of this approach is warranted. The 2002 World Congress on Drowning recommended further studies to identify the best treatments for drowning victims.[3]

Summary

Prevention measures can reduce the incidence of drowning, and immediate, high-quality bystander CPR and early BLS care can improve survival. Rescue breathing should be provided even before the victim is pulled from the water if possible. Routine stabilization of the cervical spine is not needed. Further studies are necessary to improve neurologic outcome for drowning victims.

References

1. Thompson DC, Rivara FP. Pool fencing for preventing drowning in children. *Cochrane Database Syst Rev.* 2000;CD001047.
2. Quan L, Kinder D. Pediatric submersions: prehospital predictors of outcome. *Pediatrics.* 1992;90:909–913.
3. Idris AH, Berg RA, Bierens J, Bossaert L, Branche CM, Gabrielli A, Graves SA, Handley AJ, Hoelle R, Morley PT, Papa L, Pepe PE, Quan L, Szpilman D, Wigginton JG, Modell JH. Recommended guidelines for uniform reporting of data from drowning: the "Utstein style." *Resuscitation.* 2003;59:45–57.
4. Quan L, Wentz KR, Gore EJ, Copass MK. Outcome and predictors of outcome in pediatric submersion victims receiving prehospital care in King County, Washington. *Pediatrics.* 1990;86:586–593.
5. Modell JH, Davis JH. Electrolyte changes in human drowning victims. *Anesthesiology.* 1969;30:414–420.
6. Southwick FS, Dalglish PHJ. Recovery after prolonged asystolic cardiac arrest in profound hypothermia: a case report and literature review. *JAMA.* 1980;243:1250–1253.
7. Siebke H, Rod T, Breivik H, Link B. Survival after 40 minutes: submersion without cerebral sequelae. *Lancet.* 1975;1:1275–1277.
8. Bolte RG, Black PG, Bowers RS, Thorne JK, Corneli HM. The use of extracorporeal rewarming in a child submerged for 66 minutes. *JAMA.* 1988;260:377–379.
9. Watson RS, Cummings P, Quan L, Bratton S, Weiss NS. Cervical spine injuries among submersion victims. *J Trauma.* 2001;51:658–662.
10. Kyriacou DN, Arcinue EL, Peek C, Kraus JF. Effect of immediate resuscitation on children with submersion injury. *Pediatrics.* 1994;94:137–142.
11. Rosen P, Stoto M, Harley J. The use of the Heimlich maneuver in near-drowning: Institute of Medicine report. *J Emerg Med.* 1995;13:397–405.
12. Modell JH. Drowning. *N Engl J Med.* 1993;328:253–256.
13. Manolios N, Mackie I. Drowning and near-drowning on Australian beaches patrolled by life-savers: a 10-year study, 1973–1983. *Med J Aust.* 1988;148:165–167, 170–171.
14. Onarheim H, Vik V. Porcine surfactant (Curosurf) for acute respiratory failure after near-drowning in 12 year old. *Acta Anaesthesiol Scand.* 2004;48:778–781.
15. Staudinger T, Bankier A, Strohmaier W, Weiss K, Locker GJ, Knapp S, Roggla M, Laczika K, Frass M. Exogenous surfactant therapy in a patient with adult respiratory distress syndrome after near drowning. *Resuscitation.* 1997;35:179–182.
16. Suzuki H, Ohta T, Iwata K, Yamaguchi K, Sato T. Surfactant therapy for respiratory failure due to near-drowning. *Eur J Pediatr.* 1996;155:383–384.
17. Thalmann M, Trampitsch E, Haberfellner N, Eisendle E, Kraschl R, Kobinia G. Resuscitation in near drowning with extracorporeal membrane oxygenation. *Ann Thorac Surg.* 2001;72:607–608.
18. Foex BA, Boyd R. Towards evidence based emergency medicine: best BETs from the Manchester Royal Infirmary. Corticosteroids in the management of near-drowning. *Emerg Med J.* 2001;18:465–466.
19. Takano Y, Hirosako S, Yamaguchi T, Saita N, Suga M, Kukita I, Okamoto K, Ando M. [Nitric oxide inhalation as an effective therapy for

acute respiratory distress syndrome due to near-drowning: a case report.] *Nihon Kokyuki Gakkai Zasshi*. 1999;37:997–1002.

20. Williamson JP, Illing R, Gertler P, Braude S. Near-drowning treated with therapeutic hypothermia. *Med J Aust*. 2004;181:500–501.
21. Sumann G, Krismer AC, Wenzel V, Adelsmayr E, Schwarz B, Lindner KH, Mair P. Cardiopulmonary resuscitation after near drowning and hypothermia: restoration of spontaneous circulation after vasopressin. *Acta Anaesthesiol Scand*. 2003;47:363–365.
22. Hypothermia After Cardiac Arrest Study Group. Mild therapeutic hypothermia to improve the neurologic outcome after cardiac arrest. *N Engl J Med*. 2002;346:549–556.
23. Bernard SA, Gray TW, Buist MD, Jones BM, Silvester W, Gutteridge G, Smith K. Treatment of comatose survivors of out-of-hospital cardiac arrest with induced hypothermia. *N Engl J Med*. 2002;346:557–563.
24. Nolan JP, Morley PT, Vanden Hoek TL, Hickey RW. Therapeutic hypothermia after cardiac arrest. An advisory statement by the Advanced Life Support Task Force of the International Liaison Committee on Resuscitation. *Resuscitation*. 2003;57:231–235.
25. Nolan JP, Morley PT, Vanden Hoek TL, Hickey RW, Kloeck WG, Billi J, Bottiger BW, Okada K, Reyes C, Shuster M, Steen PA, Weil MH, Wenzel V, Carli P, Atkins D. Therapeutic hypothermia after cardiac arrest: an advisory statement by the Advanced Life Support Task Force of the International Liaison Committee on Resuscitation. *Circulation*. 2003;108:118–121.

Part 10.4: Hypothermia

Unintentional hypothermia is a serious and preventable health problem. Severe hypothermia (body temperature <30°C [86°F]) is associated with marked depression of critical body functions that may make the victim appear clinically dead during the initial assessment. But in some cases hypothermia may exert a protective effect on the brain and organs in cardiac arrest.[1,2] Intact neurologic recovery may be possible after hypothermic cardiac arrest, although those with nonasphyxial arrest have a better prognosis than those with asphyxial-associated hypothermic arrest.[3–5] With this in mind, lifesaving procedures should not be withheld on the basis of clinical presentation.[4] Victims should be transported as soon as possible to a center where monitored rewarming is possible.

General Care for All Victims of Hypothermia

When the victim is extremely cold but has maintained a perfusing rhythm, the rescuer should focus on interventions that prevent further heat loss and begin to rewarm the victim. These include the following:

- Prevent additional evaporative heat loss by removing wet garments and insulating the victim from further environmental exposures.
- Do not delay urgent procedures, such as intubation and insertion of vascular catheters, but perform them gently while closely monitoring cardiac rhythm. These patients are prone to develop ventricular fibrillation (VF).

For patients with moderate to severe hypothermia, therapy is determined by the presence or absence of a perfusing rhythm. We provide an overview of therapy here and give more details below. Management of the patient with moderate to severe hypothermia is as follows:

- Hypothermia with a perfusing rhythm
  - –Mild (>34°C [>93.2°F]): passive rewarming
  - –Moderate (30°C to 34°C [86°F to 93.2°F]): active external rewarming
  - –Severe (<30°C [86°F]): active internal rewarming; consider extracorporeal membrane oxygenation
- Patients in cardiac arrest will require CPR with some modifications of conventional BLS and ACLS care and will require active internal rewarming
  - –Moderate (30°C to 34°C [86°F to 93.2°F]): start CPR, attempt defibrillation, establish IV access, give IV medications spaced at longer intervals, provide active internal rewarming
  - –Severe (<30°C [86°F]): start CPR, attempt defibrillation once, withhold medications until temperature >30°C (86°F), provide active internal rewarming
  - –Patients with a core temperature of >34°C (>93.2°F) may be passively rewarmed with warmed blankets and a warm environment. This form of rewarming will not be adequate for a patient with cardiopulmonary arrest or severe hypothermia.[6]
  - –For patients with moderate hypothermia (30°C to 34°C [86°F to 93.2°F]) and a perfusing rhythm and no preceding cardiac arrest, active external warming (with heating blankets, forced air, and warmed infusion) should be considered (Class IIb). Active external rewarming uses heating methods or devices (radiant heat, forced hot air, warmed IV fluids, warm water packs) but no invasive devices. Use of these methods requires careful monitoring for hemodynamic changes and tissue injury from external heating devices. Some researchers believe that active external rewarming contributes to "afterdrop" (continued drop in core temperature when cold blood from the periphery is mobilized). But recent studies have indicated that forced air rewarming (one study used warmed IV fluids and forced air rewarming) is effective in some patients, even those with severe hypothermia.[7,8]
  - –For patients with a core body temperature <30°C (86°F) and cardiac arrest, active internal rewarming techniques (invasive) are needed. With or without return of spontaneous circulation, these patients may benefit from prolonged CPR and internal warming (peritoneal lavage, esophageal rewarming tubes, cardiopulmonary bypass, extracorporeal circulation, etc).

Modifications of BLS for Hypothermia

If the hypothermic victim has not yet developed cardiac arrest, focus attention on warming the patient with available methods. Handle the victim gently for all procedures; physical manipulations have been reported to precipitate VF.[4,9]

If the hypothermic victim is in cardiac arrest, the general approach to BLS management should still target airway, breathing, and circulation but with some modifications in approach. When the victim is hypothermic, pulse and respiratory rates may be slow or difficult to detect. For these reasons the BLS healthcare provider should assess breathing and later assess the pulse for a period of 30 to 45 seconds to confirm respiratory arrest, pulseless cardiac arrest, or bradycardia that is profound enough to require CPR.[10] If the victim is not breathing, start rescue breathing immediately. If possible, administer warmed (42°C to 46°C [108°F to 115°F]) humidified oxygen during bag-mask ventilation. If the victim is pulseless with no detectable signs of circulation, start chest compressions immediately. If there is any doubt about whether a pulse is present, begin compressions.

The temperature at which defibrillation should first be attempted in the severely hypothermic patient and the number

(*Circulation*. 2005;112:IV-136-IV-138.)

This special supplement to *Circulation* is freely available at http://www.circulationaha.org

DOI: 10.1161/CIRCULATIONAHA.105.166566

of defibrillation attempts that should be made have not been established. But if ventricular tachycardia (VT) or VF is present, defibrillation should be attempted. Automated external defibrillators (AEDs) may be used for these patients. If VF is detected, it should be treated with 1 shock then immediately followed by resumption of CPR, as outlined elsewhere in these guidelines for VF/VT (see Part 5: "Electrical Therapies: Automated External Defibrillators, Defibrillation, Cardioversion, and Pacing"). If the patient does not respond to 1 shock, further defibrillation attempts should be deferred, and the rescuer should focus on continuing CPR and rewarming the patient to a range of 30°C to 32°C (86°F to 89.6°F) before repeating the defibrillation attempt. If core temperature is <30°C (86°F), successful conversion to normal sinus rhythm may not be possible until rewarming is accomplished.[11]

To prevent further core heat loss, remove wet garments and protect the victim from further environmental exposure. Insofar as possible this should be done while providing initial BLS therapies. Beyond these critical initial steps, the treatment of severe hypothermia (temperature <30°C [86°F]) in the field remains controversial. Many providers do not have the time or equipment to assess core body temperature or to institute aggressive rewarming techniques, although these methods should be initiated when available.[4,9,12,13]

Modifications to ACLS for Hypothermia

For unresponsive patients or those in arrest, endotracheal intubation is appropriate. Intubation serves 2 purposes in the management of hypothermia: it enables provision of effective ventilation with warm, humidified oxygen, and it can isolate the airway to reduce the likelihood of aspiration.

ACLS management of cardiac arrest due to hypothermia focuses on more aggressive active core rewarming techniques as the primary therapeutic modality. The hypothermic heart may be unresponsive to cardiovascular drugs, pacemaker stimulation, and defibrillation.[9] In addition, drug metabolism is reduced. There is concern that in the severely hypothermic victim, cardioactive medications can accumulate to toxic levels in the peripheral circulation if given repeatedly. For these reasons IV drugs are often withheld if the victim's core body temperature is <30°C (86°F). If the core body temperature is >30°C, IV medications may be administered but with increased intervals between doses.

As noted previously, a defibrillation attempt is appropriate if VF/VT is present. If the patient fails to respond to the initial defibrillation attempt or initial drug therapy, defer subsequent defibrillation attempts or additional boluses of medication until the core temperature rises above 30°C (86°F).[9] Sinus bradycardia may be physiologic in severe hypothermia (ie, appropriate to maintain sufficient oxygen delivery when hypothermia is present), and cardiac pacing is usually not indicated.

In-hospital treatment of severely hypothermic (core temperature <30°C [86°F]) victims in cardiac arrest should be directed at rapid core rewarming. Techniques for in-hospital controlled rewarming include administration of warmed, humidified oxygen (42°C to 46°C [108°F to 115°F]), warmed IV fluids (normal saline) at 43°C (109°F), peritoneal lavage with warmed fluids, pleural lavage with warm saline through chest tubes, extracorporeal blood warming with partial bypass,[4,9,12,14,15] and cardiopulmonary bypass.[16]

During rewarming, patients who have been hypothermic for >45 to 60 minutes are likely to require volume administration because the vascular space expands with vasodilation. Routine administration of steroids, barbiturates, and antibiotics has not been documented to increase survival rates or decrease postresuscitation damage.[17,18]

If drowning preceded hypothermia, successful resuscitation is unlikely. Because severe hypothermia is frequently preceded by other disorders (eg, drug overdose, alcohol use, or trauma), the clinician must look for and treat these underlying conditions while simultaneously treating the hypothermia.

Withholding and Cessation of Resuscitative Efforts

In the field resuscitation may be withheld if the victim has obvious lethal injuries or if the body is frozen so that nose and mouth are blocked by ice and chest compression is impossible.[19]

Some clinicians believe that patients who appear dead after prolonged exposure to cold temperatures should not be considered dead until they are warmed to near normal core temperature.[10,11] Hypothermia may exert a protective effect on the brain and organs if the hypothermia develops rapidly in victims of cardiac arrest. When a victim of hypothermia is discovered, however, it may be impossible to distinguish primary from secondary hypothermia. When it is clinically impossible to know whether the arrest or the hypothermia occurred first, rescuers should try to stabilize the patient with CPR. Basic maneuvers to limit heat loss and begin rewarming should be started. Once the patient is in the hospital, physicians should use their clinical judgment to decide when resuscitative efforts should cease in a victim of hypothermic arrest.

References

1. Holzer M, Behringer W, Schorkhuber W, Zeiner A, Sterz F, Laggner AN, Frass M, Siostrozonek P, Ratheiser K, Kaff A. Mild hypothermia and outcome after CPR. Hypothermia for Cardiac Arrest (HACA) Study Group. *Acta Anaesthesiol Scand Suppl.* 1997;111:55–58.
2. Sterz F, Safar P, Tisherman S, Radovsky A, Kuboyama K, Oku K. Mild hypothermic cardiopulmonary resuscitation improves outcome after prolonged cardiac arrest in dogs. *Crit Care Med.* 1991;19:379–389.
3. Farstad M, Andersen KS, Koller ME, Grong K, Segadal L, Husby P. Rewarming from accidental hypothermia by extracorporeal circulation: a retrospective study. *Eur J Cardiothorac Surg.* 2001;20:58–64.
4. Schneider SM. Hypothermia: from recognition to rewarming. *Emerg Med Rep.* 1992;13:1–20.
5. Gilbert M, Busund R, Skagseth A, Nilsen PÅ, Solbø JP. Resuscitation from accidental hypothermia of 13.7°C with circulatory arrest. *Lancet.* 2000;355:375–376.
6. Larach MG. Accidental hypothermia. *Lancet.* 1995;345:493–498.
7. Kornberger E, Schwarz B, Lindner KH, Mair P. Forced air surface rewarming in patients with severe accidental hypothermia. *Resuscitation.* 1999;41:105–111.
8. Roggla M, Frossard M, Wagner A, Holzer M, Bur A, Roggla G. Severe accidental hypothermia with or without hemodynamic instability: rewarming without the use of extracorporeal circulation. *Wien Klin Wochenschr.* 2002;114:315–320.
9. Reuler JB. Hypothermia: pathophysiology, clinical settings, and management. *Ann Intern Med.* 1978;89:519–527.

10. Steinman AM. Cardiopulmonary resuscitation and hypothermia. *Circulation.* 1986;74(pt 2):IV29-IV32.
11. Southwick FS, Dalglish PH Jr. Recovery after prolonged asystolic cardiac arrest in profound hypothermia: a case report and literature review. *JAMA.* 1980;243:1250–1253.
12. Weinberg AD, Hamlet MP, Paturas JL, White RD, McAninch GW. *Cold Weather Emergencies: Principles of Patient Management.* Branford, CT: American Medical Publishing Co; 1990:10–30.
13. Romet TT. Mechanism of afterdrop after cold water immersion. *J Appl Physiol.* 1988;65:1535–1538.
14. Zell SC, Kurtz KJ. Severe exposure hypothermia: a resuscitation protocol. *Ann Emerg Med.* 1985;14:339–345.
15. Althaus U, Aeberhard P, Schupbach P, Nachbur BH, Muhlemann W. Management of profound accidental hypothermia with cardiorespiratory arrest. *Ann Surg.* 1982;195:492–495.
16. Silfvast T, Pettila V. Outcome from severe accidental hypothermia in Southern Finland—a 10-year review. *Resuscitation.* 2003;59:285–290.
17. Moss J. Accidental severe hypothermia. *Surg Gynecol Obstet.* 1986;162: 501–513.
18. Safar P. Cerebral resuscitation after cardiac arrest: research initiatives and future directions [published correction appears in *Ann Emerg Med.* 1993; 22:759]. *Ann Emerg Med.* 1993;22:324–349.
19. Danzl DF, Pozos RS, Auerbach PS, Glazer S, Goetz W, Johnson E, Jui J, Lilja P, Marx JA, Miller J. Multicenter hypothermia survey. *Ann Emerg Med.* 1987;16:1042–1055.

Part 10.5: Near-Fatal Asthma

Asthma accounts for >2 million emergency department visits and 5000 to 6000 deaths annually in the United States, many occurring in the prehospital setting.[1] Severe asthma accounts for approximately 2% to 20% of admissions to intensive care units, with up to one third of these patients requiring intubation and mechanical ventilation.[2] This section focuses on the evaluation and treatment of patients with near-fatal asthma.

Pathophysiology

The pathophysiology of asthma consists of 3 key abnormalities:

- Bronchoconstriction
- Airway inflammation
- Mucous impaction

Complications of severe asthma, such as tension pneumothorax, lobar atelectasis, pneumonia, and pulmonary edema, can contribute to fatalities. Cardiac causes of death are less common.

Clinical Aspects of Severe Asthma

Wheezing is a common physical finding, but severity does not correlate with the degree of airway obstruction. The absence of wheezing may indicate critical airway obstruction, whereas increased wheezing may indicate a positive response to bronchodilator therapy.

Oxygen saturation (Sa_{O_2}) levels may not reflect progressive alveolar hypoventilation, particularly if O_2 is being administered. Note that the Sa_{O_2} may initially fall during therapy because β-agonists produce both bronchodilation and vasodilation and may initially increase intrapulmonary shunting.

Other causes of wheezing are pulmonary edema, chronic obstructive pulmonary disease (COPD), pneumonia, anaphylaxis,[3] foreign bodies, pulmonary embolism, bronchiectasis, and subglottic mass.[4]

Initial Stabilization

Patients with severe life-threatening asthma require urgent and aggressive treatment with simultaneous administration of oxygen, bronchodilators, and steroids. Healthcare providers must monitor these patients closely for deterioration. Although the pathophysiology of life-threatening asthma consists of bronchoconstriction, inflammation, and mucous impaction, only bronchoconstriction and inflammation are amenable to drug treatment. If the patient does not respond to therapy, consultation or transfer to a pulmonologist or intensivist is appropriate.

(*Circulation.* 2005;112:IV-139-IV-142.)

DOI: 10.1161/CIRCULATIONAHA.105.166567

Primary Therapy

Oxygen

Provide oxygen to all patients with severe asthma, even those with normal oxygenation. Titrate to maintain Sa_{O_2} >92%. As noted above, successful treatment with β-agonists may initially cause a decrease in oxygen saturation because the resultant bronchodilation may initially increase the ventilation-perfusion mismatch.

Inhaled β_2-Agonists

Albuterol (or salbutamol) provides rapid, dose-dependent bronchodilation with minimal side effects. Because the administered dose depends on the patient's lung volume and inspiratory flow rates, the same dose can be used in most patients regardless of age or size. Although 6 adult studies[5] and 1 pediatric study[6] showed no difference in the effects of continuous versus intermittent administration of nebulized albuterol, continuous administration was more effective in the subset of patients with severe exacerbations of asthma,[7,8] and it was more cost-effective in a pediatric trial.[6] A Cochrane meta-analysis showed no overall difference between the effects of albuterol delivered by metered dose inhaler (MDI)-spacer or nebulizer,[9] but MDI-spacer administration can be difficult in patients in severe distress. The typical dose of albuterol by nebulizer is 2.5 or 5 mg every 15 to 20 minutes intermittently or continuous nebulization in a dose of 10 to 15 mg/h.

Levalbuterol is the R-isomer of albuterol. It has recently become available in the United States for treatment of acute asthma. Some studies have shown equivalent or slight improvement in bronchodilation when compared with albuterol in the emergency department.[10] Further studies are needed before a definitive recommendation can be made.

Corticosteroids

Systemic corticosteroids are the only proven treatment for the inflammatory component of asthma, but the onset of their anti-inflammatory effects is 6 to 12 hours after administration. A comprehensive search of the literature by the Cochrane approach (including pediatric and adult patients) determined that the early use of systemic steroids reduced rates of admission to the hospital.[11] Thus, providers should administer steroids as early as possible to all asthma patients but should not expect effects for several hours. Although there is no difference in clinical effects between oral and intravenous (IV) formulations of corticosteroids,[12] the IV route is preferable because patients with near-fatal asthma may vomit or be unable to swallow. A typical initial adult dose of methylprednisolone is 125 mg (dose range: 40 to 250 mg).

Incorporation or substitution of inhaled steroids into this scheme remains controversial. A Cochrane meta-analysis of 7 randomized trials (4 adult and 3 pediatric) of inhaled corticosteroids concluded that steroids significantly reduced the likelihood of admission to the hospital, particularly in patients who were not receiving concomitant systemic steroids. But the meta-analysis concluded that there is insufficient evidence that inhaled corticosteroids alone are as effective as systemic steroids.[13]

Adjunctive Therapies

Anticholinergics

Ipratropium bromide is an anticholinergic bronchodilator that is pharmacologically related to atropine. It can produce a clinically modest improvement in lung function compared with albuterol alone.[14,15] The nebulizer dose is 0.5 mg. It has a slow onset of action (approximately 20 minutes), with peak effectiveness at 60 to 90 minutes and no systemic side effects. It is typically given only once because of its prolonged onset of action, but some studies have shown clinical improvement only with repeated doses.[16] Given the few side effects, ipratropium should be considered an adjunct to albuterol. Tiotropium is a new, longer-acting anticholinergic that is currently undergoing clinical testing for use in acute asthma.[17]

Magnesium Sulfate

IV magnesium sulfate can modestly improve pulmonary function in patients with asthma when combined with nebulized β-adrenergic agents and corticosteroids.[18] Magnesium causes bronchial smooth muscle relaxation independent of the serum magnesium level, with only minor side effects (flushing, lightheadedness). A Cochrane meta-analysis of 7 studies concluded that IV magnesium sulfate improves pulmonary function and reduces hospital admissions, particularly for patients with the most severe exacerbations of asthma.[19] The typical adult dose is 1.2 to 2 g IV given over 20 minutes. When given with a β_2-agonist, nebulized magnesium sulfate also improved pulmonary function during acute asthma but did not reduce rate of hospitalization.[20]

Parenteral Epinephrine or Terbutaline

Epinephrine and terbutaline are adrenergic agents that can be given subcutaneously to patients with acute severe asthma. The dose of subcutaneous epinephrine (concentration of 1:1000) is 0.01 mg/kg divided into 3 doses of approximately 0.3 mg given at 20-minute intervals. The nonselective adrenergic properties of epinephrine may cause an increase in heart rate, myocardial irritability, and increased oxygen demand. But its use (even in patients >35 years of age) is well-tolerated.[21] Terbutaline is given in a dose of 0.25 mg subcutaneously and can be repeated in 30 to 60 minutes. These drugs are more commonly administered to children with acute asthma. Although most studies have shown them to be equally efficacious,[22] one study concluded that terbutaline was superior.[23]

Ketamine

Ketamine is a parenteral dissociative anesthetic that has bronchodilatory properties. Ketamine may also have indirect effects in patients with asthma through its sedative properties. One case series[24] suggested substantial effectiveness, but the single randomized trial published to date[25] showed no benefit of ketamine when compared with standard care. Ketamine will stimulate copious bronchial secretions.

Heliox

Heliox is a mixture of helium and oxygen (usually a 70:30 helium to oxygen ratio mix) that is less viscous than ambient air. Heliox has been shown to improve the delivery and deposition of nebulized albuterol.[26] Although recent meta-analysis of 4 clinical trials did not support the use of heliox in the initial treatment of patients with acute asthma,[27] it may be useful for asthma that is refractory to conventional therapy.[28] The heliox mixture requires at least 70% helium for effect, so if the patient requires >30% oxygen, the heliox mixture cannot be used.

Methylxanthines

Although previously a mainstay in the treatment of acute asthma, methylxanthines are infrequently used because of erratic pharmacokinetics and known side effects.

Leukotriene Antagonists

Leukotriene antagonists improve lung function and decrease the need for short-acting β-agonists during long-term asthma therapy, but their effectiveness during acute exacerbations of asthma is unproven. One study showed improvement in lung function with the addition of IV montelukast to standard therapy,[29] but further research is needed.

Inhaled Anesthetics

Case reports in adults[30] and children[31] suggest a benefit of inhalation anesthetics for patients with status asthmaticus unresponsive to maximal conventional therapy. These anesthetic agents may work directly as bronchodilators and may have indirect effects by enhancing patient-ventilator synchrony and reducing oxygen demand and carbon dioxide production. This therapy, however, requires an ICU setting, and there have been no randomized studies to evaluate its effectiveness.

Assisted Ventilation

Noninvasive Positive-Pressure Ventilation

Noninvasive positive-pressure ventilation (NIPPV) may offer short-term support to patients with acute respiratory failure and may delay or eliminate the need for endotracheal intubation.[32,33] This therapy requires an alert patient with adequate spontaneous respiratory effort. Bi-level positive airway pressure (BiPAP), the most common way of delivering NIPPV, allows for separate control of inspiratory and expiratory pressures.

Endotracheal Intubation With Mechanical Ventilation

Endotracheal intubation does not solve the problem of small airway constriction in patients with severe asthma. In addition, intubation and positive-pressure ventilation can trigger further bronchoconstriction and complications such as breath stacking (auto-PEEP [positive end-expiratory pressure]) and barotrauma. Although endotracheal intubation introduces risks, elective intubation should be performed if the asthmatic patient deteriorates despite aggressive management.

Rapid sequence intubation is the technique of choice. The provider should use the largest endotracheal tube available (usually 8 or 9 mm) to decrease airway resistance. Immediately after intubation, confirm endotracheal tube placement by clinical examination and a device (eg, exhaled CO_2 detector) and obtain a chest radiograph.

Troubleshooting After Intubation

When severe bronchoconstriction is present, breath stacking (so-called auto-PEEP) can develop during positive-pressure ventilation, leading to complications such as hyperinflation, tension pneumothorax, and hypotension. During manual or mechanical ventilation use a slower respiratory rate (eg, 6 to 10 breaths per minute) with smaller tidal volumes (eg, 6 to 8 mL/kg),[34] shorter inspiratory time (eg, adult inspiratory flow rate 80 to 100 mL/min), and longer expiratory time (eg, inspiratory to expiratory ratio 1:4 or 1:5) than would typically be provided to nonasthmatic patients.

Mild hypoventilation (permissive hypercapnia) reduces the risk of barotrauma. Hypercapnia is typically well tolerated.[35] Sedation is often required to optimize ventilation and minimize barotrauma after intubation. Delivery of inhaled medications may be inadequate before intubation, so continue to administer inhaled albuterol treatments through the endotracheal tube.

Four common causes of acute deterioration in any intubated patient are recalled by the mnemonic DOPE (tube **D**isplacement, tube **O**bstruction, **P**neumothorax, and **E**quipment failure). This mnemonic still holds in the patient with severe asthma.

If the patient with asthma deteriorates or is difficult to ventilate, verify endotracheal tube position, eliminate tube obstruction (eliminate any mucous plugs and kinks), and rule out (or decompress) a pneumothorax. Only experienced providers should perform needle decompression or insertion of a chest tube for pneumothorax.

Check the ventilator circuit for leaks or malfunction. High end-expiratory pressure can be quickly reduced by separating the patient from the ventilator circuit; this will allow PEEP to dissipate during passive exhalation. To minimize auto-PEEP, decrease inhalation time (this increases exhalation time), decrease the respiratory rate by 2 breaths per minute, and reduce the tidal volume to 3 to 5 mL/kg. Continue treatment with inhaled albuterol.

Cardiac Arrest in the Asthmatic Patient

When the asthmatic patient experiences a cardiac arrest, the provider may be concerned about modifications to the ACLS guidelines. There is inadequate evidence to recommend for or against the use of heliox during cardiac arrest (Class Indeterminate).[36] There is insufficient evidence to recommend compression of the chest wall to relieve gas trapping if dynamic hyperinflation occurs.[37]

Summary

When treating patients with severe asthma, providers should closely monitor patients to detect further deterioration or development of complications. When there is no improvement and intubation is required, these patients require the care of experienced providers in an intensive care setting. Some tertiary centers can offer experimental therapies as a last resort, and transfer should be considered for patients with near-fatal asthma that is refractory to aggressive medical management.

References

1. Division of Data Services. *New Asthma Estimates: Tracking Prevalence, Health Care, and Mortality*. Hyattsville, Md: National Center for Health Statistics; 2001.
2. McFadden ER Jr. Acute severe asthma. *Am J Respir Crit Care Med*. 2003;168:740–759.
3. Rainbow J, Browne GJ. Fatal asthma or anaphylaxis? *Emerg Med J*. 2002;19:415–417.
4. Kokturk N, Demir N, Kervan F, Dinc E, Koybasioglu A, Turktas H. A subglottic mass mimicking near-fatal asthma: a challenge of diagnosis. *J Emerg Med*. 2004;26:57–60.
5. Rodrigo GJ, Rodrigo C. Continuous vs intermittent beta-agonists in the treatment of acute adult asthma: a systematic review with meta-analysis. *Chest*. 2002;122:160–165.
6. Khine H, Fuchs SM, Saville AL. Continuous vs intermittent nebulized albuterol for emergency management of asthma. *Acad Emerg Med*. 1996; 3:1019–1024.
7. Lin RY, Sauter D, Newman T, Sirleaf J, Walters J, Tavakol M. Continuous versus intermittent albuterol nebulization in the treatment of acute asthma. *Ann Emerg Med*. 1993;22:1847–1853.
8. Rudnitsky GS, Eberlein RS, Schoffstall JM, Mazur JE, Spivey WH. Comparison of intermittent and continuously nebulized albuterol for treatment of asthma in an urban emergency department. *Ann Emerg Med*. 1993;22:1842–1846.
9. Newman KB, Milne S, Hamilton C, Hall K. A comparison of albuterol administered by metered-dose inhaler and spacer with albuterol by nebulizer in adults presenting to an urban emergency department with acute asthma. *Chest*. 2002;121:1036–1041.
10. Nowak R. Single-isomer levalbuterol: a review of the acute data. *Curr Allergy Asthma Rep*. 2003;3:172–178.
11. Gibbs MA, Camargo CA Jr, Rowe BH, Silverman RA. State of the art: therapeutic controversies in severe acute asthma. *Acad Emerg Med*. 2000;7:800–815.
12. Ratto D, Alfaro C, Sipsey J, Glovsky MM, Sharma OP. Are intravenous corticosteroids required in status asthmaticus? *JAMA*. 1988;260:527–529.
13. Rowe BH, Spooner CH, Ducharme FM, Bretzlaff JA, Bota GW. Early emergency department treatment of acute asthma with systemic corticosteroids. *Cochrane Database Syst Rev*. 2000;CD002178.
14. Aaron SD. The use of ipratropium bromide for the management of acute asthma exacerbation in adults and children: a systematic review. *J Asthma*. 2001;38:521–530.
15. Rodrigo G, Rodrigo C, Burschtin O. A meta-analysis of the effects of ipratropium bromide in adults with acute asthma. *Am J Med*. 1999;107: 363–370.
16. Plotnick LH, Ducharme FM. Acute asthma in children and adolescents: should inhaled anticholinergics be added to beta(2)-agonists? *Am J Respir Med*. 2003;2:109–115.
17. Keam SJ, Keating GM. Tiotropium bromide. A review of its use as maintenance therapy in patients with COPD. *Treat Respir Med*. 2004;3: 247–268.
18. Silverman RA, Osborn H, Runge J, Gallagher EJ, Chiang W, Feldman J, Gaeta T, Freeman K, Levin B, Mancherje N, Scharf S. IV magnesium sulfate in the treatment of acute severe asthma: a multicenter randomized controlled trial. *Chest*. 2002;122:489–497.
19. Rowe BH, Bretzlaff JA, Bourdon C, Bota GW, Camargo CA Jr. Magnesium sulfate for treating exacerbations of acute asthma in the emergency department. *Cochrane Database Syst Rev*. 2000;CD001490.
20. Blitz M, Blitz S, Beasely R, Diner B, Hughes R, Knopp J, Rowe B. Inhaled magnesium sulfate in the treatment of acute asthma. *Cochrane Database Syst Rev*. 2005;CD003898.
21. Cydulka R, Davison R, Grammer L, Parker M, Mathews J IV. The use of epinephrine in the treatment of older adult asthmatics. *Ann Emerg Med*. 1988;17:322–326.
22. Victoria MS, Battista CJ, Nangia BS. Comparison of subcutaneous terbutaline with epinephrine in the treatment of asthma in children. *J Allergy Clin Immunol*. 1977;59:128–135.

23. Victoria MS, Battista CJ, Nangia BS. Comparison between epinephrine and terbutaline injections in the acute management of asthma. *J Asthma.* 1989;26:287–290.
24. Petrillo TM, Fortenberry JD, Linzer JF, Simon HK. Emergency department use of ketamine in pediatric status asthmaticus. *J Asthma.* 2001;38:657–664.
25. Howton JC, Rose J, Duffy S, Zoltanski T, Levitt MA. Randomized, double-blind, placebo-controlled trial of intravenous ketamine in acute asthma. *Ann Emerg Med.* 1996;27:170–175.
26. Hess DR, Acosta FL, Ritz RH, Kacmarek RM, Camargo CA Jr. The effect of heliox on nebulizer function using a beta-agonist bronchodilator. *Chest.* 1999;115:184–189.
27. Rodrigo GJ, Rodrigo C, Pollack CV, Rowe B. Use of helium-oxygen mixtures in the treatment of acute asthma: a systematic review. *Chest.* 2003;123:891–896.
28. Reuben AD, Harris AR. Heliox for asthma in the emergency department: a review of the literature. *Emerg Med J.* 2004;21:131–135.
29. Camargo CA Jr, Smithline HA, Malice MP, Green SA, Reiss TF. A randomized controlled trial of intravenous montelukast in acute asthma. *Am J Respir Crit Care Med.* 2003;167:528–533.
30. Schultz TE. Sevoflurane administration in status asthmaticus: a case report. *AANA J.* 2005;73:35–36.
31. Wheeler DS, Clapp CR, Ponaman ML, Bsn HM, Poss WB. Isoflurane therapy for status asthmaticus in children: a case series and protocol. *Pediatr Crit Care Med.* 2000;1:55–59.
32. Non-invasive ventilation in acute respiratory failure. *Thorax.* 2002;57:192–211.
33. Soroksky A, Stav D, Shpirer I. A pilot prospective, randomized, placebo-controlled trial of bilevel positive airway pressure in acute asthmatic attack. *Chest.* 2003;123:1018–1025.
34. Marik PE, Varon J, Fromm R Jr. The management of acute severe asthma. *J Emerg Med.* 2002;23:257–268.
35. Mazzeo AT, Spada A, Pratico C, Lucanto T, Santamaria LB. Hypercapnia: what is the limit in paediatric patients? A case of near-fatal asthma successfully treated by multipharmacological approach. *Paediatr Anaesth.* 2004;14:596–603.
36. Rodrigo G, Pollack C, Rodrigo C, Rowe BH. Heliox for nonintubated acute asthma patients. *Cochrane Database Syst Rev.* 2003;CD002884.
37. Van der Touw T, Mudaliar Y, Nayyar V. Cardiorespiratory effects of manually compressing the rib cage during tidal expiration in mechanically ventilated patients recovering from acute severe asthma. *Crit Care Med.* 1998;26:1361–1367.

Part 10.6: Anaphylaxis

Anaphylaxis is a severe, systemic allergic reaction characterized by multisystem involvement, including the skin, airway, vascular system, and gastrointestinal tract. Severe cases may result in complete obstruction of the airway, cardiovascular collapse, and death. The term *classic anaphylaxis* refers to hypersensitivity reactions mediated by the subclass of antibodies immunoglobulins IgE and IgG. Prior sensitization to an allergen has occurred, producing antigen-specific immunoglobulins. Subsequent reexposure to the allergen provokes the anaphylactic reaction. Many anaphylactic reactions, however, occur without a documented prior exposure.

Anaphylactoid or *pseudoanaphylactic* reactions display a similar clinical syndrome, but they are not immune-mediated. Treatment for the two conditions is similar.

Pathophysiology

The inciting allergen binds to antigen-specific IgE that has accumulated on previously sensitized basophils and mast cells. These cells almost immediately release a series of mediators, including histamines, leukotrienes, prostaglandins, thromboxanes, and bradykinins. When released locally and systemically, these mediators cause increased mucous membrane secretions, increased capillary permeability and leak, and markedly reduced smooth muscle tone in blood vessels (vasodilation) and bronchioles.

Etiology

Any antigen capable of activating IgE can be a trigger for anaphylaxis. In terms of etiology, researchers generally list the following categories of causes: pharmacologic agents, latex, stinging insects, and foods. In up to 5% of cases the antigenic agent cannot be identified.

Pharmacologic agents. Antibiotics (especially parenteral penicillins and other β-lactams), aspirin and nonsteroidal anti-inflammatory drugs, and intravenous (IV) contrast agents are the most frequent medications associated with life-threatening anaphylaxis.

Latex. Much attention has focused on latex-induced anaphylaxis, but it is actually quite rare.[1,2] A decade-long registry of anaphylactic deaths in England has not registered any latex-associated deaths.[3,4]

Stinging insects. Fatal anaphylaxis has long been associated with stings from hymenoptera (membrane-winged insects), including ants, bees, hornets, wasps, and yellow jackets. Fatal anaphylaxis can develop when a person with IgE antibodies induced by a previous sting is stung again. A fatal reaction occurs within 10 to 15 minutes. Cardiovascular collapse is the most common mechanism.[3–5]

Foods. Peanuts, tree-grown nuts, seafood, and wheat are the foods most frequently associated with life-threatening anaphylaxis.[6] Bronchospasm and asphyxia are the most frequent mechanisms.[3–5]

Signs and Symptoms

Consider anaphylaxis when responses from 2 or more body systems (cutaneous, respiratory, cardiovascular, neurologic, or gastrointestinal) are noted; the cardiovascular and respiratory systems may not be involved. The shorter the interval between exposure and reaction, the more likely the reaction is to be severe. Signs and symptoms include the following:

- Serious upper airway (laryngeal) edema, lower airway edema (asthma), or both may develop, causing stridor and wheezing. Rhinitis is often an early sign of respiratory involvement.
- *Cardiovascular collapse* is the most common periarrest manifestation. Vasodilation produces a relative hypovolemia. Increased capillary permeability contributes to further intravascular volume loss. The patient may be agitated or anxious and may appear either flushed or pale. Additional cardiac dysfunction may result from underlying disease or the development of myocardial ischemia from administration of epinephrine.[3–5]
- Gastrointestinal signs and symptoms of anaphylaxis include abdominal pain, vomiting, and diarrhea.

Differential Diagnoses

A number of disease processes produce some of the signs and symptoms of anaphylaxis. Only after the clinician eliminates anaphylaxis as a diagnosis should the other conditions be considered, because failure to identify and appropriately treat anaphylaxis can be fatal.[7,8]

- *Scombroid poisoning* often develops within 30 minutes of eating spoiled fish, including tuna, mackerel, or dolphin (mahi-mahi). Typically scombroid poisoning presents with urticaria, nausea, vomiting, diarrhea, and headache. It is treated with antihistamines.
- *Angioedema* that seems to occur in families is termed *hereditary angioedema.* This hereditary form is indistinguishable from the early angioedema of anaphylaxis or medication-related angioedema. Urticaria does not occur with *hereditary angioedema*, however. Angioedema is treated with C1 esterase inhibitor replacement concentrate if available. Otherwise, fresh frozen plasma may be used.
- *Angiotensin-converting enzyme (ACE) inhibitors* are associated with a reactive angioedema predominantly of the upper airway. This reaction can develop days or years after ACE inhibitor therapy is begun. The best treatment for this form of angioedema is unclear, but aggressive early airway management is critical.[9]

(*Circulation.* 2005;000:IV-143-IV-145.)

This special supplement to *Circulation* is freely available at http://www.circulationaha.org

DOI: 10.1161/CIRCULATIONAHA.105.166568

- Severe, near-fatal asthma attacks can present with bronchospasm and stridor. In general, asthma attacks do not present with urticaria or angioedema. Asthma treatment is very different from treatment of anaphylaxis even though the mechanism of immunologic hypersensitivity may be common to both.
- In some forms of *panic disorder,* functional stridor develops as a result of forced adduction of the vocal cords. In a panic attack there is no urticaria, angioedema, hypoxia, or hypotension.
- Along with anaphylaxis, consider *vasovagal reactions.* Urticaria, angioedema, and bronchospasm are not present in vasovagal reactions.

Interventions to Prevent Cardiopulmonary Arrest

Recommendations to prevent cardiopulmonary arrest are difficult to standardize because etiology, clinical presentation (including severity and course), and organ involvement vary widely. Few randomized trials of treatment approaches have been reported. Providers, however, must be aware that the patient can deteriorate quickly and that urgent support of airway, breathing, and circulation are essential. The following therapies are commonly used and widely accepted but are based more on consensus than evidence:

- *Oxygen.* Administer oxygen at high flow rates.
- *Epinephrine*

  –Absorption and subsequent achievement of maximum plasma concentration after subcutaneous administration is slower and may be significantly delayed with shock.[10,11] Thus, intramuscular (IM) administration is favored.
    - Administer epinephrine by IM injection early to all patients with signs of a systemic reaction, especially hypotension, airway swelling, or definite difficulty breathing.
    - Use an IM dose of 0.3 to 0.5 mg (1:1000) repeated every 15 to 20 minutes if there is no clinical improvement.

  –Administer IV epinephrine if anaphylaxis appears to be severe with immediate life-threatening manifestations.[12]
    - Use epinephrine (1:10 000) 0.1 mg IV slowly over 5 minutes. Epinephrine may be diluted to a 1:10 000 solution before infusion.
    - An IV infusion at rates of 1 to 4 μg/min may prevent the need to repeat epinephrine injections frequently.[13]

  –Close monitoring is critical because fatal overdose of epinephrine has been reported.[3,14]

  –Patients who are taking β-blockers have increased incidence and severity of anaphylaxis and can develop a paradoxical response to epinephrine.[15] Consider glucagon as well as ipratropium for these patients (see below).

Aggressive fluid resuscitation. Give isotonic crystalloid (eg, normal saline) if hypotension is present and does not respond rapidly to epinephrine. A rapid infusion of 1 to 2 L or even 4 L may be needed initially.

Antihistamines. Administer antihistamines slowly IV or IM (eg, 25 to 50 mg of diphenhydramine).

H_2 blockers. Administer H_2 blockers such as cimetidine (300 mg orally, IM, or IV).[16]

Inhaled β-adrenergic agents. Provide inhaled albuterol if bronchospasm is a major feature. Inhaled ipratropium may be especially useful for treatment of bronchospasm in patients receiving β-blockers. Note that some patients treated for near-fatal asthma actually had anaphylaxis, so they received repeated doses of conventional bronchodilators rather than epinephrine.[17]

Corticosteroids. Infuse high-dose IV corticosteroids early in the course of therapy. Beneficial effects are delayed at least 4 to 6 hours.

Removal of venom sac. Insect envenomation by bees (but not wasps) may leave a venom sac attached to the victim's skin. At some point during initial assessment, look at the sting site, and if you see a stinger, immediately scrape it or any insect parts at the site of the sting, using the dull edge of a knife.[18] Avoid compressing or squeezing any insect parts near the skin because squeezing may increase envenomation.

Potential Therapies

- *Vasopressin.* There are case reports that vasopressin may benefit severely hypotensive patients.[19,20]
- *Atropine.* Case reports suggest that when relative or severe bradycardia is present, there may be a role for administration of atropine.[8]
- *Glucagon.* For patients who are unresponsive to epinephrine, especially those receiving β-blockers, glucagon may be effective. This agent is short-acting; give 1 to 2 mg every 5 minutes IM or IV. Nausea, vomiting, and hyperglycemia are common side effects.

Observation

Patients who respond to therapy require observation, but there is no evidence to suggest the length of observation time needed. Symptoms may recur in some patients (up to 20%) within 1 to 8 hours (biphasic response) despite an intervening asymptomatic period. Biphasic responses have been reported to occur up to 36 hours after the initial reaction.[15,16,21–24] A patient who remains symptom-free for 4 hours after treatment may be discharged.[25] Severity of reaction or other problems, however, may necessitate longer periods of observation.

Airway Obstruction

Early elective intubation is recommended for patients observed to develop hoarseness, lingual edema, stridor, or oropharyngeal swelling. Patients with angioedema pose a particularly worrisome problem because they are at high risk for rapid deterioration. Most will present with some degree of labial or facial swelling. Patients with hoarseness, lingual edema, and oropharyngeal swelling are at particular risk for respiratory compromise.

Patients can deteriorate over a brief period of time (½ to 3 hours), with progressive development of stridor, dysphonia or aphonia, laryngeal edema, massive lingual swelling, facial and neck swelling, and hypoxemia. This may occur when patients have a delayed presentation to the hospital or fail to respond to therapy.

At this point use of either the laryngeal mask airway or the Combitube will be ineffective, and endotracheal intubation and cricothyrotomy may be difficult or impossible. Attempts at endotracheal intubation may only further increase laryngeal edema or cause trauma to the airway. Early recognition of the potentially difficult airway allows planning for alternative airway management by those who are trained in these techniques, including consultation with anesthesia and an ear, nose, and throat specialist if the provider is unfamiliar with advanced airway techniques.

Cardiac Arrest

If cardiac arrest develops, CPR, volume administration, and adrenergic drugs are the cornerstones of therapy. Critical therapies are as follows:

- *Aggressive volume expansion.* Near-fatal anaphylaxis produces profound vasodilation that significantly increases intravascular capacity. Massive volume replacement is needed. Use at least 2 large-bore IVs with pressure bags to administer large volumes (typically between 4 and 8 L) of isotonic crystalloid as quickly as possible.
- *High-dose epinephrine IV.* Use a rapid progression to high dose without hesitation in patients in full cardiac arrest. A commonly used sequence is 1 to 3 mg IV (3 minutes), 3 to 5 mg IV (3 minutes), then 4 to 10 μg/min infusion.
- *Antihistamine IV.* There is little data about the value of antihistamines in anaphylactic cardiac arrest, but it is reasonable to assume that little additional harm could result.[16]
- *Steroid therapy.* Steroids given during a cardiac arrest will have little effect, but they may have value in the early hours of any postresuscitation period.
- *Asystole/Pulseless Electrical Activity (PEA) Algorithms.* The arrest rhythm in anaphylaxis is often PEA or asystole. See the ACLS Pulseless Arrest Algorithm in Part 7.2: "Management of Cardiac Arrest."
- *Prolonged CPR.* Patients with anaphylaxis are often young with healthy hearts and cardiovascular systems, and they may respond to rapid correction of vasodilation and low intravascular volume. Effective CPR may maintain sufficient oxygen delivery until the catastrophic effects of the anaphylactic reaction resolve.

Summary

The management of anaphylaxis includes early recognition, anticipation of deterioration, and aggressive support of airway, oxygenation, ventilation, and circulation. Potential fatal complications include airway obstruction and cardiovascular collapse. Prompt, aggressive therapy may succeed even if cardiac arrest develops.

References

1. Dreyfus DH, Fraser B, Randolph CC. Anaphylaxis to latex in patients without identified risk factors for latex allergy. *Conn Med.* 2004;68: 217–222.
2. Ownby DR. A history of latex allergy. *J Allergy Clin Immunol.* 2002; 110:S27–S32.
3. Pumphrey RS. Lessons for management of anaphylaxis from a study of fatal reactions. *Clin Exp Allergy.* 2000;30:1144–1150.
4. Pumphrey RS. Fatal anaphylaxis in the UK, 1992–2001. *Novartis Found Symp.* 2004;257:116–128; discussion 128–132, 157–160, 276–185.
5. Pumphrey RS, Roberts IS. Postmortem findings after fatal anaphylactic reactions. *J Clin Pathol.* 2000;53:273–276.
6. Mullins RJ. Anaphylaxis: risk factors for recurrence. *Clin Exp Allergy.* 2003;33:1033–1040.
7. Brown AF. Anaphylaxis: quintessence, quarrels, and quandaries. *Emerg Med J.* 2001;18:328.
8. Brown AFT. Anaphylaxis gets the adrenaline going. *Emerg Med J.* 2004;21:128–129.
9. Ishoo E, Shah UK, Grillone GA, Stram JR, Fuleiham NS. Predicting airway risk in angioedema: staging system based on presentation. *Otolaryngol Head Neck Surg.* 1999;121:263–268.
10. Simons FE, Gu X, Simons KJ. Epinephrine absorption in adults: intramuscular versus subcutaneous injection. *J Allergy Clin Immunol.* 2001; 108:871–873.
11. Simons FE, Chan ES, Gu X, Simons KJ. Epinephrine for the out-of-hospital (first-aid) treatment of anaphylaxis in infants: is the ampule/syringe/needle method practical? *J Allergy Clin Immunol.* 2001;108: 1040–1044.
12. Brown SG, Blackman KE, Stenlake V, Heddle RJ. Insect sting anaphylaxis; prospective evaluation of treatment with intravenous adrenaline and volume resuscitation. *Emerg Med J.* 2004;21:149–154.
13. Barach EM, Nowak RM, Lee TG, Tomlanovich MM. Epinephrine for treatment of anaphylactic shock. *JAMA.* 1984;251:2118–2122.
14. Pumphrey R. Anaphylaxis: can we tell who is at risk of a fatal reaction? *Curr Opin Allergy Clin Immunol.* 2004;4:285–290.
15. Ellis AK, Day JH. Diagnosis and management of anaphylaxis. *CMAJ.* 2003;169:307–311.
16. Winbery SL, Lieberman PL. Histamine and antihistamines in anaphylaxis. *Clin Allergy Immunol.* 2002;17:287–317.
17. Rainbow J, Browne GJ. Fatal asthma or anaphylaxis? *Emerg Med J.* 2002;19:415–417.
18. Visscher PK, Vetter RS, Camazine S. Removing bee stings. *Lancet.* 1996;348:301–302.
19. Kill C, Wranze E, Wulf H. Successful treatment of severe anaphylactic shock with vasopressin: two case reports. *Int Arch Allergy Immunol.* 2004;134:260–261.
20. Williams SR, Denault AY, Pellerin M, Martineau R. Vasopressin for treatment of shock following aprotinin administration. *Can J Anaesth.* 2004;51:169–172.
21. Yocum MW, Butterfield JH, Klein JS, Volcheck GW, Schroeder DR, Silverstein MD. Epidemiology of anaphylaxis in Olmsted County: a population-based study. *J Allergy Clin Immunol.* 1999;104(pt 1):452–456.
22. Smith PL, Kagey-Sobotka A, Bleecker ER, Traystman R, Kaplan AP, Gralnick H, Valentine MD, Permutt S, Lichtenstein LM. Physiologic manifestations of human anaphylaxis. *J Clin Invest.* 1980;66:1072–1080.
23. Stark BJ, Sullivan TJ. Biphasic and protracted anaphylaxis. *J Allergy Clin Immunol.* 1986;78:76–83.
24. Brazil E, MacNamara AF. 'Not so immediate' hypersensitivity: the danger of biphasic anaphylactic reactions. *J Accid Emerg Med.* 1998;15: 252–253.
25. Brady WJ Jr, Luber S, Carter CT, Guertter A, Lindbeck G. Multiphasic anaphylaxis: an uncommon event in the emergency department. *Acad Emerg Med.* 1997;4:193–197.

Part 10.7: Cardiac Arrest Associated With Trauma

Basic and advanced life support for the trauma patient are fundamentally the same as that for the patient with a primary cardiac arrest, with focus on support of airway, breathing, and circulation. In trauma resuscitation providers perform the Primary Survey (called the initial assessment in the National Highway Traffic Safety Administration [NHTSA] EMS Curricula), with rapid evaluation and stabilization of the airway, breathing, and circulation. This is followed by the Secondary Survey (called the focused history and detailed physical examination in the NHTSA courses), which detects more subtle but potentially lethal injuries.

Cardiopulmonary deterioration associated with trauma has several possible causes:

- Hypoxia secondary to respiratory arrest, airway obstruction, large open pneumothorax, tracheobronchial injury, or thoracoabdominal injury
- Injury to vital structures, such as the heart, aorta, or pulmonary arteries
- Severe head injury with secondary cardiovascular collapse
- Underlying medical problems or other conditions that led to the injury, such as sudden cardiac arrest (eg, ventricular fibrillation [VF]) in the driver of a motor vehicle or in the victim of an electric shock)
- Diminished cardiac output or pulseless arrest (pulseless electrical activity [PEA]) from tension pneumothorax or pericardial tamponade
- Extreme blood loss leading to hypovolemia and diminished delivery of oxygen

Despite a rapid and effective out-of-hospital and trauma center response, patients with out-of-hospital cardiac arrest due to trauma rarely survive.[1–4] Those patients with the best outcome from trauma arrest generally are young, have treatable penetrating injuries, have received early (out-of-hospital) endotracheal intubation, and undergo prompt transport (typically ≤10 minutes) to a trauma care facility.[3–6] Cardiac arrest in the field due to blunt trauma is fatal in all age groups.[7–9]

Extrication and Initial Evaluation

For years there has been a debate over whether ACLS providers should deploy a full armamentarium of interventions when treating victims of severe trauma at the scene. A number of studies have questioned the clinical effectiveness of on-site advanced airway management via endotracheal intubation as well as circulatory support with rapid intravenous (IV) infusions. The case against these interventions centers on 2 arguments: whether they are truly safe and effective and whether they adversely delay transport to, and definitive management at, a hospital or emergency department (ED).

There is considerable evidence that out-of-hospital endotracheal intubation is either harmful or at best ineffective for most EMS patients.[10–13] Researchers and emergency medical services (EMS) leaders have also questioned the safety and effectiveness of aggressive out-of-hospital IV fluid resuscitation in an urban environment.[14–17] In addition, field ACLS interventions unquestionably prolong time at the scene, delay transport to the ED or trauma center, and thereby delay essential interventions, such as surgical control of life-threatening bleeding.[17–20]

With the above discussion in mind, the focus of prehospital resuscitation should be to safely extricate and attempt to stabilize the patient and to minimize interventions that will delay transport to definitive care. Strict attention should be paid to stabilizing the spine during care. Patients suspected of having severe traumatic injuries should be transported or receive early transfer to a facility that can provide definitive trauma care. Attempts to stabilize the patient are typically performed during transport to avoid delay.

BLS for Cardiac Arrest Associated With Trauma

Airway

When multisystem trauma is present or trauma involves the head and neck, rescuers must stabilize the spine during all BLS maneuvers. A jaw thrust is used instead of a head tilt–chin lift to open the airway, with the priority to establish a patent airway. If at all possible, a second rescuer should be responsible for manually stabilizing the head and neck during BLS maneuvers and until spinal immobilization equipment is applied by trained providers. When the airway is open, clear the mouth of blood, vomitus, and other secretions.

Breathing/Ventilation

Once a patent airway is established, assess for breathing. If breathing is absent, agonal, or slow and extremely shallow, manual ventilation is needed. When ventilation is provided with a barrier device, a pocket mask, or a bag-mask device, the rescuer must still maintain cervical spine stabilization if cervical spine injury is suspected. Deliver breaths slowly to reduce risk of gastric inflation. If the chest does not expand during ventilation despite the presence of an adequate and patent airway, rule out tension pneumothorax or hemothorax.

Circulation

The provider should stop any visible hemorrhage using direct compression and appropriate dressings. After opening the airway and delivering 2 effective rescue breaths, the healthcare provider should attempt to feel a carotid pulse. If the healthcare provider does not definitely feel a pulse within 10 seconds, the provider should begin chest compressions and

(*Circulation*. 2005;112:IV-146-IV-149.)

DOI: 10.1161/CIRCULATIONAHA.105.166569

provide cycles of compressions and ventilations. During CPR, rescuers should provide compressions of adequate number and depth (rescuers should push hard and fast), allow full chest recoil after each compression, and minimize interruptions in chest compressions.

When CPR is provided for a victim with an advanced airway in place, 2 rescuers no longer deliver cycles of compressions interrupted with pauses for ventilation. Instead, the compressing rescuer should deliver 100 compressions per minute continuously, without pauses for ventilation. The rescuer delivering the ventilations should give 8 to 10 breaths per minute and should be careful to avoid delivering an excessive number of ventilations. The 2 rescuers should change compressor and ventilator roles approximately every 2 minutes to prevent compressor fatigue and deterioration in quality and rate of chest compressions. When multiple rescuers are present, they should rotate the compressor role about every 2 minutes.

If an automated external defibrillator (AED) is available, turn it on and attach it. The AED will evaluate the victim's cardiac rhythm and advise delivery of a shock if appropriate. If VF is present, note that the VF may have been the cause rather than the consequence of the trauma (eg, an automobile driver develops VF sudden cardiac arrest and when he loses consciousness he crashes the car). The victim may require further cardiac evaluation following resuscitation.

Disability

Throughout all interventions, assess the victim's response and monitor closely for signs of deterioration.

Exposure

To define the extent of injury, remove the victim's clothing. When the assessment for injuries is complete, cover the patient to prevent the development of hypothermia.

ACLS for Cardiac Arrest Associated With Trauma

ACLS includes continued assessment and support of the airway, oxygenation and ventilation (breathing), and circulation. Some of these procedures may be performed only after the patient has arrived at the hospital.

Airway

Indications for immediate intubation of the trauma patient include

- Respiratory arrest or apnea
- Respiratory failure, including severe hypoventilation or hypoxemia despite oxygen therapy
- Severe head injury (eg, Glasgow Coma Scale score [GCS] <8)
- Inability to protect the upper airway (eg, loss of gag reflex, depressed level of consciousness)
- Thoracic injuries (eg, flail chest, pulmonary contusion, penetrating trauma)
- Injuries associated with potential airway obstruction (eg, crushing facial or neck injuries)

Endotracheal intubation is performed while maintaining cervical spine stabilization. If intubation is performed in the field, it should be done during transport. Generally orotracheal intubation is performed. Avoid nasotracheal intubation in the presence of severe maxillofacial injuries. Confirm proper tube placement by clinical examination and use of a confirmation device (eg, an exhaled CO_2 monitor) immediately after intubation, during transport, and after any transfer of the patient (eg, from ambulance to hospital stretcher). Unsuccessful endotracheal intubation for the patient with massive facial injury and edema is an indication for cricothyrotomy by experienced providers.

When an endotracheal tube or other advanced airway is in place during CPR, simultaneous ventilations and compressions may result in a tension pneumothorax in an already damaged lung, especially if fractured ribs or a fractured sternum is present. Providers should suspect the development of a tension pneumothorax if there is a decrease in chest expansion and breath sounds, increased resistance to hand (bag-tube) ventilation, or if the patient's oxygen saturation falls.

Ventilation

Provide high inspired concentrations of oxygen even if the victim's oxygenation appears adequate. Once a patent airway is established, assess breath sounds and chest expansion. A unilateral decrease in breath sounds associated with inadequate chest expansion during positive-pressure ventilation should be presumed to be caused by *tension pneumothorax* or hemothorax until those complications can be ruled out. Healthcare providers will perform needle aspiration of the pneumothorax followed by insertion of a chest tube (this procedure typically is performed in the hospital).

Rescuers should look for and seal any significant open pneumothorax, allowing an exhalation port so that tension pneumothorax will not occur.

Hemothorax may also interfere with ventilation and chest expansion. Treat hemothorax with blood replacement and insertion of a chest tube, and check the initial volume of blood that comes out of the chest tube. Ongoing hemorrhage from the chest tube is an indication for surgical exploration.

Circulation

When the airway, oxygenation, and ventilation are adequate, evaluate and support circulation. Immediately control obvious visible bleeding. Volume resuscitation is an important but controversial part of trauma resuscitation. ACLS providers should establish large-bore IV access while en route to the ED or trauma center, limiting attempts to two. Isotonic crystalloid is the resuscitation fluid of choice because research has not clearly established any specific type of solution as superior.[21] When replacement of blood loss is required in the hospital, it is accomplished with a combination of packed red blood cells and isotonic crystalloid.

Aggressive fluid resuscitation is not required for trauma patients who have no evidence of hemodynamic compromise. Recommendations for volume resuscitation in trauma patients with signs of hypovolemic shock are determined by the type of trauma (penetrating vs blunt) and the setting (urban vs

TABLE. Suggested Indications for Resuscitative Thoracotomy: Patients With Traumatic Cardiac Arrest

Type of Injury	Assessment
Blunt trauma	• Patient arrives at ED or trauma center with pulse, blood pressure, and spontaneous respirations, *and* • then experiences witnessed cardiac arrest
Penetrating cardiac trauma	• Patient experiences a witnessed cardiac arrest in ED or trauma center *or* • Patient arrives in ED or trauma center after <5 minutes of out-of-hospital CPR and with positive secondary signs of life (eg, pupillary reflexes, spontaneous movement, organized ECG activity)
Penetrating thoracic (noncardiac) trauma	• Patient experiences a witnessed cardiac arrest in ED or trauma center *or* • Patient arrives in ED or trauma center after <15 minutes of out-of-hospital CPR and with positive secondary signs of life (eg, pupillary reflexes, spontaneous movement, organized ECG activity)
Exsanguinating abdominal vascular trauma	• Patient experiences a witnessed cardiac arrest in ED or trauma center *or* • Patient arrives in ED or trauma center with positive secondary signs of life (eg, pupillary reflexes, spontaneous movement, organized ECG activity) *plus* • Resources available for definitive repair of abdominal-vascular injuries

rural). A high rate of volume infusion with the therapeutic goal of a systolic blood pressure ≥100 mm Hg is now recommended only for patients with isolated head or extremity trauma, either blunt or penetrating. In the urban setting, aggressive prehospital volume resuscitation for penetrating trauma is no longer recommended because it is likely to increase blood pressure and consequently accelerate the rate of blood loss, delay arrival at the trauma center, and delay surgical intervention to repair or ligate bleeding vessels.[4,14,22] Such delay cannot be justified when the patient can be delivered to a trauma center within a few minutes. In rural settings, transport times to trauma centers will be longer, so volume resuscitation for blunt or penetrating trauma is provided during transport to maintain a systolic blood pressure of 90 mm Hg.

As noted above, if pulseless arrest develops, outcome is poor unless a reversible cause can be immediately identified and treated. Successful trauma resuscitation often depends on restoration of an adequate circulating blood volume.

The most common terminal cardiac rhythms observed in victims of trauma are PEA, bradyasystolic rhythms, and occasionally VF/ventricular tachycardia (VT). Treatment of PEA requires CPR and identification and treatment of reversible causes, such as severe hypovolemia, hypothermia, cardiac tamponade, or tension pneumothorax.[23] Development of bradyasystolic rhythms often indicates the presence of severe hypovolemia, severe hypoxemia, or cardiorespiratory failure. VF and pulseless VT are treated with CPR and attempted defibrillation. Although epinephrine is typically administered during the ACLS treatment of these arrhythmias, it will likely be ineffective in the presence of uncorrected severe hypovolemia.

Since publication of the *ECC Guidelines 2000* several centers have reported their retrospective observations about resuscitative thoracotomies for patients in traumatic cardiac arrest.[24–27] For example, one series reported 49 patients with *penetrating* chest trauma who underwent resuscitative thoracotomy in the ED.[27] None of the patients in cardiac arrest or without signs of life *before* thoracotomy survived to hospital discharge.

In a 2002 report of resuscitative thoracotomies for trauma patients in the ED,[24] the 3 survivors of 10 victims of penetrating trauma all had signs of life and vital signs on arrival at the ED. In contrast, all 19 patients with blunt trauma died, despite the fact that 14 of the 19 "had vital signs" at the time of the thoracotomy. In a database of 959 resuscitative thoracotomies,[26] 22 victims of penetrating trauma and 4 victims of blunt trauma survived to hospital discharge after receiving prehospital CPR (overall survival rate of 3%).

In 2001 the Committee on Trauma of the American College of Surgeons published a systematic review of 42 studies of ED thoracotomies involving nearly 7000 patients, published from 1966 to 1999.[28] In this database, survival was 11% (500 of 4482) for victims of penetrating trauma and 1.6% (35 of 2193) for victims of blunt trauma.

These studies suggest that there may be a role for open thoracotomy in specific patients or situations. The Table describes conditions under which an open thoracotomy may be considered. Open thoracotomy does not improve outcome from out-of-hospital blunt trauma arrest but can be lifesaving for patients with penetrating chest trauma if the patient has an arrest immediately before arrival at the ED or while in the ED. During concurrent volume resuscitation for penetrating trauma, prompt emergency thoracotomy will permit direct massage of the heart, relief of cardiac tamponade, control of thoracic and extrathoracic hemorrhage, and aortic cross-clamping.[2,4] This procedure should be performed only by experienced providers.

Cardiac contusions causing significant arrhythmias or impaired cardiac function are present in approximately 10% to 20% of victims of severe blunt chest trauma.[29] Myocardial contusion should be suspected if the trauma victim has extreme tachycardia, arrhythmias, and ST–T-wave changes. Cardiac biomarkers (see Part 8: "Stabilization of the Patient With Acute Coronary Syndromes") are not sensitive indicators of cardiac contusion.[30] The diagnosis of myocardial contusion is confirmed by echocardiography or radionuclide angiography.

Transfer

If a patient arrives at a facility with limited trauma capability, hospital staff should treat identifiable and reversible injuries to their capability. The patient should then be rapidly transferred to a facility that can provide definitive trauma care.

References

1. Pepe PE. Emergency medical services systems and prehospital management of patients requiring critical care. In: Carlson R, Geheb M, eds. *Principles and Practice of Medical Intensive Care*. Philadelphia, Pa: WB Saunders Co; 1993:9–24.
2. Rozycki GS, Adams C, Champion HR, Kihn R. Resuscitative thoracotomy—trends in outcome [abstract]. *Ann Emerg Med*. 1990;19:462.
3. Copass MK, Oreskovich MR, Bladergroen MR, Carrico CJ. Prehospital cardiopulmonary resuscitation of the critically injured patient. *Am J Surg*. 1984;148:20–26.
4. Durham LA III, Richardson RJ, Wall MJ Jr, Pepe PE, Mattox KL. Emergency center thoracotomy: impact of prehospital resuscitation. *J Trauma*. 1992;32:775–779.
5. Kloeck W. Prehospital advanced CPR in the trauma patient. *Trauma Emerg Med*. 1993;10:772–776.
6. Schmidt U, Frame SB, Nerlich ML, Rowe DW, Enderson BL, Maull KI, Tscherne H. On-scene helicopter transport of patients with multiple injuries—comparison of a German and an American system. *J Trauma*. 1992;33:548–553.
7. Rosemurgy AS, Norris PA, Olson SM, Hurst JM, Albrink MH. Prehospital traumatic cardiac arrest: the cost of futility. *J Trauma*. 1993;35:468–473.
8. Bouillon B, Walther T, Kramer M, Neugebauer E. Trauma and circulatory arrest: 224 preclinical resuscitations in Cologne in 1987–1990 [in German]. *Anaesthesist*. 1994;43:786–790.
9. Hazinski MF, Chahine AA, Holcomb GW III, Morris JA Jr. Outcome of cardiovascular collapse in pediatric blunt trauma. *Ann Emerg Med*. 1994;23:1229–1235.
10. Cummins RO, Hazinski MF. Guidelines based on the principle 'First, do no harm': new guidelines on tracheal tube confirmation and prevention of dislodgment. *Resuscitation*. 2000;46:443–447.
11. Katz SH, Falk JL. Misplaced endotracheal tubes by paramedics in an urban emergency medical services system. *Ann Emerg Med*. 2001;37:32–37.
12. Gausche M, Lewis RJ, Stratton SJ, Haynes BE, Gunter CS, Goodrich SM, Poore PD, McCollough MD, Henderson DP, Pratt FD, Seidel JS. Effect of out-of-hospital pediatric endotracheal intubation on survival and neurological outcome: a controlled clinical trial. *JAMA*. 2000;283:783–790.
13. Dutton RP, Mackenzie CF, Scalea TM. Hypotensive resuscitation during active hemorrhage: impact on in-hospital mortality. *J Trauma*. 2002;52:1141–1146.
14. Bickell WH, Wall MJ Jr, Pepe PE, Martin RR, Ginger VF, Allen MK, Mattox KL. Immediate versus delayed fluid resuscitation for hypotensive patients with penetrating torso injuries. *N Engl J Med*. 1994;331:1105–1109.
15. Dretzke J, Sandercock J, Bayliss S, Burls A. Clinical effectiveness and cost-effectiveness of prehospital intravenous fluids in trauma patients. *Health Technol Assess*. 2004;8:iii-1–iii-103.
16. Dula DJ, Wood GC, Rejmer AR, Starr M, Leicht M. Use of prehospital fluids in hypotensive blunt trauma patients. *Prehosp Emerg Care*. 2002;6:417–420.
17. Greaves I, Porter KM, Revell MP. Fluid resuscitation in pre-hospital trauma care: a consensus view. *J R Coll Surg Edinb*. 2002;47:451–457.
18. Koenig KL. Quo vadis: "scoop and run," "stay and treat," or "treat and street"? *Acad Emerg Med*. 1995;2:477–479.
19. Deakin CD, Allt-Graham J. Pre-hospital management of trauma patients: field stabilisation or scoop and run? *Clin Intensive Care*. 1993;4:24–27.
20. Nolan J. Advanced life support training. *Resuscitation*. 2001;50:9–11.
21. Moore FA, McKinley BA, Moore EE. The next generation in shock resuscitation. *Lancet*. 2004;363:1988–1996.
22. Solomonov E, Hirsh M, Yahiya A, Krausz MM. The effect of vigorous fluid resuscitation in uncontrolled hemorrhagic shock after massive splenic injury. *Crit Care Med*. 2000;28:749–754.
23. Kloeck WG. A practical approach to the aetiology of pulseless electrical activity: a simple 10-step training mnemonic. *Resuscitation*. 1995;30:157–159.
24. Grove CA, Lemmon G, Anderson G, McCarthy M. Emergency thoracotomy: appropriate use in the resuscitation of trauma patients. *Am Surg*. 2002;68:313–316; discussion 316.
25. Ladd AP, Gomez GA, Jacobson LE, Broadie TA, Scherer LR III, Solotkin KC. Emergency room thoracotomy: updated guidelines for a level I trauma center. *Am Surg*. 2002;68:421–424.
26. Powell DW, Moore EE, Cothren CC, Ciesla DJ, Burch JM, Moore JB, Johnson JL. Is emergency department resuscitative thoracotomy futile care for the critically injured patient requiring prehospital cardiopulmonary resuscitation? *J Am Coll Surg*. 2004;199:211–215.
27. Aihara R, Millham FH, Blansfield J, Hirsch EF. Emergency room thoracotomy for penetrating chest injury: effect of an institutional protocol. *J Trauma*. 2001;50:1027–1030.
28. Practice management guidelines for emergency department thoracotomy. Working Group, Ad Hoc Subcommittee on Outcomes, American College of Surgeons-Committee on Trauma. *J Am Coll Surg*. 2001;193:303–309.
29. McLean RF, Devitt JH, Dubbin J, McLellan BA. Incidence of abnormal RNA studies and dysrhythmias in patients with blunt chest trauma. *J Trauma*. 1991;31:968–970.
30. Paone RF, Peacock JB, Smith DL. Diagnosis of myocardial contusion. *South Med J*. 1993;86:867–870.

Part 10.8: Cardiac Arrest Associated With Pregnancy

During attempted resuscitation of a pregnant woman, providers have two potential patients, the mother and the fetus. The best hope of fetal survival is maternal survival. For the critically ill patient who is pregnant, rescuers must provide appropriate resuscitation, with consideration of the physiologic changes due to pregnancy.

Key Interventions to Prevent Arrest

To treat the critically ill pregnant patient:

- Place the patient in the left lateral position (see below).
- Give 100% oxygen.
- Establish intravenous (IV) access and give a fluid bolus.
- Consider reversible causes of cardiac arrest and identify any preexisting medical conditions that may be complicating the resuscitation.

Resuscitation of the Pregnant Woman in Cardiac Arrest

Modifications of Basic Life Support

Several modifications to standard BLS approaches are appropriate for the pregnant woman in cardiac arrest (Table). At a gestational age of 20 weeks and beyond, the pregnant uterus can press against the inferior vena cava and the aorta, impeding venous return and cardiac output. Uterine obstruction of venous return can produce prearrest hypotension or shock and in the critically ill patient may precipitate arrest.[1,2] In cardiac arrest the compromise in venous return and cardiac output by the gravid uterus limits the effectiveness of chest compressions. The gravid uterus may be shifted away from the inferior vena cava and the aorta by placing the patient 15° to 30° back from the left lateral position (Class IIa) or by pulling the gravid uterus to the side.[3] This may be accomplished manually or by placement of a rolled blanket or other object under the right hip and lumbar area. Other modifications are discussed below.

- Airway and breathing
  - Hormonal changes promote insufficiency of the gastroesophageal sphincter, increasing the risk of regurgitation. Apply continuous cricoid pressure during positive-pressure ventilation for any unconscious pregnant woman.
- Circulation
  - Perform chest compressions higher on the sternum, slightly above the center of the sternum. This will adjust for the elevation of the diaphragm and abdominal contents caused by the gravid uterus.[4]

(*Circulation.* 2005;112:IV-150-IV-153.)

This special supplement to *Circulation* is freely available at http://www.circulationaha.org

DOI: 10.1161/CIRCULATIONAHA.105.166570

- Defibrillation
  - Defibrillate using standard ACLS defibrillation doses (Class IIa).[5] Review the ACLS Pulseless Arrest Algorithm (see Part 7.2: "Management of Cardiac Arrest"). There is no evidence that shocks from a direct current defibrillator have adverse effects on the heart of the fetus.
  - If fetal or uterine monitors are in place, remove them before delivering shocks.

Modifications of Advanced Cardiovascular Life Support

The treatments listed in the standard ACLS Pulseless Arrest Algorithm, including recommendations and doses for defibrillation, medications, and intubation, apply to cardiac arrest in the pregnant woman (see the Table). There are important considerations to keep in mind, however, about airway, breathing, circulation, and the differential diagnosis.

- Airway
  - Secure the airway early in resuscitation. Because of the potential for gastroesophageal sphincter insufficiency with an increased risk of regurgitation, use continuous cricoid pressure before and during attempted endotracheal intubation.
  - Be prepared to use an endotracheal tube 0.5 to 1 mm smaller in internal diameter than that used for a nonpregnant woman of similar size because the airway may be narrowed from edema.[6]
- Breathing
  - Pregnant patients can develop hypoxemia rapidly because they have decreased functional residual capacity and increased oxygen demand, so rescuers should be prepared to support oxygenation and ventilation.
  - Verify correct endotracheal tube placement using clinical assessment and a device such as an exhaled CO_2 detector. In late pregnancy the esophageal detector device is more likely to suggest esophageal placement (the aspirating bulb does not reinflate after compression) when the tube is actually in the trachea. This could lead to the removal of a properly placed endotracheal tube.
  - Ventilation volumes may need to be reduced because the mother's diaphragm is elevated.
- Circulation
  - Follow the ACLS guidelines for resuscitation medications.
  - Vasopressor agents such as epinephrine, vasopressin, and dopamine will decrease blood flow to the uterus. There are no alternatives, however, to using all indicated medications in recommended doses. The mother must be resuscitated or the chances of fetal resuscitation vanish.
- Differential diagnoses. The same reversible causes of cardiac arrest that occur in nonpregnant women can occur during pregnancy. But providers should be familiar with

Primary and Secondary ABCD Surveys: Modifications for Pregnant Women

ACLS Approach	Modifications to BLS and ACLS Guidelines
Primary ABCD Survey	**Airway** • No modifications. **Breathing** • No modifications. **Circulation** • Place the woman on her left side with her back angled 15° to 30° back from the left lateral position. Then start chest compressions. **or** • Place a wedge under the woman's right side (so that she tilts toward her left side). **or** • Have one rescuer kneel next to the woman's left side and pull the gravid uterus laterally. This maneuver will relieve pressure on the inferior vena cava. **Defibrillation** • No modifications in dose or pad position. • Defibrillation shocks transfer no significant current to the fetus. • Remove any fetal or uterine monitors before shock delivery.
Secondary ABCD Survey	**Airway** • Insert an advanced airway early in resuscitation to reduce the risk of regurgitation and aspiration. • Airway edema and swelling may reduce the diameter of the trachea. Be prepared to use a tracheal tube that is slightly smaller than the one you would use for a nonpregnant woman of similar size. • Monitor for excessive bleeding following insertion of any tube into the oropharynx or nasopharynx. • No modifications to intubation techniques. A provider experienced in intubation should insert the tracheal tube. • Effective preoxygenation is critical because hypoxia can develop quickly. • Rapid sequence intubation with continuous cricoid pressure is the preferred technique. • Agents for anesthesia or deep sedation should be selected to minimize hypotension. **Breathing** • No modifications of confirmation of tube placement. Note that the esophageal detector device may suggest esophageal placement despite correct tracheal tube placement. • The gravid uterus elevates the diaphragm: —Patients can develop hypoxemia if either oxygen demand or pulmonary function is compromised. They have less reserve because functional residual capacity and functional residual volume are decreased. Minute ventilation and tidal volume are increased. —Tailor ventilatory support to produce effective oxygenation and ventilation. **Circulation** • Follow standard ACLS recommendations for administration of all resuscitation medications. • Do not use the femoral vein or other lower extremity sites for venous access. Drugs administered through these sites may not reach the maternal heart unless or until the fetus is delivered. **Differential Diagnosis and Decisions** • Decide whether to perform emergency hysterotomy. • Identify and treat reversible causes of the arrest. Consider causes related to pregnancy and causes considered for all ACLS patients (see the 6 H's and 6 T's, in Part 7.2: "Management of Cardiac Arrest").

pregnancy-specific diseases and procedural complications. Providers should try to identify these common and reversible causes of cardiac arrest in pregnancy during resuscitation attempts.[7] The use of abdominal ultrasound by a skilled operator should be considered in detecting pregnancy and possible causes of the cardiac arrest, but this should not delay other treatments.

– *Excess magnesium sulfate.* Iatrogenic overdose is possible in women with eclampsia who receive magnesium sulfate, particularly if the woman becomes oliguric. Administration of calcium gluconate (1 ampule or 1 g) is the treatment of choice for magnesium toxicity. Empiric calcium administration may be lifesaving.[8,9]
– *Acute coronary syndromes.* Pregnant women may experience acute coronary syndromes, typically in association with other medical conditions. Because fibrinolytics are relatively contraindicated in pregnancy, percutaneous coronary intervention is the reperfusion strategy of choice for ST-elevation myocardial infarction.[10]
– *Pre-eclampsia/eclampsia.* Pre-eclampsia/eclampsia develops after the 20th week of gestation and can produce severe hypertension and ultimate diffuse organ system

failure. If untreated it may result in maternal and fetal morbidity and mortality.
- *Aortic dissection.* Pregnant women are at increased risk for spontaneous aortic dissection.
- *Life-threatening pulmonary embolism and stroke.* Successful use of fibrinolytics for a massive, life-threatening pulmonary embolism[11–13] and ischemic stroke[14] have been reported in pregnant women.
- *Amniotic fluid embolism.* Clinicians have reported successful use of cardiopulmonary bypass for women with life-threatening amniotic fluid embolism during labor and delivery.[15]
- *Trauma and drug overdose.* Pregnant women are not exempt from the accidents and mental illnesses that afflict much of society. Domestic violence also increases during pregnancy; in fact, homicide and suicide are leading causes of mortality during pregnancy.[6,7]

Emergency Hysterotomy (Cesarean Delivery) for the Pregnant Woman in Cardiac Arrest

Maternal Cardiac Arrest Not Immediately Reversed by BLS and ACLS

The resuscitation team leader should consider the need for an emergency hysterotomy (cesarean delivery) protocol as soon as a pregnant woman develops cardiac arrest.[4,16–18] The best survival rate for infants >24 to 25 weeks in gestation occurs when the delivery of the infant occurs no more than 5 minutes after the mother's heart stops beating.[16,19–21] This typically requires that the provider begin the hysterotomy about 4 minutes after cardiac arrest.

Emergency hysterotomy is an aggressive procedure. It may seem counterintuitive given that the *key to salvage of a potentially viable infant is resuscitation of the mother.*[6,10,22–24] But the mother cannot be resuscitated until venous return and aortic output are restored. Delivery of the baby empties the uterus, relieving both the venous obstruction and the aortic compression. The hysterotomy also allows access to the infant so that newborn resuscitation can begin.

The critical point to remember is that you will lose both mother and infant if you cannot restore blood flow to the mother's heart.[4,18,25,26] Note that 4 to 5 minutes is the maximum time rescuers will have to determine if the arrest can be reversed by BLS and ACLS interventions. The rescue team is not required to wait for this time to elapse before initiating emergency hysterotomy.[27] Recent reports document long intervals between an urgent decision for hysterotomy and actual delivery of the infant, far exceeding the obstetrical guideline of 30 minutes.[28,29]

Establishment of IV access and an advanced airway typically requires several minutes. In most cases the actual cesarean delivery cannot proceed until after administration of IV medications and endotracheal intubation. Resuscitation team leaders should activate the protocol for an emergency cesarean delivery as soon as cardiac arrest is identified in the pregnant woman. By the time the team leader is poised to deliver the baby, IV access has been established, initial medications have been administered, an advanced airway is in place, and the immediate reversibility of the cardiac arrest has been determined.

Decision Making for Emergency Hysterotomy

The resuscitation team should consider several maternal and fetal factors in determining the need for an emergency hysterotomy.

- *Consider gestational age.* Although the gravid uterus reaches a size that will begin to compromise aortocaval blood flow at approximately 20 weeks of gestation, fetal viability begins at approximately 24 to 25 weeks. Portable ultrasonography, available in some emergency departments, may aid in determination of gestational age (in experienced hands) and positioning. However, the use of ultrasound should not delay the decision to perform emergency hysterotomy.[30]
  - Gestational age <20 weeks. Urgent cesarean delivery need not be considered because a gravid uterus of this size is unlikely to significantly compromise maternal cardiac output.
  - Gestational age approximately 20 to 23 weeks. Perform an emergency hysterotomy to enable successful resuscitation of the mother, not the survival of the delivered infant, which is unlikely at this gestational age.
  - Gestational age approximately ≥24 to 25 weeks. Perform an emergency hysterotomy to save the life of both the mother and the infant.
- *Consider features of the cardiac arrest.* The following features of the cardiac arrest can increase the infant's chance for survival:
  - Short interval between the mother's arrest and the infant's delivery[19]
  - No sustained prearrest hypoxia in the mother
  - Minimal or no signs of fetal distress before the mother's cardiac arrest[31]
  - Aggressive and effective resuscitative efforts for the mother
  - The hysterotomy is performed in a medical center with a neonatal intensive care unit
- *Consider the professional setting.*
  - Are appropriate equipment and supplies available?
  - Is emergency hysterotomy within the rescuer's procedural range of experience and skills?
  - Are skilled neonatal/pediatric support personnel available to care for the infant, especially if the infant is not full term?
  - Are obstetric personnel immediately available to support the mother after delivery?

Advance Preparation

Experts and organizations have emphasized the importance of advance preparation.[4,18,26] Medical centers must review whether performance of an emergency hysterotomy is feasible at their center, and if so, they must identify the best means of rapidly accomplishing this procedure. The plans should be made in collaboration with the obstetric and pediatric services.

Summary

Successful resuscitation of a pregnant woman and survival of the fetus require prompt and excellent CPR with some modifications in basic and advanced cardiovascular life support techniques. By the 20th week of gestation, the gravid uterus can compress the inferior vena cava and the aorta, obstructing venous return and arterial blood flow. Rescuers can relieve this compression by positioning the woman on her side or by pulling the gravid uterus to the side. Defibrillation and medication doses used for resuscitation of the pregnant woman are the same as those used for other adults in pulseless arrest. Rescuers should consider the need for emergency hysterotomy as soon as the pregnant woman develops cardiac arrest because rescuers should be prepared to proceed with the hysterotomy if the resuscitation is not successful within minutes.

References

1. Page-Rodriguez A, Gonzalez-Sanchez JA. Perimortem cesarean section of twin pregnancy: case report and review of the literature. *Acad Emerg Med.* 1999;6:1072–1074.
2. Cardosi RJ, Porter KB. Cesarean delivery of twins during maternal cardiopulmonary arrest. *Obstet Gynecol.* 1998;92:695–697.
3. Goodwin AP, Pearce AJ. The human wedge. A manoeuvre to relieve aortocaval compression during resuscitation in late pregnancy. *Anaesthesia.* 1992;47:433–434.
4. Morris S, Stacey M. Resuscitation in pregnancy. *BMJ.* 2003;327: 1277–1279.
5. Nanson J, Elcock D, Williams M, Deakin CD. Do physiological changes in pregnancy change defibrillation energy requirements? *Br J Anaesth.* 2001;87:237–239.
6. Johnson MD, Luppi CJ, Over DC. Cardiopulmonary Resuscitation. In: Gambling DR, Douglas MJ, eds. *Obstetric Anesthesia and Uncommon Disorders.* Philadelphia: WB Saunders; 1998:51–74.
7. Department of Health, Welsh Office, Scottish Office Department of Health, Department of Health and Social Services, Northern Ireland. *Why mothers die. Report on confidential enquiries into maternal deaths in the United Kingdom 2000–2002.* London, England: The Stationery Office; 2004.
8. Poole JH, Long J. Maternal mortality—a review of current trends. *Crit Care Nurs Clin North Am.* 2004;16:227–230.
9. Munro PT. Management of eclampsia in the accident and emergency department. *J Accid Emerg Med.* 2000;17:7–11.
10. Doan-Wiggins L. Resuscitation of the pregnant patient suffering sudden death. In: Paradis NA, Halperin HR, Nowak RM, eds. *Cardiac Arrest: The Science and Practice of Resuscitation Medicine.* Baltimore, Md: Williams & Wilkins; 1997:812–819.
11. Turrentine MA, Braems G, Ramirez MM. Use of thrombolytics for the treatment of thromboembolic disease during pregnancy. *Obstet Gynecol Surv.* 1995;50:534–541.
12. Thabut G, Thabut D, Myers RP, Bernard-Chabert B, Marrash-Chahla R, Mal H, Fournier M. Thrombolytic therapy of pulmonary embolism: a meta-analysis. *J Am Coll Cardiol.* 2002;40:1660–1667.
13. Patel RK, Fasan O, Arya R. Thrombolysis in pregnancy. *Thromb Haemost.* 2003;90:1216–1217.
14. Dapprich M, Boessenecker W. Fibrinolysis with alteplase in a pregnant woman with stroke. *Cerebrovasc Dis.* 2002;13:290.
15. Stanten RD, Iverson LI, Daugharty TM, Lovett SM, Terry C, Blumenstock E. Amniotic fluid embolism causing catastrophic pulmonary vasoconstriction: diagnosis by transesophageal echocardiogram and treatment by cardiopulmonary bypass. *Obstet Gynecol.* 2003;102: 496–498.
16. Katz VL, Dotters DJ, Droegemueller W. Perimortem cesarean delivery. *Obstet Gynecol.* 1986;68:571–576.
17. American Heart Association in collaboration with International Liaison Committee on Resuscitation. Guidelines 2000 for Cardiopulmonary Resuscitation and Emergency Cardiovascular Care: International Consensus on Science, Part 8: Advanced Challenges in Resuscitation: Section 3: Advanced Challenges in ECC. *Circulation.* 2000;102(suppl I):I229–I252.
18. Cummins RO, Hazinski MF, Zelop CM. Cardiac Arrest Associated with Pregnancy. In: Cummins R, Hazinski M, Field J, eds. *ACLS—The Reference Textbook.* Dallas: American Heart Association; 2003:143–158.
19. Oates S, Williams GL, Rees GA. Cardiopulmonary resuscitation in late pregnancy. *BMJ.* 1988;297:404–405.
20. Strong THJ, Lowe RA. Perimortem cesarean section. *Am J Emerg Med.* 1989;7:489–494.
21. Boyd R, Teece S. Towards evidence based emergency medicine: best BETs from the Manchester Royal Infirmary. Perimortem caesarean section. *Emerg Med J.* 2002;19:324–325.
22. Datner EM, Promes SB. Resuscitation issues in pregnancy. In: Rosen P, Barkin R, eds. *Emergency Medicine: Concepts and Clinical Practice.* 4th ed. St Louis, Mo: Mosby; 1998:71–76.
23. Whitten M, Irvine LM. Postmortem and perimortem caesarean section: what are the indications? *J R Soc Med.* 2000;93:6–9.
24. Kupas DF, Harter SC, Vosk A. Out-of-hospital perimortem cesarean section. *Prehosp Emerg Care.* 1998;2:206–208.
25. Lanoix R, Akkapeddi V, Goldfeder B. Perimortem cesarean section: case reports and recommendations. *Acad Emerg Med.* 1995;2:1063–1067.
26. Part 8: advanced challenges in resuscitation. Section 3: special challenges in ECC. 3F: cardiac arrest associated with pregnancy. European Resuscitation Council. *Resuscitation.* 2000;46:293–295.
27. Stallard TC, Burns B. Emergency delivery and perimortem C-section. *Emerg Med Clin North Am.* 2003;21:679–693.
28. MacKenzie IZ, Cooke I. What is a reasonable time from decision-to-delivery by caesarean section? Evidence from 415 deliveries. *BJOG.* 2002;109:498–504.
29. Helmy WH, Jolaoso AS, Ifaturoti OO, Afify SA, Jones MH. The decision-to-delivery interval for emergency caesarean section: is 30 minutes a realistic target? *BJOG.* 2002;109:505–508.
30. Moore C, Promes SB. Ultrasound in pregnancy. *Emerg Med Clin North Am.* 2004;22:697–722.
31. Morris JA Jr, Rosenbower TJ, Jurkovich GJ, Hoyt DB, Harviel JD, Knudson MM, Miller RS, Burch JM, Meredith JW, Ross SE, Jenkins JM, Bass JG. Infant survival after cesarean section for trauma. *Ann Surg.* 1996;223:481–488; discussion 488–491.

Part 10.9: Electric Shock and Lightning Strikes

Electric shock and lightning strike injuries result from the direct effects of current on the heart and brain and on cell membranes and vascular smooth muscle. Additional injuries result from the conversion of electric energy into heat energy as current passes through body tissues.

Background

Electric Shock

Factors that determine the site and severity of electric trauma are the magnitude of energy delivered, voltage, resistance to current flow, type of current, duration of contact with the current source, and current pathway.

High-tension current generally causes the most serious injuries, although fatal electrocutions may occur with household current (eg, 110 V in the United States and Canada and 220 V in Europe, Australia, and Asia).[1] Contact with alternating current at 60 cycles per second (the frequency used in most US household and commercial sources of electricity) may cause tetanic skeletal muscle contractions, preventing self-release from the source of the electricity and thereby leading to prolonged exposure. The repetitive frequency of alternating current also increases the likelihood of current flow through the heart during the relative refractory period (the "vulnerable period") of the cardiac cycle. This exposure can precipitate ventricular fibrillation (VF), which is analogous to the R-on-T phenomenon.[2]

Lightning Strike

The mortality rate from lightning injuries is 30%, and up to 70% of survivors sustain significant morbidity.[3–5] The presentation of lightning strike injuries varies widely, even among groups of people struck at the same time.[6] In some victims symptoms are mild and require little medical attention, whereas fatal injuries occur in others.[7,8]

The primary cause of death in victims of lightning strike is cardiac arrest, which may be associated with primary VF or asystole.[7–10] Lightning acts as an instantaneous, massive direct current shock, simultaneously depolarizing the entire myocardium.[8,11] In many cases intrinsic cardiac automaticity may spontaneously restore organized cardiac activity and a perfusing rhythm. But concomitant respiratory arrest due to thoracic muscle spasm and suppression of the respiratory center may continue after return of spontaneous circulation. Unless ventilation is supported, a secondary hypoxic (asphyxial) cardiac arrest will develop.[12]

(*Circulation.* 2005;112:IV-154-IV-155.)

This special supplement to *Circulation* is freely available at http://www.circulationaha.org

DOI: 10.1161/CIRCULATIONAHA.105.166571

Lightning can also have widespread effects on the cardiovascular system, producing extensive catecholamine release or autonomic stimulation. The victim may develop hypertension, tachycardia, nonspecific electrocardiographic changes (including prolongation of the QT interval and transient T-wave inversion), and myocardial necrosis with release of creatine kinase-MB fraction.

Lightning can produce a wide spectrum of peripheral and central neurologic injuries. The current can produce brain hemorrhages, edema, and small-vessel and neuronal injury. Hypoxic encephalopathy can result from cardiac arrest.

Victims are most likely to die of lightning injury if they experience immediate respiratory or cardiac arrest and no treatment is provided. Patients who do not suffer respiratory or cardiac arrest and those who respond to immediate treatment have an excellent chance of recovery. Therefore, when multiple victims are struck simultaneously by lightning, rescuers should give the highest priority to patients in respiratory or cardiac arrest.

Victims with respiratory arrest may require only ventilation and oxygenation to avoid secondary hypoxic cardiac arrest. For victims in cardiac arrest, treatment should be early, aggressive, and persistent. Resuscitative attempts may have higher success rates in lightning victims than in patients with cardiac arrest from other causes, and efforts may be effective even when the interval before the resuscitative attempt is prolonged.[12]

Modifications to Basic Life Support

The rescuer must first be certain that rescue efforts will not put him or her in danger of electric shock. When the scene is safe (the danger of shock has been removed), determine the victim's cardiorespiratory status. Immediately after electrocution, respiration or circulation or both may fail. Vigorous resuscitative measures are indicated even for those who appear dead on initial evaluation. Because many victims are young, without preexisting cardiopulmonary disease, they have a good chance for survival if immediate support of cardiopulmonary function is provided.

If spontaneous respiration or circulation is absent, initiate immediate BLS, including activation of the emergency medical services (EMS) system, provision of prompt CPR, and use of a defibrillator when available. Immediate provision of ventilation and compressions (if needed) is essential. In addition, use the automated external defibrillator (AED) to identify and treat ventricular tachycardia or VF.

Maintain spinal stabilization during extrication and treatment if there is a likelihood of head or neck trauma.[13,14] Both lightning and electrical trauma often cause multiple trauma, including injury to the spine[14] and muscular strains, internal injuries from being thrown, and fractures caused by the tetanic response of skeletal muscles.[15] Remove smoldering clothing, shoes, and belts to prevent further thermal damage.

Modifications to Advanced Cardiovascular Life Support

Rescuers must be sure that the scene is safe. Patients who are unresponsive after an electrical injury may be in either respiratory or cardiac arrest. Thus, airway control, prompt CPR, and attempts at defibrillation (if indicated) are critically important. Treat VF, asystole, and other serious arrhythmias with the ACLS techniques outlined in these guidelines. Quickly start CPR and attempt defibrillation at the scene if needed. Then take steps to manage the airway, including early placement of an advanced airway (eg, endotracheal intubation). Establishing an airway may be difficult for patients with electric burns of the face, mouth, or anterior neck. Extensive soft-tissue swelling may develop rapidly, complicating airway control measures. Thus, early intubation should be performed for patients with evidence of extensive burns even if the patient has begun to breathe spontaneously.

For victims with hypovolemic shock or significant tissue destruction, rapid intravenous fluid administration is indicated to counteract shock and correct ongoing fluid losses due to third spacing. Fluid administration should be adequate to maintain diuresis to facilitate excretion of myoglobin, potassium, and other byproducts of tissue destruction (this is particularly true for patients with electrical injury).[11] As significant as the external injuries may appear after electrothermal shock, the underlying tissue damage is far more extensive. Early consultation with or transfer to a physician and a facility (eg, burn center) familiar with treatment of these injuries is recommended. Survivors may have permanent neurologic and cardiac sequelae.

Summary

Although morbidity and mortality from electric shock and lightning strike is high, patients who respond to immediate treatment have an excellent chance of recovery. Once the scene is safe, rescuers should provide prompt CPR and early defibrillation even when the victim appears dead. Electric shock and lightning injuries can cause ventricular fibrillation or asystole, musculoskeletal injuries, organ damage, and internal and external burns. Early insertion of an advanced airway and volume administration are often required, and early consultation with experts in these injuries is recommended.

References

1. Budnick LD. Bathtub-related electrocutions in the United States, 1979 to 1982. *JAMA*. 1984;252:918–920.
2. Geddes LA, Bourland JD, Ford G. The mechanism underlying sudden death from electric shock. *Med Instrum*. 1986;20:303–315.
3. Cooper MA. Lightning injuries: prognostic signs for death. *Ann Emerg Med*. 1980;9:134–138.
4. Kleinschmidt-DeMasters BK. Neuropathology of lightning strike injuries. *Semin Neurol*. 1995;15:323–328.
5. Stewart CE. When lightning strikes. *Emerg Med Serv*. 2000;29:57–67; quiz 103.
6. Fahmy FS, Brinsden MD, Smith J, Frame JD. Lightning: the multisystem group injuries. *J Trauma*. 1999;46:937–940.
7. Patten BM. Lightning and electrical injuries. *Neurol Clin*. 1992;10: 1047–1058.
8. Browne BJ, Gaasch WR. Electrical injuries and lightning. *Emerg Med Clin North Am*. 1992;10:211–229.
9. Kleiner JP, Wilkin JH. Cardiac effects of lightning strike. *JAMA*. 1978; 240:2757–2759.
10. Lichtenberg R, Dries D, Ward K, Marshall W, Scanlon P. Cardiovascular effects of lightning strikes. *J Am Coll Cardiol*. 1993;21:531–536.
11. Cooper MA. Emergent care of lightning and electrical injuries. *Semin Neurol*. 1995;15:268–278.
12. Milzman DP, Moskowitz L, Hardel M. Lightning strikes at a mass gathering. *South Med J*. 1999;92:708–710.
13. Duclos PJ, Sanderson LM. An epidemiological description of lightning-related deaths in the United States. *Int J Epidemiol*. 1990;19:673–679.
14. Epperly TD, Stewart JR. The physical effects of lightning injury. *J Fam Pract*. 1989;29:267–272.
15. Whitcomb D, Martinez JA, Daberkow D. Lightning injuries. *South Med J*. 2002;95:1331–1334.

Part 11: Pediatric Basic Life Support

For best survival and quality of life, pediatric basic life support (BLS) should be part of a community effort that includes prevention, basic CPR, prompt access to the emergency medical services (EMS) system, and prompt pediatric advanced life support (PALS). These 4 links form the American Heart Association (AHA) pediatric Chain of Survival (Figure 1). The first 3 links constitute pediatric BLS.

Rapid and effective bystander CPR is associated with successful return of spontaneous circulation and neurologically intact survival in children.[1,2] The greatest impact occurs in respiratory arrest,[3] in which neurologically intact survival rates of >70% are possible,[4–6] and in ventricular fibrillation (VF), in which survival rates of 30% have been documented.[7] But only 2% to 10% of all children who develop out-of-hospital cardiac arrest survive, and most are neurologically devastated.[7–13] Part of the disparity is that bystander CPR is provided for less than half of the victims of out-of-hospital arrest.[8,11,14] Some studies show that survival and neurologic outcome can be improved with prompt CPR.[6,15–17]

Prevention of Cardiopulmonary Arrest

The major causes of death in infants and children are respiratory failure, sudden infant death syndrome (SIDS), sepsis, neurologic diseases, and injuries.[18]

Injuries

Injuries, the leading cause of death in children and young adults, cause more childhood deaths than all other causes combined.[18] Many injuries are preventable. The most common fatal childhood injuries amenable to prevention are motor vehicle passenger injuries, pedestrian injuries, bicycle injuries, drowning, burns, and firearm injuries.[19]

Motor Vehicle Injuries

Motor vehicle–related injuries account for nearly half of all pediatric deaths in the United States.[18] Contributing factors include failure to use proper passenger restraints, inexperienced adolescent drivers, and alcohol.

Appropriate restraints include properly installed, rear-facing infant seats for infants <20 pounds (<9 kg) and <1 year of age, child restraints for children 1 to 4 years of age, and booster seats with seat belts for children 4 to 7 years of age.[20] The lifesaving benefit of air bags for older children and adults far outweighs their risk. Most pediatric air bag–related fatalities occur when children <12 years of age are in the vehicle's front seat or are improperly restrained for their age. For additional information consult the website of the National Highway Traffic Safety Administration (NHTSA): *http://nhtsa.gov*. Look for the Comprehensive Child Passenger Safety Information.

(*Circulation*. **2005;112:IV-156-IV-166.**)

This special supplement to *Circulation* is freely available at http://www.circulationaha.org

DOI: 10.1161/CIRCULATIONAHA.105.166572

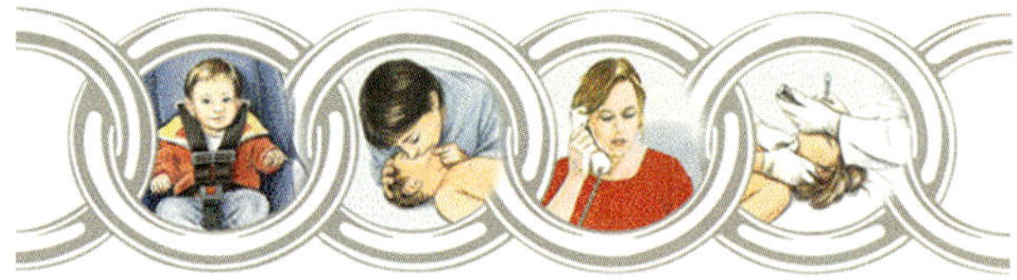

Figure 1. Pediatric Chain of Survival.

Adolescent drivers are responsible for a disproportionate number of motor vehicle–related injuries; the risk is highest in the first 2 years of driving. Driving with teen passengers and driving at night dramatically increase the risk. Additional risks include not wearing a seat belt, drinking and driving, speeding, and aggressive driving.[21]

Pedestrian Injuries

Pedestrian injuries account for a third of motor vehicle-related injuries. Adequate supervision of children in the street is important because injuries typically occur when a child darts out mid-block, dashes across intersections, or gets off a bus.[22]

Bicycle Injuries

Bicycle crashes are responsible for approximately 200 000 injuries and nearly 150 deaths per year in children and adolescents.[23] Head injuries are a major cause of bicycle-related morbidity and mortality. It is estimated that bicycle helmets can reduce the severity of head injuries by >80%.[24]

Burns

Approximately 80% of fire-related and burn-related deaths result from house fires and smoke inhalation.[25,26] Smoke detectors are the most effective way to prevent deaths and injuries; 70% of deaths occur in homes without functioning smoke alarms.[27]

Firearm Injuries

The United States has the highest firearm-related injury rate of any industrialized nation—more than twice that of any other country.[28] The highest number of deaths is in adolescents and young adults, but firearm injuries are more likely to be fatal in young children.[29] The presence of a gun in the home is associated with an increased likelihood of adolescent[30,31] and adult suicides or homicides.[32] Although overall firearm-related deaths declined from 1995 to 2002, firearm homicide remains the leading cause of death among African-American adolescents and young adults.[18]

Sudden Infant Death Syndrome

SIDS is "the sudden death of an infant under 1 year of age, which remains unexplained after a thorough case investigation, including performance of a complete autopsy, examination of the death scene, and review of the clinical history."[33] The peak incidence of SIDs occurs in infants 2 to 4 months of age.[34] The etiology of SIDS remains unknown, but risk factors include prone sleeping position, sleeping on a soft surface,[35–37] and second-hand smoke.[38,39] The incidence of SIDS has declined 40%[40] since the "Back to Sleep" public education campaign was introduced in the United States in 1992. This campaign aims to educate parents about placing an infant on the back rather than the abdomen or side to sleep.

Drowning

Drowning is the second major cause of death from unintentional injury in children <5 years of age and the third major cause of death in adolescents. Most young children drown after falling into swimming pools while unsupervised; adolescents more commonly drown in lakes and rivers while swimming or boating. Drowning can be prevented by installing isolation fencing around swimming pools (gates should be self-closing and self-latching)[41] and wearing personal flotation devices (life jackets) while in, around, or on water.

The BLS Sequence for Infants and Children

For the purposes of these guidelines, an "infant" is less than approximately 1 year of age. This section does not deal with newborn infants (see Part 13: "Neonatal Resuscitation Guidelines"). For lay rescuers the "child" BLS guidelines should be applied when performing CPR for a child from about 1 year of age to about 8 years of age. For a healthcare provider, the pediatric ("child") guidelines apply from about 1 year to about the start of puberty. For an explanation of the differences in etiology of arrest and elaboration of the differences in the recommended sequence for lay rescuer and healthcare provider CPR for infants, children, and adults, see Part 3: "Overview of CPR."

These guidelines delineate a series of skills as a *sequence* of distinct steps, but they are often performed simultaneously (eg, starting CPR and activating the EMS system), especially when more than one rescuer is present. This sequence is depicted in the Pediatric Healthcare Provider BLS Algorithm (Figure 2). The numbers listed with the headings below refer to the corresponding box in that algorithm.

Safety of Rescuer and Victim

Always make sure that the area is safe for you and the victim. Move a victim only to ensure the victim's safety. Although exposure to a victim while providing CPR carries a theoretical risk of infectious disease transmission, the risk is very low.[42]

Check for Response (Box 1)

- Gently tap the victim and ask loudly, "Are you okay?" Call the child's name if you know it.
- Look for movement. If the child is *responsive*, he or she will answer or move. Quickly check to see if the child has any injuries or needs medical assistance. If necessary, leave the child to phone EMS, but return quickly and recheck the child's condition frequently. Children with respiratory distress often assume a position that maintains airway patency and optimizes ventilation. Allow the child with respiratory distress to remain in a position that is most comfortable.
- If the child is *unresponsive* and is not moving, shout for help and start CPR. If you are alone, continue CPR for 5 cycles (about 2 minutes). One cycle of CPR for the lone rescuer is 30 compressions and 2 breaths (see below). Then activate the EMS system and get an automated external defibrillator (AED) (see below). If you are alone and there is no evidence of trauma, you may carry a small child with you to the telephone. The EMS dispatcher can guide you through the steps of CPR. If a second rescuer is present, that rescuer should immediately activate the EMS system and get an AED (if the child is 1 year of age or older) while you continue CPR. If you suspect trauma, the second rescuer may assist by stabilizing the child's cervical spine (see below). If the child must be moved for safety reasons, support the head and body to minimize turning, bending, or twisting of the head and neck.

Activate the EMS System and Get the AED (Box 2)

If the arrest is witnessed and sudden[2,7,43] (eg, an athlete who collapses on the playing field), a lone healthcare provider should activate the EMS system (by telephoning 911 in most locales) and get an AED (if the child is 1 year of age or older) before starting CPR. It would be ideal for the lone lay rescuer who witnesses the sudden collapse of a child to also activate the EMS system and get an AED and return to the child to begin CPR and use the AED. But for simplicity of lay rescuer education it is acceptable for the lone lay rescuer to provide about 5 cycles (about 2 minutes) of CPR for any infant or child victim before leaving to phone 911 and get an AED (if appropriate). This sequence may be tailored for some learners (eg, the mother of a child at high risk for a sudden arrhythmia). If two rescuers are present, one rescuer should begin CPR while the other rescuer activates the EMS system and gets the AED.

Position the Victim

If the victim is unresponsive, make sure that the victim is in a supine (face up) position on a flat, hard surface, such as a sturdy table, the floor, or the ground. If you must turn the victim, minimize turning or twisting of the head and neck.

Open the Airway and Check Breathing (Box 3)

In an unresponsive infant or child, the tongue may obstruct the airway, so the rescuer should open the airway.[44–47]

Open the Airway: Lay Rescuer

If you are a lay rescuer, open the airway using a head tilt–chin lift maneuver for both injured and noninjured victims (Class IIa). The jaw thrust is no longer recommended for lay rescuers because it is difficult to learn and perform, is often not an effective way to open the airway, and may cause spinal movement (Class IIb).

Open the Airway: Healthcare Provider

A healthcare provider should use the head tilt–chin lift maneuver to open the airway of a victim without evidence of head or neck trauma.

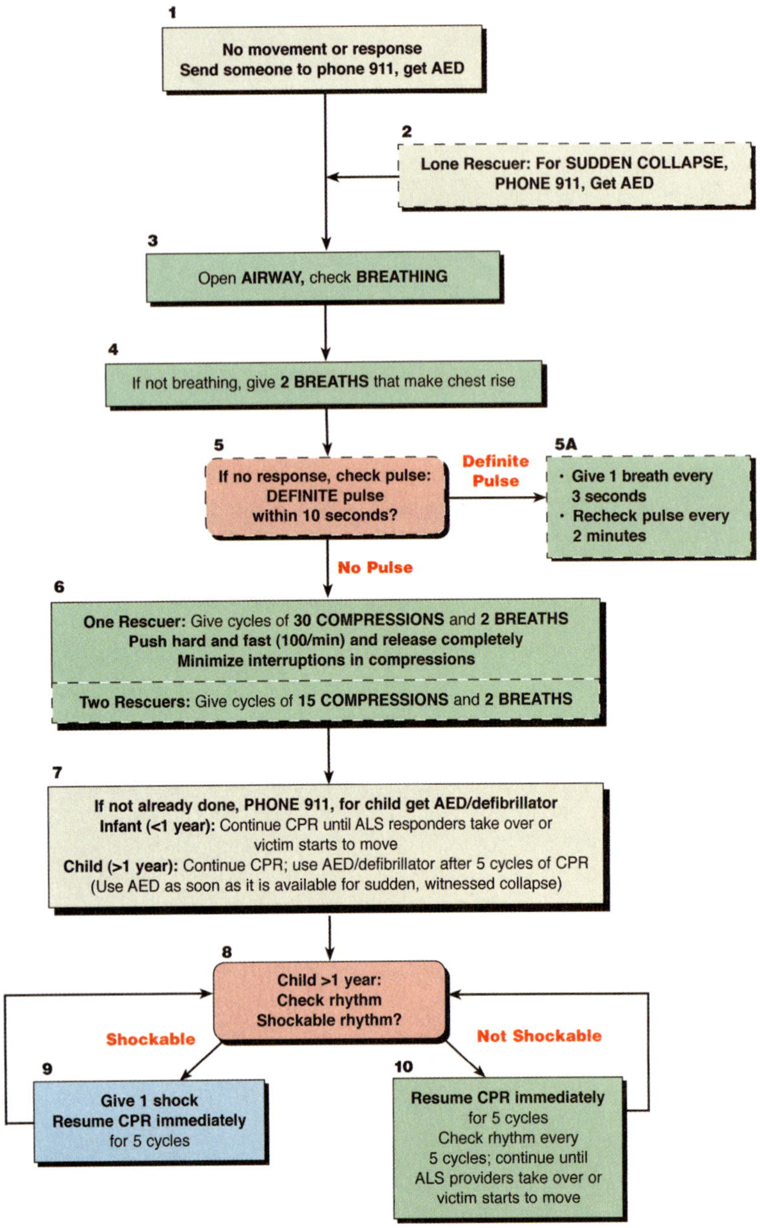

Figure 2. Pediatric Healthcare Provider BLS Algorithm. Note that the boxes bordered by dotted lines are performed by healthcare providers and not by lay rescuers.

Approximately 2% of all victims with blunt trauma requiring spinal imaging in an emergency department have a spinal injury. This risk is tripled if the victim has craniofacial injury,[48] a Glasgow Coma Scale score of <8,[49] or both.[48,50] If you are a healthcare provider and suspect that the victim may have a cervical spine injury, open the airway using a jaw thrust without head tilt (Class IIb).[46,51,52] Because maintaining a patent airway and providing adequate ventilation is a priority in CPR (Class I), use a head tilt–chin lift maneuver if the jaw thrust does not open the airway.

Check Breathing (Box 3)

While maintaining an open airway, take no more than 10 seconds to check whether the victim is breathing: *Look* for rhythmic chest and abdominal movement, *listen* for exhaled breath sounds at the nose and mouth, and *feel* for exhaled air on your cheek. Periodic gasping, also called *agonal gasps,* is not breathing.[53,54]

- If the child is *breathing* and there is no evidence of trauma: turn the child onto the side (recovery position, Figure 3). This helps maintain a patent airway and decreases risk of aspiration.

Give Rescue Breaths (Box 4)

If the child is *not breathing or has only occasional gasps:*

- For the lay rescuer: maintain an open airway and give 2 breaths.
- For the healthcare provider: maintain an open airway and give 2 breaths. Make sure that the breaths are effective (ie, the chest rises). If the chest does not rise, reposition the head, make a better seal, and try again.[55] It may be necessary to move the child's head through a range of positions to obtain optimal airway patency and effective rescue breathing.

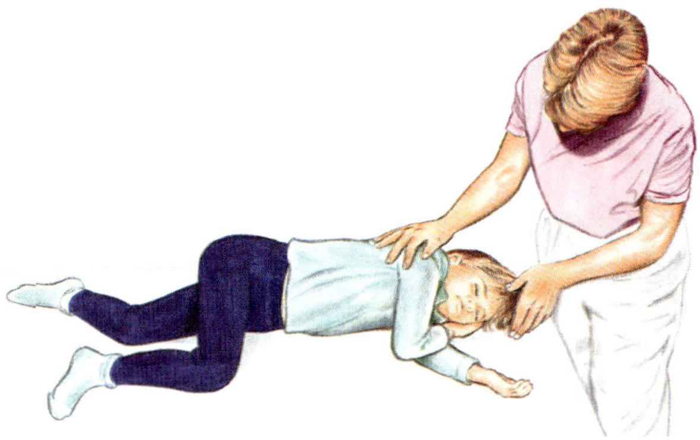

Figure 3. Recovery position.

In an infant, use a mouth-to–mouth-and-nose technique (LOE 7; Class IIb); in a child, use a mouth-to-mouth technique.[55]

Comments on Technique

In an infant, if you have difficulty making an effective seal over the mouth and nose, try either mouth-to-mouth or mouth-to-nose ventilation (LOE 5; Class IIb).[56–58] If you use the mouth-to-mouth technique, pinch the nose closed. If you use the mouth-to-nose technique, close the mouth. In either case make sure the chest rises when you give a breath.

Barrier Devices

Despite its safety,[42] some healthcare providers[59–61] and lay rescuers[8,62,63] may hesitate to give mouth-to-mouth rescue breathing and prefer to use a barrier device. Barrier devices have not reduced the risk of transmission of infection,[42] and some may increase resistance to air flow.[64,65] If you use a barrier device, do not delay rescue breathing.

Bag-Mask Ventilation (Healthcare Providers)

Bag-mask ventilation can be as effective as endotracheal intubation and safer when providing ventilation for short periods.[66–69] But bag-mask ventilation requires training and periodic retraining in the following skills: selecting the correct mask size, opening the airway, making a tight seal between the mask and face, delivering effective ventilation, and assessing the effectiveness of that ventilation. In the out-of-hospital setting, preferentially ventilate and oxygenate infants and children with a bag and mask rather than attempt intubation if transport time is short (Class IIa; LOE 1[66]; 3[67]; 4[68,69]).

Ventilation Bags

Use a self-inflating bag with a volume of at least 450 to 500 mL[70]; smaller bags may not deliver an effective tidal volume or the longer inspiratory times required by full-term neonates and infants.[71]

A self-inflating bag delivers only room air unless supplementary oxygen is attached, but even with an oxygen inflow of 10 L/min, the concentration of delivered oxygen varies from 30% to 80% and depends on the tidal volume and peak inspiratory flow rate.[72] To deliver a high oxygen concentration (60% to 95%), attach an oxygen reservoir to the self-inflating bag. You must maintain an oxygen flow of 10 to 15 L/min into a reservoir attached to a pediatric bag[72] and a flow of at least 15 L/min into an adult bag.

Precautions

Avoid hyperventilation; use only the force and tidal volume necessary to make the chest rise. Give each breath over 1 second.

- In a victim of cardiac arrest with no advanced airway in place, pause after 30 compressions (1 rescuer) or 15 compressions (2 rescuers) to give 2 ventilations when using either mouth-to-mouth or bag-mask technique.
- During CPR for a victim with an advanced airway (eg, endotracheal tube, esophageal-tracheal combitube [Combitube], or laryngeal mask airway [LMA]) in place, rescuers should no longer deliver "cycles" of CPR. The compressing rescuer should compress the chest at a rate of 100 times per minute without pauses for ventilations, and the rescuer providing the ventilation should deliver 8 to 10 breaths per minute. Two or more rescuers should change the compressor role approximately every 2 minutes to prevent compressor fatigue and deterioration in quality and rate of chest compressions.
- If the victim has a perfusing rhythm (ie, pulses are present) but no breathing, give 12 to 20 breaths per minute (1 breath every 3 to 5 seconds).

Healthcare providers often deliver excessive ventilation during CPR,[73–75] particularly when an advanced airway is in place. Excessive ventilation is detrimental because it

- Impedes venous return and therefore decreases cardiac output, cerebral blood flow, and coronary perfusion by increasing intrathoracic pressure[74]
- Causes air trapping and barotrauma in patients with small-airway obstruction
- Increases the risk of regurgitation and aspiration

Rescuers should provide the recommended number of rescue breaths per minute.

You may need high pressures to ventilate patients with airway obstruction or poor lung compliance. A pressure-relief valve can prevent delivery of sufficient tidal volume.[72] Make sure that the manual bag allows you to use high pressures if necessary to achieve visible chest expansion.[76]

Two-Person Bag-Mask Ventilation

A 2-person technique may be necessary to provide effective bag-mask ventilation when there is significant airway obstruction, poor lung compliance,[76] or difficulty in creating a tight seal between the mask and the face. One rescuer uses both hands to open the airway and maintain a tight mask-to-face seal while the other compresses the ventilation bag. Both rescuers should observe the chest to ensure chest rise.

Gastric Inflation and Cricoid Pressure

Gastric inflation may interfere with effective ventilation[77] and cause regurgitation. To minimize gastric inflation:

- Avoid excessive peak inspiratory pressures (eg, ventilate slowly).[66]

- Apply cricoid pressure. Do this only in an unresponsive victim and if there is a second rescuer.[78–80] Avoid excessive pressure so as not to obstruct the trachea.[81]

Oxygen

Despite animal and theoretic data suggesting possible adverse effects of 100% oxygen,[82–85] there are no studies comparing various concentrations of oxygen during resuscitation beyond the newborn period. Until additional information becomes available, healthcare providers should use 100% oxygen during resuscitation (Class Indeterminate). Once the patient is stable, wean supplementary oxygen but ensure adequate oxygen delivery by appropriate monitoring. Whenever possible, humidify oxygen to prevent mucosal drying and thickening of pulmonary secretions.

Masks

Masks provide an oxygen concentration of 30% to 50% to a victim with spontaneous breathing. For a higher concentration of oxygen, use a tight-fitting nonrebreathing mask with an oxygen inflow rate of approximately 15 L/min that maintains inflation of the reservoir bag.

Nasal Cannulas

Infant and pediatric size nasal cannulas are suitable for children with spontaneous breathing. The concentration of delivered oxygen depends on the child's size, respiratory rate, and respiratory effort.[86] For example, a flow rate of only 2 L/min can provide young infants with an inspired oxygen concentration >50%.

Pulse Check (for Healthcare Providers) (Box 5)

If you are a healthcare provider, you should try to palpate a pulse (brachial in an infant and carotid or femoral in a child). Take no more than 10 seconds. Studies show that healthcare providers[87–93] as well as lay rescuers[94–96] are unable to reliably detect a pulse and at times will think a pulse is present when there is no pulse. For this reason, if you do not definitely feel a pulse (eg, there is no pulse or you are not sure you feel a pulse) within 10 seconds, proceed with chest compressions.

If despite oxygenation and ventilation the pulse is <60 beats per minute (bpm) and there are signs of poor perfusion (ie, pallor, cyanosis), begin chest compressions. Profound bradycardia in the presence of poor perfusion is an indication for chest compressions because an inadequate heart rate with poor perfusion indicates that cardiac arrest is imminent. Cardiac output in infancy and childhood largely depends on heart rate. No scientific data has identified an absolute heart rate at which chest compressions should be initiated; the recommendation to provide cardiac compression for a heart rate <60 bpm with signs of poor perfusion is based on ease of teaching and skills retention. For additional information see "Bradycardia" in Part 12: "Pediatric Advanced Life Support."

If the pulse is ≥60 bpm but the infant or child is not breathing, provide rescue breathing without chest compressions (see below).

Lay rescuers are not taught to check for a pulse. The lay rescuer should immediately begin chest compressions after delivering 2 rescue breaths.

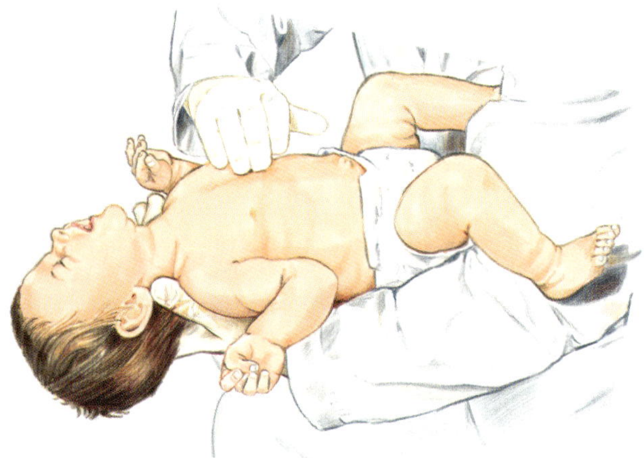

Figure 4. Two-finger chest compression technique in infant (1 rescuer).

Rescue Breathing Without Chest Compressions (for Healthcare Providers Only) (Box 5A)

If the pulse is ≥60 bpm but there is no spontaneous breathing or inadequate breathing, give rescue breaths at a rate of about 12 to 20 breaths per minute (1 breath every 3 to 5 seconds) until spontaneous breathing resumes (Box 5A). Give each breath over 1 second. Each breath should cause visible chest rise.

During delivery of rescue breaths, reassess the pulse about every 2 minutes (Class IIa), but spend no more than 10 seconds doing so.

Chest Compressions (Box 6)

To give chest compressions, compress the lower half of the sternum but do not compress over the xiphoid. After each compression allow the chest to recoil fully (Class IIb) because complete chest reexpansion improves blood flow into the heart.[97] A manikin study[97] showed that one way to ensure complete recoil is to lift your hand slightly off the chest at the end of each compression, but this has not been studied in humans (Class Indeterminate). The following are characteristics of good compressions:

- "Push hard": push with sufficient force to depress the chest approximately one third to one half the anterior-posterior diameter of the chest.
- "Push fast": push at a rate of approximately 100 compressions per minute.
- Release completely to allow the chest to fully recoil.
- Minimize interruptions in chest compressions.

In an *infant victim,* lay rescuers and lone rescuers should compress the sternum with 2 fingers (Figure 4) placed just below the intermammary line (Class IIb; LOE 5, 6).[98–102]

The 2 thumb–encircling hands technique (Figure 5) is recommended for healthcare providers when 2 rescuers are present. Encircle the infant's chest with both hands; spread your fingers around the thorax, and place your thumbs together over the lower half of the sternum.[98–102] Forcefully compress the sternum with your thumbs as you squeeze the thorax with your fingers for counterpressure (Class IIa; LOE

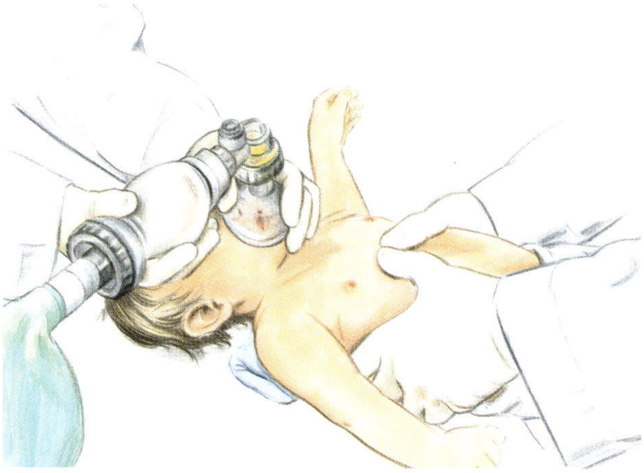

Figure 5. Two thumb–encircling hands chest compression in infant (2 rescuers).

5[103,104]; 6[105,106]). If you are alone or you cannot physically encircle the victim's chest, compress the chest with 2 fingers (as above). The 2 thumb–encircling hands technique is preferred because it produces higher coronary artery perfusion pressure, more consistently results in appropriate depth or force of compression,[105–108] and may generate higher systolic and diastolic pressures.[103,104,109,110]

In a *child,* lay rescuers and healthcare providers should compress the lower half of the sternum with the heel of 1 hand or with 2 hands (as used for adult victims) but should not press on the xiphoid or the ribs. There is no outcome data that shows a 1-hand or 2-hand method to be superior; higher compression pressures can be obtained on a child manikin with 2 hands.[111] Because children and rescuers come in all sizes, rescuers may use either 1 or 2 hands to compress the child's chest. It is most important that the chest be compressed about one third to one half the anterior-posterior depth of the chest.

Coordinate Chest Compressions and Breathing (Box 6)

The ideal compression-ventilation ratio is unknown, but studies have emphasized the following:

- In 2000[112] a compression-ventilation ratio of 5:1 and a compression rate of 100 per minute were recommended. But at that ratio and compression rate, fewer than 50 compressions per minute were performed in an adult manikin, and fewer than 60 compressions per minute were performed in a pediatric manikin even under ideal circumstances.[113–115]
- It takes a number of chest compressions to raise coronary perfusion pressure, which drops with each pause (eg, to provide rescue breathing, check for a pulse, attach an AED).[116,117]
- Long and frequent interruptions in chest compressions have been documented during CPR by lay rescuers[118,119] and by healthcare providers[75,120] in the out-of-hospital and in-hospital settings. Interruptions in chest compressions are associated with decreased rate of return of spontaneous circulation.[121–123]
- Ventilations are relatively less important during the first minutes of CPR for victims of a sudden arrhythmia-induced cardiac arrest (VF or pulseless ventricular tachycardia [VT]) than they are after asphyxia-induced arrest,[116,117,124–127] but even in asphyxial arrest, a minute ventilation that is lower than normal is likely to maintain an adequate ventilation-perfusion ratio because cardiac output and, therefore, pulmonary blood flow produced by chest compressions is quite low.
- For lay rescuers, a single compression-ventilation ratio (30:2) for all age groups may increase the number of bystanders who perform CPR because it is easier to remember.

If you are the only rescuer, perform cycles of 30 chest compressions (Class Indeterminate) followed by 2 effective ventilations with as short a pause in chest compressions as possible (Class IIb). Make sure to open the airway before giving ventilations.

For 2-rescuer CPR (eg, by healthcare providers or others, such as lifeguards, who are trained in this technique), one provider should perform chest compressions while the other maintains the airway and performs ventilations at a ratio of 15:2 with as short a pause in compressions as possible. Do not ventilate and compress the chest simultaneously with either mouth-to-mouth or bag-mask ventilation. The 15:2 ratio for 2 rescuers is applicable in children up to the start of puberty.

Rescuer fatigue can lead to inadequate compression rate and depth and may cause the rescuer to fail to allow complete chest wall recoil between compressions.[128] The quality of chest compressions deteriorates within minutes even when the rescuer denies feeling fatigued.[129,130] Once an advanced airway is in place for infant, child, or adult victims, 2 rescuers no longer deliver cycles of compressions interrupted with pauses for ventilation. Instead, the compressing rescuer should deliver 100 compressions per minute continuously without pauses for ventilation. The rescuer delivering the ventilations should give 8 to 10 breaths per minute and should be careful to avoid delivering an excessive number of ventilations. Two or more rescuers should rotate the compressor role approximately every 2 minutes to prevent compressor fatigue and deterioration in quality and rate of chest compressions. The switch should be accomplished as quickly as possible (ideally in less than 5 seconds) to minimize interruptions in chest compressions.

Compression-Only CPR

Ventilation may not be essential in the first minutes of VF cardiac arrest,[116,124,127,131] during which periodic gasps and passive chest recoil may provide some ventilation if the airway is open.[124] This, however, is not true for most cardiac arrests in infants and children, which are more likely to be asphyxial cardiac arrest. These victims require both prompt ventilations and chest compressions for optimal resuscitation. If a rescuer is unwilling or unable to provide ventilations, chest compressions alone are better than no resuscitation at all (LOE 5 through 7; Class IIb).[125,126]

Activate the EMS System and Get the AED (Box 7)

In the majority of infants and children with cardiac arrest, the arrest is asphyxial.[8,11,17,132,133] Lone rescuers (with the exception of healthcare providers who witness sudden collapse) should perform CPR for 5 cycles (about 2 minutes) before activating EMS, then start CPR again with as few interruptions of chest compressions as possible. If there are more rescuers present, one rescuer should begin the steps of CPR as soon as the infant or child is found to be unresponsive and a second rescuer should activate the EMS system and get an AED. Minimize interruption of chest compressions.

Defibrillation (Box 8)

VF can be the cause of sudden collapse, or it may develop during resuscitation attempts.[7,134] Children with sudden witnessed collapse (eg, a child collapsing during an athletic event) are likely to have VF or pulseless VT and need immediate CPR and rapid defibrillation. VF and pulseless VT are referred to as "shockable rhythms" because they respond to electric shocks (defibrillation).

Many AEDs have high specificity in recognizing pediatric shockable rhythms, and some are equipped to decrease the delivered energy to make it suitable for children 1 to 8 years of age.[134,135] Since the publication of the *ECC Guidelines 2000*,[112] data has shown that AEDs can be safely and effectively used in children 1 to 8 years of age.[136–138] However, there is insufficient data to make a recommendation for or against using an AED in infants <1 year of age (Class Indeterminate).[136–138]

In systems and institutions that care for children and have an AED program, it is recommended that the AED have both a high specificity in recognizing pediatric shockable rhythms and a pediatric dose-attenuating system to reduce the dose delivered by the device. In an emergency if an AED with a pediatric attenuating system is not available, use a standard AED. Turn the AED on, follow the AED prompts, and resume chest compressions immediately after the shock. Minimize interruptions in chest compressions.

CPR Techniques and Adjuncts

There is insufficient data in infants and children to recommend for or against the use of mechanical devices to compress the sternum, active compression-decompression CPR, interposed abdominal compression CPR (IAC-CPR), or the impedance threshold device (Class Indeterminate). See Part 6: "CPR Techniques and Devices" for adjuncts in adults.

Foreign-Body Airway Obstruction (Choking)

Epidemiology and Recognition

More than 90% of deaths from foreign-body aspiration occur in children <5 years of age; 65% of the victims are infants. Liquids are the most common cause of choking in infants,[139] whereas balloons, small objects, and foods (eg, hot dogs, round candies, nuts, and grapes) are the most common causes of foreign-body airway obstruction (FBAO) in children.[140–142] Signs of FBAO include a *sudden* onset of respiratory distress with coughing, gagging, stridor (a high-pitched, noisy sound), or wheezing. The characteristics that distinguish FBAO from other causes (eg, croup) are sudden onset in a proper setting and the absence of antecedent fever or respiratory symptoms.

Relief of FBAO

FBAO may cause mild or severe airway obstruction. When the airway obstruction is mild, the child can cough and make some sounds. When the airway obstruction is severe, the victim cannot cough or make any sound.

- If FBAO is mild, do not interfere. Allow the victim to clear the airway by coughing while you observe for signs of severe FBAO.
- If the FBAO is severe (ie, the victim is unable to make a sound):
  - — For a child, perform subdiaphragmatic abdominal thrusts (Heimlich maneuver)[143,144] until the object is expelled or the victim becomes unresponsive. For an infant, deliver 5 back blows (slaps) followed by 5 chest thrusts[145–149] repeatedly until the object is expelled or the victim becomes unresponsive. Abdominal thrusts are not recommended for infants because they may damage the relatively large and unprotected liver.[150–152]
  - — If the victim becomes unresponsive, lay rescuers and healthcare providers should perform CPR but should look into the mouth before giving breaths. If you see a foreign body, remove it. Healthcare providers should not perform blind finger sweeps because they may push obstructing objects further into the pharynx and may damage the oropharynx.[153,154] Healthcare providers should attempt to remove an object only if they can see it in the pharynx. Then rescuers should attempt ventilation and follow with chest compressions.

Special Resuscitation Situations

Children With Special Healthcare Needs

Children with special healthcare needs[155–157] may require emergency care for complications of chronic conditions (eg, obstruction of a tracheostomy), failure of support technology (eg, ventilator failure), progression of underlying disease, or events unrelated to those special needs.[158] Care is often complicated by a lack of medical information, plan of medical care, list of current medications, and Do Not Attempt Resuscitation (DNAR) orders. Parents and child-care providers are encouraged to keep copies of medical information at home, with the child, and at the child's school or child-care facility. School nurses should have copies and should maintain a readily available list of children with DNAR orders.[158,159] An Emergency Information Form (EIF) was developed by the American Academy of Pediatrics and the American College of Emergency Physicians[157] and is available on the Worldwide Web at *http://www.pediatrics.org/cgi/content/full/104/4/e53.*

If a decision to limit or withhold resuscitative efforts is made, the physician must write an order clearly detailing the limits of any attempted resuscitation. A separate order must be written for the out-of-hospital setting. Regulations regarding out-of-hospital "do not attempt resuscitation" (DNAR or so-called "no-CPR") directives vary from state to state. For further information about ethical issues of resuscitation, see Part 2: "Ethical Issues."

When a child with a chronic or potentially life-threatening condition is discharged from the hospital, parents, school nurses, and home healthcare providers should be informed about the reason for hospitalization, hospital course, and how to recognize signs of deterioration. They should receive specific instructions about CPR and whom to contact.[159]

Ventilation With a Tracheostomy or Stoma

Everyone involved with the care of a child with a tracheostomy (parents, school nurses, and home healthcare providers) should know how to assess patency of the airway, clear the airway, and perform CPR using the artificial airway.

Use the tracheostomy tube for ventilation and verify adequacy of airway and ventilation by watching for chest expansion. If the tracheostomy tube does not allow effective ventilation even after suctioning, replace it. Alternative ventilation methods include mouth-to-stoma ventilation and bag-mask ventilation through the nose and mouth while you or someone else occludes the tracheal stoma.

Trauma

The principles of BLS resuscitation for the injured child are the same as those for the ill child, but some aspects require emphasis; improper resuscitation is a major cause of preventable pediatric trauma death.[160] Errors include failure to properly open and maintain the airway and failure to recognize and treat internal bleeding.

The following are important aspects of resuscitation of pediatric victims of trauma:

- Anticipate airway obstruction by dental fragments, blood, or other debris. Use a suction device if necessary.
- Stop all external bleeding with pressure.
- When the mechanism of injury is compatible with spinal injury, minimize motion of the cervical spine and avoid traction or movement of the head and neck. Open and maintain the airway with a jaw thrust and try not to tilt the head. If a jaw thrust does not open the airway, use a head tilt–chin lift. If there are 2 rescuers, the first opens the airway while the second restricts cervical spine motion. To limit spine motion, secure at least the thighs, pelvis, and shoulders to the immobilization board. Because of the disproportionately large size of the head in infants and young children, optimal positioning may require recessing the occiput[161] or elevating the torso to avoid undesirable backboard-induced cervical flexion.[161,162]
- If possible, transport children with multisystem trauma to a trauma center with pediatric expertise.

Drowning

Outcome after drowning depends on the duration of submersion, the water temperature, and how promptly CPR is started.[1,16,163] An excellent outcome can occur after prolonged submersion in icy waters.[164,165] Start resuscitation by safely removing the victim from the water as rapidly as possible. If you have special training, start rescue breathing while the victim is still in the water[166] if doing so will not delay removing the victim from the water. Do not attempt chest compressions in the water, however.

There is no evidence that water acts as an obstructive foreign body; don't waste time trying to remove water from the victim. Start CPR by opening the airway and giving 2 *effective* breaths followed by chest compressions; if you are alone, continue with 5 cycles (about 2 minutes) of compressions and ventilations before activating EMS and (for children 1 year of age and older) getting an AED. If 2 rescuers are present, send the second rescuer to activate the EMS system immediately and get an AED (if appropriate), while you continue CPR.

Summary: The Quality of BLS

Immediate CPR can improve survival from cardiorespiratory arrest in children, but not enough children receive high-quality CPR. We must increase the number of laypersons who learn, remember, and perform CPR and must improve the quality of CPR provided by lay rescuers and healthcare providers alike.

Systems that deliver professional CPR should implement processes of continuous quality improvement that include monitoring the quality of CPR delivered at the scene of cardiac arrest, other process-of-care measures (eg, initial rhythm, bystander CPR, and response intervals), and patient outcome up to hospital discharge (see Part 3: "Overview of CPR"). This evidence should be used to optimize the quality of CPR delivered (Class Indeterminate).

References

1. Kyriacou DN, Arcinue EL, Peek C, Kraus JF. Effect of immediate resuscitation on children with submersion injury. *Pediatrics*. 1994;94(pt 1):137–142.
2. Hickey RW, Cohen DM, Strausbaugh S, Dietrich AM. Pediatric patients requiring CPR in the prehospital setting. *Ann Emerg Med*. 1995;25:495–501.
3. Kuisma M, Alaspaa A. Out-of-hospital cardiac arrests of non-cardiac origin: epidemiology and outcome. *Eur Heart J*. 1997;18:1122–1128.
4. Friesen RM, Duncan P, Tweed WA, Bristow G. Appraisal of pediatric cardiopulmonary resuscitation. *Can Med Assoc J*. 1982;126:1055–1058.
5. Zaritsky A, Nadkarni V, Getson P, Kuehl K. CPR in children. *Ann Emerg Med*. 1987;16:1107–1111.
6. Lopez-Herce J, Garcia C, Rodriguez-Nunez A, Dominguez P, Carrillo A, Calvo C, Delgado MA. Long-term outcome of paediatric cardiorespiratory arrest in Spain. *Resuscitation*. 2005;64:79–85.
7. Mogayzel C, Quan L, Graves JR, Tiedeman D, Fahrenbruch C, Herndon P. Out-of-hospital ventricular fibrillation in children and adolescents: causes and outcomes. *Ann Emerg Med*. 1995;25:484–491.
8. Sirbaugh PE, Pepe PE, Shook JE, Kimball KT, Goldman MJ, Ward MA, Mann DM. A prospective, population-based study of the demographics, epidemiology, management, and outcome of out-of-hospital pediatric cardiopulmonary arrest [published correction appears in *Ann Emerg Med*. 1999;33:358]. *Ann Emerg Med*. 1999;33:174–184.
9. Schindler MB, Bohn D, Cox PN, McCrindle BW, Jarvis A, Edmonds J, Barker G. Outcome of out-of-hospital cardiac or respiratory arrest in children. *N Engl J Med*. 1996;335:1473–1479.
10. O'Rourke PP. Outcome of children who are apneic and pulseless in the emergency room. *Crit Care Med*. 1986;14:466–468.
11. Young KD, Seidel JS. Pediatric cardiopulmonary resuscitation: a collective review. *Ann Emerg Med*. 1999;33:195–205.
12. Dieckmann R, Vardis R. High-dose epinephrine in pediatric out-of-hospital cardiopulmonary arrest. *Pediatrics*. 1995;95:901–913.
13. Herlitz J, Engdahl J, Svensson L, Young M, Angquist KA, Holmberg S. Characteristics and outcome among children suffering from out of hospital cardiac arrest in Sweden. *Resuscitation*. 2005;64:37–40.
14. Pell JP, Sirel JM, Marsden AK, Ford I, Walker NL, Cobbe SM. Presentation, management, and outcome of out of hospital cardiopulmonary arrest: comparison by underlying aetiology. *Heart (British Cardiac Society)*. 2003;89:839–842.
15. Lopez-Herce J, Garcia C, Dominguez P, Carrillo A, Rodriguez-Nunez A, Calvo C, Delgado MA. Characteristics and outcome of cardiorespiratory arrest in children. *Resuscitation*. 2004;63:311–320.
16. Suominen P, Baillie C, Korpela R, Rautanen S, Ranta S, Olkkola KT. Impact of age, submersion time and water temperature on outcome in near-drowning. *Resuscitation*. 2002;52:247–254.

17. Kuisma M, Suominen P, Korpela R. Paediatric out-of-hospital cardiac arrests: epidemiology and outcome. *Resuscitation*. 1995;30:141–150.
18. Centers for Disease Control and Prevention. Web-based Injury Statistics Query and Reporting System (WISQARS) (Online). National Center for Injury Prevention and Control, Centers for Disease Control and Prevention (producer). Available from: *URL: www.cdc.gov/ncipc/wisqars (February 3, 2005)*. 2005.
19. Pressley JC, Barlow B. Preventing injury and injury-related disability in children and adolescents. *Semin Pediatr Surg*. 2004;13:133–140.
20. Durbin DR, Elliott MR, Winston FK. Belt-positioning booster seats and reduction in risk of injury among children in vehicle crashes. *Jama*. 2003; 289:2835–2840.
21. Foss RD, Feaganes JR, Rodgman EA. Initial effects of graduated driver licensing on 16-year-old driver crashes in North Carolina. *Jama*. 2001;286: 1588–1592.
22. Schieber RA, Vegega ME. Reducing childhood pedestrian injuries. *Inj Prev*. 2002;8 Suppl 1:i1–10.
23. *National SAFE KIDS Campaign (NSKC) Bicycle Injury Fact Sheet*. Washington, DC: NSKC; 2004.
24. Thompson DC, Thompson RS, Rivara FP, Wolf ME. A case-control study of the effectiveness of bicycle safety helmets in preventing facial injury. *Am J Public Health*. 1990;80:1471–1474.
25. Karter M. Fire Loss in the United States During 2003. Quincy, Mass: National Fire Protection Agency Association; 2004.
26. *National SAFE KIDS Campaign (NSKC) Injury Facts: Fire Injury (Residential)*. Washington, DC: NSKC; 2004.
27. Ahrens M. *U.S. Experience with Smoke Alarms and Other Fire Detection/Alarm Equipment*. Quincy, MA: National Fire Protection Agency Association; 2004.
28. Hemenway D. *Private Guns, Public Health 2004*. Ann Arbor, MI: The University of Michigan Press; 2004.
29. Beaman V, Annest JL, Mercy JA, Kresnow Mj, Pollock DA. Lethality of firearm-related injuries in the United States population. *Ann Emerg Med*. 2000;35:258–266.
30. Brent DA, Perper JA, Allman CJ, Moritz GM, Wartella ME, Zelenak JP. The presence and accessibility of firearms in the homes of adolescent suicides: a case-control study. *JAMA*. 1991;266:2989–2995.
31. Svenson JE, Spurlock C, Nypaver M. Pediatric firearm-related fatalities: not just an urban problem. *Arch Pediatr Adolesc Med*. 1996;150:583–587.
32. Dahlberg LL, Ikeda RM, Kresnow MJ. Guns in the home and risk of a violent death in the home: findings from a national study. *Am J Epidemiol*. 2004;160:929–936.
33. Willinger M, James LS, Catz C. Defining the sudden infant death syndrome (SIDS): deliberations of an expert panel convened by the National Institute of Child Health and Human Development. *Pediatr Pathol*. 1991;11: 677–684.
34. Changing concepts of sudden infant death syndrome: implications for infant sleeping environment and sleep position. American Academy of Pediatrics. Task Force on Infant Sleep Position and Sudden Infant Death Syndrome. *Pediatrics*. 2000;105:650–656.
35. Positioning and sudden infant death syndrome (SIDS): update. American Academy of Pediatrics Task Force on Infant Positioning and SIDS. *Pediatrics*. 1996;98:1216–1218.
36. American Academy of Pediatrics AAP Task Force on Infant Positioning and SIDS: Positioning and SIDS. *Pediatrics*. 1992;89:1120–1126.
37. Willinger M, Hoffman HJ, Hartford RB. Infant sleep position and risk for sudden infant death syndrome: report of meeting held January 13 and 14, 1994, National Institutes of Health, Bethesda, MD. *Pediatrics*. 1994;93: 814–819.
38. Tong EK, England L, Glantz SA. Changing conclusions on secondhand smoke in a sudden infant death syndrome review funded by the tobacco industry. *Pediatrics*. 2005;115:e356–e366.
39. Anderson ME, Johnson DC, Batal HA. Sudden Infant Death Syndrome and prenatal maternal smoking: rising attributed risk in the Back to Sleep era. *BMC Med*. 2005;3:4.
40. Hoyert DL, Kochanek KD, Murphy SL. Deaths: final data for 1997. *Natl Vital Stat Rep*. 1999;47:1–104.
41. Prevention of drowning in infants, children, and adolescents. *Pediatrics*. 2003;112:437–439.
42. Mejicano GC, Maki DG. Infections acquired during cardiopulmonary resuscitation: estimating the risk and defining strategies for prevention. *Ann Intern Med*. 1998;129:813–828.
43. Appleton GO, Cummins RO, Larson MP, Graves JR. CPR and the single rescuer: at what age should you "call first" rather than "call fast"? *Ann Emerg Med*. 1995;25:492–494.
44. Ruben HM, Elam JO, Ruben AM, Greene DG. Investigation of upper airway problems in resuscitation, 1: studies of pharyngeal x-rays and performance by laymen. *Anesthesiology*. 1961;22:271–279.
45. Safar P, Aguto-Escarraga L. Compliance in apneic anesthetized adults. *Anesthesiology*. 1959;20:283–289.
46. Elam JO, Greene DG, Schneider MA, Ruben HM, Gordon AS, Hustead RF, Benson DW, Clements JA, Ruben A. Head-tilt method of oral resuscitation. *JAMA*. 1960;172:812–815.
47. Guildner CW. Resuscitation: opening the airway. A comparative study of techniques for opening an airway obstructed by the tongue. *JACEP*. 1976; 5:588–590.
48. Hackl W, Hausberger K, Sailer R, Ulmer H, Gassner R. Prevalence of cervical spine injuries in patients with facial trauma. *Oral Surg Oral Med Oral Pathol Oral Radiol Endod*. 2001;92:370–376.
49. Demetriades D, Charalambides K, Chahwan S, Hanpeter D, Alo K, Velmahos G, Murray J, Asensio J. Nonskeletal cervical spine injuries: epidemiology and diagnostic pitfalls. *J Trauma*. 2000;48:724–727.
50. Holly LT, Kelly DF, Counelis GJ, Blinman T, McArthur DL, Cryer HG. Cervical spine trauma associated with moderate and severe head injury: incidence, risk factors, and injury characteristics. *J Neurosurg Spine*. 2002; 96:285–291.
51. Roth B, Magnusson J, Johansson I, Holmberg S, Westrin P. Jaw lift: a simple and effective method to open the airway in children. *Resuscitation*. 1998;39:171–174.
52. Bruppacher H, Reber A, Keller JP, Geiduschek J, Erb TO, Frei FJ. The effects of common airway maneuvers on airway pressure and flow in children undergoing adenoidectomies. *Anesth Analg*. 2003;97:29–34, table of contents.
53. Clark JJ, Larsen MP, Culley LL, Graves JR, Eisenberg MS. Incidence of agonal respirations in sudden cardiac arrest. *Ann Emerg Med*. 1992;21: 1464–1467.
54. Poets CF, Meny RG, Chobanian MR, Bonofiglo RE. Gasping and other cardiorespiratory patterns during sudden infant deaths. *Pediatr Res*. 1999; 45:350–354.
55. Zideman DA. Paediatric and neonatal life support. *Br J Anaesth*. 1997;79: 178–187.
56. Tonkin SL, Davis SL, Gunn TR. Nasal route for infant resuscitation by mothers. *Lancet*. 1995;345:1353–1354.
57. Segedin E, Torrie J, Anderson B. Nasal airway versus oral route for infant resuscitation. *Lancet*. 1995;346:382.
58. Tonkin SL, Gunn AJ. Failure of mouth-to-mouth resuscitation in cases of sudden infant death. *Resuscitation*. 2001;48:181–184.
59. Ornato JP, Hallagan LF, McMahan SB, Peeples EH, Rostafinski AG. Attitudes of BCLS instructors about mouth-to-mouth resuscitation during the AIDS epidemic. *Ann Emerg Med*. 1990;19:151–156.
60. Brenner BE, Van DC, Cheng D, Lazar EJ. Determinants of reluctance to perform CPR among residents and applicants: the impact of experience on helping behavior. *Resuscitation*. 1997;35:203–211.
61. Hew P, Brenner B, Kaufman J. Reluctance of paramedics and emergency medical technicians to perform mouth-to-mouth resuscitation. *J Emerg Med*. 1997;15:279–284.
62. Locke CJ, Berg RA, Sanders AB, Davis MF, Milander MM, Kern KB, Ewy GA. Bystander cardiopulmonary resuscitation. Concerns about mouth-to-mouth contact. *Arch Intern Med*. 1995;155:938–943.
63. Shibata K, Taniguchi T, Yoshida M, Yamamoto K. Obstacles to bystander cardiopulmonary resuscitation in Japan. *Resuscitation*. 2000;44:187–193.
64. Terndrup TE, Warner DA. Infant ventilation and oxygenation by basic life support providers: comparison of methods. *Prehospital Disaster Med*. 1992; 7:35–40.
65. Hess D, Ness C, Oppel A, Rhoads K. Evaluation of mouth-to-mask ventilation devices. *Respir Care*. 1989;34:191–195.
66. Gausche M, Lewis RJ, Stratton SJ, Haynes BE, Gunter CS, Goodrich SM, Poore PD, McCollough MD, Henderson DP, Pratt FD, Seidel JS. Effect of out-of-hospital pediatric endotracheal intubation on survival and neurological outcome: a controlled clinical trial. *JAMA*. 2000;283:783–790.
67. Cooper A, DiScala C, Foltin G, Tunik M, Markenson D, Welborn C. Prehospital endotracheal intubation for severe head injury in children: a reappraisal. *Semin Pediatr Surg*. 2001;10:3–6.
68. Stockinger ZT, McSwain NE, Jr. Prehospital endotracheal intubation for trauma does not improve survival over bag-valve-mask ventilation. *J Trauma*. 2004;56:531–536.
69. Pitetti R, Glustein JZ, Bhende MS. Prehospital care and outcome of pediatric out-of-hospital cardiac arrest. *Prehosp Emerg Care*. 2002;6: 283–290.

70. Terndrup TE, Kanter RK, Cherry RA. A comparison of infant ventilation methods performed by prehospital personnel. *Ann Emerg Med.* 1989;18:607–611.
71. Field D, Milner AD, Hopkin IE. Efficiency of manual resuscitators at birth. *Arch Dis Child.* 1986;61:300–302.
72. Finer NN, Barrington KJ, Al-Fadley F, Peters KL. Limitations of self-inflating resuscitators. *Pediatrics.* 1986;77:417–420.
73. Kern KB, Sanders AB, Raife J, Milander MM, Otto CW, Ewy GA. A study of chest compression rates during cardiopulmonary resuscitation in humans: the importance of rate-directed chest compressions. *Arch Intern Med.* 1992;152:145–149.
74. Aufderheide TP, Sigurdsson G, Pirrallo RG, Yannopoulos D, McKnite S, von Briesen C, Sparks CW, Conrad CJ, Provo TA, Lurie KG. Hyperventilation-induced hypotension during cardiopulmonary resuscitation. *Circulation.* 2004;109:1960–1965.
75. Abella BS, Alvarado JP, Myklebust H, Edelson DP, Barry A, O'Hearn N, Vanden Hoek TL, Becker LB. Quality of cardiopulmonary resuscitation during in-hospital cardiac arrest. *JAMA.* 2005;293:305–310.
76. Hirschman AM, Kravath RE. Venting vs ventilating. A danger of manual resuscitation bags. *Chest.* 1982;82:369–370.
77. Berg MD, Idris AH, Berg RA. Severe ventilatory compromise due to gastric distention during pediatric cardiopulmonary resuscitation. *Resuscitation.* 1998;36:71–73.
78. Moynihan RJ, Brock-Utne JG, Archer JH, Feld LH, Kreitzman TR. The effect of cricoid pressure on preventing gastric insufflation in infants and children. *Anesthesiology.* 1993;78:652–656.
79. Salem MR, Wong AY, Mani M, Sellick BA. Efficacy of cricoid pressure in preventing gastric inflation during bag- mask ventilation in pediatric patients. *Anesthesiology.* 1974;40:96–98.
80. Sellick BA. Cricoid pressure to control regurgitation of stomach contents during induction of anaesthesia. *Lancet.* 1961;2:404–406.
81. Hartsilver EL, Vanner RG. Airway obstruction with cricoid pressure. *Anaesthesia.* 2000;55:208–211.
82. Lipinski CA, Hicks SD, Callaway CW. Normoxic ventilation during resuscitation and outcome from asphyxial cardiac arrest in rats. *Resuscitation.* 1999;42:221–229.
83. Liu Y, Rosenthal RE, Haywood Y, Miljkovic-Lolic M, Vanderhoek JY, Fiskum G. Normoxic ventilation after cardiac arrest reduces oxidation of brain lipids and improves neurological outcome. *Stroke.* 1998;29:1679–1686.
84. Lefkowitz W. Oxygen and resuscitation: beyond the myth. *Pediatrics.* 2002;109:517–519.
85. Zwemer CF, Whitesall SE, D'Alecy LG. Cardiopulmonary-cerebral resuscitation with 100% oxygen exacerbates neurological dysfunction following nine minutes of normothermic cardiac arrest in dogs. *Resuscitation.* 1994;27:159–170.
86. Finer NN, Bates R, Tomat P. Low flow oxygen delivery via nasal cannula to neonates. *Pediatr Pulmonol.* 1996;21:48–51.
87. Inagawa G, Morimura N, Miwa T, Okuda K, Hirata M, Hiroki K. A comparison of five techniques for detecting cardiac activity in infants. *Paediatr Anaesth.* 2003;13:141–146.
88. Eberle B, Dick WF, Schneider T, Wisser G, Doetsch S, Tzanova I. Checking the carotid pulse check: diagnostic accuracy of first responders in patients with and without a pulse. *Resuscitation.* 1996;33:107–116.
89. Graham CA, Lewis NF. Evaluation of a new method for the carotid pulse check in cardiopulmonary resuscitation. *Resuscitation.* 2002;53:37–40.
90. Ochoa FJ, Ramalle-Gomara E, Carpintero JM, Garcia A, Saralegui I. Competence of health professionals to check the carotid pulse. *Resuscitation.* 1998;37:173–175.
91. Mather C, O'Kelly S. The palpation of pulses. *Anaesthesia.* 1996;51:189–191.
92. Lapostolle F, Le Toumelin P, Agostinucci JM, Catineau J, Adnet F. Basic cardiac life support providers checking the carotid pulse: performance, degree of conviction, and influencing factors. *Acad Emerg Med.* 2004;11:878–880.
93. Moule P. Checking the carotid pulse: diagnostic accuracy in students of the healthcare professions. *Resuscitation.* 2000;44:195–201.
94. Bahr J, Klingler H, Panzer W, Rode H, Kettler D. Skills of lay people in checking the carotid pulse. *Resuscitation.* 1997;35:23–26.
95. Cavallaro DL, Melker RJ. Comparison of two techniques for detecting cardiac activity in infants. *Crit Care Med.* 1983;11:189–190.
96. Lee CJ, Bullock LJ. Determining the pulse for infant CPR: time for a change? *Mil Med.* 1991;156:190–193.
97. Aufderheide TP, Pirrallo RG, Yannopoulos D, Klein JP, von Briesen C, Sparks CW, Deja KA, Conrad CJ, Kitscha DJ, Provo TA, Lurie KG. Incomplete chest wall decompression: a clinical evaluation of CPR performance by EMS personnel and assessment of alternative manual chest compression-decompression techniques. *Resuscitation.* 2005;64:353–362.
98. Clements F, McGowan J. Finger position for chest compressions in cardiac arrest in infants. *Resuscitation.* 2000;44:43–46.
99. Finholt DA, Kettrick RG, Wagner HR, Swedlow DB. The heart is under the lower third of the sternum: implications for external cardiac massage. *Am J Dis Child.* 1986;140:646–649.
100. Phillips GW, Zideman DA. Relation of infant heart to sternum: its significance in cardiopulmonary resuscitation. *Lancet.* 1986;1:1024–1025.
101. Orlowski JP. Optimum position for external cardiac compression in infants and young children. *Ann Emerg Med.* 1986;15:667–673.
102. Shah NM, Gaur HK. Position of heart in relation to sternum and nipple line at various ages. *Indian Pediatr.* 1992;29:49–53.
103. David R. Closed chest cardiac massage in the newborn infant. *Pediatrics.* 1988;81:552–554.
104. Todres ID, Rogers MC. Methods of external cardiac massage in the newborn infant. *J Pediatr.* 1975;86:781–782.
105. Menegazzi JJ, Auble TE, Nicklas KA, Hosack GM, Rack L, Goode JS. Two-thumb versus two-finger chest compression during CRP in a swine infant model of cardiac arrest. *Ann Emerg Med.* 1993;22:240–243.
106. Houri PK, Frank LR, Menegazzi JJ, Taylor R. A randomized, controlled trial of two-thumb vs two-finger chest compression in a swine infant model of cardiac arrest. *Prehosp Emerg Care.* 1997;1:65–67.
107. Dorfsman ML, Menegazzi JJ, Wadas RJ, Auble TE. Two-thumb vs two-finger chest compression in an infant model of prolonged cardiopulmonary resuscitation. *Acad Emerg Med.* 2000;7:1077–1082.
108. Whitelaw CC, Slywka B, Goldsmith LJ. Comparison of a two-finger versus two-thumb method for chest compressions by healthcare providers in an infant mechanical model. *Resuscitation.* 2000;43:213–216.
109. Thaler MM, Stobie GH. An improved technique of external caridac compression in infants and young children. *N Engl J Med.* 1963;269:606–610.
110. Ishimine P, Menegazzi J, Weinstein D. Evaluation of two-thumb chest compression with thoracic squeeze in a swine model of infant cardiac arrest. *Acad Emerg Med.* 1998;5:397.
111. Stevenson AG, McGowan J, Evans AL, Graham CA. CPR for children: one hand or two? *Resuscitation.* 2005;64:205–208.
112. American Heart Association in collaboration with International Liaison Committee on Resuscitation. Guidelines 2000 for Cardiopulmonary Resuscitation and Emergency Cardiovascular Care: International Consensus on Science, Part 9: Pediatric Basic Life Support. *Circulation.* 2000;102(suppl I):I-253–I-290.
113. Dorph E, Wik L, Steen PA. Effectiveness of ventilation-compression ratios 1:5 and 2:15 in simulated single rescuer paediatric resuscitation. *Resuscitation.* 2002;54:259–264.
114. Greingor JL. Quality of cardiac massage with ratio compression-ventilation 5/1 and 15/2. *Resuscitation.* 2002;55:263–267.
115. Srikantan S, Berg RA, Cox T, Tice L, Nadkarni VM. Effect of 1-rescuer compression: ventilation ratios on CPR in infant, pediatric and adult manikins. *Crit Care Med.* In Press.
116. Berg RA, Sanders AB, Kern KB, Hilwig RW, Heidenreich JW, Porter ME, Ewy GA. Adverse hemodynamic effects of interrupting chest compressions for rescue breathing during cardiopulmonary resuscitation for ventricular fibrillation cardiac arrest. *Circulation.* 2001;104:2465–2470.
117. Kern KB, Hilwig RW, Berg RA, Ewy GA. Efficacy of chest compression-only BLS CPR in the presence of an occluded airway. *Resuscitation.* 1998;39:179–188.
118. Assar D, Chamberlain D, Colquhoun M, Donnelly P, Handley AJ, Leaves S, Kern KB. Randomised controlled trials of staged teaching for basic life support, 1: skill acquisition at bronze stage. *Resuscitation.* 2000;45:7–15.
119. Heidenreich JW, Higdon TA, Kern KB, Sanders AB, Berg RA, Niebler R, Hendrickson J, Ewy GA. Single-rescuer cardiopulmonary resuscitation: 'two quick breaths'—an oxymoron. *Resuscitation.* 2004;62:283–289.
120. Wik L, Kramer-Johansen J, Myklebust H, Sorebo H, Svensson L, Fellows B, Steen PA. Quality of cardiopulmonary resuscitation during out-of-hospital cardiac arrest. *JAMA.* 2005;293:299–304.
121. Eftestol T, Sunde K, Steen PA. Effects of interrupting precordial compressions on the calculated probability of defibrillation success during out-of-hospital cardiac arrest. *Circulation.* 2002;105:2270–2273.
122. Yu T, Weil MH, Tang W, Sun S, Klouche K, Povoas H, Bisera J. Adverse outcomes of interrupted precordial compression during automated defibrillation. *Circulation.* 2002;106:368–372.
123. Abella BS, Sandbo N, Vassilatos P, Alvarado JP, O'Hearn N, Wigder HN, Hoffman P, Tynus K, Vanden Hoek TL, Becker LB. Chest compression

rates during cardiopulmonary resuscitation are suboptimal: a prospective study during in-hospital cardiac arrest. *Circulation.* 2005;111:428–434.

124. Becker LB, Berg RA, Pepe PE, Idris AH, Aufderheide TP, Barnes TA, Stratton SJ, Chandra NC. A reappraisal of mouth-to-mouth ventilation during bystander-initiated cardiopulmonary resuscitation. A statement for healthcare professionals from the Ventilation Working Group of the Basic Life Support and Pediatric Life Support Subcommittees, American Heart Association. *Resuscitation.* 1997;35:189–201.
125. Berg RA, Hilwig RW, Kern KB, Babar I, Ewy GA. Simulated mouth-to-mouth ventilation and chest compressions (bystander cardiopulmonary resuscitation) improves outcome in a swine model of prehospital pediatric asphyxial cardiac arrest. *Crit Care Med.* 1999;27:1893–1899.
126. Berg RA, Hilwig RW, Kern KB, Ewy GA. "Bystander" chest compressions and assisted ventilation independently improve outcome from piglet asphyxial pulseless "cardiac arrest". *Circulation.* 2000;101:1743–1748.
127. Kern KB, Hilwig RW, Berg RA, Sanders AB, Ewy GA. Importance of continuous chest compressions during cardiopulmonary resuscitation: improved outcome during a simulated single lay-rescuer scenario. *Circulation.* 2002;105:645–649.
128. Ashton A, McCluskey A, Gwinnutt CL, Keenan AM. Effect of rescuer fatigue on performance of continuous external chest compressions over 3 min. *Resuscitation.* 2002;55:151–155.
129. Ochoa FJ, Ramalle-Gomara E, Lisa V, Saralegui I. The effect of rescuer fatigue on the quality of chest compressions. *Resuscitation.* 1998;37: 149–152.
130. Hightower D, Thomas SH, Stone CK, Dunn K, March JA. Decay in quality of closed-chest compressions over time. *Ann Emerg Med.* 1995;26: 300–303.
131. Sanders AB, Kern KB, Berg RA, Hilwig RW, Heidenrich J, Ewy GA. Survival and neurologic outcome after cardiopulmonary resuscitation with four different chest compression-ventilation ratios. *Ann Emerg Med.* 2002; 40:553–562.
132. Young KD, Gausche-Hill M, McClung CD, Lewis RJ. A prospective, population-based study of the epidemiology and outcome of out-of-hospital pediatric cardiopulmonary arrest. *Pediatrics.* 2004;114:157–164.
133. Reis AG, Nadkarni V, Perondi MB, Grisi S, Berg RA. A prospective investigation into the epidemiology of in-hospital pediatric cardiopulmonary resuscitation using the international Utstein reporting style. *Pediatrics.* 2002;109:200–209.
134. Atkins DL, Jorgenson DB. Attenuated pediatric electrode pads for automated external defibrillator use in children. *Resuscitation.* 2005;66: 31–37.
135. Berg RA, Chapman FW, Berg MD, Hilwig RW, Banville I, Walker RG, Nova RC, Sherrill D, Kern KB. Attenuated adult biphasic shocks compared with weight-based monophasic shocks in a swine model of prolonged pediatric ventricular fibrillation. *Resuscitation.* 2004;61:189–197.
136. Atkinson E, Mikysa B, Conway JA, Parker M, Christian K, Deshpande J, Knilans TK, Smith J, Walker C, Stickney RE, Hampton DR, Hazinski MF. Specificity and sensitivity of automated external defibrillator rhythm analysis in infants and children. *Ann Emerg Med.* 2003;42:185–196.
137. Cecchin F, Jorgenson DB, Berul CI, Perry JC, Zimmerman AA, Duncan BW, Lupinetti FM, Snyder D, Lyster TD, Rosenthal GL, Cross B, Atkins DL. Is arrhythmia detection by automatic external defibrillator accurate for children? Sensitivity and specificity of an automatic external defibrillator algorithm in 696 pediatric arrhythmias. *Circulation.* 2001;103:2483–2488.
138. Samson RA, Berg RA, Bingham R, Biarent D, Coovadia A, Hazinski MF, Hickey RW, Nadkarni V, Nichol G, Tibballs J, Reis AG, Tse S, Zideman D, Potts J, Uzark K, Atkins D. Use of automated external defibrillators for children: an update: an advisory statement from the pediatric advanced life support task force, International Liaison Committee on Resuscitation. *Circulation.* 2003;107:3250–3255.
139. Vilke GM, Smith AM, Ray LU, Steen PJ, Murrin PA, Chan TC. Airway obstruction in children aged less than 5 years: the prehospital experience. *Prehosp Emerg Care.* 2004;8:196–199.
140. Morley RE, Ludemann JP, Moxham JP, Kozak FK, Riding KH. Foreign body aspiration in infants and toddlers: recent trends in British Columbia. *J Otolaryngol.* 2004;33:37–41.
141. Harris CS, Baker SP, Smith GA, Harris RM. Childhood asphyxiation by food. A national analysis and overview. *Jama.* 1984;251:2231–2235.
142. Rimell FL, Thome AJ, Stool S, Reilly JS, Rider G, Stool D, Wilson CL. Characteristics of objects that cause choking in children. *JAMA.* 1995;274: 1763–1766.
143. Heimlich HJ. A life-saving maneuver to prevent food-choking. *Jama.* 1975; 234:398–401.
144. Day RL, Crelin ES, DuBois AB. Choking: the Heimlich abdominal thrust vs back blows: an approach to measurement of inertial and aerodynamic forces. *Pediatrics.* 1982;70:113–119.
145. Langhelle A, Sunde K, Wik L, Steen PA. Airway pressure with chest compressions versus Heimlich manoeuvre in recently dead adults with complete airway obstruction. *Resuscitation.* 2000;44:105–108.
146. Sternbach G, Kiskaddon RT. Henry Heimlich: a life-saving maneuver for food choking. *J Emerg Med.* 1985;3:143–148.
147. Redding JS. The choking controversy: critique of evidence on the Heimlich maneuver. *Crit Care Med.* 1979;7:475–479.
148. Gordon AS, Belton MK, Ridolpho PF. Emergency management of foreign body obstruction. In: Safar P, Elam JO, eds. *Advances in Cardiopulmonary Resuscitation.* New York: Springer-Verlag, Inc.; 1977:39–50.
149. Guildner CW, Williams D, Subitch T. Airway obstructed by foreign material: the Heimlich maneuver. *JACEP.* 1976;5:675–677.
150. Rosen P, Stoto M, Harley J. The use of the Heimlich maneuver in near-drowning: Institute of Medicine report. *J Emerg Med.* 1995;13:397–405.
151. Majumdar A, Sedman PC. Gastric rupture secondary to successful Heimlich manoeuvre. *Postgrad Med J.* 1998;74:609–610.
152. Fink JA, Klein RL. Complications of the Heimlich maneuver. *J Pediatr Surg.* 1989;24:486–487.
153. Kabbani M, Goodwin SR. Traumatic epiglottis following blind finger sweep to remove a pharyngeal foreign body. *Clin Pediatr (Phila).* 1995;34: 495–497.
154. Hartrey R, Bingham RM. Pharyngeal trauma as a result of blind finger sweeps in the choking child. *J Accid Emerg Med.* 1995;12:52–54.
155. McPherson M, Arango P, Fox H, Lauver C, McManus M, Newacheck PW, Perrin JM, Shonkoff JP, Strickland B. A new definition of children with special health care needs. *Pediatrics.* 1998;102:137–140.
156. Newacheck PW, Strickland B, Shonkoff JP, Perrin JM, McPherson M, McManus M, Lauver C, Fox H, Arango P. An epidemiologic profile of children with special health care needs. *Pediatrics.* 1998;102:117–123.
157. Emergency preparedness for children with special health care needs. Committee on Pediatric Emergency Medicine. American Academy of Pediatrics. *Pediatrics.* 1999;104:e53.
158. Spaite DW, Conroy C, Tibbitts M, Karriker KJ, Seng M, Battaglia N, Criss EA, Valenzuela TD, Meislin HW. Use of emergency medical services by children with special health care needs. *Prehosp Emerg Care.* 2000;4: 19–23.
159. Schultz-Grant LD, Young-Cureton V, Kataoka-Yahiro M. Advance directives and do not resuscitate orders: nurses' knowledge and the level of practice in school settings. *J Sch Nurs.* 1998;14:4–10, 12–13.
160. Dykes EH, Spence LJ, Young JG, Bohn DJ, Filler RM, Wesson DE. Preventable pediatric trauma deaths in a metropolitan region. *J Pediatr Surg.* 1989;24:107–110.
161. Herzenberg JE, Hensinger RN, Dedrick DK, Phillips WA. Emergency transport and positioning of young children who have an injury of the cervical spine. The standard backboard may be hazardous. *J Bone Joint Surg Am.* 1989;71:15–22.
162. Nypaver M, Treloar D. Neutral cervical spine positioning in children. *Ann Emerg Med.* 1994;23:208–211.
163. Graf WD, Cummings P, Quan L, Brutocao D. Predicting outcome in pediatric submersion victims. *Ann Emerg Med.* 1995;26:312–319.
164. Modell JH, Idris AH, Pineda JA, Silverstein JH. Survival after prolonged submersion in freshwater in Florida. *Chest.* 2004;125:1948–1951.
165. Mehta SR, Srinivasan KV, Bindra MS, Kumar MR, Lahiri AK. Near drowning in cold water. *J Assoc Physicians India.* 2000;48:674–676.
166. Szpilman D, Soares M. In-water resuscitation—is it worthwhile? *Resuscitation.* 2004;63:25–31.

Part 12: Pediatric Advanced Life Support

In contrast to adults, sudden cardiac arrest in children is uncommon, and cardiac arrest does not usually result from a primary cardiac cause.[1] More often it is the terminal event of progressive respiratory failure or shock, also called an asphyxial arrest.

Respiratory Failure

Respiratory failure is characterized by inadequate ventilation or oxygenation. Anticipate respiratory failure and possible respiratory arrest if you see any of the following:

- An increased respiratory rate, particularly with signs of distress (eg, increased effort, nasal flaring, retractions, or grunting)
- An inadequate respiratory rate, effort, or chest excursion (eg, diminished breath sounds, gasping, and cyanosis), especially if mental status is depressed

Shock

Shock results from inadequate blood flow and oxygen delivery to meet tissue metabolic demands. Shock progresses over a continuum of severity, from a compensated to a decompensated state. Attempts to compensate include tachycardia and increased systemic vascular resistance (vasoconstriction) in an effort to maintain cardiac output and blood pressure. Although decompensation can occur rapidly, it is usually preceded by a period of inadequate end-organ perfusion.

Signs of compensated shock include

- Tachycardia
- Cool extremities
- Prolonged capillary refill (despite warm ambient temperature)
- Weak peripheral pulses compared with central pulses
- Normal blood pressure

As compensatory mechanisms fail, signs of inadequate end-organ perfusion develop. In addition to the above, these signs include

- Depressed mental status
- Decreased urine output
- Metabolic acidosis
- Tachypnea
- Weak central pulses

Signs of decompensated shock include the signs listed above plus hypotension. In the absence of blood pressure measurement, decompensated shock is indicated by the nondetectable distal pulses with weak central pulses in an infant or child with other signs and symptoms consistent with inadequate tissue oxygen delivery.

The most common cause of shock is hypovolemia, one form of which is hemorrhagic shock. Distributive and cardiogenic shock are seen less often.

Learn to integrate the signs of shock because no single sign confirms the diagnosis. For example:

- Capillary refill time alone is not a good indicator of circulatory volume, but a capillary refill time of >2 seconds is a useful indicator of moderate dehydration when combined with a decreased urine output, absent tears, dry mucous membranes, and a generally ill appearance (Class IIb; LOE 3[2]). It is influenced by ambient temperature,[3] lighting,[4] site, and age.
- Tachycardia also results from other causes (eg, pain, anxiety, fever).
- Pulses may be bounding in anaphylactic, neurogenic, and septic shock.

In compensated shock, blood pressure remains normal; it is low in decompensated shock. Hypotension is a *systolic* blood pressure less than the 5th percentile of normal for age, namely:

- <60 mm Hg in term neonates (0 to 28 days)
- <70 mm Hg in infants (1 month to 12 months)
- <70 mm Hg + (2 × age in years) in children 1 to 10 years
- <90 mm Hg in children ≥10 years of age

Airway

Oropharyngeal and Nasopharyngeal Airways

Oropharyngeal and nasopharyngeal airways are adjuncts for maintaining an open airway. Oropharyngeal airways are used in unconscious victims (ie, with no gag reflex). Select the correct size: an oropharyngeal airway that is too small will not keep the tongue from obstructing the pharynx; one that is too large may obstruct the airway.

Nasopharyngeal airways will be better tolerated than oral airways by patients who are not deeply unconscious. Small nasopharyngeal tubes (for infants) may be easily obstructed by secretions.

Laryngeal Mask Airway

There is insufficient evidence to recommend for or against the routine use of a laryngeal mask airway (LMA) during cardiac arrest (Class Indeterminate). When endotracheal intubation is not possible, the LMA is an acceptable adjunct for experienced providers (Class IIb; LOE 7),[5] but it is associated with a higher incidence of complications in young children.[6]

Breathing: Oxygenation and Assisted Ventilation

For information about the role of ventilation during CPR, see Part 11: "Pediatric Basic Life Support."

(*Circulation.* 2005;112:IV-167-IV-187.)

This special supplement to *Circulation* is freely available at http://www.circulationaha.org

DOI: 10.1161/CIRCULATIONAHA.105.166573

Oxygen

There are no studies comparing various concentrations of oxygen during resuscitation beyond the perinatal period. Use 100% oxygen during resuscitation (Class Indeterminate). Monitor the patient's oxygen level. When the patient is stable, wean the supplementary oxygen if the oxygen saturation is maintained.

Pulse Oximetry

If the patient has a perfusing rhythm, monitor oxygen saturation continuously with a pulse oximeter because clinical recognition of hypoxemia is not reliable.[7] Pulse oximetry, however, may be unreliable in a patient with poor peripheral perfusion.

Bag-Mask Ventilation

Bag-mask ventilation can be as effective as ventilation through an endotracheal tube for short periods and may be safer.[8–11] In the prehospital setting ventilate and oxygenate infants and children with a bag-mask device, especially if transport time is short (Class IIa; LOE 1[8]; 3[10]; 4[9,11]). Bag-mask ventilation requires training and periodic retraining on how to select a correct mask size, open the airway, make a tight seal between mask and face, ventilate, and assess effectiveness of ventilation (see Part 11: "Pediatric Basic Life Support").

Precautions

Victims of cardiac arrest are frequently overventilated during resuscitation.[12–14] Excessive ventilation increases intrathoracic pressure and impedes venous return, reducing cardiac output, cerebral blood flow, and coronary perfusion.[13] Excessive ventilation also causes air trapping and barotrauma in patients with small-airway obstruction and increases the risk of stomach inflation, regurgitation, and aspiration.

Minute ventilation is determined by the tidal volume and ventilation rate. Use only the force and tidal volume needed to make the chest rise visibly. During CPR for the patient with no advanced airway (eg, endotracheal tube, esophageal-tracheal combitube [Combitube], LMA) in place, ventilation rate is determined by the compression-ventilation ratio. Pause after 30 compressions (1 rescuer) or after 15 compressions (2 rescuers) to give 2 ventilations with mouth-to-mouth, mouth-to-mask, or bag-mask techniques. Give each breath over 1 second.

If an advanced airway is in place during CPR (eg, endotracheal tube, Combitube, LMA), ventilate at a rate of 8 to 10 times per minute without pausing chest compressions. In the victim with a perfusing rhythm but absent or inadequate respiratory effort, give 12 to 20 breaths per minute. One way to achieve this rate with a ventilating bag is to use the mnemonic "squeeze-release-release" at a normal speaking rate.[8,15]

Two-Person Bag-Mask Ventilation

A 2-person technique may be more effective than ventilation by a single rescuer if the patient has significant airway obstruction, poor lung compliance, or difficulty in creating a tight mask-to-face seal.[16,17] One rescuer uses both hands to maintain an open airway with a jaw thrust and a tight mask-to-face seal while the other compresses the ventilation bag. Both rescuers should observe the victim's chest to ensure chest rise.

Gastric Inflation

Gastric inflation may interfere with effective ventilation[18] and cause regurgitation. You can minimize gastric inflation by doing the following:

- Avoid excessive peak inspiratory pressures (eg, by ventilating slowly and watching chest rise).[8] To avoid use of excessive volume, deliver only the volume needed to produce visible chest rise.
- Apply cricoid pressure. You should do so only in an unresponsive victim. This technique may require an additional (third) rescuer if the cricoid pressure cannot be applied by the rescuer who is securing the bag to the face.[19–21] Avoid excessive pressure so as not to obstruct the trachea.[22]
- If you intubate the patient, pass a nasogastric or orogastric tube *after* you intubate because a gastric tube interferes with the gastroesophageal sphincter, allowing possible regurgitation.

Ventilation Through an Endotracheal Tube

Endotracheal intubation in infants and children requires special training because the pediatric airway anatomy differs from adult airway anatomy. Success and a low complication rate are related to the length of training, supervised experience in the operating room and in the field,[23,24] adequate ongoing experience,[25] and the use of rapid sequence intubation (RSI).[23,26,27]

Rapid Sequence Intubation

To facilitate emergency intubation and reduce the incidence of complications, skilled, experienced providers may use sedatives, neuromuscular blocking agents, and other medications to rapidly sedate and paralyze the victim.[28] Use RSI only if you are trained and have experience using these medications and are proficient in the evaluation and management of the pediatric airway. If you use RSI you must have a secondary plan to manage the airway in the event that you cannot achieve intubation.

Cuffed Versus Uncuffed Tubes

In the in-hospital setting a cuffed endotracheal tube is as safe as an uncuffed tube for infants beyond the newborn period and in children.[29–31] In certain circumstances (eg, poor lung compliance, high airway resistance, or a large glottic air leak) a cuffed tube may be preferable provided that attention is paid to endotracheal tube size, position, and cuff inflation pressure (Class IIa; LOE 2[30]; 3[29,31]). Keep cuff inflation pressure <20 cm H_2O.[32]

Endotracheal Tube Size

The internal diameter of the appropriate endotracheal tube for a child will roughly equal the size of that child's little finger, but this estimation may be difficult and unreliable.[33,34] Several formulas such as the ones below allow estimation of proper endotracheal tube size (ID, internal diameter) for children 1 to 10 years of age, based on the child's age:

Uncuffed endotracheal tube size (mm ID)
=(age in years/4) + 4

In general, during preparation for intubation using the above formula, providers should have the estimated tube size available, as well as uncuffed endotracheal tubes that have internal diameters that are 0.5 mm smaller and 0.5 mm larger than the size estimated ready at the bedside for use.

The formula for estimation of a cuffed endotracheal tube size is as follows[30]:

Cuffed endotracheal tube size (mm ID)
= (age in years/4) + 3

Endotracheal tube size, however, is more reliably based on a child's *body length.* Length-based resuscitation tapes are helpful for children up to approximately 35 kg.[35]

Verification of Endotracheal Tube Placement

There is a high risk that an endotracheal tube will be misplaced (ie, placed in the esophagus or in the pharynx above the vocal chords), displaced, or become obstructed,[8,36] especially when the patient is moved.[37] No single confirmation technique, including clinical signs[38] or the presence of water vapor in the tube,[39] is completely reliable, so providers must use both clinical assessment and confirmatory devices to verify proper tube placement immediately after intubation, during transport, and when the patient is moved (ie, from gurney to bed).

Immediately after intubation and again after securing the tube, confirm correct tube position with the following techniques while you provide positive-pressure ventilation with a bag:

- Look for bilateral chest movement and listen for equal breath sounds over both lung fields, especially over the axillae.
- Listen for gastric insufflation sounds over the stomach (they should not be present if the tube is in the trachea).[38]
- Use a device to evaluate placement. Check for exhaled CO_2 (see below) if there is a perfusing rhythm. If the child has a perfusing rhythm and is >20 kg, you may use an esophageal detector device to check for evidence of esophageal placement (see below).
- Check oxygen saturation with a pulse oximeter. Following hyperoxygenation, the oxyhemoglobin saturation detected by pulse oximetry may not demonstrate a fall indicative of incorrect endotracheal tube position (ie, tube misplacement or displacement) for as long as 3 minutes.[40,41]
- If you are still uncertain, perform direct laryngoscopy and look to see if the tube goes between the cords.
- In hospital settings perform a chest x-ray to verify that the tube is not in the right main bronchus and to identify a high tube position at risk of easy displacement.

After intubation secure the tube. There is insufficient evidence to recommend any one method (Class Indeterminate). After you secure the tube, maintain the patient's head in a neutral position; neck flexion pushes the tube farther into the airway, and extension pulls the tube out of the airway.[42,43]

If an intubated patient's condition deteriorates, consider the following possibilities (**DOPE**):

- **D**isplacement of the tube from the trachea
- **O**bstruction of the tube
- **P**neumothorax
- **E**quipment failure

Exhaled or End-Tidal CO_2 Monitoring

In infants and children with a perfusing rhythm, use a colorimetric detector or capnography to detect exhaled CO_2 to confirm endotracheal tube position in the prehospital and in-hospital settings (Class IIa; LOE 5[44]) and during intrahospital and interhospital transport (Class IIb; LOE 5[45]). A color change or the presence of a capnography waveform confirms tube position in the trachea but does not rule out right main bronchus intubation. During cardiac arrest, if exhaled CO_2 is not detected, confirm tube position with direct laryngoscopy (Class IIa; LOE 5[46–49]; 6[50]) because the absence of CO_2 may be a reflection of low pulmonary blood flow.

You may also detect a low end-tidal CO_2 in the following circumstances:

- If the detector is contaminated with gastric contents or acidic drugs (eg, endotracheally administered epinephrine), you may see a constant color rather than breath-to-breath color change.
- An intravenous (IV) bolus of epinephrine may transiently reduce pulmonary blood flow and exhaled CO_2 below the limits of detection.[51]
- Severe airway obstruction (eg, status asthmaticus) and pulmonary edema may impair CO_2 elimination.[49,52–54]

Esophageal Detector Devices

The self-inflating bulb (esophageal detector device) may be considered to confirm endotracheal tube placement in children weighing >20 kg with a perfusing rhythm (Class IIb; LOE 2[55,56]). There is insufficient data to make a recommendation for or against its use in children during cardiac arrest (Class Indeterminate).

Transtracheal Catheter Ventilation

Transtracheal catheter ventilation may be considered for support of oxygenation in the patient with severe airway obstruction if you cannot provide oxygen or ventilation any other way. Try transtracheal ventilation only if you are properly trained and have appropriate equipment.[57]

Suction Devices

A suction device with an adjustable suction regulator should be available. Use a maximum suction force of 80 to 120 mm Hg for suctioning the airway via an endotracheal tube.[58] You will need higher suction pressures and large-bore noncollapsible suction tubing as well as semirigid pharyngeal tips to suction the mouth and pharynx.

Circulation

Advanced cardiovascular life support techniques are useless without effective circulation, which is supported by good chest compressions during cardiac arrest. Good chest compressions require an adequate compression rate (100 compressions per minute), an adequate compression depth (about one third to one half of the anterior-posterior diameter), full recoil of the chest after each compression, and minimal interruptions in compressions. Unfortunately, good compressions are not always performed for many reasons,[14] including rescuer fatigue and long or frequent interruptions to secure the airway, check the heart rhythm, and move the patient.

Backboard

A firm surface that extends from the shoulders to the waist and across the full width of the bed provides optimal support for effective chest compressions. In ambulances and mobile life support units, use a spine board.[59,60]

CPR Techniques and Adjuncts

There is insufficient data to make a recommendation for or against the use of mechanical devices to compress the sternum, active compression-decompression CPR, interposed abdominal compression CPR, pneumatic antishock garment during resuscitation from cardiac arrest, and open-chest direct heart compression (Class Indeterminate). For further information see Part 6: "CPR Techniques and Devices."

Extracorporeal Membrane Oxygenation

Consider extracorporeal CPR for in-hospital cardiac arrest refractory to initial resuscitation attempts if the condition leading to cardiac arrest is reversible or amenable to heart transplantation, if excellent conventional CPR has been performed after no more than several minutes of no-flow cardiac arrest (arrest time without CPR), and if the institution is able to rapidly perform extracorporeal membrane oxygenation (Class IIb; LOE 5[61,62]). Long-term survival is possible even after >50 minutes of CPR in selected patients.[61,62]

Cardiovascular Monitoring

Attach electrocardiographic (ECG) monitoring leads or defibrillator pads as soon as possible and monitor blood pressure. If the patient has an indwelling arterial catheter, use the waveform to guide your technique in compressing the chest. A minor adjustment of your hand position or depth of compression can significantly improve the waveform.

Vascular Access

Vascular access is essential for administering medications and drawing blood samples. Venous access can be challenging in infants and children during an emergency, whereas intraosseous (IO) access can be easily achieved. Limit the time you attempt venous access,[63] and if you cannot achieve reliable access quickly, establish IO access. In cardiac arrest immediate IO access is recommended if no other IV access is already in place.

Intraosseous Access

IO access is a rapid, safe, and effective route for the administration of medications and fluids,[64,65] and it may be used for obtaining an initial blood sample during resuscitation (Class IIa; LOE 3[65,66]). You can safely administer epinephrine, adenosine, fluids, blood products,[64,66] and catecholamines.[67] Onset of action and drug levels achieved are comparable to venous administration.[68] You can also obtain blood specimens for type and crossmatch and for chemical and blood gas analysis even during cardiac arrest,[69] but acid-base analysis is inaccurate after sodium bicarbonate administration via the IO cannula.[70] Use manual pressure or an infusion pump to administer viscous drugs or rapid fluid boluses,[71,72] and follow each medication with a saline flush to promote entry into the central circulation.

Venous Access

A central intravenous line (IV) provides more secure long-term access, but central drug administration does not achieve higher drug levels or a substantially more rapid response than peripheral administration.[73]

Endotracheal Drug Administration

Any vascular access, IO or IV, is preferable, but if you cannot establish vascular access, you can give lipid-soluble drugs such as lidocaine, epinephrine, atropine, and naloxone ("LEAN")[74,75] via the endotracheal tube,[76] although optimal endotracheal doses are unknown (Table 1). Flush with a minimum of 5 mL normal saline followed by 5 assisted manual ventilations.[77] If CPR is in progress, stop chest compressions briefly during administration of medications. Although naloxone and vasopressin may be given by the endotracheal route, there are no human studies to support a specific dose. Non–lipid-soluble drugs (eg, sodium bicarbonate and calcium) may injure the airway and should not be administered via the endotracheal route.

Administration of resuscitation drugs into the trachea results in lower blood concentrations than the same dose given intravascularly. Furthermore, recent animal studies suggest that the lower epinephrine concentrations achieved when the drug is delivered by the endotracheal route may produce transient β-adrenergic effects. These effects can be detrimental, causing hypotension, lower coronary artery perfusion pressure and flow, and reduced potential for return of spontaneous circulation. Thus, although endotracheal administration of some resuscitation drugs is possible, IV or IO drug administration is preferred because it will provide a more predictable drug delivery and pharmacologic effect.

Emergency Fluids and Medications

Estimating Weight

In the out-of-hospital setting a child's weight is often unknown, and even experienced personnel may not be able to estimate it accurately.[78] Tapes with precalculated doses printed at various patient lengths are helpful and have been clinically validated.[35,78,79] Hospitalized patients should have weights and precalculated emergency drug doses recorded and readily available.

Fluids

Use an isotonic crystalloid solution (eg, lactated Ringer's solution or normal saline)[80,81] to treat shock; there is no benefit in using colloid (eg, albumin) during initial resuscitation.[82] Use bolus therapy with a glucose-containing solution to only treat documented hypoglycemia (Class IIb; LOE 2[83]; 6[84]). There is insufficient data to make a recommendation for

TABLE 1. Medications for Pediatric Resuscitation and Arrhythmias

Medication	Dose	Remarks
Adenosine	0.1 mg/kg (maximum 6 mg) Repeat: 0.2 mg/kg (maximum 12 mg)	Monitor ECG Rapid IV/IO bolus
Amiodarone	5 mg/kg IV/IO; repeat up to 15 mg/kg Maximum: 300 mg	Monitor ECG and blood pressure Adjust administration rate to urgency (give more slowly when perfusing rhythm present) Use caution when administering with other drugs that prolong QT (consider expert consultation)
Atropine	0.02 mg/kg IV/IO 0.03 mg/kg ET* Repeat once if needed Minimum dose: 0.1 mg Maximum single dose: Child 0.5 mg Adolescent 1 mg	Higher doses may be used with organophosphate poisoning
Calcium chloride (10%)	20 mg/kg IV/IO (0.2 mL/kg)	Slowly Adult dose: 5–10 mL
Epinephrine	0.01 mg/kg (0.1 mL/kg 1:10 000) IV/IO 0.1 mg/kg (0.1 mL/kg 1:1000) ET* Maximum dose: 1 mg IV/IO; 10 mg ET	May repeat q 3–5 min
Glucose	0.5–1 g/kg IV/IO	$D_{10}W$: 5–10 mL/kg $D_{25}W$: 2–4 mL/kg $D_{50}W$: 1–2 mL/kg
Lidocaine	Bolus: 1 mg/kg IV/IO Maximum dose: 100 mg Infusion: 20–50 μg/kg per minute ET*: 2–3 mg	
Magnesium sulfate	25–50 mg/kg IV/IO over 10–20 min; faster in torsades Maximum dose: 2g	
Naloxone	$<$5 y or $\leq$20 kg: 0.1 mg/kg IV/IO/ET* $\geq$5 y or $>$20 kg: 2 mg IV/IO/ET*	Use lower doses to reverse respiratory depression associated with therapeutic opioid use (1–15 μg/kg)
Procainamide	15 mg/kg IV/IO over 30–60 min Adult dose: 20 mg/min IV infusion up to total maximum dose 17 mg/kg	Monitor ECG and blood pressure Use caution when administering with other drugs that prolong QT (consider expert consultation)
Sodium bicarbonate	1 mEq/kg per dose IV/IO slowly	After adequate ventilation

IV indicates intravenous; IO, intraosseous; and ET, via endotracheal tube.
*Flush with 5 mL of normal saline and follow with 5 ventilations.

or against hypertonic saline for shock associated with head injuries or hypovolemia (Class Indeterminate).[85,86]

Medications (See Table 1)

Adenosine

Adenosine causes a temporary atrioventricular (AV) nodal conduction block and interrupts reentry circuits that involve the AV node. It has a wide safety margin because of its short half-life.

A higher dose may be required for peripheral administration than central venous administration.[87,88] Based on experimental data[89] and a case report,[90] adenosine may also be given by IO route. Administer adenosine and follow with a rapid saline flush to promote flow toward the central circulation.

Amiodarone

Amiodarone slows AV conduction, prolongs the AV refractory period and QT interval, and slows ventricular conduction (widens the QRS).

Precautions

Monitor blood pressure and administer as slowly as the patient's clinical condition allows; it should be administered slowly to a patient with a pulse but may be given rapidly to a patient with cardiac arrest or ventricular fibrillation (VF). Amiodarone causes hypotension through its vasodilatory property. The severity of the hypotension is related to the infusion rate and is less common with the aqueous form of amiodarone.[91]

Monitor the ECG because complications may include bradycardia, heart block, and torsades de pointes ventricular tachycardia (VT). Use extreme caution when administering with another drug causing QT prolongation, such as procainamide. Consider obtaining expert consultation. Adverse effects may be long lasting because the half-life is up to 40 days.[92]

Atropine

Atropine sulfate is a parasympatholytic drug that accelerates sinus or atrial pacemakers and increases AV conduction.

Precautions
Small doses of atropine (<0.1 mg) may produce paradoxical bradycardia.[93] Larger than recommended doses may be required in special circumstances (eg, organophosphate poisoning[94] or exposure to nerve gas agents).

Calcium
Routine administration of calcium does not improve outcome of cardiac arrest.[95] In critically ill children, calcium chloride may provide greater bioavailability than calcium gluconate.[96] Preferably administer calcium chloride via a central venous catheter because of the risk of sclerosis or infiltration with a peripheral venous line.

Epinephrine
The α-adrenergic-mediated vasoconstriction of epinephrine increases aortic diastolic pressure and thus coronary perfusion pressure, a critical determinant of successful resuscitation.[97,98]

Precautions
Administer all catecholamines through a secure line, preferably into the central circulation; local ischemia, tissue injury, and ulceration may result from tissue infiltration.

Do not mix catecholamines with sodium bicarbonate; alkaline solutions inactivate them.

In patients with a perfusing rhythm, epinephrine causes tachycardia and may cause ventricular ectopy, tachyarrhythmias, hypertension, and vasoconstriction.[99]

Glucose
Infants have high glucose requirements and low glycogen stores and develop hypoglycemia when energy requirements rise.[100] Check blood glucose concentrations during and after arrest and treat hypoglycemia promptly (Class IIb; LOE 1[101]; 7 [most extrapolated from neonates and adult ICU studies]).

Lidocaine
Lidocaine decreases automaticity and suppresses ventricular arrhythmias[102] but is not as effective as amiodarone for improving intermediate outcomes (ie, return of spontaneous circulation or survival to hospital admission) among adult patients with VF refractory to a shock and epinephrine.[103] Neither lidocaine nor amiodarone has been shown to improve survival to hospital discharge among patients with VF cardiac arrest.

Precautions
Lidocaine toxicity includes myocardial and circulatory depression, drowsiness, disorientation, muscle twitching, and seizures, especially in patients with poor cardiac output and hepatic or renal failure.[104,105]

Magnesium
There is insufficient evidence to recommend for or against the routine administration of magnesium during cardiac arrest (Class Indeterminate).[106–108] Magnesium is indicated for the treatment of documented hypomagnesemia or for torsades de pointes (polymorphic VT associated with long QT interval). Magnesium produces vasodilation and may cause hypotension if administered rapidly.

Procainamide
Procainamide prolongs the refractory period of the atria and ventricles and depresses conduction velocity.

Precautions
There is little clinical data on using procainamide in infants and children.[109,110] Infuse procainamide very slowly while you monitor for hypotension, prolongation of the QT interval, and heart block. Stop the infusion if the QRS widens to >50% of baseline or if hypotension develops. Use extreme caution when administering with another drug causing QT prolongation, such as amiodarone. Consider obtaining expert consultation.

Sodium Bicarbonate
The routine administration of sodium bicarbonate has not been shown to improve outcome of resuscitation (Class Indeterminate). After you have provided effective ventilation and chest compressions and administered epinephrine, you may consider sodium bicarbonate for prolonged cardiac arrest (Class IIb; LOE 6). Sodium bicarbonate administration may be used for treatment of some toxidromes (see "Toxicologic Emergencies," below) or special resuscitation situations.

During cardiac arrest or severe shock, arterial blood gas analysis may not accurately reflect tissue and venous acidosis.[111,112]

Precautions
Excessive sodium bicarbonate may impair tissue oxygen delivery[113]; cause hypokalemia, hypocalcemia, hypernatremia, and hyperosmolality[114,115]; decrease the VF threshold[116]; and impair cardiac function.

Vasopressin
There is limited experience with the use of vasopressin in pediatric patients,[117] and the results of its use in the treatment of adults with VF cardiac arrest have been inconsistent.[118–121] There is insufficient evidence to make a recommendation for or against the routine use of vasopressin during cardiac arrest (Class Indeterminate; LOE 5[117]; 6[121], 7[118–120] [extrapolated from adult literature]).

Pulseless Arrest

In the text below, box numbers identify the corresponding box in the algorithm (Figure 1.)

If a victim becomes unresponsive (Box 1), start CPR immediately (with supplementary oxygen if available) and send for a defibrillator (manual or automated external defibrillator [AED]). Asystole and bradycardia with a wide QRS complex are most common in asphyxial cardiac arrest.[1,23] VF and pulseless electrical activity (PEA) are less common[122] and more likely to be observed in children with sudden arrest. If you are using an ECG monitor, determine the rhythm (Box 2); if you are using an AED, the device will tell you whether the rhythm is "shockable" (ie, VF or rapid VT), but it may not display the rhythm.

"Shockable Rhythm": VF/Pulseless VT (Box 3)

VF occurs in 5% to 15% of all pediatric victims of out-of-hospital cardiac arrest[123–125] and is reported in up to 20% of

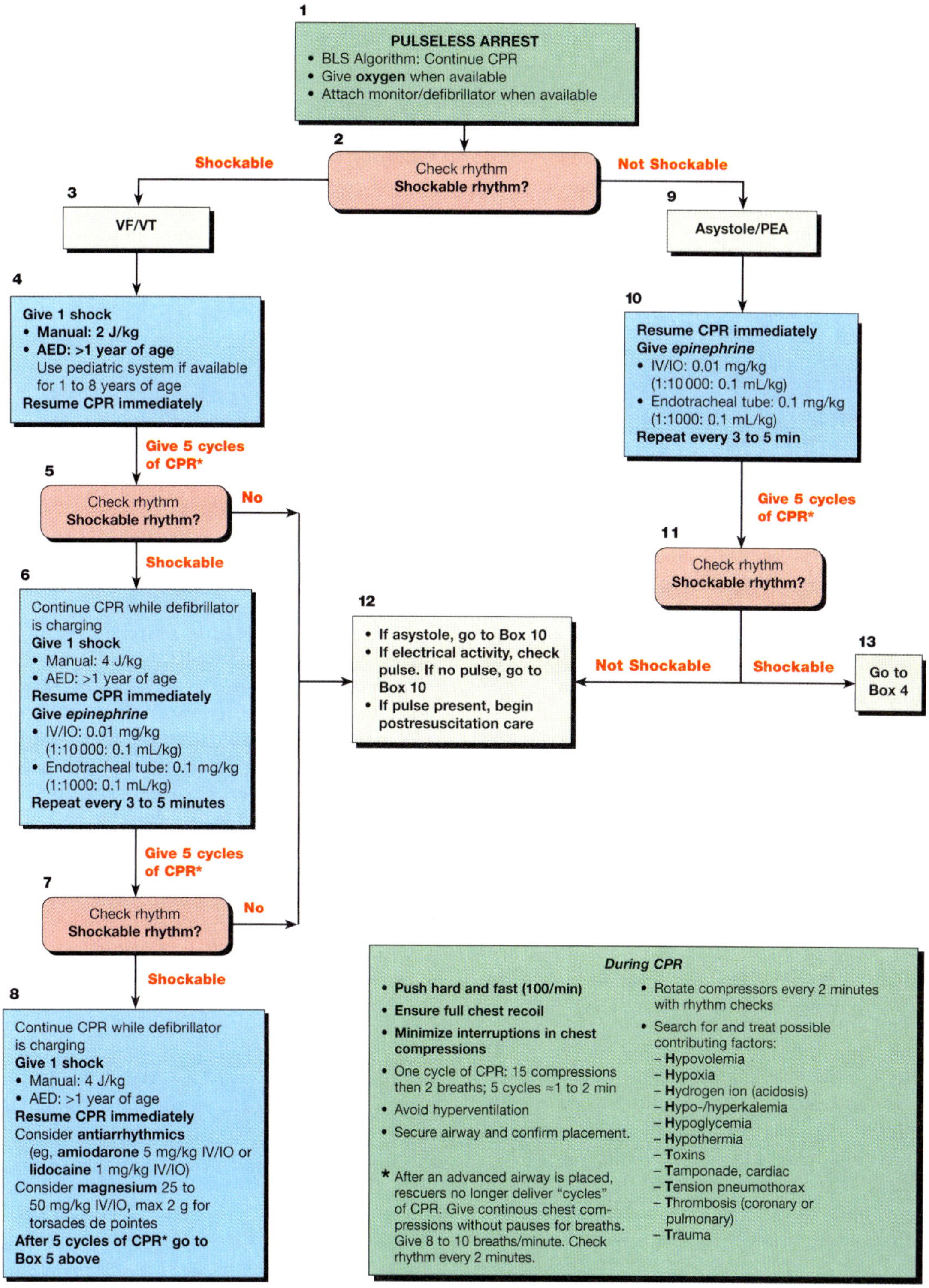

Figure 1. PALS Pulseless Arrest Algorithm.

pediatric in-hospital arrests at some point during the resuscitation. The incidence increases with age.[123,125] Defibrillation is the definitive treatment for VF (Class I) with an overall survival rate of 17% to 20%,[125–127] but in adults the probability of survival declines by 7% to 10% for each minute of arrest without CPR and defibrillation.[128] The decline in survival is more gradual when early CPR is provided.

Defibrillators

Defibrillators are either manual or automated (AED), with monophasic or biphasic waveforms. For further information see Part 5: "Electrical Therapies: Automated External Defibrillators, Defibrillation, Cardioversion, and Pacing."

Institutions that care for children at risk for arrhythmias and cardiac arrest (eg, hospitals, emergency departments) ideally should have defibrillators available that are capable of energy adjustment that is appropriate for children. Many AED parameters are set automatically. When using a manual defibrillator, several elements should be considered, and they are highlighted below.

Paddle Size
Use the largest paddles or self-adhering electrodes[129–131] that will fit on the chest wall without touching (leave about 3 cm between the paddles). The best paddle size is

- Adult paddles (8 to 10 cm) for children >10 kg (more than approximately 1 year of age)
- Infant paddles for infants weighing <10 kg

Interface
The electrode–chest wall interface can be gel pads, electrode cream, paste, or self-adhesive monitoring-defibrillation pads. Do not use saline-soaked pads, ultrasound gel, bare paddles, or alcohol pads.

Paddle Position
Apply firm pressure on the paddles (manual) placed over the right side of the upper chest and the apex of the heart (to the left of the nipple over the left lower ribs). Alternatively place one electrode on the front of the chest just to the left of the sternum and the other over the upper back below the scapula.[132]

Energy Dose
The lowest energy dose for effective defibrillation and the upper limit for safe defibrillation in infants and children are not known. Energy doses >4 J/kg (up to 9 J/kg) have effectively defibrillated children[133–135] and pediatric animal models[136] with negligible adverse effects. Based on data from adult studies[137,138] and pediatric animal models,[139–141] biphasic shocks appear to be at least as effective as monophasic shocks and less harmful. With a manual defibrillator (monophasic or biphasic), use a dose of 2 J/kg for the first attempt (Class IIa; LOE 5[142]; 6[136]) and 4 J/kg for subsequent attempts (Class Indeterminate).

AEDs
Many AEDs can accurately detect VF in children of all ages[143–145] and differentiate shockable from nonshockable rhythms with a high degree of sensitivity and specificity.[143,144] Since publication of the *ECC Guidelines 2000*, data has shown that AEDs can be safely and effectively used in children 1 to 8 years of age.[143–146] There is insufficient data to make a recommendation for or against using an AED in infants <1 year of age (Class Indeterminate).[146] When using an AED for children about 1 to 8 years old, use a pediatric attenuator system, which decreases the delivered energy to a dose suitable for children (Class IIb; LOE 5[136]; 6[139,141]). If an AED with a pediatric attenuating system is not available, use a standard AED, preferably one with sensitivity and specificity for pediatric shockable rhythms. It is recommended that systems and institutions caring for children and having AED programs should use AEDs with both a high specificity to recognize pediatric shockable rhythms and a pediatric attenuating system.

Defibrillation Sequence (Boxes 4, 5, 6, 7, 8)
The following are important considerations:

- Attempt defibrillation immediately. The earlier you attempt defibrillation, the more likely the attempt will be successful.
- Provide CPR until the defibrillator is ready to deliver a shock, and resume CPR, beginning with chest compressions, immediately after shock delivery. Minimize interruptions of chest compressions. In adults with a prolonged arrest[147,148] and animal models,[134,149] defibrillation is more likely to be successful after a period of effective chest compressions. Ideally, chest compressions should be interrupted only for ventilations (until an advanced airway is in place), rhythm check, and shock delivery. Rescuers should provide chest compressions after a rhythm check (when possible) while the defibrillator is charging.
- Give 1 shock (2 J/kg) as quickly as possible and immediately resume CPR, beginning with chest compressions (Box 4). Biphasic defibrillators have a first shock success rate that exceeds 90%.[150] If 1 shock fails to eliminate VF, the incremental benefit of another shock is low, and resumption of CPR is likely to confer a greater value than another shock. CPR may provide some coronary perfusion with oxygen and substrate delivery, increasing the likelihood of defibrillation with a subsequent shock. It is important to minimize the time between any interruption in chest compressions and shock delivery and between shock delivery and resumption of postshock compressions. Check the rhythm (Box 5). Continue CPR for about 5 cycles (about 2 minutes). In in-hospital settings with continuous monitoring (eg, electrocardiographic, hemodynamic) in place, this sequence may be modified at the physician's discretion (see Part 7.2: "Management of Cardiac Arrest").
- Check the rhythm (Box 5). If a shockable rhythm persists, give 1 shock (4 J/kg), resume compressions immediately. Give a dose of epinephrine. The drug should be administered as soon as possible after the rhythm check. It is helpful if a third rescuer prepares the drug doses *before* the rhythm is checked so a drug can be administered as soon as possible after the rhythm is checked. A drug should be administered during the CPR that is performed while the defibrillator is charging or immediately after shock delivery. However, the timing of drug administration is less important than the need to minimize interruptions in chest compressions.

  Use a standard dose of epinephrine for the first and subsequent doses (Class IIa; LOE 4).[151] There is no survival benefit from routine use of high-dose epinephrine, and it may be harmful, particularly in asphyxia (Class III; LOE 2, 4).[151] High-dose epinephrine may be considered in exceptional circumstances, such as β-blocker overdose (Class IIb). Give the standard dose of epinephrine about every 3 to 5 minutes during cardiac arrest.
- After 5 cycles (approximately 2 minutes) of CPR, check the rhythm (Box 7). If the rhythm continues to be "shockable," deliver a shock (4 J/kg), resume CPR (beginning with chest compressions) immediately, and give amiodarone (Class IIb; LOE 3, 7)[103, 152–154] or lidocaine if you

do not have amiodarone (Box 8) while CPR is provided. Continue CPR for 5 cycles (about 2 minutes) before again checking the rhythm and attempting to defibrillate if needed with 4 J/kg (you now have returned to Box 6).

- Once an advanced airway is in place, 2 rescuers no longer deliver cycles of CPR (ie, compressions interrupted by pauses for ventilation). Instead, the compressing rescuer should give continuous chest compressions at a rate of 100 per minute without pauses for ventilation. The rescuer delivering ventilation provides 8 to 10 breaths per minute. Two or more rescuers should rotate the compressor role approximately every 2 minutes to prevent compressor fatigue and deterioration in quality and rate of chest compressions.
- If you have a monitor or an AED with a rhythm display and there is an organized rhythm at any time, check for a pulse and proceed accordingly (Box 12).
- If defibrillation is successful but VF recurs, continue CPR while you give another bolus of amiodarone before you try to defibrillate with the previously successful shock dose (see Box 8).
- Search for and treat reversible causes (see green "During CPR" box).

Torsades de Pointes

This polymorphic VT is seen in patients with a long QT interval, which may be congenital or may result from toxicity with type I_A antiarrhythmics (eg, procainamide, quinidine, and disopyramide) or type III antiarrhythmics (eg, sotalol and amiodarone), tricyclic antidepressants (see below), digitalis, or drug interactions.[155,156] These are examples of contributing factors listed in the green box in the algorithm.

Treatment

Regardless of the cause, treat torsades de pointes with a rapid (over several minutes) IV infusion of magnesium sulfate.

"Nonshockable Rhythm": Asystole/PEA (Box 9)

The most common ECG findings in infants and children in cardiac arrest are asystole and PEA. PEA is organized electrical activity—most commonly slow, wide QRS complexes—without palpable pulses. Less frequently there is a sudden impairment of cardiac output with an initially normal rhythm but without pulses and with poor perfusion. This subcategory (formerly known as electromechanical dissociation [EMD]) is more likely to be treatable. For asystole and PEA:

- Resume CPR and continue with as few interruptions in chest compressions as possible (Box 10). A second rescuer gives epinephrine while the first continues CPR. As with VF/pulseless VT, there is no survival benefit from routine high-dose epinephrine, and it may be harmful, particularly in asphyxia (Class III; LOE 2[151]; 6[99,157,158]; 7[159]). Use a standard dose for the first and subsequent doses (Class IIa; LOE 4).[151] High-dose epinephrine may be considered in exceptional circumstances such as β-blocker overdose (Class IIb).
- Search for and treat reversible causes (see the green box).

Bradycardia

Box numbers in the text below refer to the corresponding boxes in the PALS Bradycardia Algorithm (Figure 2).

The emergency treatment of bradycardia depends on its hemodynamic consequences.

- This algorithm applies to the care of the patient with bradycardia that is causing cardiorespiratory compromise (Box 1). If at any time the patient develops pulseless arrest, see the PALS Pulseless Arrest Algorithm.
- Support airway, breathing, and circulation as needed, administer oxygen, and attach a monitor/defibrillator (Box 2).
- Reassess the patient to determine if bradycardia is still causing cardiorespiratory symptoms despite support of adequate oxygenation and ventilation (Box 3).
- If pulses, perfusion, and respirations are normal, no emergency treatment is necessary. Monitor and proceed with evaluation (Box 5A).
- If heart rate is <60 beats per minute with poor perfusion despite effective ventilation with oxygen, start chest compressions (Box 6).
- Reevaluate the patient to determine if signs of hemodynamic compromise persist despite the support of adequate oxygenation and ventilation and compressions if indicated (Box 5). Verify that the support is adequate—eg, check airway and oxygen source and effectiveness of ventilation.
- Medications and pacing (Box 6)
  —Continue to support airway, ventilation, oxygenation (and provide compressions as needed) and give epinephrine (Class IIa; LOE 7, 8). If bradycardia persists or responds only transiently, consider a continuous infusion of epinephrine or isoproterenol.
  —If bradycardia is due to vagal stimulation, give atropine (Class I) (Box 6). Emergency transcutaneous pacing may be lifesaving if the bradycardia is due to complete heart block or sinus node dysfunction unresponsive to ventilation, oxygenation, chest compressions, and medications, especially if it is associated with congenital or acquired heart disease (Class IIb; LOE 5, 7).[160] Pacing is not useful for asystole[160,161] or bradycardia due to postarrest hypoxic/ischemic myocardial insult or respiratory failure.

Tachycardia and Hemodynamic Instability

The box numbers in the text below correspond to the numbered boxes in the Tachycardia Algorithm (Figure 3)

If there are no palpable pulses, proceed with the PALS Pulseless Arrest Algorithm. If pulses are palpable and the patient has signs of hemodynamic compromise (poor perfusion, tachypnea, weak pulses), ensure that the airway is patent, assist ventilations if necessary, administer supplementary oxygen, and attach an ECG monitor or defibrillator (Box 1). Assess QRS duration (Box 2): determine if the QRS duration is ≤0.08 second (narrow-complex tachycardia) or >0.08 second (wide-complex tachycardia).

Narrow-Complex (≤0.08 Second) Tachycardia

Evaluation of a 12-lead ECG (Box 3) and the patient's clinical presentation and history (Boxes 4 and 5) should help

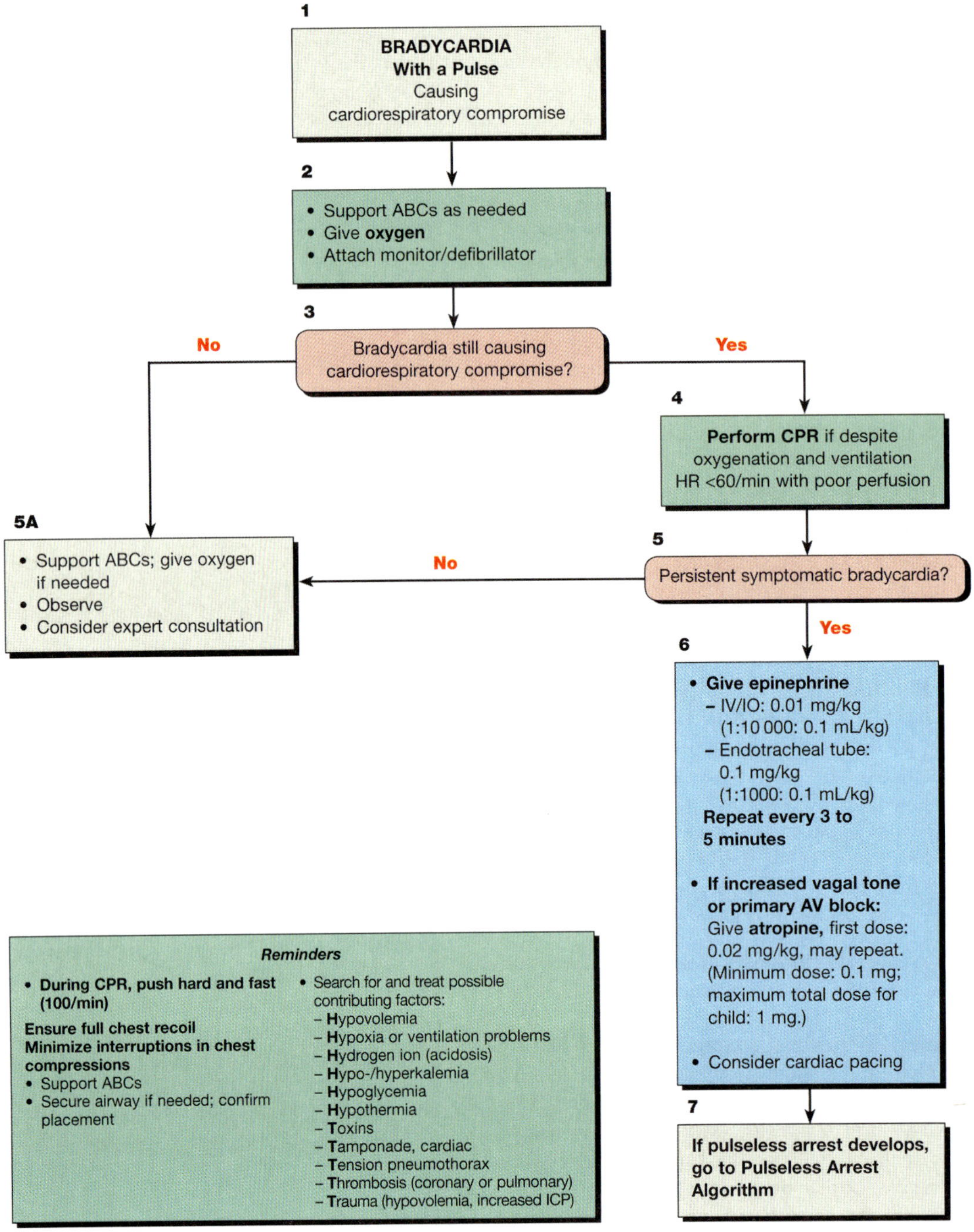

Figure 2. PALS Bradycardia Algorithm.

you differentiate probable sinus tachycardia from probable supraventricular tachycardia (SVT). If the rhythm is sinus tachycardia, search for and treat reversible causes.

Probable Supraventricular Tachycardia (Box 5)

Monitor rhythm during therapy to evaluate effect. The choice of therapy depends on the patient's degree of hemodynamic instability.

- Attempt *vagal stimulation* (Box 7) first unless the patient is very unstable and if it does not unduly delay chemical or electrical cardioversion (Class IIa; LOE 4, 5, 7, 8). In infants and young children, apply ice to the face without occluding the airway.[162,163] In older children, carotid sinus massage or Valsalva maneuvers are safe (Class IIb; LOE 5, 7).[164–166] One method of a Valsalva maneuver is to have the child blow through an obstructed straw.[165] Do not apply pressure to the eye because this can damage the retina.
- Chemical cardioversion with adenosine (Box 8) is very effective (Class IIa; LOE 2[87]; 3[88]; 7 [extrapolation from adult studies]). If IV access is readily available administer adenosine using 2 syringes connected to a T-connector or stopcock; give adenosine rapidly with one syringe and immediately flush with ≥5 mL of normal saline with the other.

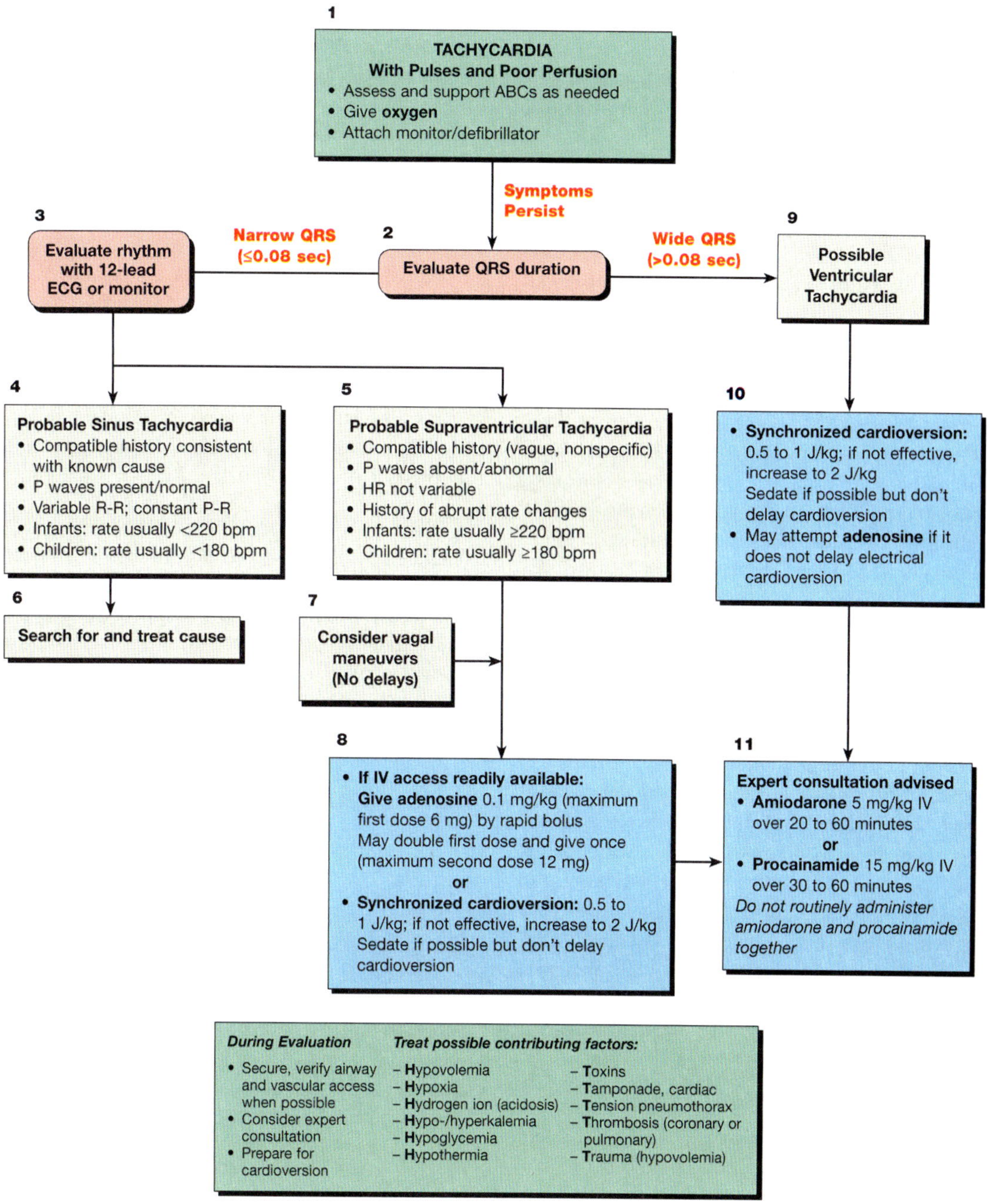

Figure 3. PALS Tachycardia Algorithm.

- If the patient is very unstable or IV access is not readily available, provide electrical (synchronized) cardioversion (Box 8). Consider sedation if possible. Start with a dose of 0.5 to 1 J/kg. If unsuccessful, repeat using a dose of 2 J/kg. If a second shock is unsuccessful or the tachycardia recurs quickly, consider antiarrhythmic therapy (amiodarone or procainamide) before a third shock.
- Consider amiodarone or procainamide (Box 11) for SVT unresponsive to vagal maneuvers and adenosine (Class IIb; 5[153, 154]; 6[167–169]; 7 [extrapolated from LOE 2 adult studies][103,152]). Use extreme caution when administering more than one drug that causes QT prolongation (eg, amiodarone and procainamide). Consider obtaining expert consultation. Give an infusion of amiodarone or procainamide slowly (over several minutes to an hour), depending on the urgency, while you monitor the ECG and blood pressure. If there is no effect and there are no signs of toxicity, give additional doses (Table 1).
- Do not use verapamil in infants because it may cause refractory hypotension and cardiac arrest (Class III; LOE 5[170,171]), and use with caution in children because it may cause hypotension and myocardial depression.[172]

Wide-Complex (>0.08 Second) Tachycardia (Box 9)

Wide-complex tachycardia with poor perfusion is probably ventricular in origin but may be supraventricular with aberrancy.[173]

- Treat with synchronized electrical cardioversion (0.5 J to 1 J/kg). If it does not delay cardioversion, try a dose of adenosine first to determine if the rhythm is SVT with aberrant conduction (Box 10).

- If a second shock (2 J/kg) is unsuccessful or if the tachycardia recurs quickly, consider antiarrhythmic therapy (amiodarone or procainamide) before a third shock (see above) (Box 11).

Tachycardia With Hemodynamic Stability

Because all arrhythmia therapies have the potential for serious adverse effects, consider consulting an expert in pediatric arrhythmias before treating children who are hemodynamically stable.

- For SVT, see above.
- For VT, give an infusion of amiodarone slowly (minutes to an hour depending on the urgency) (Class IIb; LOE 7 [extrapolated from adult studies]) while you monitor the ECG and blood pressure. If there is no effect and there are no signs of toxicity, give additional doses (Table 1). If amiodarone is not available, consider giving procainamide slowly (over 30 to 60 minutes) while you monitor the ECG and blood pressure (Class IIb; LOE 5, 6, 7). Do not administer amiodarone and procainamide together without expert consultation.

Special Resuscitation Situations

Trauma

Some aspects of trauma resuscitation require emphasis because improperly performed resuscitation is a major cause of preventable pediatric death.[174] Common errors in pediatric trauma resuscitation include failure to open and maintain the airway, failure to provide appropriate fluid resuscitation, and failure to recognize and treat internal bleeding. Involve a qualified surgeon early, and if possible, transport a child with multisystem trauma to a trauma center with pediatric expertise.

The following are special aspects of trauma resuscitation:

- When the mechanism of injury is compatible with spinal injury, restrict motion of the cervical spine and avoid traction or movement of the head and neck. Open and maintain the airway with a jaw thrust, and do not tilt the head.

  If you cannot open the airway with a jaw thrust, use head tilt–chin lift, because you must establish a patent airway. Because of the disproportionately large head size in infants and young children, optimal positioning may require recessing the occiput[60] or elevating the torso to avoid undesirable backboard-induced cervical flexion.[59,60]
- Do not overventilate (Class III; LOE 3[175]; 5, 6) even in case of head injury.[176] Intentional brief hyperventilation may be used as a temporizing rescue therapy when you observe signs of impending brain herniation (eg, sudden rise in measured intracranial pressure, dilated pupil[s] not responsive to light, bradycardia, hypertension).
- Suspect thoracic injury in all thoracoabdominal trauma, even in the absence of external injuries. Tension pneumothorax, hemothorax, or pulmonary contusion may impair breathing.
- If the patient has maxillofacial trauma or if you suspect a basilar skull fracture, insert an orogastric rather than a nasogastric tube.[177]
- Treat signs of shock with a bolus of 20 mL/kg of an isotonic crystalloid (eg, normal saline or lactated Ringer's solution) even if blood pressure is normal. Give additional boluses (20 mL/kg) if systemic perfusion fails to improve. If signs of shock persist after administration of 40 to 60 mL/kg of isotonic crystalloid, give 10 to 15 mL/kg of blood. Although type-specific crossmatched blood is preferred, in an emergency use O-negative blood in females and O-positive or O-negative in males. If possible warm the blood before rapid infusion.[178,179]
- Consider intra-abdominal hemorrhage, tension pneumothorax, pericardial tamponade, spinal cord injury in infants and children, and intracranial hemorrhage in infants with signs of shock.[180,181]

Children With Special Healthcare Needs

Children with special healthcare needs[182–184] may require emergency care for their chronic conditions (eg, obstruction of a tracheostomy), failure of support technology (eg, ventilator failure), progression of their underlying disease, or events unrelated to those special needs.[185] For additional information about CPR see Part 11: "Pediatric Basic Life Support."

Ventilation With a Tracheostomy or Stoma

Parents, school nurses, and home healthcare providers should know how to assess patency of the airway, clear the airway, and perform CPR using the artificial airway in a child with a tracheostomy.

Parents and providers should be able to provide ventilation via the tracheostomy tube and verify effectiveness by chest expansion. If you cannot ventilate after suctioning the tube, replace it. If a clean tube is unavailable, perform mouth-to-stoma or mask-to-stoma ventilations. If the upper airway is patent, you may be able to provide effective bag-mask ventilation through the nose and mouth while you or someone else occludes the tracheal stoma.

Toxicologic Emergencies

Overdose with cocaine, narcotics, tricyclic antidepressants, calcium channel blockers, and β-adrenergic blockers poses some unique resuscitation problems in addition to the usual resuscitative measures.

Cocaine

Acute coronary syndrome, manifested by chest pain and cardiac rhythm disturbances (including VT and VF), is the most frequent cocaine-related reason for hospitalization in adults.[186,187] Cocaine prolongs the action potential and QRS duration and impairs myocardial contractility.[188,189]

Treatment

- Cool aggressively; hyperthermia is associated with an increase in toxicity.[190]
- For coronary vasospasm, consider nitroglycerin (Class IIa; LOE 5, 6),[191,192] a benzodiazepine, and phentolamine[193,194] (Class IIb; LOE 5, 6).

- Do not give β-adrenergic blockers.[190]
- For ventricular arrhythmia, consider sodium bicarbonate (1 to 2 mEq/kg)[195,196] (Class IIb; LOE 5, 6, 7) in addition to standard treatments.
- To prevent arrhythmia secondary to myocardial infarction, consider a lidocaine bolus followed by a lidocaine infusion (Class IIb; LOE 5, 6).

Tricyclic Antidepressants and Other Sodium Channel Blockers
Toxic doses cause cardiovascular abnormalities, including intraventricular conduction delays, heart block, bradycardia, prolongation of the QT interval, ventricular arrhythmias (including torsades de pointes, VT, and VF), hypotension,[189,197] seizures, and a depressed level of consciousness.

Treatment

- Give 1 to 2 mEq/kg boluses of sodium bicarbonate until arterial pH is >7.45, and then infuse 150 mEq $NaHCO_3$ per liter of D_5W to maintain alkalosis. In severe intoxication, increase the pH to 7.50 to 7.55.[189,198] Do not administer Class I_A (quinidine, procainamide), Class I_C (flecainide, propafenone), or Class III (amiodarone and sotalol) antiarrhythmics, which may exacerbate cardiac toxicity (Class III; LOE 6, 8).[198]
- For hypotension, give boluses (10 mL/kg each) of normal saline. If you need a vasopressor, epinephrine and norepinephrine have been shown to be more effective than dopamine in raising blood pressure.[199,200]
- Consider extracorporeal membrane oxygenation if high-dose vasopressors do not maintain blood pressure.[201,202]

Calcium Channel Blockers
Manifestations of toxicity include hypotension, ECG changes (prolongation of the QT interval, widening of the QRS, and right bundle branch block), arrhythmias (bradycardia, SVT, VT, torsades de pointes, and VF),[203] and altered mental status.

Treatment

- Treat mild hypotension with small boluses (5 to 10 mL/kg) of normal saline because myocardial depression may limit the amount of fluid the patient can tolerate.
- The effectiveness of calcium administration is variable (Class IIb; LOE 7, 8).[203–207] Try giving 20 mg/kg (0.2 mL/kg) of 10% calcium chloride over 5 to 10 minutes; if there is a beneficial effect, give an infusion of 20 to 50 mg/kg per hour. Monitor ionized calcium concentration to prevent hypercalcemia. It is preferable to administer calcium chloride via a central venous catheter; use caution when infusing into a peripheral IV because of the risk for sclerosis or infiltration.
- For bradycardia and hypotension, consider a high-dose vasopressor such as norepinephrine or epinephrine (Class IIb; LOE 5).[206]
- There is insufficient data to recommend for or against an infusion of insulin and glucose[208–211] or sodium bicarbonate (Class Indeterminate).

β-Adrenergic Blockers
Toxic doses of β-adrenergic blockers cause bradycardia, heart block, and decreased cardiac contractility, and some (eg, propranolol and sotalol) may also prolong the QRS and the QT intervals.[211–214]

Treatment

- High-dose epinephrine infusion may be effective[214,215] (Class Indeterminate; LOE 5, 6).
- Consider glucagon (Class IIb; LOE 5, 6).[211,214,216,217] In adolescents, infuse 5 to 10 mg of glucagon over several minutes followed by an IV infusion of 1 to 5 mg/h. If you are giving >2 mg of glucagon, reconstitute it in sterile water (<1 mg/mL) rather than the diluent supplied by the manufacturer.[217]
- Consider an infusion of glucose and insulin (Class Indeterminate; LOE 6).[208]
- There is insufficient data to make a recommendation for or against using calcium (Class Indeterminate; LOE 5, 6).[204,218,219] Calcium may be considered if glucagon and catecholamine are ineffective (Class IIb; LOE 5, 6).

Opioids
Narcotics may cause hypoventilation, apnea, bradycardia, and hypotension.

Treatment

- Ventilation is the initial treatment for severe respiratory depression from any cause (Class I).
- Naloxone reverses the respiratory depression of narcotic overdose (Class I; LOE: 1[220]; LOE 2[221]; LOE 3[222]; 5, 6[223,224]), but in persons with long-term addictions or those with cardiovascular disease, naloxone may increase heart rate and blood pressure and cause acute pulmonary edema, cardiac arrhythmias (including asystole), and seizures. Ventilation before administration of naloxone appears to reduce these adverse effects.[225] Intramuscular administration of naloxone may lower the risk.

Postresuscitation Stabilization

The goals of postresuscitation care are to preserve brain function, avoid secondary organ injury, diagnose and treat the cause of illness, and enable the patient to arrive at a pediatric tertiary-care facility in an optimal physiological state. Reassess frequently because cardiorespiratory status may deteriorate.

Respiratory System

Continue supplementary oxygen until you confirm adequate blood oxygenation and oxygen delivery. Monitor by continuous pulse oximetry.

Intubate and mechanically ventilate the patient if there is significant respiratory compromise (tachypnea, respiratory distress with agitation or decreased responsiveness, poor air exchange, cyanosis, hypoxemia). If the patient is already intubated, verify tube position, patency, and security. In the hospital setting, obtain arterial blood gases 10 to 15 minutes after establishing the initial ventilatory settings and make appropriate adjustments. Ideally correlate blood gases with capnographic end-tidal CO_2 concentration to enable noninvasive monitoring of ventilation.

Control pain and discomfort with analgesics (eg, fentanyl or morphine) and sedatives (eg, lorazepam, midazolam). In very agitated patients, neuromuscular blocking agents (eg,

TABLE 2. Medications to Maintain Cardiac Output and for Postresuscitation Stabilization

Medication	Dose Range	Comment
Inamrinone	0.75–1 mg/kg IV/IO over 5 minutes; may repeat × 2; then: 2–20 μg/kg per minute	Inodilator
Dobutamine	2–20 μg/kg per minute IV/IO	Inotrope; vasodilator
Dopamine	2–20 μg/kg per minute IV/IO	Inotrope; chronotrope; renal and splanchnic vasodilator in low doses; pressor in high doses
Epinephrine	0.1–1 μg/kg per minute IV/IO	Inotrope; chronotrope; vasodilator in low doses; pressor in higher doses
Milrinone	50–75 μg/kg IV/IO over 10–60 min then 0.5–0.75 μg/kg per minute	Inodilator
Norepinephrine	0.1–2 μg/kg per minute	Inotrope; vasopressor
Sodium nitroprusside	1–8 μg/kg per minute	Vasodilator; prepare only in D_5W

IV indicates intravenous; and IO, intraosseous.
Alternative formula for calculating an infusion:
Infusion rate (mL/h) = [weight (kg) × dose (μg/kg/min) × 60 (min/h)]/concentration μg/mL).

vecuronium or pancuronium) with analgesia or sedation, or both, may improve ventilation and minimize the risk of tube displacement. Neuromuscular blockers, however, will mask seizures.

Monitor exhaled CO_2, especially during transport and diagnostic procedures.[226] Insert a gastric tube to relieve and help prevent gastric inflation.

Cardiovascular System

Continuously monitor heart rate, blood pressure (by direct arterial line if possible), and oxygen saturation. Repeat clinical evaluations at least every 5 minutes until the patient is stable. Monitor urine output with an indwelling catheter.

Remove the IO access after you have alternate (preferably 2) secure venous lines. As a minimum, perform the following laboratory tests: central venous or arterial blood gas analysis and measurement of serum electrolytes, glucose, and calcium levels. A chest x-ray may help you evaluate endotracheal tube position, heart size, and pulmonary status.

Drugs Used to Maintain Cardiac Output (Table 2)

Myocardial dysfunction is common after cardiac arrest.[227,228] Systemic and pulmonary vascular resistance are increased except in some cases of septic shock.[229] Vasoactive agents may improve hemodynamics, but each drug and dose must be tailored to the patient (Class IIa; LOE 5, 6, 7) because clinical response is variable. Infuse all vasoactive drugs into a secure IV line. The potential adverse effects of catecholamines include local ischemia and ulceration, tachycardia, atrial and ventricular tachyarrhythmias, hypertension, and metabolic changes (hyperglycemia, increased lactate concentration,[230] and hypokalemia).

Epinephrine

Low-dose infusions (<0.3 μg/kg per minute) generally produce β-adrenergic action (potent inotropy and decreased systemic vascular resistance), and higher-dose infusions (>0.3 μg/kg per minute) cause α-adrenergic vasoconstriction.[231] Because there is great interpatient variability,[232,233] titrate the drug to the desired effect. Epinephrine may be preferable to dopamine in patients (especially infants) with marked circulatory instability and decompensated shock.

Dopamine

Titrate dopamine to treat shock that is unresponsive to fluid and when systemic vascular resistance is low (Class IIb; LOE 5, 6, 7).[229,234] Typically a dose of 2 to 20 μg/kg per minute is used. Although low-dose dopamine infusion has been frequently recommended to maintain renal blood flow or improve renal function, more recent data has failed to show a beneficial effect from such therapy. At higher doses (>5 μg/kg per minute), dopamine stimulates cardiac β-adrenergic receptors, but this effect may be reduced in infants and in chronic congestive heart failure.[231] Infusion rates >20 μg/kg per minute may result in excessive vasoconstriction.[231]

Dobutamine Hydrochloride

Dobutamine has a selective effect on β_1- and β_2-adrenergic receptors; it increases myocardial contractility and usually decreases peripheral vascular resistance. Titrate an infusion[232,235,236] to improve cardiac output and blood pressure, especially due to poor myocardial function.[236]

Norepinephrine

Norepinephrine is a potent inotropic and peripheral vasoconstricting agent. Titrate an infusion to treat shock with low systemic vascular resistance (septic, anaphylactic, spinal, or vasodilatory) unresponsive to fluid.

Sodium Nitroprusside

Sodium nitroprusside increases cardiac output by decreasing vascular resistance (afterload). If hypotension is related to poor myocardial function, consider using a combination of sodium nitroprusside to reduce afterload and an inotrope to improve contractility.

Inodilators

Inodilators (inamrinone and milrinone) augment cardiac output with little effect on myocardial oxygen demand. Use an inodilator for treatment of myocardial dysfunction with increased systemic or pulmonary vascular resistance.[237–239]

Administration of fluids may be required because of the vasodilatory effects.

Inodilators have a long half-life with a long delay in reaching a new steady-state hemodynamic effect after changing the infusion rate (18 hours with inamrinone and 4.5 hours with milrinone). In case of toxicity, if you stop the infusion the adverse effects may persist for several hours.

Neurologic System

One goal of resuscitation is to preserve brain function. Prevent secondary neuronal injury by adhering to the following precautions:

- Do not provide routine hyperventilation. Hyperventilation has no benefit and may impair neurologic outcome, most likely by adversely affecting cardiac output and cerebral perfusion.[175] Intentional brief hyperventilation may be used as temporizing rescue therapy in response to signs of impending cerebral herniation (eg, sudden rise in measured intracranial pressure, dilated pupil[s] not responsive to light, bradycardia, hypertension).
- When patients remain comatose after resuscitation, consider cooling them to a temperature of 32°C to 34°C for 12 to 24 hours because cooling may aid brain recovery (Class IIb). Evidence in support of hypothermia is LOE 7 (extrapolated from LOE 1[240] and LOE 2[241] studies in adults following resuscitation from VF sudden cardiac arrest and 2 LOE 2 neonatal studies[242,243]). The ideal method and duration of cooling and rewarming are not known. Prevent shivering by providing sedation and, if needed, neuromuscular blockade. Closely watch for signs of infection. Other complications of hypothermia include diminished cardiac output, arrhythmia, pancreatitis, coagulopathy, thrombocytopenia, hypophosphatemia, and hypomagnesemia. Neuromuscular blockade can mask seizures.
- Monitor temperature and treat fever aggressively with antipyretics and cooling devices because fever adversely influences recovery from ischemic brain injury (Class IIb; LOE 4, 5, 6).[244–248]
- Treat postischemic seizures aggressively; search for a correctable metabolic cause such as hypoglycemia or electrolyte imbalance.

Renal System

Decreased urine output (<1 mL/kg per hour in infants and children or <30 mL/h in adolescents) may be caused by prerenal conditions (eg, dehydration, inadequate systemic perfusion), renal ischemic damage, or a combination of factors. Avoid nephrotoxic medications and adjust the dose of medications excreted by the kidneys until you have checked renal function.

Interhospital Transport

Ideally postresuscitation care should be provided by a trained team in a pediatric intensive care facility. Contact such a unit as early into the resuscitation attempt as possible and coordinate transportation with the receiving unit.[249] Transport team members should be trained and experienced in the care of critically ill and injured children[37,250] and supervised by a pediatric emergency medicine or pediatric critical care physician. The mode of transport and composition of the team should be established for each system based on the care required by an individual patient.[251] Monitor exhaled CO_2 (qualitative colorimetric detector or capnography) during interhospital or intrahospital transport of intubated patients (Class IIa).

Family Presence During Resuscitation

Most family members would like to be present during resuscitation.[252–257] Parents and care providers of chronically ill children are often knowledgeable about and comfortable with medical equipment and emergency procedures. Family members with no medical background report that being at the side of a loved one and saying goodbye during the final moments of life is comforting[254,258] and helps in their adjustment,[252] and most would participate again.[254] Standardized psychological examinations suggest that, compared with those not present, family members who were present during attempted resuscitation have less anxiety and depression and more constructive grieving behavior.[257] Parents or family members often fail to ask, but healthcare providers should offer the opportunity whenever possible.[256,258,259] If the presence of family members proves detrimental to the resuscitation, they should be gently asked to leave. Members of the resuscitation team must be sensitive to the presence of family members, and one person should be assigned to comfort, answer questions, and discuss the needs of the family.[260]

Termination of Resuscitative Efforts

Unfortunately there are no reliable predictors of outcome during resuscitation to guide when to terminate resuscitative efforts. Witnessed collapse, bystander CPR, and a short time interval from collapse to arrival of professionals improve the chances of a successful resuscitation. In the past, children who underwent prolonged resuscitation and absence of return of spontaneous circulation after 2 doses of epinephrine were considered unlikely to survive,[1,23,261] but intact survival after unusually prolonged in-hospital resuscitation has been documented.[61,122,262–265] Prolonged efforts should be made for infants and children with recurring or refractory VF or VT, drug toxicity, or a primary hypothermic insult. For further discussion on the ethics of resuscitation, see Part 2: "Ethical Issues."

References

1. Young KD, Seidel JS. Pediatric cardiopulmonary resuscitation: a collective review. *Ann Emerg Med.* 1999;33:195–205.
2. Gorelick MH, Shaw KN, Murphy KO. Validity and reliability of clinical signs in the diagnosis of dehydration in children. *Pediatrics.* 1997; 99:E6.
3. Raju NV, Maisels MJ, Kring E, Schwarz-Warner L. Capillary refill time in the hands and feet of normal newborn infants. *Clin Pediatr.* 1999; 38:139–144.
4. Brown LH, Prasad NH, Whitley TW. Adverse lighting condition effects on the assessment of capillary refill. *Am J Emerg Med.* 1994;12:46–47.
5. Park C, Bahk JH, Ahn WS, Do SH, Lee KH. The laryngeal mask airway in infants and children. *Can J Anaesth.* 2001;48:413–417.
6. Bagshaw O. The size 1.5 laryngeal mask airway (LMA) in paediatric anaesthetic practice. *Paediatr Anaesth.* 2002;12:420–423.

7. Brown LH, Manring EA, Kornegay HB, Prasad NH. Can prehospital personnel detect hypoxemia without the aid of pulse oximeters? *Am J Emerg Med.* 1996;14:43–44.
8. Gausche M, Lewis RJ, Stratton SJ, Haynes BE, Gunter CS, Goodrich SM, Poore PD, McCollough MD, Henderson DP, Pratt FD, Seidel JS. Effect of out-of-hospital pediatric endotracheal intubation on survival and neurological outcome: a controlled clinical trial. *JAMA.* 2000;283: 783–790.
9. Cooper A, DiScala C, Foltin G, Tunik M, Markenson D, Welborn C. Prehospital endotracheal intubation for severe head injury in children: a reappraisal. *Semin Pediatr Surg.* 2001;10:3–6.
10. Stockinger ZT, McSwain NE Jr. Prehospital endotracheal intubation for trauma does not improve survival over bag-valve-mask ventilation. *J Trauma.* 2004;56:531–536.
11. Pitetti R, Glustein JZ, Bhende MS. Prehospital care and outcome of pediatric out-of-hospital cardiac arrest. *Prehosp Emerg Care.* 2002;6: 283–290.
12. Kern KB, Sanders AB, Raife J, Milander MM, Otto CW, Ewy GA. A study of chest compression rates during cardiopulmonary resuscitation in humans: the importance of rate-directed chest compressions. *Arch Intern Med.* 1992;152:145–149.
13. Aufderheide TP, Sigurdsson G, Pirrallo RG, Yannopoulos D, McKnite S, von Briesen C, Sparks CW, Conrad CJ, Provo TA, Lurie KG. Hyperventilation-induced hypotension during cardiopulmonary resuscitation. *Circulation.* 2004;109:1960–1965.
14. Abella BS, Alvarado JP, Myklebust H, Edelson DP, Barry A, O'Hearn N, Vanden Hoek TL, Becker LB. Quality of cardiopulmonary resuscitation during in-hospital cardiac arrest. *JAMA.* 2005;293:305–310.
15. Gausche-Hill M, Lewis RJ, Gunter CS, Henderson DP, Haynes BE, Stratton SJ. Design and implementation of a controlled trial of pediatric endotracheal intubation in the out-of-hospital setting. *Ann Emerg Med.* 2000;36:356–365.
16. Jesudian MC, Harrison RR, Keenan RL, Maull KI. Bag-valve-mask ventilation; two rescuers are better than one: preliminary report. *Crit Care Med.* 1985;13:122–123.
17. Davidovic L, LaCovey D, Pitetti R. Comparison of 1- vs 2-person bag-valve-mask techniques for manikin ventilation of infants and children. *Ann Emerg Med.* In press.
18. Berg MD, Idris AH, Berg RA. Severe ventilatory compromise due to gastric distention during pediatric cardiopulmonary resuscitation. *Resuscitation.* 1998;36:71–73.
19. Moynihan RJ, Brock-Utne JG, Archer JH, Feld LH, Kreitzman TR. The effect of cricoid pressure on preventing gastric insufflation in infants and children. *Anesthesiology.* 1993;78:652–656.
20. Salem MR, Wong AY, Mani M, Sellick BA. Efficacy of cricoid pressure in preventing gastric inflation during bag-mask ventilation in pediatric patients. *Anesthesiology.* 1974;40:96–98.
21. Sellick BA. Cricoid pressure to control regurgitation of stomach contents during induction of anaesthesia. *Lancet.* 1961;2:404–406.
22. Hartsilver EL, Vanner RG. Airway obstruction with cricoid pressure. *Anaesthesia.* 2000;55:208–211.
23. Sirbaugh PE, Pepe PE, Shook JE, Kimball KT, Goldman MJ, Ward MA, Mann DM. A prospective, population-based study of the demographics, epidemiology, management, and outcome of out-of-hospital pediatric cardiopulmonary arrest [published correction appears in *Ann Emerg Med.* 1999;33:358]. *Ann Emerg Med.* 1999;33:174–184.
24. Brownstein DR, Quan L, Orr R, Wentz KR, Copass MK. Paramedic intubation training in a pediatric operating room. *Am J Emerg Med.* 1992;10:418–420.
25. Vilke GM, Steen PJ, Smith AM, Chan TC. Out-of-hospital pediatric intubation by paramedics: the San Diego experience. *J Emerg Med.* 2002;22:71–74.
26. Ma OJ, Atchley RB, Hatley T, Green M, Young J, Brady W. Intubation success rates improve for an air medical program after implementing the use of neuromuscular blocking agents. *Am J Emerg Med.* 1998;16: 125–127.
27. Sing RF, Rotondo MF, Zonies DH, Schwab CW, Kauder DR, Ross SE, Brathwaite CC. Rapid sequence induction for intubation by an aeromedical transport team: a critical analysis. *Am J Emerg Med.* 1998;16: 598–602.
28. Sagarin MJ, Chiang V, Sakles JC, Barton ED, Wolfe RE, Vissers RJ, Walls RM. Rapid sequence intubation for pediatric emergency airway management. *Pediatr Emerg Care.* 2002;18:417–423.
29. Deakers TW, Reynolds G, Stretton M, Newth CJ. Cuffed endotracheal tubes in pediatric intensive care. *J Pediatr.* 1994;125:57–62.
30. Khine HH, Corddry DH, Kettrick RG, Martin TM, McCloskey JJ, Rose JB, Theroux MC, Zagnoev M. Comparison of cuffed and uncuffed endotracheal tubes in young children during general anesthesia. *Anesthesiology.* 1997;86:627–631; discussion 27A.
31. Newth CJ, Rachman B, Patel N, Hammer J. The use of cuffed versus uncuffed endotracheal tubes in pediatric intensive care. *J Pediatr.* 2004; 144:333–337.
32. Parwani V HI-H, Hsu B, Hoffman RJ. Experienced emergency physicians cannot safely or accurately inflate endotracheal tube cuffs or estimate endotracheal tube cuff pressure using standard technique. *Acad Emerg Med.* 2004;11:490–491.
33. King BR, Baker MD, Braitman LE, Seidl-Friedman J, Schreiner MS. Endotracheal tube selection in children: a comparison of four methods. *Ann Emerg Med.* 1993;22:530–534.
34. van den Berg AA, Mphanza T. Choice of tracheal tube size for children: finger size or age-related formula? *Anaesthesia.* 1997;52:701–703.
35. Luten RC, Wears RL, Broselow J, Zaritsky A, Barnett TM, Lee T, Bailey A, Vally R, Brown R, Rosenthal B. Length-based endotracheal tube and emergency equipment in pediatrics. *Ann Emerg Med.* 1992;21: 900–904.
36. Katz SH, Falk JL. Misplaced endotracheal tubes by paramedics in an urban emergency medical services system. *Ann Emerg Med.* 2001;37: 32–37.
37. Beyer AJ III, Land G, Zaritsky A. Nonphysician transport of intubated pediatric patients: a system evaluation. *Crit Care Med.* 1992;20: 961–966.
38. Andersen KH, Schultz-Lebahn T. Oesophageal intubation can be undetected by auscultation of the chest. *Acta Anaesthesiol Scand.* 1994;38: 580–582.
39. Kelly JJ, Eynon CA, Kaplan JL, de Garavilla L, Dalsey WC. Use of tube condensation as an indicator of endotracheal tube placement. *Ann Emerg Med.* 1998;31:575–578.
40. Poirier MP, Gonzalez Del-Rey JA, McAneney CM, DiGiulio GA. Utility of monitoring capnography, pulse oximetry, and vital signs in the detection of airway mishaps: a hyperoxemic animal model. *Am J Emerg Med.* 1998;16:350–352.
41. Birmingham PK, Cheney FW, Ward RJ. Esophageal intubation: a review of detection techniques. *Anesth Analg.* 1986;65:886–891.
42. Donn SM, Kuhns LR. Mechanism of endotracheal tube movement with change of head position in the neonate. *Pediatr Radiol.* 1980;9:37–40.
43. Hartrey R, Kestin IG. Movement of oral and nasal tracheal tubes as a result of changes in head neck position. *Anaesthesia.* 1995;50:682–687.
44. Bhende MS, Thompson AE, Cook DR, Saville AL. Validity of a disposable end-tidal CO2 detector in verifying endotracheal tube placement in infants and children. *Ann Emerg Med.* 1992;21:142–145.
45. Campbell RC, Boyd CR, Shields RO, Odom JW, Corse KM. Evaluation of an end-tidal carbon dioxide detector in the aeromedical setting. *J Air Med Transp.* 1990;9:13–15.
46. Bhende MS, Thompson AE, Orr RA. Utility of an end-tidal carbon dioxide detector during stabilization and transport of critically ill children. *Pediatrics.* 1992;89(pt 1):1042–1044.
47. Bhende MS, Thompson AE. Evaluation of an end-tidal CO2 detector during pediatric cardiopulmonary resuscitation. *Pediatrics.* 1995;95: 395–399.
48. Cardoso MM, Banner MJ, Melker RJ, Bjoraker DG. Portable devices used to detect endotracheal intubation during emergency situations: a review. *Crit Care Med.* 1998;26:957–964.
49. Ornato JP, Shipley JB, Racht EM, Slovis CM, Wrenn KD, Pepe PE, Almeida SL, Ginger VF, Fotre TV. Multicenter study of a portable, hand-size, colorimetric end-tidal carbon dioxide detection device. *Ann Emerg Med.* 1992;21:518–523.
50. Bhende MS, Karasic DG, Karasic RB. End-tidal carbon dioxide changes during cardiopulmonary resuscitation after experimental asphyxial cardiac arrest. *Am J Emerg Med.* 1996;14:349–350.
51. Cantineau JP, Merckx P, Lambert Y, Sorkine M, Bertrand C, Duvaldestin P. Effect of epinephrine on end-tidal carbon dioxide pressure during prehospital cardiopulmonary resuscitation. *Am J Emerg Med.* 1994;12:267–270.
52. Ward KR, Yealy DM. End-tidal carbon dioxide monitoring in emergency medicine. Part 2: clinical applications. *Acad Emerg Med.* 1998;5:637–646.
53. Hand IL, Shepard EK, Krauss AN, Auld PA. Discrepancies between transcutaneous and end-tidal carbon dioxide monitoring in the critically ill neonate with respiratory distress syndrome. *Crit Care Med.* 1989;17: 556–559.

54. Tobias JD, Meyer DJ. Noninvasive monitoring of carbon dioxide during respiratory failure in toddlers and infants: end-tidal versus transcutaneous carbon dioxide. *Anesth Analg*. 1997;85:55–58.
55. Sharieff GQ, Rodarte A, Wilton N, Bleyle D. The self-inflating bulb as an airway adjunct: is it reliable in children weighing less than 20 kilograms? *Acad Emerg Med*. 2003;10:303–308.
56. Sharieff GQ, Rodarte A, Wilton N, Silva PD, Bleyle D. The self-inflating bulb as an esophageal detector device in children weighing more than twenty kilograms: a comparison of two techniques. *Ann Emerg Med*. 2003;41:623–629.
57. Klain M, Keszler H, Brader E. High frequency jet ventilation in CPR. *Crit Care Med*. 1981;9:421–422.
58. Zander J, Hazinski MF. Pulmonary disorders: airway obstructions. In: Hazinski MF, ed. *Nursing Care of the Critically Ill Child*. St. Louis, Mo: Mosby-Year Book; 1992.
59. Nypaver M, Treloar D. Neutral cervical spine positioning in children. *Ann Emerg Med*. 1994;23:208–211.
60. Herzenberg JE, Hensinger RN, Dedrick DK, Phillips WA. Emergency transport and positioning of young children who have an injury of the cervical spine. The standard backboard may be hazardous. *J Bone Joint Surg Am*. 1989;71:15–22.
61. Duncan BW, Ibrahim AE, Hraska V, del Nido PJ, Laussen PC, Wessel DL, Mayer JE Jr, Bower LK, Jonas RA. Use of rapid-deployment extracorporeal membrane oxygenation for the resuscitation of pediatric patients with heart disease after cardiac arrest. *J Thorac Cardiovasc Surg*. 1998;116:305–311.
62. Morris MC, Wernovsky G, Nadkarni VM. Survival outcomes after extracorporeal cardiopulmonary resuscitation instituted during active chest compressions following refractory in-hospital pediatric cardiac arrest. *Pediatr Crit Care Med*. 2004;5:440–446.
63. Kanter RK, Zimmerman JJ, Strauss RH, Stoeckel KA. Pediatric emergency intravenous access. Evaluation of a protocol. *Am J Dis Child*. 1986;140:132–134.
64. Fiser DH. Intraosseous infusion. *N Engl J Med*. 1990;322:1579–1581.
65. Banerjee S, Singhi SC, Singh S, Singh M. The intraosseous route is a suitable alternative to intravenous route for fluid resuscitation in severely dehydrated children. *Indian Pediatr*. 1994;31:1511–1520.
66. Guy J, Haley K, Zuspan SJ. Use of intraosseous infusion in the pediatric trauma patient. *J Pediatr Surg*. 1993;28:158–161.
67. Berg RA. Emergency infusion of catecholamines into bone marrow. *Am J Dis Child*. 1984;138:810–811.
68. Andropoulos DB, Soifer SJ, Schreiber MD. Plasma epinephrine concentrations after intraosseous and central venous injection during cardiopulmonary resuscitation in the lamb. *J Pediatr*. 1990;116:312–315.
69. Johnson L, Kissoon N, Fiallos M, Abdelmoneim T, Murphy S. Use of intraosseous blood to assess blood chemistries and hemoglobin during cardiopulmonary resuscitation with drug infusions. *Crit Care Med*. 1999;27:1147–1152.
70. Abdelmoneim T, Kissoon N, Johnson L, Fiallos M, Murphy S. Acid-base status of blood from intraosseous and mixed venous sites during prolonged cardiopulmonary resuscitation and drug infusions. *Crit Care Med*. 1999;27:1923–1928.
71. Orlowski JP, Porembka DT, Gallagher JM, Lockrem JD, VanLente F. Comparison study of intraosseous, central intravenous, and peripheral intravenous infusions of emergency drugs. *Am J Dis Child*. 1990;144: 112–117.
72. Warren DW, Kissoon N, Sommerauer JF, Rieder MJ. Comparison of fluid infusion rates among peripheral intravenous and humerus, femur, malleolus, and tibial intraosseous sites in normovolemic and hypovolemic piglets. *Ann Emerg Med*. 1993;22:183–186.
73. Fleisher G, Caputo G, Baskin M. Comparison of external jugular and peripheral venous administration of sodium bicarbonate in puppies. *Crit Care Med*. 1989;17:251–254.
74. Ward JTJ. Endotracheal drug therapy. *Am J Emerg Med*. 1983;1:71–82.
75. Johnston C. Endotracheal drug delivery. *Pediatr Emerg Care*. 1992;8: 94–97.
76. Efrati O, Ben-Abraham R, Barak A, Modan-Moses D, Augarten A, Manisterski Y, Barzilay Z, Paret G. Endobronchial adrenaline: should it be reconsidered? Dose response and haemodynamic effect in dogs. *Resuscitation*. 2003;59:117–122.
77. Jasani MS, Nadkarni VM, Finkelstein MS, Mandell GA, Salzman SK, Norman ME. Effects of different techniques of endotracheal epinephrine administration in pediatric porcine hypoxic-hypercarbic cardiopulmonary arrest. *Crit Care Med*. 1994;22:1174–1180.
78. Lubitz DS, Seidel JS, Chameides L, Luten RC, Zaritsky AL, Campbell FW. A rapid method for estimating weight and resuscitation drug dosages from length in the pediatric age group. *Ann Emerg Med*. 1988; 17:576–581.
79. Hofer CK, Ganter M, Tucci M, Klaghofer R, Zollinger A. How reliable is length-based determination of body weight and tracheal tube size in the paediatric age group? The Broselow tape reconsidered. *Br J Anaesth*. 2002;88:283–285.
80. Schierhout G, Roberts I. Fluid resuscitation with colloid or crystalloid solutions in critically ill patients: a systematic review of randomised trials. *BMJ*. 1998;316:961–964.
81. Human albumin administration in critically ill patients: systematic review of randomised controlled trials. Cochrane Injuries Group Albumin Reviewers. *BMJ*. 1998;317:235–240.
82. Alderson P, Schierhout G, Roberts I, Bunn F. Colloids versus crystalloids for fluid resuscitation in critically ill patients. In: *The Cochrane Library*. Oxford: England: Update Software. 2003.
83. Longstreth WT Jr, Copass MK, Dennis LK, Rauch-Matthews ME, Stark MS, Cobb LA. Intravenous glucose after out-of-hospital cardiopulmonary arrest: a community-based randomized trial. *Neurology*. 1993;43: 2534–2541.
84. Cherian L, Goodman JC, Robertson CS. Hyperglycemia increases brain injury caused by secondary ischemia after cortical impact injury in rats. *Crit Care Med*. 1997;25:1378–1383.
85. Simma B, Burger R, Falk M, Sacher P, Fanconi S. A prospective, randomized, and controlled study of fluid management in children with severe head injury: lactated Ringer's solution versus hypertonic saline. *Crit Care Med*. 1998;26:1265–1270.
86. Bunn F, Roberts I, Tasker R, Akpa E. Hypertonic versus isotonic crystalloid for fluid resuscitation in critically ill patients. In: *The Cochrane Library*. Oxford, England: Update Software. 2003.
87. Losek JD, Endom E, Dietrich A, Stewart G, Zempsky W, Smith K. Adenosine and pediatric supraventricular tachycardia in the emergency department: multicenter study and review. *Ann Emerg Med*. 1999;33: 185–191.
88. Overholt ED, Rheuban KS, Gutgesell HP, Lerman BB, DiMarco JP. Usefulness of adenosine for arrhythmias in infants and children. *Am J Cardiol*. 1988;61:336–340.
89. Getschman SJ, Dietrich AM, Franklin WH, Allen HD. Intraosseous adenosine: as effective as peripheral or central venous administration? *Arch Pediatr Adolesc Med*. 1994;148:616–619.
90. Friedman FD. Intraosseous adenosine for the termination of supraventricular tachycardia in an infant. *Ann Emerg Med*. 1996;28:356–358.
91. Somberg JC, Bailin SJ, Haffajee CI, Paladino WP, Kerin NZ, Bridges D, Timar S, Molnar J. Intravenous lidocaine versus intravenous amiodarone (in a new aqueous formulation) for incessant ventricular tachycardia. *Am J Cardiol*. 2002;90:853–859.
92. Holt DW, Tucker GT, Jackson PR, Storey GC. Amiodarone pharmacokinetics. *Am Heart J*. 1983;106:840–847.
93. Dauchot P, Gravenstein JS. Effects of atropine on the electrocardiogram in different age groups. *Clin Pharmacol Ther*. 1971;12:274–280.
94. Zwiener RJ, Ginsburg CM. Organophosphate and carbamate poisoning in infants and children [published correction appears in *Pediatrics*. 1988;81:683]. *Pediatrics*. 1988;81:121–126.
95. Stueven HA, Thompson B, Aprahamian C, Tonsfeldt DJ, Kastenson EH. Lack of effectiveness of calcium chloride in refractory asystole. *Ann Emerg Med*. 1985;14:630–632.
96. Broner CW, Stidham GL, Westenkirchner DF, Watson DC. A prospective, randomized, double-blind comparison of calcium chloride and calcium gluconate therapies for hypocalcemia in critically ill children. *J Pediatr*. 1990;117:986–989.
97. Niemann JT, Criley JM, Rosborough JP, Niskanen RA, Alferness C. Predictive indices of successful cardiac resuscitation after prolonged arrest and experimental cardiopulmonary resuscitation. *Ann Emerg Med*. 1985;14:521–528.
98. Sanders A, Ewy G, Taft T. Prognostic and therapeutic importance of the aortic diastolic pressure in resuscitation from cardiac arrest. *Crit Care Med*. 1984;12:871–873.
99. Berg RA, Otto CW, Kern KB, Sanders AB, Hilwig RW, Hansen KK, Ewy GA. High-dose epinephrine results in greater early mortality after resuscitation from prolonged cardiac arrest in pigs: a prospective, randomized study. *Crit Care Med*. 1994;22:282–290.
100. Losek JD. Hypoglycemia and the ABC'S (sugar) of pediatric resuscitation. *Ann Emerg Med*. 2000;35:43–46.

101. Agus MSD, Jaksic T. Nutritional support of the critically ill child (review). *Curr Opin Pediat.* 2002;14:470–481.
102. Bigger JT Jr, Mandel WJ. Effect of lidocaine on the electrophysiological properties of ventricular muscle and purkinje fibers. *J Clin Invest.* 1970;49:63–77.
103. Dorian P, Cass D, Schwartz B, Cooper R, Gelaznikas R, Barr A. Amiodarone as compared with lidocaine for shock-resistant ventricular fibrillation. *N Engl J Med.* 2002;346:884–890.
104. Wilson FC, Harpur J, Watson T, Morrow JI. Adult survivors of severe cerebral hypoxia–case series survey and comparative analysis. *Neuro Rehabilitation.* 2003;18:291–298.
105. Thomson PD, Melmon KL, Richardson JA, Cohn K, Steinbrunn W, Cudihee R, Rowland M. Lidocaine pharmacokinetics in advanced heart failure, liver disease, and renal failure in humans. *Ann Intern Med.* 1973;78:499–508.
106. Allegra J, Lavery R, Cody R, Birnbaum G, Brennan J, Hartman A, Horowitz M, Nashed A, Yablonski M. Magnesium sulfate in the treatment of refractory ventricular fibrillation in the prehospital setting. *Resuscitation.* 2001;49:245–249.
107. Hassan TB, Jagger C, Barnett DB. A randomised trial to investigate the efficacy of magnesium sulphate for refractory ventricular fibrillation. *Emerg Med J.* 2002;19:57–62.
108. Thel MC, Armstrong AL, McNulty SE, Califf RM, O'Connor CM. Randomised trial of magnesium in in-hospital cardiac arrest. Duke Internal Medicine Housestaff. *Lancet.* 1997;350:1272–1276.
109. Luedtke SA, Kuhn RJ, McCaffrey FM. Pharmacologic management of supraventricular tachycardias in children. Part 1: Wolff-Parkinson-White and atrioventricular nodal reentry. *Ann Pharmacother.* 1997;31:1227–1243.
110. Luedtke SA, Kuhn RJ, McCaffrey FM. Pharmacologic management of supraventricular tachycardias in children, part 2: atrial flutter, atrial fibrillation, and junctional and atrial ectopic tachycardia. *Ann Pharmacother.* 1997;31:1347–1359.
111. Weil MH, Rackow EC, Trevino R, Grundler W, Falk JL, Griffel MI. Difference in acid-base state between venous and arterial blood during cardiopulmonary resuscitation. *N Engl J Med.* 1986;315:153–156.
112. Steedman DJ, Robertson CE. Acid-base changes in arterial and central venous blood during cardiopulmonary resuscitation. *Arch Emerg Med.* 1992;9:169–176.
113. Wayne MA, Delbridge TR, Ornato JP, Swor RA, Blackwell T. Concepts and application of prehospital ventilation. *Prehosp Emerg Care.* 2001;5:73–78.
114. Mattar JA, Weil MH, Shubin H, Stein L. Cardiac arrest in the critically ill. II. Hyperosmolal states following cardiac arrest. *Am J Med.* 1974;56:162–168.
115. Aufderheide TP, Martin DR, Olson DW, Aprahamian C, Woo JW, Hendley GE, Hargarten KM, Thompson B. Prehospital bicarbonate use in cardiac arrest: a 3-year experience. *Am J Emerg Med.* 1992;10:4–7.
116. Bishop RL, Weisfeldt ML. Sodium bicarbonate administration during cardiac arrest. Effect on arterial pH PCO2, and osmolality. *JAMA.* 1976;235:506–509.
117. Mann K, Berg RA, Nadkarni V. Beneficial effects of vasopressin in prolonged pediatric cardiac arrest: a case series. *Resuscitation.* 2002;52:149–156.
118. Wenzel V, Krismer AC, Arntz HR, Sitter H, Stadlbauer KH, Lindner KH. A comparison of vasopressin and epinephrine for out-of-hospital cardiopulmonary resuscitation. *N Engl J Med.* 2004;350:105–113.
119. Stiell IG, Hebert PC, Wells GA, Vandemheen KL, Tang AS, Higginson LA, Dreyer JF, Clement C, Battram E, Watpool I, Mason S, Klassen T, Weitzman BN. Vasopressin versus epinephrine for inhospital cardiac arrest: a randomised controlled trial. *Lancet.* 2001;358:105–109.
120. Lindner KH, Dirks B, Strohmenger HU, Prengel AW, Lindner IM, Lurie KG. Randomised comparison of epinephrine and vasopressin in patients with out-of-hospital ventricular fibrillation. *Lancet.* 1997;349:535–537.
121. Guyette FX, Guimond GE, Hostler D, Callaway CW. Vasopressin administered with epinephrine is associated with a return of a pulse in out-of-hospital cardiac arrest. *Resuscitation.* 2004;63:277–282.
122. Reis AG, Nadkarni V, Perondi MB, Grisi S, Berg RA. A prospective investigation into the epidemiology of in-hospital pediatric cardiopulmonary resuscitation using the international Utstein reporting style. *Pediatrics.* 2002;109:200–209.
123. Appleton GO, Cummins RO, Larson MP, Graves JR. CPR and the single rescuer: at what age should you "call first" rather than "call fast"? *Ann Emerg Med.* 1995;25:492–494.
124. Hickey RW, Cohen DM, Strausbaugh S, Dietrich AM. Pediatric patients requiring CPR in the prehospital setting. *Ann Emerg Med.* 1995;25:495–501.
125. Mogayzel C, Quan L, Graves JR, Tiedeman D, Fahrenbruch C, Herndon P. Out-of-hospital ventricular fibrillation in children and adolescents: causes and outcomes. *Ann Emerg Med.* 1995;25:484–491.
126. Herlitz J, Engdahl J, Svensson L, Young M, Angquist KA, Holmberg S. Characteristics and outcome among children suffering from out of hospital cardiac arrest in Sweden. *Resuscitation.* 2005;64:37–40.
127. Safranek DJ, Eisenberg MS, Larsen MP. The epidemiology of cardiac arrest in young adults. *Ann Emerg Med.* 1992;21:1102–1106.
128. Larsen MP, Eisenberg MS, Cummins RO, Hallstrom AP. Predicting survival from out-of-hospital cardiac arrest: a graphic model. *Ann Emerg Med.* 1993;22:1652–1658.
129. Atkins DL, Sirna S, Kieso R, Charbonnier F, Kerber RE. Pediatric defibrillation: importance of paddle size in determining transthoracic impedance. *Pediatrics.* 1988;82:914–918.
130. Atkins DL, Kerber RE. Pediatric defibrillation: current flow is improved by using "adult" electrode paddles. *Pediatrics.* 1994;94:90–93.
131. Samson RA, Atkins DL, Kerber RE. Optimal size of self-adhesive preapplied electrode pads in pediatric defibrillation. *Am J Cardiol.* 1995;75:544–545.
132. Garcia LA, Kerber RE. Transthoracic defibrillation: does electrode adhesive pad position alter transthoracic impedance? *Resuscitation.* 1998;37:139–143.
133. Gurnett CA, Atkins DL. Successful use of a biphasic waveform automated external defibrillator in a high-risk child. *Am J Cardiol.* 2000;86:1051–1053.
134. Rossano JQ, Schiff L, Kenney MA, Atkins DL. Survival is not correlated with defibrillation dosing in pediatric out-of-hospital ventricular fibrillation. *Circulation.* 2003;108:IV320–IV321.
135. Atkins D, Jorgenson D. Attenuated pediatric electrode pads for automated external defibrillator use in children. *Resuscitation.* 2005;66:31–37.
136. Berg RA, Chapman FW, Berg MD, Hilwig RW, Banville I, Walker RG, Nova RC, Sherrill D, Kern KB. Attenuated adult biphasic shocks compared with weight-based monophasic shocks in a swine model of prolonged pediatric ventricular fibrillation. *Resuscitation.* 2004;61:189–197.
137. Schneider T, Martens PR, Paschen H, Kuisma M, Wolcke B, Gliner BE, Russell JK, Weaver WD, Bossaert L, Chamberlain D. Multicenter, randomized, controlled trial of 150-J biphasic shocks compared with 200- to 360-J monophasic shocks in the resuscitation of out-of-hospital cardiac arrest victims. *Circulation.* 2000;102:1780–1787.
138. van Alem AP, Chapman FW, Lank P, Hart AA, Koster RW. A prospective, randomised and blinded comparison of first shock success of monophasic and biphasic waveforms in out-of-hospital cardiac arrest. *Resuscitation.* 2003;58:17–24.
139. Berg RA, Samson RA, Berg MD, Chapman FW, Hilwig RW, Banville I, Walker RG, Nova RC, Anavy N, Kern KB. Better outcome after pediatric defibrillation dosage than adult dosage in a swine model of pediatric ventricular fibrillation. *J Am Coll Cardiol.* 2005;45:786–789.
140. Clark CB, Zhang Y, Davies LR, Karlsson G, Kerber RE. Pediatric transthoracic defibrillation: biphasic versus monophasic waveforms in an experimental model. *Resuscitation.* 2001;51:159–163.
141. Tang W, Weil MH, Jorgenson D, Klouche K, Morgan C, Yu T, Sun S, Snyder D. Fixed-energy biphasic waveform defibrillation in a pediatric model of cardiac arrest and resuscitation. *Crit Care Med.* 2002;30:2736–2741.
142. Gutgesell HP, Tacker WA, Geddes LA, Davis S, Lie JT, McNamara DG. Energy dose for ventricular defibrillation of children. *Pediatrics.* 1976;58:898–901.
143. Atkinson E, Mikysa B, Conway JA, Parker M, Christian K, Deshpande J, Knilans TK, Smith J, Walker C, Stickney RE, Hampton DR, Hazinski MF. Specificity and sensitivity of automated external defibrillator rhythm analysis in infants and children. *Ann Emerg Med.* 2003;42:185–196.
144. Cecchin F, Jorgenson DB, Berul CI, Perry JC, Zimmerman AA, Duncan BW, Lupinetti FM, Snyder D, Lyster TD, Rosenthal GL, Cross B, Atkins DL. Is arrhythmia detection by automatic external defibrillator accurate for children? Sensitivity and specificity of an automatic external defibrillator algorithm in 696 pediatric arrhythmias. *Circulation.* 2001;103:2483–2488.

145. Atkins DL, Hartley LL, York DK. Accurate recognition and effective treatment of ventricular fibrillation by automated external defibrillators in adolescents. *Pediatrics.* 1998;101(pt 1):393–397.
146. Samson RA, Berg RA, Bingham R, Biarent D, Coovadia A, Hazinski MF, Hickey RW, Nadkarni V, Nichol G, Tibballs J, Reis AG, Tse S, Zideman D, Potts J, Uzark K, Atkins D. Use of automated external defibrillators for children: an update: an advisory statement from the pediatric advanced life support task force, International Liaison Committee on Resuscitation. *Circulation.* 2003;107:3250–3255.
147. Cobb LA, Fahrenbruch CE, Walsh TR, Copass MK, Olsufka M, Breskin M, Hallstrom AP. Influence of cardiopulmonary resuscitation prior to defibrillation in patients with out-of-hospital ventricular fibrillation. *JAMA.* 1999;281:1182–1188.
148. Wik L, Hansen TB, Fylling F, Steen T, Vaagenes P, Auestad BH, Steen PA. Delaying defibrillation to give basic cardiopulmonary resuscitation to patients with out-of-hospital ventricular fibrillation: a randomized trial. *JAMA.* 2003;289:1389–1395.
149. Yakaitis RW, Ewy GA, Otto CW, Taren DL, Moon TE. Influence of time and therapy on ventricular defibrillation in dogs. *Crit Care Med.* 1980;8:157–163.
150. Martens PR, Russell JK, Wolcke B, Paschen H, Kuisma M, Gliner BE, Weaver WD, Bossaert L, Chamberlain D, Schneider T. Optimal Response to Cardiac Arrest study: defibrillation waveform effects. *Resuscitation.* 2001;49:233–243.
151. Perondi M, Reis A, Paiva E, Nadkarni V, Berg RA. A comparison of high-dose and standard-dose epinephrine in children with cardiac arrest. *N Engl J Med.* 2004;350:1722–1730.
152. Kudenchuk PJ, Cobb LA, Copass MK, Cummins RO, Doherty AM, Fahrenbruch CE, Hallstrom AP, Murray WA, Olsufka M, Walsh T. Amiodarone for resuscitation after out-of-hospital cardiac arrest due to ventricular fibrillation. *N Engl J Med.* 1999;341:871–878.
153. Perry JC, Fenrich AL, Hulse JE, Triedman JK, Friedman RA, Lamberti JJ. Pediatric use of intravenous amiodarone: efficacy and safety in critically ill patients from a multicenter protocol. *J Am Coll Cardiol.* 1996;27:1246–1250.
154. Perry JC, Knilans TK, Marlow D, Denfield SW, Fenrich AL, Friedman RA. Intravenous amiodarone for life-threatening tachyarrhythmias in children and young adults. *J Am Coll Cardiol.* 1993;22:95–98.
155. van Haarst AD, van't Klooster GA, van Gerven JM, Schoemaker RC, van Oene JC, Burggraaf J, Coene MC, Cohen AF. The influence of cisapride and clarithromycin on QT intervals in healthy volunteers. *Clin Pharmacol Ther.* 1998;64:542–546.
156. Ray WA, Murray KT, Meredith S, Narasimhulu SS, Hall K, Stein CM. Oral erythromycin and the risk of sudden death from cardiac causes. *N Engl J Med.* 2004;351:1089–1096.
157. Berg RA, Otto CW, Kern KB, Hilwig RW, Sanders AB, Henry CP, Ewy GA. A randomized, blinded trial of high-dose epinephrine versus standard-dose epinephrine in a swine model of pediatric asphyxial cardiac arrest. *Crit Care Med.* 1996;24:1695–1700.
158. Tang W, Weil MH, Sun S, Noc M, Yang L, Gazmuri RJ. Epinephrine increases the severity of postresuscitation myocardial dysfunction. *Circulation.* 1995;92:3089–3093.
159. Rivers EP, Wortsman J, Rady MY, Blake HC, McGeorge FT, Buderer NM. The effect of the total cumulative epinephrine dose administered during human CPR on hemodynamic, oxygen transport, and utilization variables in the postresuscitation period. *Chest.* 1994;106:1499–1507.
160. Beland MJ, Hesslein PS, Finlay CD, Faerron-Angel JE, Williams WG, Rowe RD. Noninvasive transcutaneous cardiac pacing in children. *Pacing Clin Electrophysiol.* 1987;10:1262–1270.
161. Quan L, Graves JR, Kinder DR, Horan S, Cummins RO. Transcutaneous cardiac pacing in the treatment of out-of-hospital pediatric cardiac arrests. *Ann Emerg Med.* 1992;21:905–909.
162. Sreeram N, Wren C. Supraventricular tachycardia in infants: response to initial treatment. *Arch Dis Child.* 1990;65:127–129.
163. Aydin M, Baysal K, Kucukoduk S, Cetinkaya F, Yaman S. Application of ice water to the face in initial treatment of supraventricular tachycardia. *Turk J Pediatr.* 1995;37:15–17.
164. Ornato JP, Hallagan LF, Reese WA, Clark RF, Tayal VS, Garnett AR, Gonzalez ER. Treatment of paroxysmal supraventricular tachycardia in the emergency department by clinical decision analysis [published correction appears in *Am J Emerg Med.* 1990;8:85]. *Am J Emerg Med.* 1988;6:555–560.
165. Lim SH, Anantharaman V, Teo WS, Goh PP, Tan AT. Comparison of treatment of supraventricular tachycardia by Valsalva maneuver and carotid sinus massage. *Ann Emerg Med.* 1998;31:30–35.
166. Waxman MB, Wald RW, Sharma AD, Huerta F, Cameron DA. Vagal techniques for termination of paroxysmal supraventricular tachycardia. *Am J Cardiol.* 1980;46:655–664.
167. Gouin S, Ali S. A patient with chaotic atrial tachycardia. *Pediatr Emerg Care.* 2003;19:95–98.
168. Mandapati R, Byrum CJ, Kavey RE, Smith FC, Kveselis DA, Hannan WP, Brandt B III, Gaum WE. Procainamide for rate control of postsurgical junctional tachycardia. *Pediatr Cardiol.* 2000;21:123–128.
169. Wang JN, Wu JM, Tsai YC, Lin CS. Ectopic atrial tachycardia in children. *J Formos Med Assoc.* 2000;99:766–770.
170. Epstein ML, Kiel EA, Victorica BE. Cardiac decompensation following verapamil therapy in infants with supraventricular tachycardia. *Pediatrics.* 1985;75:737–740.
171. Kirk CR, Gibbs JL, Thomas R, Radley-Smith R, Qureshi SA. Cardiovascular collapse after verapamil in supraventricular tachycardia. *Arch Dis Child.* 1987;62:1265–1266.
172. Rankin AC, Rae AP, Oldroyd KG, Cobbe SM. Verapamil or adenosine for the immediate treatment of supraventricular tachycardia. *Q J Med.* 1990;74:203–208.
173. Benson D Jr, Smith W, Dunnigan A, Sterba R, Gallagher J. Mechanisms of regular wide QRS tachycardia in infants and children. *Am J Cardiol.* 1982;49:1778–1788.
174. Dykes EH, Spence LJ, Young JG, Bohn DJ, Filler RM, Wesson DE. Preventable pediatric trauma deaths in a metropolitan region. *J Pediatr Surg.* 1989;24:107–110.
175. Buunke G, van der Hoeveen JG, Meinders AE. Cerebrovascular reactivity in comatose patients resuscitated from a cardiac arrest. *Stroke.* 1997;28:1569–1573.
176. Muizelaar JP, Marmarou A, Ward JD, Kontos HA, Choi SC, Becker DP, Gruemer H, Young HF. Adverse effects of prolonged hyperventilation in patients with severe head injury: a randomized clinical trial. *J Neurosurg.* 1991;75:731–739.
177. Baskaya MK. Inadvertent intracranial placement of a nasogastric tube in patients with head injuries. *Surg Neurol.* 1999;52:426–427.
178. Rutledge R, Sheldon GF, Collins ML. Massive transfusion. *Crit Care Clin.* 1986;2:791–805.
179. Niven MJ, Zohar M, Shimoni Z, Glick J. Symptomatic hypocalcemia precipitated by small-volume blood transfusion. *Ann Emerg Med.* 1998;32:498–501.
180. Ramenofsky ML, Luterman A, Quindlen E, Riddick L, Curreri PW. Maximum survival in pediatric trauma: the ideal system. *J Trauma.* 1984;24:818–823.
181. Luterman A, Ramenofsky M, Berryman C, Talley MA, Curreri PW. Evaluation of prehospital emergency medical service (EMS): defining areas for improvement. *J Trauma.* 1983;23:702–707.
182. McPherson M, Arango P, Fox H, Lauver C, McManus M, Newacheck PW, Perrin JM, Shonkoff JP, Strickland B. A new definition of children with special health care needs. *Pediatrics.* 1998;102:137–140.
183. Newacheck PW, Strickland B, Shonkoff JP, Perrin JM, McPherson M, McManus M, Lauver C, Fox H, Arango P. An epidemiologic profile of children with special health care needs. *Pediatrics.* 1998;102:117–123.
184. Emergency preparedness for children with special health care needs. Committee on Pediatric Emergency Medicine. American Academy of Pediatrics. *Pediatrics.* 1999;104:e53.
185. Spaite DW, Conroy C, Tibbitts M, Karriker KJ, Seng M, Battaglia N, Criss EA, Valenzuela TD, Meislin HW. Use of emergency medical services by children with special health care needs. *Prehosp Emerg Care.* 2000;4:19–23.
186. Hollander JE, Hoffman RS, Gennis P, Fairweather P, DiSano MJ, Schumb DA, Feldman JA, Fish SS, Dyer S, Wax P, et al. Prospective multicenter evaluation of cocaine-associated chest pain. Cocaine Associated Chest Pain (COCHPA) Study Group. *Acad Emerg Med.* 1994;1:330–339.
187. Brody SL, Slovis CM, Wrenn KD. Cocaine-related medical problems: consecutive series of 233 patients. *Am J Med.* 1990;88:325–331.
188. Bauman JL, Grawe JJ, Winecoff AP, Hariman RJ. Cocaine-related sudden cardiac death: a hypothesis correlating basic science and clinical observations. *J Clin Pharmacol.* 1994;34:902–911.
189. Kolecki PF, Curry SC. Poisoning by sodium channel blocking agents. *Crit Care Clin.* 1997;13:829–848.
190. Lange RA, Cigarroa RG, Flores ED, McBride W, Kim AS, Wells PJ, Bedotto JB, Danziger RS, Hillis LD. Potentiation of cocaine-induced coronary vasoconstriction by beta-adrenergic blockade. *Ann Intern Med.* 1990;112:897–903.

191. Brogan WCI, Lange RA, Kim AS, Moliterno DJ, Hillis LD. Alleviation of cocaine-induced coronary vasoconstriction by nitroglycerin. *J Am Coll Cardiol*. 1991;18:581–586.
192. Hollander JE, Hoffman RS, Gennis P, Fairweather P, DiSano MJ, Schumb DA, Feldman JA, Fish SS, Dyer S, Wax P, et al. Nitroglycerin in the treatment of cocaine associated chest pain–clinical safety and efficacy. *J Toxicol Clin Toxicol*. 1994;32:243–256.
193. Hoffman RS, Hollander JE. Evaluation of patients with chest pain after cocaine use. *Crit Care Clin*. 1997;13:809–828.
194. Lange RA, Cigarroa RG, Yancy CW Jr, Willard JE, Popma JJ, Sills MN, McBride W, Kim AS, Hillis LD. Cocaine-induced coronary-artery vasoconstriction. *N Engl J Med*. 1989;321:1557–1562.
195. Kerns W II, Garvey L, Owens J. Cocaine-induced wide complex dysrhythmia. *J Emerg Med*. 1997;15:321–329.
196. Beckman KJ, Parker RB, Hariman RJ, Gallastegui JL, Javaid JI, Bauman JL. Hemodynamic and electrophysiological actions of cocaine: effects of sodium bicarbonate as an antidote in dogs. *Circulation*. 1991; 83:1799–1807.
197. Dziukas LJ, Vohra J. Tricyclic antidepressant poisoning. *Med J Aust*. 1991;154:344–350.
198. Liebelt EL. Targeted management strategies for cardiovascular toxicity from tricyclic antidepressant overdose: the pivotal role for alkalinization and sodium loading. *Pediatr Emerg Care*. 1998;14:293–298.
199. Teba L, Schiebel F, Dedhia HV, Lazzell VA. Beneficial effect of norepinephrine in the treatment of circulatory shock caused by tricyclic antidepressant overdose. *Am J Emerg Med*. 1988;6:566–568.
200. Tran TP, Panacek EA, Rhee KJ, Foulke GE. Response to dopamine vs norepinephrine in tricyclic antidepressant-induced hypotension. *Acad Emerg Med*. 1997;4:864–868.
201. Williams JM, Hollingshed MJ, Vasilakis A, Morales M, Prescott JE, Graeber GM. Extracorporeal circulation in the management of severe tricyclic antidepressant overdose. *Am J Emerg Med*. 1994;12:456–458.
202. Larkin GL, Graeber GM, Hollingshed MJ. Experimental amitriptyline poisoning: treatment of severe cardiovascular toxicity with cardiopulmonary bypass. *Ann Emerg Med*. 1994;23:480–486.
203. Ramoska EA, Spiller HA, Winter M, Borys D. A one-year evaluation of calcium channel blocker overdoses: toxicity and treatment. *Ann Emerg Med*. 1993;22:196–200.
204. Henry M, Kay MM, Viccellio P. Cardiogenic shock associated with calcium-channel and beta blockers: reversal with intravenous calcium chloride. *Am J Emerg Med*. 1985;3:334–336.
205. Howarth DM, Dawson AH, Smith AJ, Buckley N, Whyte IM. Calcium channel blocking drug overdose: an Australian series. *Hum Exp Toxicol*. 1994;13:161–166.
206. Horowitz BZ, Rhee KJ. Massive verapamil ingestion: a report of two cases and a review of the literature. *Am J Emerg Med*. 1989;7:624–631.
207. Watling SM, Crain JL, Edwards TD, Stiller RA. Verapamil overdose: case report and review of the literature. *Ann Pharmacother*. 1992;26: 1373–1378.
208. Kerns W II, Schroeder D, Williams C, Tomaszewski C, Raymond R. Insulin improves survival in a canine model of acute beta-blocker toxicity. *Ann Emerg Med*. 1997;29:748–757.
209. Kline JA, Tomaszewski CA, Schroeder JD, Raymond RM. Insulin is a superior antidote for cardiovascular toxicity induced by verapamil in the anesthetized canine. *J Pharmacol Exp Ther*. 1993;267:744–750.
210. Yuan TH, Kerns WP II, Tomaszewski CA, Ford MD, Kline JA. Insulin-glucose as adjunctive therapy for severe calcium channel antagonist poisoning. *J Toxicol Clin Toxicol*. 1999;37:463–474.
211. Kerns W II, Kline J, Ford MD. Beta-blocker and calcium channel blocker toxicity. *Emerg Med Clin North Am*. 1994;12:365–390.
212. Lewis M, Kallenbach J, Germond C, Zaltzman M, Muller F, Steyn J, Zwi S. Survival following massive overdose of adrenergic blocking agents (acebutolol and labetalol). *Eur Heart J*. 1983;4:328–332.
213. Cruickshank JM, Neil-Dwyer G, Cameron MM, McAinsh J. Beta-adrenoreceptor-blocking agents and the blood-brain barrier. *Clin Sci*. 1980; 59(suppl 6):453s–455s.
214. Weinstein RS. Recognition and management of poisoning with beta-adrenergic blocking agents. *Ann Emerg Med*. 1984;13:1123–1131.
215. Avery GJD, Spotnitz HM, Rose EA, Malm JR, Hoffman BF. Pharmacologic antagonism of beta-adrenergic blockade in dogs, I: hemodynamic effects of isoproterenol, dopamine, and epinephrine in acute propranolol administration. *J Thorac Cardiovasc Surg*. 1979;77:267–276.
216. Zaritsky AL, Horowitz M, Chernow B. Glucagon antagonism of calcium channel blocker-induced myocardial dysfunction. *Crit Care Med*. 1988; 16:246–251.
217. Mofenson HC, Caraccio TR, Laudano J. Glucagon for propranolol overdose. *JAMA*. 1986;255:2025–2026.
218. Love JN, Hanfling D, Howell JM. Hemodynamic effects of calcium chloride in a canine model of acute propranolol intoxication. *Ann Emerg Med*. 1996;28:1–6.
219. Haddad LM. Resuscitation after nifedipine overdose exclusively with intravenous calcium chloride. *Am J Emerg Med*. 1996;14:602–603.
220. Mc Guire W, Fowlie PW. Naloxone for narcotic exposed newborn infants: systematic review. *Arch Dis Child Fetal Neonatal Ed*. 2003;88: F308–F311.
221. Chernick V, Manfreda J, DeBooy V, Davi M, Rigalto H, Seshia M. Clinical trial of naloxone in birth asphyxia. *J Pediatr*. 1988;113: 519–525.
222. Fischer CG, Cook DR. The respiratory and narcotic antagonistic effects of naloxone in infants. *Anesth Analg*. 1974;53:849–852.
223. Kattwinkel J, Niermeyer S, Nadkarni V, Tibballs J, Phillips B, Zideman D, Van Reempts P, Osmond M. An advisory statement from the Pediatric Working Group of the International Liaison Committee on Resuscitation. *Middle East J Anesthesiol*. 2001;16:315–351.
224. American Academy of Pediatrics Committee on Drugs. Naloxone dosage and route of administration for infants and children: addendum to emergency drug doses for infants and children. *Pediatrics*. 1990;86: 484–485.
225. Mills CA, Flacke JW, Flacke WE, Bloor BC, Liu MD. Narcotic reversal in hypercapnic dogs: comparison of naloxone and nalbuphine. *Can J Anaesth*. 1990;37:238–244.
226. Tobias JD, Lynch A, Garrett J. Alterations of end-tidal carbon dioxide during the intrahospital transport of children. *Pediatr Emerg Care*. 1996;12:249–251.
227. Kern KB, Hilwig RW, Berg RA, Rhee KH, Sanders AB, Otto CW, Ewy GA. Postresuscitation left ventricular systolic and diastolic dysfunction: treatment with dobutamine. *Circulation*. 1997;95:2610–2613.
228. Meyer RJ, Kern KB, Berg RA, Hilwig RW, Ewy GA. Post-resuscitation right ventricular dysfunction: delineation and treatment with dobutamine. *Resuscitation*. 2002;55:187–191.
229. Ceneviva G, Paschall JA, Maffei F, Carcillo JA. Hemodynamic support in fluid-refractory pediatric septic shock. *Pediatrics*. 1998;102:e19.
230. Levy B, Bollaert PE, Charpentier C, Nace L, Audibert G, Bauer P, Nabet P, Larcan A. Comparison of norepinephrine and dobutamine to epinephrine for hemodynamics, lactate metabolism, and gastric tonometric variables in septic shock: a prospective, randomized study. *Intensive Care Med*. 1997;23:282–287.
231. Zaritsky AL. Catecholamines, inotropic medications, and vasopressor agents. In: Chernow B, ed. *The Pharmacologic Approach to the Critically Ill Patient*. 3rd ed. Baltimore, Md: Williams & Wilkins; 1994: 387–404.
232. Berg RA, Padbury JF. Sulfoconjugation and renal excretion contribute to the interpatient variation of exogenous catecholamine clearance in critically ill children. *Crit Care Med*. 1997;25:1247–1251.
233. Fisher DG, Schwartz PH, Davis AL. Pharmacokinetics of exogenous epinephrine in critically ill children. *Crit Care Med*. 1993;21:111–117.
234. Ushay HM, Notterman DA. Pharmacology of pediatric resuscitation. *Pediatr Clin North Am*. 1997;44:207–233.
235. Habib DM, Padbury JF, Anas NG, Perkin RM, Minegar C. Dobutamine pharmacokinetics and pharmacodynamics in pediatric intensive care patients. *Crit Care Med*. 1992;20:601–608.
236. Martinez AM, Padbury JF, Thio S. Dobutamine pharmacokinetics and cardiovascular responses in critically ill neonates. *Pediatrics*. 1992;89: 47–51.
237. Barton P, Garcia J, Kouatli A, Kitchen L, Zorka A, Lindsay C, Lawless S, Giroir B. Hemodynamic effects of i.v. milrinone lactate in pediatric patients with septic shock: a prospective, double-blinded, randomized, placebo-controlled, interventional study. *Chest*. 1996;109:1302–1312.
238. Bailey JM, Miller BE, Lu W, Tosone SR, Kanter KR, Tam VK. The pharmacokinetics of milrinone in pediatric patients after cardiac surgery. *Anesthesiology*. 1999;90:1012–1018.
239. Abdallah I, Shawky H. A randomised controlled trial comparing milrinone and epinephrine as inotropes in paediatric patients undergoing total correction of tetralogy of Fallot. *Egyptian J Anaesthesia*. 2003;19: 323–329.
240. Hypothermia After Cardiac Arrest Study Group. Mild therapeutic hypothermia to improve the neurologic outcome after cardiac arrest. *N Engl J Med*. 2002;346:549–556.

241. Bernard SA, Gray TW, Buist MD, Jones BM, Silvester W, Gutteridge G, Smith K. Treatment of comatose survivors of out-of-hospital cardiac arrest with induced hypothermia. *N Engl J Med.* 2002;346:557–563.
242. Gluckman PD, Wyatt JS, Azzopardi D, Ballard R, Edwards AD, Ferriero DM, Polin RA, Robertson CM, Thoresen M, Whitelaw A, Gunn AJ. Selective head cooling with mild systemic hypothermia after neonatal encephalopathy: multicentre randomised trial. *Lancet.* 2005;365: 663–670.
243. Shankaran S, Laptook AR, Ehrenkranz RA, Tyson JE, McDonald SA, Donovan EF, Fanaroff AA, Poole WK, Wright LL, Higgins RD, Finer NN, Carlo WA, Duara S, Oh W, Cotten CM, Stevenson DK, Stoll BJ, Lemons JA, Guillet R, Jobe AH. Whole-body hypothermia for neonates with hypoxic-ischemic encephalopathy. *N Engl J Med.* 2005;353: 1574–1584.
244. Zeiner A, Holzer M, Sterz F, Schorkhuber W, Eisenburger P, Havel C, Kliegel A, Laggner AN. Hyperthermia after cardiac arrest is associated with an unfavorable neurologic outcome. *Arch Intern Med.* 2001;161: 2007–2012.
245. Takasu A, Saitoh D, Kaneko N, Sakamoto T, Okada Y. Hyperthermia: is it an ominous sign after cardiac arrest? *Resuscitation.* 2001;49: 273–277.
246. Ginsberg MD, Busto R. Combating hyperthermia in acute stroke: a significant clinical concern. *Stroke.* 1998;29:529–534.
247. Hickey RW, Kochanek PM, Ferimer H, Alexander HL, Garman RH, Graham SH. Induced hyperthermia exacerbates neurologic neuronal histologic damage after asphyxial cardiac arrest in rats. *Crit Care Med.* 2003;31:531–535.
248. Shum-Tim D, Nagashima M, Shinoka T, Bucerius J, Nollert G, Lidov HG, du Plessis A, Laussen PC, Jonas RA. Postischemic hyperthermia exacerbates neurologic injury after deep hypothermic circulatory arrest. *J Thorac Cardiovasc Surg.* 1998;116:780–792.
249. Henning R. Emergency transport of critically ill children: stabilisation before departure. *Med J Aust.* 1992;156:117–124.
250. Edge WE, Kanter RK, Weigle CG, Walsh RF. Reduction of morbidity in interhospital transport by specialized pediatric staff. *Crit Care Med.* 1994;22:1186–1191.
251. Guidelines for the transfer of critically ill patients. Guidelines Committee of the American College of Critical Care Medicine; Society of Critical Care Medicine and American Association of Critical-Care Nurses Transfer Guidelines Task Force. *Crit Care Med.* 1993;21: 931–937.
252. Barratt F, Wallis DN. Relatives in the resuscitation room: their point of view. *J Accid Emerg Med.* 1998;15:109–111.
253. Boie ET, Moore GP, Brummett C, Nelson DR. Do parents want to be present during invasive procedures performed on their children in the emergency department? A survey of 400 parents. *Ann Emerg Med.* 1999;34:70–74.
254. Doyle CJ, Post H, Burney RE, Maino J, Keefe M, Rhee KJ. Family participation during resuscitation: an option. *Ann Emerg Med.* 1987;16:673–675.
255. Hanson C, Strawser D. Family presence during cardiopulmonary resuscitation: Foote Hospital emergency department's nine-year perspective. *J Emerg Nurs.* 1992;18:104–106.
256. Meyers TA, Eichhorn DJ, Guzzetta CE. Do families want to be present during CPR? A retrospective survey. *J Emerg Nurs.* 1998;24:400–405.
257. Robinson SM, Mackenzie-Ross S, Campbell Hewson GL, Egleston CV, Prevost AT. Psychological effect of witnessed resuscitation on bereaved relatives.[comment]. *Lancet.* 1998;352:614–617.
258. Boyd R. Witnessed resuscitation by relatives. *Resuscitation.* 2000;43:171–176.
259. Offord RJ. Should relatives of patients with cardiac arrest be invited to be present during cardiopulmonary resuscitation? *Intensive Crit Care Nurs.* 1998;14:288–293.
260. Eichhorn DJ, Meyers TA, Mitchell TG, Guzzetta CE. Opening the doors: family presence during resuscitation. *J Cardiovasc Nurs.* 1996; 10:59–70.
261. Zaritsky A, Nadkarni V, Getson P, Kuehl K. CPR in children. *Ann Emerg Med.* 1987;16:1107–1111.
262. Lopez-Herce J, Garcia C, Dominguez P, Carrillo A, Rodriguez-Nunez A, Calvo C, Delgado MA. Characteristics and outcome of cardiorespiratory arrest in children. *Resuscitation.* 2004;63:311–320.
263. Lopez-Herce J, Garcia C, Rodriguez-Nunez A, Dominguez P, Carrillo A, Calvo C, Delgado MA. Long-term outcome of paediatric cardiorespiratory arrest in Spain. *Resuscitation.* 2005;64:79–85.
264. del Nido PJ, Dalton HJ, Thompson AE, Siewers RD. Extracorporeal membrane oxygenator rescue in children during cardiac arrest after cardiac surgery. *Circulation.* 1992;86(suppl):II-300–II-304.
265. Parra DA, Totapally BR, Zahn E, Jacobs J, Aldousany A, Burke RP, Chang AC. Outcome of cardiopulmonary resuscitation in a pediatric cardiac intensive care unit. *Crit Care Med.* 2000;28:3296–3300.

Part 13: Neonatal Resuscitation Guidelines

The following guidelines are intended for practitioners responsible for resuscitating neonates. They apply primarily to neonates undergoing transition from intrauterine to extrauterine life. The recommendations are also applicable to neonates who have completed perinatal transition and require resuscitation during the first few weeks to months following birth. Practitioners who resuscitate infants at birth or at any time during the initial hospital admission should consider following these guidelines. The terms *newborn* and *neonate* are intended to apply to any infant during the initial hospitalization. The term *newly born* is intended to apply specifically to an infant at the time of birth.

Approximately 10% of newborns require some assistance to begin breathing at birth. About 1% require extensive resuscitative measures. Although the vast majority of newly born infants do not require intervention to make the transition from intrauterine to extrauterine life, because of the large number of births, a sizable number will require some degree of resuscitation.

Those newly born infants who do not require resuscitation can generally be identified by a rapid assessment of the following 4 characteristics:

- Was the baby born after a full-term gestation?
- Is the amniotic fluid clear of meconium and evidence of infection?
- Is the baby breathing or crying?
- Does the baby have good muscle tone?

If the answer to all 4 of these questions is "yes," the baby does not need resuscitation and should not be separated from the mother. The baby can be dried, placed directly on the mother's chest, and covered with dry linen to maintain temperature. Observation of breathing, activity, and color should be ongoing.

If the answer to any of these assessment questions is "no," there is general agreement that the infant should receive one or more of the following 4 categories of action in sequence:

A. Initial steps in stabilization (provide warmth, position, clear airway, dry, stimulate, reposition)
B. Ventilation
C. Chest compressions
D. Administration of epinephrine and/or volume expansion

The decision to progress from one category to the next is determined by the simultaneous assessment of 3 vital signs: respirations, heart rate, and color. Approximately 30 seconds is allotted to complete each step, reevaluate, and decide whether to progress to the next step (see the Figure).

(*Circulation.* **2005;112:IV-188-IV-195.**)

DOI: 10.1161/CIRCULATIONAHA.105.166574

Anticipation of Resuscitation Need

Anticipation, adequate preparation, accurate evaluation, and prompt initiation of support are critical for successful neonatal resuscitation. At every delivery there should be at least one person whose primary responsibility is the newly born. This person must be capable of initiating resuscitation, including administration of positive-pressure ventilation and chest compressions. Either that person or someone else who is immediately available should have the skills required to perform a complete resuscitation, including endotracheal intubation and administration of medications.[1]

With careful consideration of risk factors, the majority of newborns who will need resuscitation can be identified before birth. If the possible need for resuscitation is anticipated, additional skilled personnel should be recruited and the necessary equipment prepared. Identifiable risk factors and the necessary equipment for resuscitation are listed on the Neonatal Resuscitation Program website: *www.aap.org/NRP.* If a preterm delivery (<37 weeks of gestation) is expected, special preparations will be required. Preterm babies have immature lungs that may be more difficult to ventilate and are also more vulnerable to injury by positive-pressure ventilation. Preterm babies also have immature blood vessels in the brain that are prone to hemorrhage; thin skin and a large surface area, which contribute to rapid heat loss; increased susceptibility to infection; and increased risk of hypovolemic shock caused by small blood volume.

Initial Steps

The initial steps of resuscitation are to provide warmth by placing the baby under a radiant heat source, position the head in a "sniffing" position to open the airway, clear the airway with a bulb syringe or suction catheter, and dry the baby and stimulate breathing. Recent studies have examined several aspects of these initial steps. These studies are summarized below.

Temperature Control

Very low birth weight (<1500 g) preterm babies are likely to become hypothermic despite the use of traditional techniques for decreasing heat loss (LOE 5).[2] For this reason it is recommended that additional warming techniques be used, such as covering the baby in plastic wrapping (food-grade, heat-resistant plastic) and placing him or her under radiant heat (Class IIa; LOE 2[3,4]; LOE 4[5,6]; LOE 5[7]). Temperature must be monitored closely because of the slight but described (LOE 2)[4] risk of hyperthermia with this technique. Other techniques to maintain temperature during stabilization of the baby in the delivery room (eg, drying and swaddling, warming pads, increased environmental temperature, placing the baby skin-to-skin with the mother and covering both with a blanket) have been used (LOE 8),[8,9] but they have not been

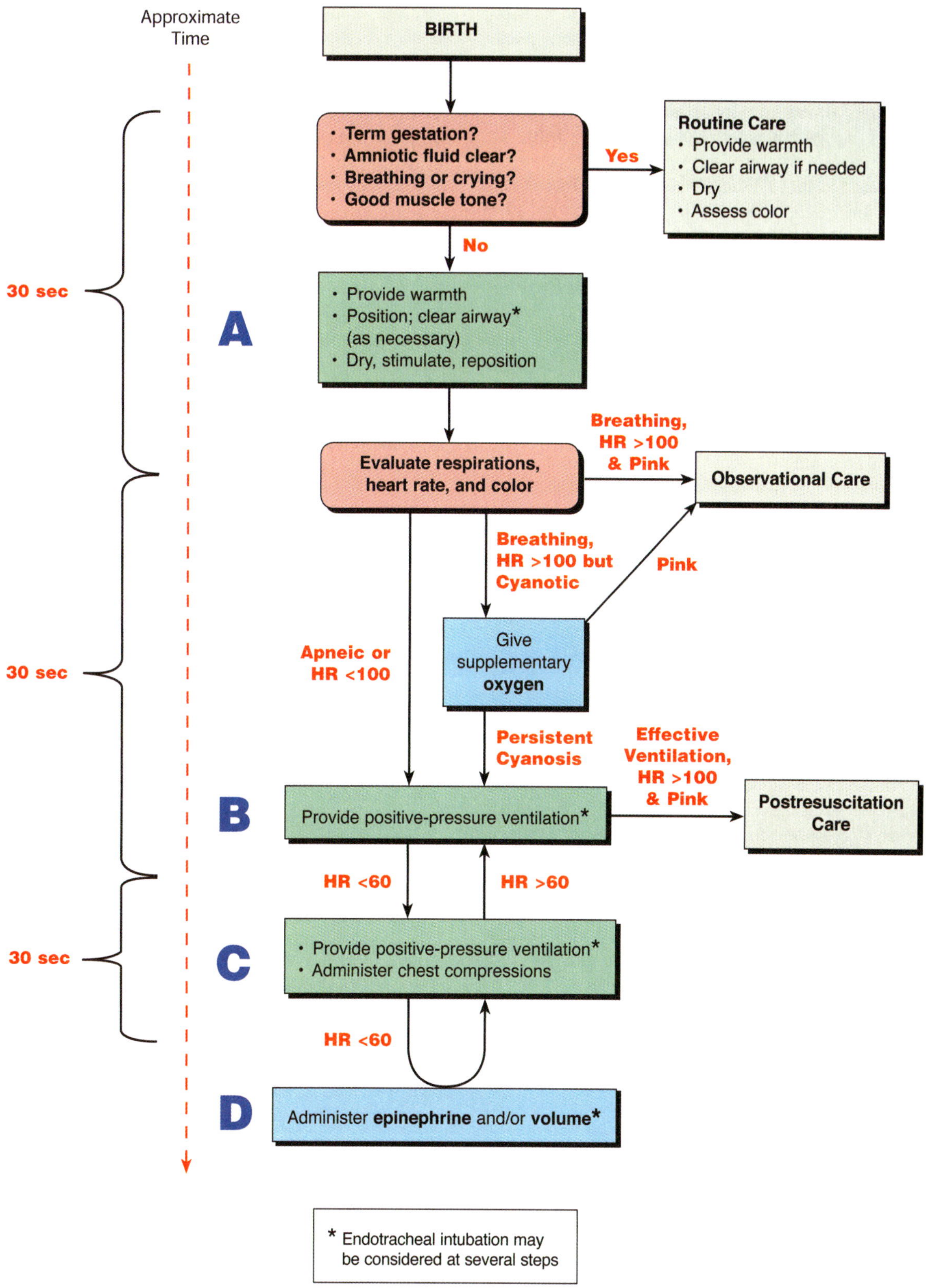

Figure. Neonatal Flow Algorithm.

evaluated in controlled trials nor compared with the plastic wrap technique for premature babies. All resuscitation procedures, including endotracheal intubation, chest compression, and insertion of lines, can be performed with these temperature-controlling interventions in place.

Infants born to febrile mothers have been reported (LOE 4)[10–12] to have a higher incidence of perinatal respiratory depression, neonatal seizures, and cerebral palsy and increased risk of mortality. Animal studies (LOE 6)[13,14] indicate that hyperthermia during or after ischemia is associated with progression of cerebral injury. Hyperthermia should be avoided (Class IIb). The goal is to achieve normothermia and avoid iatrogenic hyperthermia.

Clearing the Airway of Meconium

Aspiration of meconium before delivery, during birth, or during resuscitation can cause severe aspiration pneumonia. One obstetrical technique to try to decrease aspiration has been to suction meconium from the infant's airway after delivery of the head but before delivery of the shoulders (intrapartum suctioning). Although some studies (LOE 3[15]; 4[16,17]) suggested that intrapartum suctioning might be effective for decreasing the risk of aspiration syndrome, subsequent evidence from a large multicenter randomized trial (LOE 1)[18] did not show such an effect. Therefore, current recommendations no longer advise routine intrapartum oropharyngeal and nasopharyngeal suctioning for infants born to mothers with meconium staining of amniotic fluid (Class I).

Traditional teaching (LOE 5)[19–21] recommended that meconium-stained infants have endotracheal intubation immediately following birth and that suction be applied to the endotracheal tube as it is withdrawn. Randomized controlled trials (LOE 1)[15,22] have shown that this practice offers no benefit if the infant is vigorous (Class I). A vigorous infant is defined as one who has strong respiratory efforts, good muscle tone, and a heart rate >100 beats per minute (bpm). Endotracheal suctioning for infants who are not vigorous should be performed immediately after birth (Class Indeterminate).

Periodic Evaluation at 30-Second Intervals

After the immediate postbirth assessment and administration of initial steps, further resuscitative efforts should be guided by simultaneous assessment of respirations, heart rate, and color. After initial respiratory efforts the newly born infant should be able to establish regular respirations that are sufficient to improve color and maintain a heart rate >100 bpm. Gasping and apnea indicate the need for assisted ventilation.[23] Increasing or decreasing heart rate can also provide evidence of improvement or deterioration.

A newly born infant who is uncompromised will achieve and maintain pink mucous membranes without administration of supplementary oxygen. Evidence obtained with continuous oximetry, however, has shown that neonatal transition is a gradual process. Healthy babies born at term may take >10 minutes to achieve a preductal oxygen saturation >95% and nearly 1 hour to achieve postductal saturation >95% (LOE 5).[24–26] Central cyanosis is determined by examining the face, trunk, and mucous membranes. Acrocyanosis (blue color of hands and feet alone) is usually a normal finding at birth and is not a reliable indicator of hypoxemia but may indicate other conditions, such as cold stress. Pallor or mottling may be a sign of decreased cardiac output, severe anemia, hypovolemia, hypothermia, or acidosis.

Administration of Oxygen

There are concerns about the potential adverse effects of 100% oxygen on respiratory physiology and cerebral circulation and the potential tissue damage from oxygen free radicals. Conversely there are also concerns about tissue damage from oxygen deprivation during and after asphyxia. Studies (LOE 6)[27–31] examining blood pressure, cerebral perfusion, and various biochemical measures of cell damage in asphyxiated animals resuscitated with 100% oxygen versus 21% oxygen (room air) have shown conflicting results. One (LOE 2)[32] study of preterm infants (<33 weeks of gestation) exposed to 80% oxygen found lower cerebral blood flow when compared with those stabilized using 21% oxygen. Some animal data (LOE 6)[27] indicated the opposite effect, ie, reduced blood pressure and cerebral perfusion with 21% oxygen (room air) versus 100% oxygen. Meta-analysis of 4 human studies (LOE 1)[33,34] showed a reduction in mortality rate and no evidence of harm in infants resuscitated with room air versus those resuscitated with 100% oxygen, although these results should be viewed with caution because of significant methodological concerns.

Supplementary oxygen is recommended whenever positive-pressure ventilation is indicated for resuscitation; free-flow oxygen should be administered to babies who are breathing but have central cyanosis (Class Indeterminate). The standard approach to resuscitation is to use 100% oxygen. Some clinicians may begin resuscitation with an oxygen concentration of less than 100%, and some may start with no supplementary oxygen (ie, room air). There is evidence that employing either of these practices during resuscitation of neonates is reasonable. If the clinician begins resuscitation with room air, it is recommended that supplementary oxygen be available to use if there is no appreciable improvement within 90 seconds after birth. In situations where supplementary oxygen is not readily available, positive-pressure ventilation should be administered with room air (Class Indeterminate).

Administration of a variable concentration of oxygen guided by pulse oximetry may improve the ability to achieve normoxia more quickly. Concerns about potential oxidant injury should caution the clinician about the use of excessive oxygen, especially in the premature infant.

Positive-Pressure Ventilation

If the infant remains apneic or gasping, if the heart rate remains <100 bpm 30 seconds after administering the initial steps, or if the infant continues to have persistent central cyanosis despite administration of supplementary oxygen, start positive-pressure ventilation.

Initial Breaths and Assisted Ventilation

In term infants, initial inflations—either spontaneous or assisted—create a functional residual capacity (LOE 5).[35–41] The optimum pressure, inflation time, and flow rate required to establish an effective functional residual capacity have not been determined. Average initial peak inflating pressures of 30 to 40 cm H_2O (inflation time undefined) usually successfully ventilate unresponsive term infants (LOE 5).[36,38,40–43] Assisted ventilation rates of 40 to 60 breaths per minute are commonly used, but the relative efficacy of various rates has not been investigated.

The primary measure of adequate initial ventilation is prompt improvement in heart rate. Chest wall movement should be assessed if heart rate does not improve. The initial peak inflating pressures needed are variable and unpredictable and should be individualized to achieve an increase in heart rate and/or movement of the chest with each breath. If inflation pressure is being monitored, an initial inflation pressure of 20 cm H_2O may be effective, but $\geq$30 to 40 cm H_2O may be required in some term babies without spontaneous ventilation (Class IIb). If pressure is not monitored, the minimum inflation required to achieve an increase in heart rate should be used. There is insufficient evidence to recommend an optimum inflation time. In summary, assisted ventilation should be delivered at a rate of 40 to 60 breaths per minute (Class Indeterminate; LOE 8) to promptly achieve or maintain a heart rate >100 bpm.

Devices

Effective ventilation can be achieved with a flow-inflating bag, a self-inflating bag, or with a T-piece (LoE 4[44,45]; LOE 5[46]). A T-piece is a valved mechanical device designed to control flow and limit pressure. The pop-off valves of self-inflating bags are flow-dependent, and pressures generated may exceed the value specified by the manufacturer (LOE 6).[47] Target inflation pressures and long inspiratory times are more consistently achieved in mechanical models when T-piece devices are used rather than bags (LOE 6),[48] although the clinical implications are not clear. To provide the desired pressure, healthcare providers need more training in the use of flow-inflating bags than with self-inflating bags (LOE 6).[49] A self-inflating bag, a flow-inflating bag, or a T-piece can be used to ventilate a newborn (Class IIb).

Laryngeal mask airways (LMAs) that fit over the laryngeal inlet have been shown to be effective for ventilating newly born near-term and full-term infants (LOE 2[50] and LOE 5[51]). There is limited (LOE 5)[52,53] data on the use of these devices in small preterm infants. Data from 3 case series (LOE 5)[51,54,55] shows that the use of the LMA can provide effective ventilation in a time frame consistent with current resuscitation guidelines, although the babies being studied were not being resuscitated. A randomized controlled trial (LOE 2)[50] found no clinically significant difference between the use of the LMA and endotracheal intubation when bag-mask ventilation was unsuccessful. It is unclear whether this study can be generalized because the LMA was inserted by experienced providers. Case reports (LOE 5)[56–58] suggest that when bag-mask ventilation has been unsuccessful and endotracheal intubation is not feasible or is unsuccessful, the LMA may provide effective ventilation. There is insufficient evidence to support the routine use of the LMA as the primary airway device during neonatal resuscitation, in the setting of meconium-stained amniotic fluid, when chest compressions are required, in very low birth weight babies, or for delivery of emergency intratracheal medications (Class Indeterminate).

Assisted Ventilation of Preterm Infants

Evidence from animal studies (LOE 6)[59] indicates that preterm lungs are easily injured by large-volume inflations immediately after birth. Additional animal studies (LOE 6)[60,61] indicate that when positive-pressure ventilation is applied immediately after birth, the inclusion of positive end-expiratory pressure (PEEP) protects against lung injury and improves lung compliance and gas exchange (LOE 6).[60,61] Evidence from case series in human infants indicates that most apneic preterm infants can be ventilated with an initial inflation pressure of 20 to 25 cm H_2O, although some infants who do not respond require a higher pressure (LOE 5).[62,63]

When ventilating preterm infants after birth, excessive chest wall movement may indicate large-volume lung inflations, which should be avoided. Monitoring of pressure may help to provide consistent inflations and avoid unnecessary high pressures (Class IIb). If positive-pressure ventilation is required, an initial inflation pressure of 20 to 25 cm H_2O is adequate for most preterm infants (Class Indeterminate). If prompt improvement in heart rate or chest movement is not obtained, higher pressures may be needed. If it is necessary to continue positive-pressure ventilation, application of PEEP may be beneficial (Class Indeterminate). Continuous positive airway pressure in spontaneously breathing preterm infants after resuscitation may also be beneficial[63] (Class Indeterminate).

Endotracheal Tube Placement

Endotracheal intubation may be indicated at several points during neonatal resuscitation:

- When tracheal suctioning for meconium is required
- If bag-mask ventilation is ineffective or prolonged
- When chest compressions are performed
- When endotracheal administration of medications is desired
- For special resuscitation circumstances, such as congenital diaphragmatic hernia or extremely low birth weight (<1000 g)

The timing of endotracheal intubation may also depend on the skill and experience of the available providers.

After endotracheal intubation and administration of intermittent positive pressure, a prompt increase in heart rate is the best indicator that the tube is in the tracheobronchial tree and providing effective ventilation (LOE 5).[64] Exhaled CO_2 detection is effective for confirmation of endotracheal tube placement in infants, including very low birth weight infants (LOE 5).[65–68] A positive test result (detection of exhaled CO_2) in patients with adequate cardiac output confirms placement of the endotracheal tube within the trachea, whereas a negative test result (ie, no CO_2 detected) strongly suggests esophageal intubation (LOE 5).[65,67] Poor or absent pulmonary blood flow may give false-negative results (ie, no CO_2 detected despite tube placement in the trachea), but endotracheal tube placement is correctly identified in nearly all patients who are not in cardiac arrest (LOE 7).[69] A false-negative result may also lead to unnecessary extubation in critically ill infants with poor cardiac output.

Other clinical indicators of correct endotracheal tube placement are evaluation of condensed humidified gas during exhalation and the presence or absence of chest movement, but these have not been systematically evaluated in neonates. Endotracheal tube placement must be assessed visually during intubation and by confirmatory methods after intubation if the heart rate remains low and is not rising. Except for intubation to remove meconium, exhaled CO_2 detection is the recommended method of confirmation (Class IIa).

Chest Compressions

Chest compressions are indicated for a heart rate that is <60 bpm despite adequate ventilation with supplementary oxygen for 30 seconds. Because ventilation is the most effective action in neonatal resuscitation and because chest compressions are likely to compete with effective ventilation, rescuers should ensure that assisted ventilation is being delivered optimally before starting chest compressions.

Compressions should be delivered on the lower third of the sternum[70,71] to a depth of approximately one third of the anterior-posterior diameter of the chest. Two techniques have been described: compression with 2 thumbs with fingers encircling the chest and supporting the back[72–74] (the 2 thumb–encircling hands technique) or compression with 2 fingers with a second hand supporting the back. Because the 2 thumb–encircling hands technique may generate higher peak systolic and coronary perfusion pressure than the 2-finger technique (LOE 5[75]; LOE 6[76]), the 2 thumb–encircling hands technique is recommended for performing chest compressions in newly born infants. However, the 2-finger technique may be preferable when access to the umbilicus is required during insertion of an umbilical catheter.

A compression-relaxation ratio with a slightly shorter compression than relaxation phase offers theoretical advantages for blood flow in the very young infant.[77] Also, compressions and ventilations should be coordinated to avoid simultaneous delivery (LOE 6).[78] The chest should be permitted to fully reexpand during relaxation, but the rescuer's thumbs should not leave the chest. There should be a 3:1 ratio of compressions to ventilations with 90 compressions and 30 breaths to achieve approximately 120 events per minute to maximize ventilation at an achievable rate (Class Indeterminate). Thus, each event will be allotted approximately ½ second, with exhalation occurring during the first compression after each ventilation.

Respirations, heart rate, and color should be reassessed about every 30 seconds, and coordinated chest compressions and ventilations should continue until the spontaneous heart rate is ≥60 bpm (Class IIa; LOE 8).

Medications

Drugs are rarely indicated in resuscitation of the newly born infant.[79] Bradycardia in the newborn infant is usually the result of inadequate lung inflation or profound hypoxemia, and establishing adequate ventilation is the most important step to correct it. But if the heart rate remains <60 bpm despite adequate ventilation with 100% oxygen and chest compressions, administration of epinephrine or volume expansion, or both, may be indicated. Rarely, buffers, a narcotic antagonist, or vasopressors may be useful after resuscitation.

Route and Dose of Epinephrine Administration

Past guidelines recommended that initial doses of epinephrine be given through an endotracheal tube because the dose can be administered more quickly than when an intravenous route must be established. But animal studies (LOE 6)[80–82] that showed a positive effect of endotracheal epinephrine used considerably higher doses than are currently recommended, and the one animal study (LOE 6)[83] that used currently recommended doses given endotracheally showed no effect. Given the lack of data on endotracheal epinephrine, the IV route should be used as soon as venous access is established.

The recommended IV dose is 0.01 to 0.03 mg/kg per dose. Higher IV doses are not recommended (Class III) because animal (LOE 6)[84,85] and pediatric (LOE 7)[86] studies show exaggerated hypertension, decreased myocardial function, and worse neurologic function after administration of IV doses in the range of 0.1 mg/kg. If the endotracheal route is used, doses of 0.01 or 0.03 mg/kg will likely be ineffective. Therefore, IV administration of 0.01 to 0.03 mg/kg per dose is the preferred route (Class IIa). While access is being obtained, administration of a higher dose (up to 0.1 mg/kg) through the endotracheal tube may be considered (Class Indeterminate), but the safety and efficacy of this practice have not been evaluated. The concentration of epinephrine for either route should be 1:10 000 (0.1 mg/mL).

Volume Expansion

Consider volume expansion when blood loss is suspected or the infant appears to be in shock (pale skin, poor perfusion, weak pulse) and has not responded adequately to other resuscitative measures. An isotonic crystalloid rather than albumin is the solution of choice for volume expansion in the delivery room (Class IIb; LOE 7).[87–89] The recommended dose is 10 mL/kg, which may need to be repeated. When resuscitating premature infants, care should be taken to avoid giving volume expanders too rapidly, because rapid infusions of large volumes have been associated with intraventricular hemorrhage.

Naloxone

Administration of naloxone is not recommended as part of initial resuscitative efforts in the delivery room for newborns with respiratory depression. If administration of naloxone is considered, heart rate and color must first be restored by supporting ventilation. The preferred route is IV or intramuscular. Given the lack of clinical data in newborns, endotracheal administration of naloxone is not recommended (Class Indeterminate). The recommended dose is 0.1 mg/kg, but no studies have examined the efficacy of this dose in newborns. In one case report, naloxone given to a baby born to an opioid-addicted mother was associated with seizures (LOE 8).[90] Therefore, naloxone should be avoided in babies whose mothers are suspected of having had long-term exposure to opioids (Class Indeterminate). Naloxone may have a shorter half-life than the original maternal opioid; therefore the neonate should be monitored closely for recurrent apnea or hypoventilation, and subsequent doses of naloxone may be required.

Postresuscitation Care

Babies who require resuscitation are at risk for deterioration after their vital signs have returned to normal. Once adequate ventilation and circulation have been established, the infant should be maintained in or transferred to an environment in which close monitoring and anticipatory care can be provided.

Glucose

Low blood glucose has been associated with adverse neurologic outcome in a neonatal animal model of asphyxia and resuscitation (LOE 6).[91] Neonatal animals (LOE 6)[92,93] that were hypoglycemic at the time of an anoxic or hypoxic-ischemic insult had larger areas of cerebral infarction or decreased survival, or both, when compared with controls. One clinical study (LOE 4)[94] showed an association between hypoglycemia and poor neurologic outcome after perinatal asphyxia.

No clinical neonatal studies have investigated the relation between hyperglycemia and neurologic outcome, although hyperglycemia in adults (LOE 7 [extrapolated][95]) is associated with worse outcome. The range of blood glucose concentration associated with the least brain injury after asphyxia and resuscitation cannot be defined based on available evidence. Infants who require significant resuscitation should be monitored and treated to maintain glucose in the normal range (Class Indeterminate).

Induced Hypothermia

In a multicenter trial (LOE 2)[96] involving newborns with suspected asphyxia (indicated by need for resuscitation at birth, metabolic acidosis, and early encephalopathy), selective head cooling (34°C to 35°C) was associated with a nonsignificant reduction in the overall number of survivors with severe disability at 18 months but a significant benefit in the subgroup with moderate encephalopathy. Infants with severe electrographic suppression and seizures did not benefit from treatment with modest hypothermia (LOE 2).[96] A second large multicenter trial (LOE 2)[97] of asphyxiated newborns (indicated by need for resuscitation at birth or presence of metabolic encephalopathy) involved treatment with systemic hypothermia to 33.5°C (92.3°F) following moderate to severe encephalopathy. Hypothermia was associated with a significant (18%) decrease in death or moderate disability at 18 months.[97] A third small controlled pilot study (LOE 2)[98,99] in asphyxiated infants with early induced systemic hypothermia found fewer deaths and disability at 12 months.

Modest hypothermia is associated with bradycardia and elevated blood pressure that do not usually require treatment, but a rapid increase in body temperature may cause hypotension (LOE 5).[100] Cooling to a core temperature <33°C may cause arrhythmia, bleeding, thrombosis, and sepsis, but studies so far have not reported these complications in infants treated with modest (eg, 33°C to 34.5°C [91.4°F to 94.1°F]) hypothermia (LOE 2).[96,101]

There is insufficient data to recommend routine use of modest systemic or selective cerebral hypothermia after resuscitation of infants with suspected asphyxia (Class Indeterminate). Further clinical trials are needed to determine which infants benefit most and which method of cooling is most effective. Avoidance of hyperthermia (elevated body temperature) is particularly important in babies who may have had a hypoxic-ischemic event.

Guidelines for Withholding and Discontinuing Resuscitation

Morbidity and mortality for newborns varies according to region and availability of resources (LOE 5).[102] Social science studies[103] indicate that parents desire a larger role in decisions to initiate resuscitation and continue life support of severely compromised newborns. Opinions among neonatal providers vary widely regarding the benefits and disadvantages of aggressive therapies in such newborns (LOE 5).[104]

Withholding Resuscitation

It is possible to identify conditions associated with high mortality and poor outcome in which withholding resuscitative efforts may be considered reasonable, particularly when there has been the opportunity for parental agreement (LOE 5).[2,105]

A consistent and coordinated approach to individual cases by the obstetric and neonatal teams and the parents is an important goal. Noninitiation of resuscitation and discontinuation of life-sustaining treatment during or after resuscitation are ethically equivalent, and clinicians should not hesitate to withdraw support when functional survival is highly unlikely. The following guidelines must be interpreted according to current regional outcomes:

- When gestation, birth weight, or congenital anomalies are associated with almost certain early death and when unacceptably high morbidity is likely among the rare survivors, resuscitation is not indicated (Class IIa). Examples may include extreme prematurity (gestational age <23 weeks or birth weight <400 g), anencephaly, and chromosomal abnormalities incompatible with life, such as trisomy 13.
- In conditions associated with a high rate of survival and acceptable morbidity, resuscitation is nearly always indicated (Class IIa). This will generally include babies with gestational age ≥25 weeks (unless there is evidence of fetal compromise such as intrauterine infection or hypoxia-ischemia) and those with most congenital malformations.
- In conditions associated with uncertain prognosis in which survival is borderline, the morbidity rate is relatively high, and the anticipated burden to the child is high, parental desires concerning initiation of resuscitation should be supported (Class Indeterminate).

Discontinuing Resuscitative Efforts

Infants without signs of life (no heart beat and no respiratory effort) after 10 minutes of resuscitation show either a high mortality or severe neurodevelopmental disability (LOE 5).[106,107] After 10 minutes of continuous and adequate resuscitative efforts, discontinuation of resuscitation may be justified if there are no signs of life (Class IIb).

References

1. American Academy of Pediatrics, American College of Obstetricians and Gynecologists. In: Gilstrap LC, Oh W, eds. *Guidelines for Perinatal Care.* 5th ed. Elk Grove Village, Ill: American Academy of Pediatrics. 2002:187.
2. Costeloe K, Hennessy E, Gibson AT, Marlow N, Wilkinson AR. The EPICure study: outcomes to discharge from hospital for infants born at the threshold of viability. *Pediatrics.* 2000;106:659–671.
3. Vohra S, Frent G, Campbell V, Abbott M, Whyte R. Effect of polyethylene occlusive skin wrapping on heat loss in very low birth weight infants at delivery: a randomized trial. *J Pediatr.* 1999;134:547–551.
4. Vohra S, Roberts RS, Zhang B, Janes M, Schmidt B. Heat Loss Prevention (HeLP) in the delivery room: a randomized controlled trial of polyethylene occlusive skin wrapping in very preterm infants. *J Pediatr.* 2004;145: 750–753.
5. Lyon AJ, Stenson B. Cold comfort for babies. *Arch Dis Child Fetal Neonatal Ed.* 2004;89:F93–F94.

6. Lenclen R, Mazraani M, Jugie M, Couderc S, Hoenn E, Carbajal R, Blanc P, Paupe A. Use of a polyethylene bag: a way to improve the thermal environment of the premature newborn at the delivery room. *Arch Pediatr.* 2002;9:238–244.
7. Bjorklund LJ, Hellstrom-Westas L. Reducing heat loss at birth in very preterm infants. *J Pediatr.* 2000;137:739–740.
8. Baum JD, Scopes JW. The silver swaddler: device for preventing hypothermia in the newborn. *Lancet.* 1968;1:672–673.
9. Besch NJ, Perlstein PH, Edwards NK, Keenan WJ, Sutherland JM. The transparent baby bag: a shield against heat loss. *N Engl J Med.* 1971;284:121–124.
10. Petrova A, Demissie K, Rhoads GG, Smulian JC, Marcella S, Ananth CV. Association of maternal fever during labor with neonatal and infant morbidity and mortality. *Obstet Gynecol.* 2001;98:20–27.
11. Lieberman E, Lang J, Richardson DK, Frigoletto FD, Heffner LJ, Cohen A. Intrapartum maternal fever and neonatal outcome. *Pediatrics.* 2000;105:8–13.
12. Grether JK, Nelson KB. Maternal infection and cerebral palsy in infants of normal birth weight. *JAMA.* 1997;278:207–211.
13. Coimbra C, Boris-Moller F, Drake M, Wieloch T. Diminished neuronal damage in the rat brain by late treatment with the antipyretic drug dipyrone or cooling following cerebral ischemia. *Acta Neuropathol (Berl).* 1996;92:447–453.
14. Dietrich WD, Alonso O, Halley M, Busto R. Delayed posttraumatic brain hyperthermia worsens outcome after fluid percussion brain injury: a light and electron microscopic study in rats. *Neurosurgery.* 1996;38:533–541; discussion 541.
15. Wiswell TE, Gannon CM, Jacob J, Goldsmith L, Szyld E, Weiss K, Schutzman D, Cleary GM, Filipov P, Kurlat I, Caballero CL, Abassi S, Sprague D, Oltorf C, Padula M. Delivery room management of the apparently vigorous meconium-stained neonate: results of the multicenter, international collaborative trial. *Pediatrics.* 2000;105:1–7.
16. Falciglia HS, Henderschott C, Potter P, Helmchen R. Does DeLee suction at the perineum prevent meconium aspiration syndrome? *Am J Obstet Gynecol.* 1992;167:1243–1249.
17. Carson BS, Losey RW, Bowes WA Jr, Simmons MA. Combined obstetric and pediatric approach to prevent meconium aspiration syndrome. *Am J Obstet Gynecol.* 1976;126:712–715.
18. Vain NE, Szyld EG, Prudent LM, Wiswell TE, Aguilar AM, Vivas NI. Oropharyngeal and nasopharyngeal suctioning of meconium-stained neonates before delivery of their shoulders: multicentre, randomised controlled trial. *Lancet.* 2004;364:597–602.
19. Gregory GA, Gooding CA, Phibbs RH, Tooley WH. Meconium aspiration in infants: a prospective study. *J Pediatr.* 1974;85:848–852.
20. Rossi EM, Philipson EH, Williams TG, Kalhan SC. Meconium aspiration syndrome: intrapartum and neonatal attributes. *Am J Obstet Gynecol.* 1989;161:1106–1110.
21. Davis RO, Philips JB III, Harris BA Jr, Wilson ER, Huddleston JF. Fatal meconium aspiration syndrome occurring despite airway management considered appropriate. *Am J Obstet Gynecol.* 1985;151:731–736.
22. Halliday HL. Endotracheal intubation at birth for preventing morbidity and mortality in vigorous, meconium-stained infants born at term. *Cochrane Database Syst Rev.* 2001;CD000500.
23. Dawes GS. *Foetal and Neonatal Physiology. A Comparative Study of the Changes at Birth.* Chicago, Ill: Year Book Medical Publishers Inc; 1968.
24. Harris AP, Sendak MJ, Donham RT. Changes in arterial oxygen saturation immediately after birth in the human neonate. *J Pediatr.* 1986;109:117–119.
25. Reddy VK, Holzman IR, Wedgwood JF. Pulse oximetry saturations in the first 6 hours of life in normal term infants. *Clin Pediatr (Phila).* 1999;38:87–92.
26. Toth B, Becker A, Seelbach-Gobel B. Oxygen saturation in healthy newborn infants immediately after birth measured by pulse oximetry. *Arch Gynecol Obstet.* 2002;266:105–107.
27. Solas AB, Kutzsche S, Vinje M, Saugstad OD. Cerebral hypoxemia-ischemia and reoxygenation with 21% or 100% oxygen in newborn piglets: effects on extracellular levels of excitatory amino acids and microcirculation. *Pediatr Crit Care Med.* 2001;2:340–345.
28. Solas AB, Munkeby BH, Saugstad OD. Comparison of short- and long-duration oxygen treatment after cerebral asphyxia in newborn piglets. *Pediatr Res.* 2004;56:125–131.
29. Solas AB, Kalous P, Saugstad OD. Reoxygenation with 100 or 21% oxygen after cerebral hypoxemia-ischemia-hypercapnia in newborn piglets. *Biol Neonate.* 2004;85:105–111.
30. Huang CC, Yonetani M, Lajevardi N, Delivoria-Papadopoulos M, Wilson DF, Pastuszko A. Comparison of postasphyxial resuscitation with 100% and 21% oxygen on cortical oxygen pressure and striatal dopamine metabolism in newborn piglets. *J Neurochem.* 1995;64:292–298.
31. Kutzsche S, Kirkeby OJ, Rise IR, Saugstad OD. Effects of hypoxia and reoxygenation with 21% and 100%-oxygen on cerebral nitric oxide concentration and microcirculation in newborn piglets. *Biol Neonate.* 1999;76:153–167.
32. Lundstrom KE, Pryds O, Greisen G. Oxygen at birth and prolonged cerebral vasoconstriction in preterm infants. *Arch Dis Child Fetal Neonatal Ed.* 1995;73:F81–F86.
33. Tan A, Schulze A, O'Donnell CP, Davis PG. Air versus oxygen for resuscitation of infants at birth. Cochrane Database Syst Rev. 2005:CD002273.
34. Davis PG, Tan A, O'Donnell CP, Schulze A. Resuscitation of newborn infants with 100% oxygen or air: a systematic review and meta-analysis. *Lancet.* 2004;364:1329–1333.
35. Karlberg P, Koch G. Respiratory studies in newborn infants, III: development of mechanics of breathing during the first week of life. A longitudinal study. *Acta Paediatr.* 1962;(suppl 135):121–129.
36. Vyas H, Milner AD, Hopkin IE, Boon AW. Physiologic responses to prolonged and slow-rise inflation in the resuscitation of the asphyxiated newborn infant. *J Pediatr.* 1981;99:635–639.
37. Vyas H, Field D, Milner AD, Hopkin IE. Determinants of the first inspiratory volume and functional residual capacity at birth. *Pediatr Pulmonol.* 1986;2:189–193.
38. Boon AW, Milner AD, Hopkin IE. Lung expansion, tidal exchange, and formation of the functional residual capacity during resuscitation of asphyxiated neonates. *J Pediatr.* 1979;95:1031–1036.
39. Mortola JP, Fisher JT, Smith JB, Fox GS, Weeks S, Willis D. Onset of respiration in infants delivered by cesarean section. *J Appl Physiol.* 1982;52:716–724.
40. Hull D. Lung expansion and ventilation during resuscitation of asphyxiated newborn infants. *J Pediatr.* 1969;75:47–58.
41. Upton CJ, Milner AD. Endotracheal resuscitation of neonates using a rebreathing bag. *Arch Dis Child.* 1991;66:39–42.
42. Boon AW, Milner AD, Hopkin IE. Physiological responses of the newborn infant to resuscitation. *Arch Dis Child.* 1979;54:492–498.
43. Milner AD, Vyas H, Hopkin IE. Efficacy of facemask resuscitation at birth. *BMJ.* 1984;289:1563–1565.
44. Allwood AC, Madar RJ, Baumer JH, Readdy L, Wright D. Changes in resuscitation practice at birth. *Arch Dis Child Fetal Neonatal Ed.* 2003;88:F375–F379.
45. Hoskyns EW, Milner AD, Hopkin IE. A simple method of face mask resuscitation at birth. *Arch Dis Child.* 1987;62:376–378.
46. Cole AF, Rolbin SH, Hew EM, Pynn S. An improved ventilator system for delivery-room management of the newborn. *Anesthesiology.* 1979;51:356–358.
47. Ganga-Zandzou PS, Diependaele JF, Storme L, Riou Y, Klosowski S, Rakza T, Logier R, Lequien P. Is Ambu ventilation of newborn infants a simple question of finger-touch? *Arch Pediatr.* 1996;3:1270–1272.
48. Finer NN, Rich W, Craft A, Henderson C. Comparison of methods of bag and mask ventilation for neonatal resuscitation. *Resuscitation.* 2001;49:299–305.
49. Kanter RK. Evaluation of mask-bag ventilation in resuscitation of infants. *Am J Dis Child.* 1987;141:761–763.
50. Esmail N, Saleh M, Ali A. Laryngeal mask airway versus endotracheal intubation for Apgar score improvement in neonatal resuscitation. *Egyptian J Anesthesiol.* 2002;18:115–121.
51. Gandini D, Brimacombe JR. Neonatal resuscitation with the laryngeal mask airway in normal and low birth weight infants. *Anesth Analg.* 1999;89:642–643.
52. Brimacombe J, Gandini D. Airway rescue and drug delivery in an 800 g neonate with the laryngeal mask airway. *Paediatr Anaesth.* 1999;9:178.
53. Lonnqvist PA. Successful use of laryngeal mask airway in low-weight expremature infants with bronchopulmonary dysplasia undergoing cryotherapy for retinopathy of the premature. *Anesthesiology.* 1995;83:422–424.
54. Paterson SJ, Byrne PJ, Molesky MG, Seal RF, Finucane BT. Neonatal resuscitation using the laryngeal mask airway. *Anesthesiology.* 1994;80:1248–1253.
55. Trevisanuto D, Ferrarese P, Zanardo V, Chiandetti L. Laryngeal mask airway in neonatal resuscitation: a survey of current practice and perceived role by anaesthesiologists and paediatricians. *Resuscitation.* 2004;60:291–296.
56. Hansen TG, Joensen H, Henneberg SW, Hole P. Laryngeal mask airway guided tracheal intubation in a neonate with the Pierre Robin syndrome. *Acta Anaesthesiol Scand.* 1995;39:129–131.
57. Osses H, Poblete M, Asenjo F. Laryngeal mask for difficult intubation in children. *Paediatr Anaesth.* 1999;9:399–401.

58. Stocks RM, Egerman R, Thompson JW, Peery M. Airway management of the severely retrognathic child: use of the laryngeal mask airway. *Ear Nose Throat J.* 2002;81:223–226.
59. Ingimarsson J, Bjorklund LJ, Curstedt T, Gudmundsson S, Larsson A, Robertson B, Werner O. Incomplete protection by prophylactic surfactant against the adverse effects of large lung inflations at birth in immature lambs. *Intensive Care Med.* 2004;30:1446–1453.
60. Nilsson R, Grossmann G, Robertson B. Bronchiolar epithelial lesions induced in the premature rabbit neonate by short periods of artificial ventilation. *Acta Pathol Microbiol Scand [A].* 1980;88:359–367.
61. Probyn ME, Hooper SB, Dargaville PA, McCallion N, Crossley K, Harding R, Morley CJ. Positive end expiratory pressure during resuscitation of premature lambs rapidly improves blood gases without adversely affecting arterial pressure. *Pediatr Res.* 2004;56:198–204.
62. Hird MF, Greenough A, Gamsu HR. Inflating pressures for effective resuscitation of preterm infants. *Early Hum Dev.* 1991;26:69–72.
63. Lindner W, Vossbeck S, Hummler H, Pohlandt F. Delivery room management of extremely low birth weight infants: spontaneous breathing or intubation? *Pediatrics.* 1999;103:961–967.
64. Palme-Kilander C, Tunell R. Pulmonary gas exchange during facemask ventilation immediately after birth. *Arch Dis Child.* 1993;68:11–16.
65. Aziz HF, Martin JB, Moore JJ. The pediatric disposable end-tidal carbon dioxide detector role in endotracheal intubation in newborns. *J Perinatol.* 1999;19:110–113.
66. Bhende MS, Thompson AE. Evaluation of an end-tidal CO2 detector during pediatric cardiopulmonary resuscitation. *Pediatrics.* 1995;95:395–399.
67. Repetto JE, Donohue P-CP, Baker SF, Kelly L, Nogee LM. Use of capnography in the delivery room for assessment of endotracheal tube placement. *J Perinatol.* 2001;21:284–287.
68. Roberts WA, Maniscalco WM, Cohen AR, Litman RS, Chhibber A. The use of capnography for recognition of esophageal intubation in the neonatal intensive care unit. *Pediatr Pulmonol.* 1995;19:262–268.
69. Bhende MS, Karasic DG, Karasic RB. End-tidal carbon dioxide changes during cardiopulmonary resuscitation after experimental asphyxial cardiac arrest. *Am J Emerg Med.* 1996;14:349–350.
70. Orlowski JP. Optimum position for external cardiac compression in infants and young children. *Ann Emerg Med.* 1986;15:667–673.
71. Phillips GW, Zideman DA. Relation of infant heart to sternum: its significance in cardiopulmonary resuscitation. *Lancet.* 1986;1:1024–1025.
72. Thaler MM, Stobie GH. An improved technique of external caridac compression in infants and young children. *N Engl J Med.* 1963;269:606–610.
73. David R. Closed chest cardiac massage in the newborn infant. *Pediatrics.* 1988;81:552–554.
74. Todres ID, Rogers MC. Methods of external cardiac massage in the newborn infant. *J Pediatr.* 1975;86:781–782.
75. Menegazzi JJ, Auble TE, Nicklas KA, Hosack GM, Rack L, Goode JS. Two-thumb versus two-finger chest compression during CRP in a swine infant model of cardiac arrest. *Ann Emerg Med.* 1993;22:240–243.
76. Houri PK, Frank LR, Menegazzi JJ, Taylor R. A randomized, controlled trial of two-thumb vs two-finger chest compression in a swine infant model of cardiac arrest. *Prehosp Emerg Care.* 1997;1:65–67.
77. Dean JM, Koehler RC, Schleien CL, Berkowitz I, Michael JR, Atchison D, Rogers MC, Traystman RJ. Age-related effects of compression rate and duration in cardiopulmonary resuscitation. *J Appl Physiol.* 1990;68:554–560.
78. Berkowitz ID, Chantarojanasiri T, Koehler RC, Schleien CL, Dean JM, Michael JR, Rogers MC, Traystman RJ. Blood flow during cardiopulmonary resuscitation with simultaneous compression and ventilation in infant pigs. *Pediatr Res.* 1989;26:558–564.
79. Perlman JM, Risser R. Cardiopulmonary resuscitation in the delivery room: associated clinical events. *Arch Pediatr Adolesc Med.* 1995;149:20–25.
80. Ralston SH, Voorhees WD, Babbs CF. Intrapulmonary epinephrine during prolonged cardiopulmonary resuscitation: improved regional blood flow and resuscitation in dogs. *Ann Emerg Med.* 1984;13:79–86.
81. Ralston SH, Tacker WA, Showen L, Carter A, Babbs CF. Endotracheal versus intravenous epinephrine during electromechanical dissociation with CPR in dogs. *Ann Emerg Med.* 1985;14:1044–1048.
82. Redding JS, Pearson JW. Metabolic acidosis: a factor in cardiac resuscitation. *South Med J.* 1967;60:926–932.
83. Kleinman ME, Oh W, Stonestreet BS. Comparison of intravenous and endotracheal epinephrine during cardiopulmonary resuscitation in newborn piglets. *Crit Care Med.* 1999;27:2748–2754.
84. Berg RA, Otto CW, Kern KB, Hilwig RW, Sanders AB, Henry CP, Ewy GA. A randomized, blinded trial of high-dose epinephrine versus standard-dose epinephrine in a swine model of pediatric asphyxial cardiac arrest. *Crit Care Med.* 1996;24:1695–1700.
85. Burchfield DJ, Preziosi MP, Lucas VW, Fan J. Effects of graded doses of epinephrine during asphxia-induced bradycardia in newborn lambs. *Resuscitation.* 1993;25:235–244.
86. Perondi MB, Reis AG, Paiva EF, Nadkarni VM, Berg RA. A comparison of high-dose and standard-dose epinephrine in children with cardiac arrest. *N Engl J Med.* 2004;350:1722–1730.
87. So KW, Fok TF, Ng PC, Wong WW, Cheung KL. Randomised controlled trial of colloid or crystalloid in hypotensive preterm infants. *Arch Dis Child Fetal Neonatal Ed.* 1997;76:F43–F46.
88. Emery EF, Greenough A, Gamsu HR. Randomised controlled trial of colloid infusions in hypotensive preterm infants. *Arch Dis Child.* 1992;67: 1185–1188.
89. Oca MJ, Nelson M, Donn SM. Randomized trial of normal saline versus 5% albumin for the treatment of neonatal hypotension. *J Perinatol.* 2003;23: 473–476.
90. Gibbs J, Newson T, Williams J, Davidson DC. Naloxone hazard in infant of opioid abuser. *Lancet.* 1989;2:159–160.
91. Brambrink AM, Ichord RN, Martin LJ, Koehler RC, Traystman RJ. Poor outcome after hypoxia-ischemia in newborns is associated with physiological abnormalities during early recovery: possible relevance to secondary brain injury after head trauma in infants. *Exp Toxicol Pathol.* 1999;51:151–162.
92. Vannucci RC, Vannucci SJ. Cerebral carbohydrate metabolism during hypoglycemia and anoxia in newborn rats. *Ann Neurol.* 1978;4:73–79.
93. Yager JY, Heitjan DF, Towfighi J, Vannucci RC. Effect of insulin-induced and fasting hypoglycemia on perinatal hypoxic-ischemic brain damage. *Pediatr Res.* 1992;31:138–142.
94. Salhab WA, Wyckoff MH, Laptook AR, Perlman JM. Initial hypoglycemia and neonatal brain injury in term infants with severe fetal acidemia. *Pediatrics.* 2004;114:361–366.
95. Kent TA, Soukup VM, Fabian RH. Heterogeneity affecting outcome from acute stroke therapy: making reperfusion worse. *Stroke.* 2001;32: 2318–2327.
96. Gluckman PD, Wyatt JS, Azzopardi D, Ballard R, Edwards AD, Ferriero DM, Polin RA, Robertson CM, Thoresen M, Whitelaw A, Gunn AJ. Selective head cooling with mild systemic hypothermia after neonatal encephalopathy: multicentre randomised trial. *Lancet.* 2005;365:663–670.
97. Donovan EF, Fanaroff AA, Poole WK, Wright LL, Higgins RD, Finer NN, Carlo WA, Duara S, Oh W, Cotten CM, Stevenson DK, Stoll BJ, Lemons JA, Guillet R, Jobe AH. Whole-body hypothermia for neonates with hypoxic-ischemic encephalopathy. *N Engl J Med.* 2005;353:1574–1584.
98. Eicher DJ, Wagner CL, Katikaneni LP, Hulsey TC, Bass WT, Kaufman DA, Horgan MJ, Languani S, Bhatia JJ, Givelichian LM, Sankaran K, Yager JY. Moderate hypothermia in neonatal encephalopathy: safety outcomes. *Pediatr Neurol.* 2005;32:18–24.
99. Eicher DJ, Wagner CL, Katikaneni LP, Hulsey TC, Bass WT, Kaufman DA, Horgan MJ, Languani S, Bhatia JJ, Givelichian LM, Sankaran K, Yager JY. Moderate hypothermia in neonatal encephalopathy: efficacy outcomes. *Pediatr Neurol.* 2005;32:11–17.
100. Thoresen M, Whitelaw A. Cardiovascular changes during mild therapeutic hypothermia and rewarming in infants with hypoxic-ischemic encephalopathy. *Pediatrics.* 2000;106:92–99.
101. Shankaran S, Laptook A, Wright LL, Ehrenkranz RA, Donovan EF, Fanaroff AA, Stark AR, Tyson JE, Poole K, Carlo WA, Lemons JA, Oh W, Stoll BJ, Papile LA, Bauer CR, Stevenson DK, Korones SB, McDonald S. Whole-body hypothermia for neonatal encephalopathy: animal observations as a basis for a randomized, controlled pilot study in term infants. *Pediatrics.* 2002;110:377–385.
102. De Leeuw R, Cuttini M, Nadai M, Berbik I, Hansen G, Kucinskas A, Lenoir S, Levin A, Persson J, Rebagliato M, Reid M, Schroell M, de Vonderweid U. Treatment choices for extremely preterm infants: an international perspective. *J Pediatr.* 2000;137:608–616.
103. Lee SK, Penner PL, Cox M. Comparison of the attitudes of health care professionals and parents toward active treatment of very low birth weight infants. *Pediatrics.* 1991;88:110–114.
104. Kopelman LM, Irons TG, Kopelman AE. Neonatologists judge the "Baby Doe" regulations. *N Engl J Med.* 1988;318:677–683.
105. Draper ES, Manktelow B, Field DJ, James D. Tables for predicting survival for preterm births are updated. *BMJ.* 2003;327:872.
106. Jain L, Ferre C, Vidyasagar D, Nath S, Sheftel D. Cardiopulmonary resuscitation of apparently stillborn infants: survival and long-term outcome. *J Pediatr.* 1991;118:778–782.
107. Haddad B, Mercer BM, Livingston JC, Talati A, Sibai BM. Outcome after successful resuscitation of babies born with apgar scores of 0 at both 1 and 5 minutes. *Am J Obstet Gynecol.* 2000;182:1210–1214.

Part 14: First Aid

The American Heart Association (AHA) and the American Red Cross (ARC) cofounded the National First Aid Science Advisory Board (Table) to review and evaluate the scientific literature on first aid. The goals of the National First Aid Science Advisory Board were to reduce morbidity and mortality due to emergency events and to analyze the scientific evidence that answers the following questions:

- What are the most common emergency conditions that lead to significant morbidity and mortality?
- In which of these emergency conditions can morbidity or mortality be reduced by the intervention of a first aid provider?
- How strong is the scientific evidence that interventions performed by a first aid provider are safe, effective, and feasible?

This critical review of the scientific literature resulted in a Consensus on Science for First Aid With Treatment Recommendations, from which these guidelines are derived.[1] The critical review and evaluation of the literature identified areas for future scientific research.

Background

From the perspective of the 21st century, the need for first aid training seems self-evident, but the history of organized first aid spans only 120 years. There is evidence, though, that Native Americans practiced first aid and taught it. For example, Sioux medicine men of the Bear Society were noted for treating battle injuries, fixing fractures, controlling bleeding, removing arrows, and using a sharp flint to cut around wounds and inflammations.[2]

Modern first aid evolved from military experience when surgeons taught soldiers how to splint and bandage battlefield wounds. Two British officers, Peter Shepherd and Francis Duncan, are said to have been the first to expand the concept to civilians and develop the first curriculum in first aid.[3] Training in first aid began in the United States in 1903 when Clara Barton, president of the ARC, formed a committee to establish instruction in first aid among the nation's industrial workers, where, under dangerous conditions, accidents and deaths were all too frequent. In 2000 the first evidence-based guidelines in first aid were developed by the AHA in collaboration with the International Liaison Committee on Resuscitation (ILCOR).[4] Many organizations have developed training programs in first aid.

(*Circulation.* 2005;112:IV-196-IV-203.)

This special supplement to *Circulation* is freely available at http://www.circulationaha.org

DOI: 10.1161/CIRCULATIONAHA.105.166575

What Really Works in First Aid?

Members of the National First Aid Science Advisory Board reviewed morbidity data from the Centers for Disease Control and Prevention and first aid texts and reviewed published studies to identify and evaluate the scientific basis for first aid recommendations. Previous studies[5–7] have noted the paucity of scientific evidence to support many interventions in prehospital emergency care. Many first aid practices rest on an equally precarious scientific foundation. The information presented here represents a consensus of evaluation of the evidence on common first aid interventions.

Definition of First Aid

The National First Aid Science Advisory Board defined first aid as assessments and interventions that can be performed by a bystander (or by the victim) with minimal or no medical equipment. A first aid provider is defined as someone with formal training in first aid, emergency care, or medicine who provides first aid. First aid assessments and interventions should be medically sound and based on scientific evidence or, in the absence of such evidence, on expert consensus. Administration of first aid must not delay activation of the emergency medical services (EMS) system or other medical assistance when required. The board recognizes that certain conditions that can be treated with first aid may not require EMS involvement or assistance by other medical professionals. The National First Aid Science Advisory Board strongly believes that education in first aid should be universal: everyone can learn first aid and everyone should.

The National First Aid Science Advisory Board recognized that the scope of first aid is not purely scientific and is related to both training and regulatory issues. The definition of scope is therefore variable, and it should be defined according to circumstances, need, and regulatory requirements.

These 2005 First Aid Guidelines differ from the recommendations in the First Aid section in the *ECC Guidelines 2000* in the increased number of topics, the inclusion of representatives from many organizations involved with First Aid education in discussions leading to the guidelines, and the cosponsorship by the AHA and ARC. An important byproduct of these discussions is to again emphasize the paucity of evidence to guide first aid interventions. Very little research is being conducted in first aid, and many of the following recommendations have had to be made by extrapolation from the experience of healthcare professionals. It is important to recognize the limitations of the evidence so that research can be undertaken and future guidelines can be based on a larger body of scientific evidence.

Calling for Help

The single most important information for a first aid provider is to know how to get help. Rescuers should learn how and when to access the EMS system, how to activate the on-site

Organizations Represented on the National First Aid Science Advisory Board

American Academy of Orthopaedic Surgeons
American Academy of Pediatrics
American Association of Poison Control Centers
American Burn Association
American College of Emergency Physicians
American College of Occupational and Environmental Medicine
American College of Surgeons
American Heart Association
The American Pediatric Surgical Association
American Red Cross
American Safety and Health Institute
Army Medical Command
Australian Resuscitation Council
Canadian Red Cross
International Association of Fire Chiefs
International Association of Fire Fighters
Medic First Aid International
Military Training Network
National Association of EMS Educators
National Association of EMS Physicians
National Association of EMTs
National Safety Council
Occupational Safety and Health Administration
Save a Life Foundation

emergency response plan (ERP), and how to contact the Poison Control Center (see below).

Positioning the Victim

As a general rule, a victim should not be moved, but there are times when you should do so:

- If the area is unsafe for you or the victim, move the victim to a safe location.
- If the victim is face down and needs CPR, turn the victim face up.
- If the victim is unresponsive, has an open airway, and is breathing spontaneously, turn the victim onto his or her side (recovery position) with the victim's hand in front (Class IIb; LOE 7[8,9]). Be aware of the potential for nerve and vessel injury if the victim lies on one arm for a prolonged period; it may be necessary to roll the victim to the other side (Class Indeterminate; LOE 7[8,9]).
- If you suspect that the victim might have a spinal injury, it is best not to move the victim. If the injured victim is unresponsive and has difficulty breathing because of copious secretions or vomiting, or if you are alone and have to leave the victim to get help, place the victim in a modified HAINES recovery position by extending one of the victim's arms above the head and rolling the body to the side so that the victim's head rests on the extended arm. Bend both legs to stabilize the victim (Class IIb; LOE 7[8,9]).

Oxygen

There is insufficient evidence to recommend for or against the use of oxygen by a first aid provider (Class Indeterminate), and concern exists that oxygen administration may delay other interventions.

Medical Emergencies

Breathing Difficulties

The incidence of acute asthma is increasing, especially in urban populations.[10] Many victims with asthma have and can self-administer bronchodilator medication.[11–14] Inhaled bronchodilator medications are safe with few untoward effects. First aid providers may assist the victim in using prescribed bronchodilator medication (Class IIb; LOE 4 studies[11–14] extrapolated to first aid = LOE 7). They are not expected to make a diagnosis, but they can assist the victim under the following conditions:

- The victim states that he or she is having an asthma attack and has medications or an inhaler.
- The victim identifies the medication and is unable to administer it without assistance.[12]

Anaphylaxis

Allergies are relatively common, but only a small proportion of people with allergies develop anaphylactic reactions. An anaphylactic reaction is characterized by swelling, especially of the face, breathing difficulty, shock, and even death. Many people with a history of anaphylaxis carry a lifesaving epinephrine auto-injector. With proper training, parents can be taught to correctly use the auto-injector to administer epinephrine to their child.[15] Unfortunately all too often neither the victim nor family members know how to use an auto-injector correctly.[16–18] First aid providers should be familiar with the epinephrine auto-injector so that they can help someone having an anaphylactic reaction self-administer the epinephrine. First aid providers should be able to administer the auto-injector if the victim is unable to do so, provided that the medication has been prescribed by a physician and state law permits (Class IIb; LOE 7[15]).

Seizures

The general principles of first aid management of seizures are to (1) prevent injury, (2) ensure an open airway, and (3) ensure that the airway remains open after the seizure has ended.

The victim of a seizure must be protected from injury. Protect the head with a pillow or other soft material. Do not restrain the victim during a seizure or place any object in the victim's mouth. Restraining the victim may cause musculoskeletal or soft-tissue injury. Placing an object in the victim's mouth is futile because most tongue biting occurs at the onset of seizure activity and attempts to insert an object may cause dental damage or aspiration or may injure the rescuer's fingers.

To prevent aspiration of secretions and maintain an open airway, place the victim in a recovery position after the seizure stops. It is not unusual for the victim to be unresponsive or confused for a short time after a seizure.

Injury Emergencies

Bleeding

Control of bleeding is one of the few actions by which you can critically influence outcome. Control external bleeding by applying pressure over the bleeding area until bleeding stops or EMS rescuers arrive (Class IIb; LOE 4[19]; 5[20]; 6[21]; 7 [extrapolated from LOE 1 and 2 in the cardiac catheterization laboratory][22–25]). The important factors in successful control of bleeding are to apply pressure firmly and for a long time. Methods of applying pressure include

- Manual pressure on gauze or other cloth placed over the bleeding source.[22–25] If bleeding continues, do not remove the gauze; add more gauze on top and apply more pressure.
- An elastic bandage firmly wrapped over gauze[20] to hold it in place with pressure.

The effectiveness, feasibility, and safety of tourniquets to control bleeding by first aid providers are unknown, but the use of tourniquets is potentially dangerous (Class Indeterminate). Tourniquets are routinely used in the operating room under controlled conditions and have been effective in controlling bleeding from an extremity,[26] but potential undesired effects include temporary[27] or permanent[28] injury to the underlying nerves and muscles,[29] as well as systemic complications resulting from limb ischemia,[30] including acidemia, hyperkalemia, arrhythmias, shock, limb loss, and death. Complications are related to tourniquet pressure[31] and occlusion time.[32] Pressure has been found to be superior to tourniquets in controlling bleeding,[19] although tourniquets may be useful under some unique conditions (eg, the battlefield, when rapid evacuation is required and ischemic time is carefully monitored). The method of application and the best design of tourniquets are under investigation.[33]

There is insufficient evidence to recommend for or against the first aid use of pressure points or extremity elevation to control hemorrhage (Class Indeterminate). The efficacy, feasibility, and safety of pressure points to control bleeding have never been subjected to study, and there have been no published studies to determine if elevation of a bleeding extremity helps in bleeding control or causes harm. Using these unproven procedures has the potential to compromise the proven intervention of direct pressure.

Wounds and Abrasions

Irrigate wounds and abrasions with clean running tap water (Class IIa; LOE 1[34]; 2[35,36]; 7[37–39]) for ≥5 minutes or until there appears to be no foreign matter in the wound. If running water is unavailable, use any source of clean water. Wounds heal better and with less infection if an antibiotic ointment or cream is used (Class IIa; LOE 1[40,41]; and evidence extrapolated from LOE 2 studies to first aid = LOE 7[42–45]); triple antibiotic ointment appears to be superior to single antibiotic ointment or cream (Class IIb; LOE 1[41]). Apply antibiotic ointment or cream only if the victim's wound is an abrasion or is superficial.

Burns

Thermal Burns

Cool thermal burns with cold water as soon as possible[46,47] (Class IIa; LOE 3[48]; 4[49]; 5[50–52]; 6[46]) and continue at least until pain is relieved.[53] Cooling reduces the injury and relieves pain.[48–52] There is some evidence that brief cooling of small burns with ice water may be effective (LOE 5),[53,54] but direct application of ice to a burn may produce tissue ischemia,[55,56] and prolonged cold exposure even of small burns can lead to further injury.[52,55,57] Avoid cooling of burns with ice or ice water for longer than 10 minutes, especially if the burn is large (>20% of body surface area) (Class III; LOE 6[58]).

Burn Blisters

Loosely cover burn blisters with a sterile dressing but leave them intact (Class IIb; LOE 5[59]; 6[60–62]).

Electrocution and Electrical Burns

The severity of electrical injuries can vary widely, from an unpleasant tingling sensation caused by low-intensity current to thermal burns, cardiopulmonary arrest, and death. Thermal burns may result from burning clothing that is in contact with the skin or from electric current traversing a portion of the body. When current transverses the body, thermal burns may be present at the points where the current entered and exited the body and internally along its pathway. Cardiopulmonary arrest is the primary cause of immediate death from electrocution.[63] Cardiac arrhythmias, including ventricular fibrillation, ventricular asystole, and ventricular tachycardia that progresses to ventricular fibrillation, may result from exposure to low- or high-voltage current.[64] Respiratory arrest may result from electrical injury to the respiratory center in the brain or from tetanic contractions or paralysis of respiratory muscles.

Do not place yourself in danger by touching an electrocuted victim while the power is on. Turn off the power at its source; at home the switch is usually near the fuse box. In case of high-voltage electrocution, such as that caused by fallen power lines, immediately notify the appropriate authorities (ie, 911, fire department, etc). All materials will conduct electricity if the voltage is high enough, so do not enter the area around the victim or try to remove wires or other materials with any object, including wooden ones, until the power has been turned off by knowledgeable personnel.

Once the power is off, assess the victim, who may need CPR, defibrillation, and treatment for shock and thermal burns. All victims of electric shock require medical assessment because the extent of injury may not be apparent.

Spine Stabilization

There is an approximately 2% risk of injury to the cervical spine after blunt trauma that is serious enough to require spinal imaging in an emergency department,[65,66] and this risk is tripled in patients with craniofacial injury[67] or a Glasgow Coma Scale score of <8.[68] Most victims with spinal injuries are males between the ages of 10 and 30 years. Motor vehicles cause approximately half of the injuries; the remainder are caused by falls (especially from a height or diving), sports, and assaults.[69] A victim with a spinal injury has an increased risk of permanent neurologic damage, including quadriplegia from a secondary spinal cord injury.[70,71] First aid rescuers may not be able to conclusively identify a victim with a spinal injury, but they should suspect spinal injury if an injured victim.[66,72–75]

- Is involved in a motor vehicle, motorized cycle, or bicycle crash as an occupant, rider, or pedestrian
- Is injured as a result of a fall from greater than a standing height
- Complains of neck or back pain, tingling in the extremities, or weakness
- Is not fully alert
- Appears to be intoxicated
- Appears frail or >65 years of age
- Has a head or neck injury

In these situations or any situation in which you suspect a possible spinal injury, manually stabilize the head so that the head, neck, and spine do not move and are kept in line (Class IIa; LOE 3[65]; 7 [extrapolated from healthcare provider literature][66,73]). Do not use any immobilization devices because their benefit in first aid has not been proven[76] and may be harmful (Class III; LOE 4[77]; 6[71]; 7[78]). Immobilization devices may be needed in special circumstances when immediate extrication (ie, rescue of drowning victim) is required. First aid providers should be trained in the proper use of these devices before using them.

Musculoskeletal Trauma: Sprains, Strains, Contusions, and Fractures

Soft-tissue injuries include joint sprains and muscle contusions. Apply cold to soft-tissue injuries (Class IIa; LOE 2[79]; 6[80]; 7[81]). Cold application decreases hemorrhage, edema, pain, and disability.[79,81–83] Cooling is best accomplished with a plastic bag or damp cloth filled with a cooling modality that undergoes a phase change (eg, ice).[84] Refreezable gel packs are not as good as ice.[80,85] To prevent cold injury, limit each application of cold to periods ≤20 minutes and place a barrier, such as a thin towel, between the cold container and the skin.[86,87]

There is insufficient evidence to recommend for or against the use of a compression bandage to reduce edema following a closed soft-tissue injury such as a joint sprain (Class Indeterminate).

Assume that any injury to an extremity includes a bone fracture. Cover open wounds with a dressing if one is available. Do not move or straighten an injured extremity. If you are far from definitive health care, you may stabilize the extremity in the position found. If an injured extremity is blue or extremely pale, activate EMS immediately because this could be a medical emergency.

A victim with an injured lower extremity should not bear weight until advised by definitive health care.

Dental Injuries

Traumatic dental injuries are common. The first aid for dental injuries:

- Handle the tooth by the crown, not the root (do not handle the part that was embedded in the gum).
- Clean bleeding wounds with saline solution or tap water.
- Stop bleeding by applying pressure with a piece of cotton for 5 minutes.
- If there is an avulsed tooth, rinse it in water (do not scrub it), place it in milk, and bring it with you and consult a dentist as quickly as possible (Class IIa).[88–91]
- If there are other dental injuries, consult a dentist.

Environmental Emergencies

Snakebite

Do not apply suction as first aid for snakebite (Class III; LOE 5[92]; 6[93,94]). Suction does remove some venom,[92,94] but the amount is very small,[95] suction has no clinical benefit, and it may aggravate the injury.[96]

In case of an elapid (eg, coral) snakebite, wrap a bandage snugly (comfortably tight but loose enough to slip or fit a finger under it) around the entire length of the bitten extremity, immobilize the extremity, and get definitive medical help as rapidly as possible (Class IIa; LOE 3[97]; 6[98–100]). Wrapping the extremity slows dissemination of venom by slowing lymph flow.[97–101] There is a paucity of studies evaluating whether pressure and immobilization bandage are effective in bites by nonelapid snakes.

Cold Emergencies

Hypothermia

Hypothermia is caused by exposure to cold. The urgency of treatment depends on the length of exposure and the victim's body temperature. Immediately begin rewarming a victim of hypothermia (Class IIa; LOE 2[102,103]; 5[104–108]; 8[109,110]). Move the victim to a warm environment, remove wet clothing, and wrap all exposed body surfaces with anything at hand, including blankets, clothing, newspapers, etc. If you are far from definitive health care, you may begin active rewarming for a victim of hypothermia (Class IIb; LOE 2[102,103]; 8[109,110]). For example, active rewarming may be achieved by placing the victim near a heat source and placing containers of warm, but not hot, water in contact with the skin. Active rewarming should not delay definitive care.

Frostbite

Frostbite usually affects an exposed extremity. In case of frostbite, remove wet clothing and make sure the victim does not develop hypothermia. Get the victim to a medical facility as rapidly as possible. Do not try to rewarm the frostbite if there is any chance that it might refreeze or if you are close to a medical facility. If you are in a remote area far from a medical facility, you may slowly rewarm the frostbite using warm water (100°F to 105°F) (Class Indeterminate).

Drowning

Drowning is a major cause of unintentional death. It can be prevented with isolation fencing around swimming pools (gates should be self-closing and self-latching),[111] wearing personal flotation devices (life jackets) while in, around, or on water, and never swimming alone.

Outcome following drowning depends on the duration of the submersion, the water temperature, and how promptly CPR is started.[112,113] Case reports have documented intact neurologic survival in small children following prolonged submersion in icy waters.[114,115] Remove the victim rapidly and safely from the water, but do not place yourself in danger.

If you have special training, you can start rescue breathing while the victim is still in the water[116] if it does not delay removing the victim from the water. There is no evidence that water acts as an obstructive foreign body, so don't waste time trying to remove it. Start CPR with 2 effective ventilations and continue with 5 cycles (about 2 minutes) of chest compressions and ventilations before activating EMS. If 2 rescuers are present, send the second rescuer to activate EMS immediately.

Poison Emergencies

Poison Control Centers

There are a large number of poisonous substances in the home and worksite. It is important to understand the toxic nature of the chemical substances in your environment and the proper protective equipment and emergency procedures in case of toxic exposure. The Poison Control Center (800-222-1222) is an excellent resource for treating ingestion of, or exposure to, a potential poison. Inform the Poison Control Center of the nature of the exposure, the time of exposure, and the name of the product or toxic substance.

Chemical Burns

Brush powdered chemicals off the skin with a gloved hand or piece of cloth. Remove all contaminated clothing and make sure not to contaminate yourself in the process. In case of an acid or alkali exposure to the skin[117–123] or eye,[124–129] immediately irrigate the affected area with copious amounts of water (Class I; LOE 4[117]; 6[124–127]).

Ingested Poisons

Milk or Water

Do not administer anything by mouth unless advised to do so by a poison control center (Class IIb).

Animal studies[130,131] suggest that dilution or neutralization of a caustic agent by water or milk reduces tissue injury, but no human studies have shown a clinical benefit, and the possibility of emesis with aspiration must be considered (Class Indeterminate).

Activated Charcoal

There is insufficient evidence to recommend for or against the use of activated charcoal as first aid for ingestions (Class Indeterminate). Until more definitive evidence becomes available, do not administer activated charcoal unless you have been advised to do so by a poison control center.[132] Activated charcoal is effective for adsorbing toxins, but there is no evidence that charcoal administered by a first aid provider improves outcome.[133] Many children will not take the recommended dose (LOE 3[134]) and there are reports of harm.[135–137]

Ipecac

Do not administer syrup of ipecac for ingestions (Class III; LOE 2[138–141]; 4[142]; 7[132,143]). There are several problems with ipecac. These include questions about the amount of poison removed,[144–147] longer lengths of stay in the emergency department,[138] and lack of evidence that it improves outcome.[139,140,142] Side effects include lethargy[138,148] and the potential hazard of aspiration during emesis.[141] Syrup of ipecac is contraindicated in hydrocarbon or corrosive substance ingestion.

References

1. International Liaison Committee on Resuscitation. 2005 International Consensus on Cardiopulmonary Resuscitation and Emergency Cardiovascular Care Science with Treatment Recommendations. *Circulation.* 2005;112:III-1–III-136.
2. Lewis TH. *The Medicine Men: Oglala Sioux Ceremony and Healing.* Lincoln, NE: University of Nebraska Press; 1992.
3. Pearn J. The earliest days of first aid. *BMJ.* 1994;309:1718–1720.
4. American Heart Association in collaboration with International Liaison Committee on Resuscitation. Guidelines 2000 for Cardiopulmonary Resuscitation and Emergency Cardiovascular Care: International Consensus on Science, Part 5: New Guidelines for First Aid. *Circulation.* 2000;102(suppl I):I-77–I-85.
5. Neely KW, Drake ME, Moorhead JC, Schmidt TA, Skeen DT, Wilson EA. Multiple options and unique pathways: a new direction for EMS? *Ann Emerg Med.* 1997;30:797–799.
6. Callaham M. Quantifying the scanty science of prehospital emergency care. *Ann Emerg Med.* 1997;30:785–790.
7. Spaite DW, Criss EA, Valenzuela TD, Meislin HW. Developing a foundation for the evaluation of expanded-scope EMS: a window of opportunity that cannot be ignored. *Ann Emerg Med.* 1997;30:791–796.
8. Blake WE, Stillman BC, Eizenberg N, Briggs C, McMeeken JM. The position of the spine in the recovery position–an experimental comparison between the lateral recovery position and the modified HAINES position. *Resuscitation.* 2002;53:289–297.
9. Gunn BD, Eizenberg N, Silberstein M, McMeeken JM, Tully EA, Stillman BC, Brown DJ, Gutteridge GA. How should an unconscious person with a suspected neck injury be positioned? *Prehospital Disaster Med.* 1995;10:239–244.
10. Mannino DM, Homa DM, Pertowski CA, Ashizawa A, Nixon LL, Johnson CA, Ball LB, Jack E, Kang DS. Surveillance for asthma–United States, 1960–1995. *MMWR CDC Surveill Summ.* 1998;47:1–27.
11. Connellan SJ, Wilson RS. The use of domiciliary nebulised salbutamol in the treatment of severe emphysema. *Br J Clin Pract.* 1979;33: 135–136.
12. Hamid S, Kumaradevan J, Cochrane GM. Single centre open study to compare patient recording of PRN salbutamol use on a daily diary card with actual use as recorded by the MDI compliance monitor. *Respir Med.* 1998;92:1188–1190.
13. O'Driscoll BR, Kay EA, Taylor RJ, Weatherby H, Chetty MC, Bernstein A. A long-term prospective assessment of home nebulizer treatment. *Respir Med.* 1992;86:317–325.
14. Simon HK. Caregiver knowledge and delivery of a commonly prescribed medication (albuterol) for children. *Arch Pediatr Adolesc Med.* 1999;153:615–618.
15. Dobbie A, Robertson CM. Provision of self-injectable adrenaline for children at risk of anaphylaxis: Its source, frequency and appropriateness of use, and effect. *Ambulatory Child Health.* 1998;4:283–288.
16. Clegg SK, Ritchie JM. 'Epipen' training: A survey of the provision for parents and teachers in West Lothian. *Ambulatory Child Health.* 2001; 7:169–175.
17. Gold MS, Sainsbury R. First aid anaphylaxis management in children who were prescribed an epinephrine autoinjector device (EpiPen). *J Allergy Clin Immunol.* 2000;106:171–176.
18. Sicherer SH, Forman JA, Noone SA. Use assessment of self-administered epinephrine among food-allergic children and pediatricians. *Pediatrics.* 2000;105:359–362.
19. Pillgram-Larsen J, Mellesmo S. [Not a tourniquet, but compressive dressing. Experience from 68 traumatic amputations after injuries from mines]. *Tidsskr Nor Laegeforen.* 1992;112:2188–2190.
20. Naimer SA, Chemla F. Elastic adhesive dressing treatment of bleeding wounds in trauma victims. *Am J Emerg Med.* 2000;18:816–819.
21. Sava J, Velmahos GC, Karaiskakis M, Kirkman P, Toutouzas K, Sarkisyan G, Chan L, Demetriades D. Abdominal insufflation for prevention of exsanguination. *J Trauma.* 2003;54:590–594.
22. Lehmann KG, Heath-Lange SJ, Ferris ST. Randomized comparison of hemostasis techniques after invasive cardiovascular procedures. *Am Heart J.* 1999;138:1118–1125.
23. Walker SB, Cleary S, Higgins M. Comparison of the FemoStop device and manual pressure in reducing groin puncture site complications

following coronary angioplasty and coronary stent placement. *Int J Nurs Pract*. 2001;7:366–375.
24. Simon A, Bumgarner B, Clark K, Israel S. Manual versus mechanical compression for femoral artery hemostasis after cardiac catheterization. *Am J Crit Care*. 1998;7:308–313.
25. Koreny M, Riedmuller E, Nikfardjam M, Siostrzonek P, Mullner M. Arterial puncture closing devices compared with standard manual compression after cardiac catheterization: systematic review and meta-analysis. *JAMA*. 2004;291:350–357.
26. Lakstein D, Blumenfeld A, Sokolov T, Lin G, Bssorai R, Lynn M, Ben-Abraham R. Tourniquets for hemorrhage control on the battlefield: a 4-year accumulated experience. *J Trauma*. 2003;54:S221-S225.
27. Savvidis E, Parsch K. [Prolonged transitory paralysis after pneumatic tourniquet use on the upper arm]. *Unfallchirurg*. 1999;102:141–144.
28. Kornbluth ID, Freedman MK, Sher L, Frederick RW. Femoral, saphenous nerve palsy after tourniquet use: a case report. *Arch Phys Med Rehabil*. 2003;84:909–911.
29. Landi A, Saracino A, Pinelli M, Caserta G, Facchini MC. Tourniquet paralysis in microsurgery. *Ann Acad Med Singapore*. 1995;24(suppl): 89–93.
30. Wakai A, Wang JH, Winter DC, Street JT, O'Sullivan RG, Redmond HP. Tourniquet-induced systemic inflammatory response in extremity surgery. *J Trauma*. 2001;51:922–926.
31. Mohler LR, Pedowitz RA, Lopez MA, Gershuni DH. Effects of tourniquet compression on neuromuscular function. *Clin Orthop*. 1999: 213–220.
32. Kokki H, Vaatainen U, Penttila I. Metabolic effects of a low-pressure tourniquet system compared with a high-pressure tourniquet system in arthroscopic anterior crucial ligament reconstruction. *Acta Anaesthesiol Scand*. 1998;42:418–424.
33. Calkins D, Snow C, Costello M, Bentley TB. Evaluation of possible battlefield tourniquet systems for the far-forward setting. *Mil Med*. 2000;165:379–384.
34. Fernandez R, Griffiths R, Ussia C. Water for wound cleansing. (Cochrane Review). *The Cochrane Library*. 2004.
35. Griffiths RD, Fernandez RS, Ussia CA. Is tap water a safe alternative to normal saline for wound irrigation in the community setting? *J Wound Care*. 2001;10:407–411.
36. Valente JH, Forti RJ, Freundlich LF, Zandieh SO, Crain EF. Wound irrigation in children: saline solution or tap water? *Ann Emerg Med*. 2003;41:609–616.
37. Dire DJ, Welsh AP. A comparison of wound irrigation solutions used in the emergency department. *Ann Emerg Med*. 1990;19:704–708.
38. Moscati R, Mayrose J, Fincher L, Jehle D. Comparison of normal saline with tap water for wound irrigation. *Am J Emerg Med*. 1998;16: 379–381.
39. Moscati RM, Reardon RF, Lerner EB, Mayrose J. Wound irrigation with tap water. *Acad Emerg Med*. 1998;5:1076–1080.
40. Leyden JJ, Bartelt NM. Comparison of topical antibiotic ointments, a wound protectant, and antiseptics for the treatment of human blister wounds contaminated with Staphylococcus aureus. *J Fam Pract*. 1987; 24:601–604.
41. Maddox JS, Ware JC, Dillon HC, Jr. The natural history of streptococcal skin infection: prevention with topical antibiotics. *J Am Acad Dermatol*. 1985;13:207–212.
42. Berger RS, Pappert AS, Van Zile PS, Cetnarowski WE. A newly formulated topical triple-antibiotic ointment minimizes scarring. *Cutis*. 2000;65:401–404.
43. Atiyeh BS, Ioannovich J, Al-Amm CA, El-Musa KA, Dham R. Improving scar quality: a prospective clinical study. *Aesthetic Plast Surg*. 2002;26:470–476.
44. Hendley JO, Ashe KM. Effect of topical antimicrobial treatment on aerobic bacteria in the stratum corneum of human skin. *Antimicrob Agents Chemother*. 1991;35:627–631.
45. Hendley JO, Ashe KM. Eradication of resident bacteria of normal human skin by antimicrobial ointment. *Antimicrob Agents Chemother*. 2003;47:1988–1990.
46. King TC, Zimmerman JM. First-Aid Cooling of the Fresh Burn. *Surg Gynecol Obstet*. 1965;120:1271–1273.
47. Jandera V, Hudson DA, de Wet PM, Innes PM, Rode H. Cooling the burn wound: evaluation of different modalites. *Burns*. 2000;26:265–270.
48. Raghupati N. First-aid treatment of burns: efficacy of water cooling. *Br J Plast Surg*. 1968;21:68–72.
49. Berberian GM. Temporary regional surface cooling and long-term heparinization in the therapy of burns. *Surgery*. 1960;48:391–393.
50. Nguyen NL, Gun RT, Sparnon AL, Ryan P. The importance of immediate cooling–a case series of childhood burns in Vietnam. *Burns*. 2002;28:173–176.
51. Li C, Yu D, Li MS. [Clinical and experiment study of cooling therapy on burned wound]. *Zhonghua Yi Xue Za Zhi*. 1997;77:586–588.
52. Matthews RN, Radakrishnan T. First-aid for burns. *Lancet*. 1987; 1:1371.
53. Shulman AG. Ice water as primary treatment of burns: simple method of emergency treatment of burns to alleviate pain, reduce sequelae, and hasten healing. *JAMA*. 1960;173:1916–1919.
54. Grounds M. Immediate surface cooling in treatment of burns. *Med J Aust*. 1967;2:846–847.
55. Purdue GF, Layton TR, Copeland CE. Cold injury complicating burn therapy. *J Trauma*. 1985;25:167–168.
56. *Advanced Burn Life Support Providers Manual*. Chicago, IL: American Burn Association; 2002.
57. Sawada Y, Urushidate S, Yotsuyanagi T, Ishita K. Is prolonged and excessive cooling of a scalded wound effective? *Burns*. 1997;23:55–58.
58. Ofeigsson OJ. Observations and experiments on the immediate cold water treatment for burns and scalds. *Br J Plast Surg*. 1959;12:104–119.
59. Forage AV. The effects of removing the epidermis from burnt skin. *Lancet*. 1962;2:690–693.
60. Gimbel NS, Kapetansky DI, Weissman F, Pinkus HK. A study of epithelization in blistered burns. *AMA Arch Surg*. 1957;74:800–803.
61. Singer AJ, Thode HCJ, McClain SA. The effects of epidermal debridement of partial-thickness burns on infection and reepithelialization in swine. *Acad Emerg Med*. 2000;7:114–119.
62. Wheeler ES, Miller TA. The blister and the second degree burn in guinea pigs: the effect of exposure. *Plast Reconstr Surg*. 1976;57: 74–83.
63. Homma S, Gillam LD, Weyman AE. Echocardiographic observations in survivors of acute electrical injury. *Chest*. 1990;97:103–105.
64. Jensen PJ, Thomsen PE, Bagger JP, Norgaard A, Baandrup U. Electrical injury causing ventricular arrhythmias. *Br Heart J*. 1987;57:279–283.
65. Lowery DW, Wald MM, Browne BJ, Tigges S, Hoffman JR, Mower WR. Epidemiology of cervical spine injury victims. *Ann Emerg Med*. 2001;38:12–16.
66. Stiell IG, Wells GA, Vandemheen KL, Clement CM, Lesiuk H, De Maio VJ, Laupacis A, Schull M, McKnight RD, Verbeek R, Brison R, Cass D, Dreyer J, Eisenhauer MA, Greenberg GH, MacPhail I, Morrison L, Reardon M, Worthington J. The Canadian C-spine rule for radiography in alert and stable trauma patients. *JAMA*. 2001;286:1841–1848.
67. Hackl W, Hausberger K, Sailer R, Ulmer H, Gassner R. Prevalence of cervical spine injuries in patients with facial trauma. *Oral Surg Oral Med Oral Pathol Oral Radiol Endod*. 2001;92:370–376.
68. Demetriades D, Charalambides K, Chahwan S, Hanpeter D, Alo K, Velmahos G, Murray J, Asensio J. Nonskeletal cervical spine injuries: epidemiology and diagnostic pitfalls. *J Trauma*. 2000;48:724–727.
69. Kennedy E. Spinal Cord Injury: The facts and Figures. *Birmingham, Alabama University of Alabama*. 1986.
70. Reid DC, Henderson R, Saboe L, Miller JD. Etiology and clinical course of missed spine fractures. *J Trauma*. 1987;27:980–986.
71. Davis JW, Phreaner DL, Hoyt DB, Mackersie RC. The etiology of missed cervical spine injuries. *J Trauma*. 1993;34:342–346.
72. Hoffman JR, Mower WR, Wolfson AB, Todd KH, Zucker MI. Validity of a set of clinical criteria to rule out injury to the cervical spine in patients with blunt trauma. National Emergency X-Radiography Utilization Study Group. *N Engl J Med*. 2000;343:94–99.
73. Panacek EA, Mower WR, Holmes JF, Hoffman JR. Test performance of the individual NEXUS low-risk clinical screening criteria for cervical spine injury. *Ann Emerg Med*. 2001;38:22–25.
74. Viccellio P, Simon H, Pressman BD, Shah MN, Mower WR, Hoffman JR. A prospective multicenter study of cervical spine injury in children. *Pediatrics*. 2001;108:E20.
75. Touger M, Gennis P, Nathanson N, Lowery DW, Pollack CV, Jr., Hoffman JR, Mower WR. Validity of a decision rule to reduce cervical spine radiography in elderly patients with blunt trauma. *Ann Emerg Med*. 2002;40:287–293.
76. Hauswald M, Ong G, Tandberg D, Omar Z. Out-of-hospital spinal immobilization: its effect on neurologic injury. *Acad Emerg Med*. 1998; 5:214–219.
77. Barkana Y, Stein M, Scope A, Maor R, Abramovich Y, Friedman Z, Knoller N. Prehospital stabilization of the cervical spine for penetrating injuries of the neck—is it necessary? *Injury*. 2000;31:305–309.

78. Vickery D. The use of the spinal board after the pre-hospital phase of trauma management. *Emerg Med J.* 2001;18:51–54.
79. Cote DJ, Prentice WE, Jr., Hooker DN, Shields EW. Comparison of three treatment procedures for minimizing ankle sprain swelling. *Phys Ther.* 1988;68:1072–1076.
80. McMaster WC, Liddle S, Waugh TR. Laboratory evaluation of various cold therapy modalities. *Am J Sports Med.* 1978;6:291–294.
81. Meeusen R, Lievens P. The use of cryotherapy in sports injuries. *Sports Med.* 1986;3:398–414.
82. Hocutt JE, Jr., Jaffe R, Rylander CR, Beebe JK. Cryotherapy in ankle sprains. *Am J Sports Med.* 1982;10:316–319.
83. Airaksinen OV, Kyrklund N, Latvala K, Kouri JP, Gronblad M, Kolari P. Efficacy of cold gel for soft tissue injuries: a prospective randomized double-blinded trial. *Am J Sports Med.* 2003;31:680–684.
84. Merrick MA, Jutte LS, Smith ME. Cold modalities with different thermodynamic properties produce different surface and intramuscular temperatures. *J Athl Train.* 2003;38:28–33.
85. Chesterton LS, Foster NE, Ross L. Skin temperature response to cryotherapy. *Arch Phys Med Rehabil.* 2002;83:543–549.
86. Bassett FH, 3rd, Kirkpatrick JS, Engelhardt DL, Malone TR. Cryotherapy-induced nerve injury. *Am J Sports Med.* 1992;20:516–518.
87. Graham CA, Stevenson J. Frozen chips: an unusual cause of severe frostbite injury. *Br J Sports Med.* 2000;34:382–383.
88. Flores MT. Traumatic injuries in the primary dentition. *Dent Traumatol.* 2002;18:287–298.
89. Hiltz J, Trope M. Vitality of human lip fibroblasts in milk, Hanks balanced salt solution and Viaspan storage media. *Endod Dent Traumatol.* 1991;7:69–72.
90. Chan AW, Wong TK, Cheung GS. Lay knowledge of physical education teachers about the emergency management of dental trauma in Hong Kong. *Dent Traumatol.* 2001;17:77–85.
91. Sae-Lim V, Lim LP. Dental trauma management awareness of Singapore pre-school teachers. *Dent Traumatol.* 2001;17:71–76.
92. Bronstein A, Russell F, Sullivan J. Negative pressure suction in the field treatment of rattlesnake bite victims. *Vet Hum Toxicol.* 1986;28:485.
93. Leopold RS, Huber GS. Ineffectiveness of suction in removing snake venom from open wounds. *U S Armed Forces Med J.* 1960;11:682–685.
94. Bronstein A, Russell F, Sullivan J, Egen N, Rumack B. Negative pressure suction in field treatment of rattlesnake bite. *Vet Hum Toxicol.* 1985;28:297.
95. Alberts MB, Shalit M, LoGalbo F. Suction for venomous snakebite: a study of "mock venom" extraction in a human model. *Ann Emerg Med.* 2004;43:181–186.
96. Bush SP, Hegewald KG, Green SM, Cardwell MD, Hayes WK. Effects of a negative pressure venom extraction device (Extractor) on local tissue injury after artificial rattlesnake envenomation in a porcine model. *Wilderness Environ Med.* 2000;11:180–188.
97. Howarth DM, Southee AE, Whyte IM. Lymphatic flow rates and first-aid in simulated peripheral snake or spider envenomation. *Med J Aust.* 1994;161:695–700.
98. German B, Brewer K, Hack JB, Meggs WJ. Pressure-immobilization bandages delay toxicity in a porcine model of eastern coral snake (Micrurus fulrius fulvius) envenomation. *Ann Emerg Med.* 2005;45: 603–608.
99. Sutherland SK, Coulter AR, Harris RD. Rationalisation of first-aid measures for elapid snakebite. *Lancet.* 1979;1:183–185.
100. Sutherland SK, Coulter AR. Early management of bites by the eastern diamondback rattlesnake (Crotalus adamanteus): studies in monkeys (Macaca fascicularis). *Am J Trop Med Hyg.* 1981;30:497–500.
101. Anker RL, Straffon WG, Loiselle DS, Anker KM. Retarding the uptake of "mock venom" in humans: comparison of three first-aid treatments. *Med J Aust.* 1982;1:212–214.
102. Greif R, Rajek A, Laciny S, Bastanmehr H, Sessler DI. Resistive heating is more effective than metallic-foil insulation in an experimental model of accidental hypothermia: a randomized controlled trial. *Ann Emerg Med.* 2000;35:337–345.
103. Steele MT, Nelson MJ, Sessler DI, Fraker L, Bunney B, Watson WA, Robinson WA. Forced air speeds rewarming in accidental hypothermia. *Ann Emerg Med.* 1996;27:479–484.
104. Althaus U, Aeberhard P, Schupbach P, Nachbur BH, Muhlemann W. Management of profound accidental hypothermia with cardiorespiratory arrest. *Ann Surg.* 1982;195:492–495.
105. Kornberger E, Schwarz B, Lindner KH, Mair P. Forced air surface rewarming in patients with severe accidental hypothermia. *Resuscitation.* 1999;41:105–111.
106. Ledingham IM, Mone JG. Treatment of accidental hypothermia: a prospective clinical study. *Br Med J.* 1980;280:1102–1105.
107. Walpoth BH, Walpoth-Aslan BN, Mattle HP, Radanov BP, Schroth G, Schaeffler L, Fischer AP, von Segesser L, Althaus U. Outcome of survivors of accidental deep hypothermia and circulatory arrest treated with extracorporeal blood warming. *N Engl J Med.* 1997;337: 1500–1505.
108. Koller R, Schnider TW, Neidhart P. Deep accidental hypothermia and cardiac arrest–rewarming with forced air. *Acta Anaesthesiol Scand.* 1997;41:1359–1364.
109. Danzl DF. Accidental hypothermia. In: Auerbach PS, ed. *Wilderness Medicine.* 4th ed. St Louis, Mo: Mosby; 2001:135–177.
110. Danzl D. Hypothermia. *Seminars in Respiratory and Critical Care Medicine.* 2002;23:57–68.
111. Prevention of drowning in infants, children, and adolescents. *Pediatrics.* 2003;112:437–439.
112. Suominen P, Baillie C, Korpela R, Rautanen S, Ranta S, Olkkola KT. Impact of age, submersion time and water temperature on outcome in near-drowning. *Resuscitation.* 2002;52:247–254.
113. Graf WD, Cummings P, Quan L, Brutocao D. Predicting outcome in pediatric submersion victims. *Ann Emerg Med.* 1995;26:312–319.
114. Modell JH, Idris AH, Pineda JA, Silverstein JH. Survival after prolonged submersion in freshwater in Florida. *Chest.* 2004;125: 1948–1951.
115. Mehta SR, Srinivasan KV, Bindra MS, Kumar MR, Lahiri AK. Near drowning in cold water. *J Assoc Physicians India.* 2000;48:674–676.
116. Szpilman D, Soares M. In-water resuscitation–is it worthwhile? *Resuscitation.* 2004;63:25–31.
117. Latenser BA, Lucktong TA. Anhydrous ammonia burns: case presentation and literature review. *J Burn Care Rehabil.* 2000;21:40–42.
118. Wibbenmeyer LA, Morgan LJ, Robinson BK, Smith SK, Lewis RW, 2nd, Kealey GP. Our chemical burn experience: exposing the dangers of anhydrous ammonia. *J Burn Care Rehabil.* 1999;20:226–231.
119. Yano K, Hosokawa K, Kakibuchi M, Hikasa H, Hata Y. Effects of washing acid injuries to the skin with water: an experimental study using rats. *Burns.* 1995;21:500–502.
120. Kono K, Yoshida Y, Watanabe M, Tanioka Y, Dote T, Orita Y, Bessho Y, Yoshida J, Sumi Y, Umebayashi K. An experimental study on the treatment of hydrofluoric acid burns. *Arch Environ Contam Toxicol.* 1992;22:414–418.
121. Murao M. Studies on the treatment of hydrofluoric acid burn. *Bull Osaka Med Coll.* 1989;35:39–48.
122. Lorette JJ, Jr., Wilkinson JA. Alkaline chemical burn to the face requiring full-thickness skin grafting. *Ann Emerg Med.* 1988;17: 739–741.
123. Leonard LG, Scheulen JJ, Munster AM. Chemical burns: effect of prompt first aid. *J Trauma.* 1982;22:420–423.
124. Kompa S, Schareck B, Tympner J, Wustemeyer H, Schrage NF. Comparison of emergency eye-wash products in burned porcine eyes. *Graefes Arch Clin Exp Ophthalmol.* 2002;240:308–313.
125. McCulley JP. Ocular hydrofluoric acid burns: animal model, mechanism of injury and therapy. *Trans Am Ophthalmol Soc.* 1990;88:649–684.
126. Hojer J, Personne M, Hulten P, Ludwigs U. Topical treatments for hydrofluoric acid burns: a blind controlled experimental study. *J Toxicol Clin Toxicol.* 2002;40:861–866.
127. Herr RD, White GL, Jr., Bernhisel K, Mamalis N, Swanson E. Clinical comparison of ocular irrigation fluids following chemical injury. *Am J Emerg Med.* 1991;9:228–231.
128. Ingram TA. Response of the human eye to accidental exposure to sodium hypochlorite. *J Endod.* 1990;16:235–238.
129. Burns FR, Paterson CA. Prompt irrigation of chemical eye injuries may avert severe damage. *Occup Health Saf.* 1989;58:33–36.
130. Homan CS, Maitra SR, Lane BP, Thode HC Jr, Davidson L. Histopathologic evaluation of the therapeutic efficacy of water and milk dilution for esophageal acid injury. *Acad Emerg Med.* 1995;2:587–591.
131. Homan CS, Maitra SR, Lane BP, Thode HC Jr, Finkelshteyn J, Davidson L. Effective treatment for acute alkali injury to the esophagus using weak-acid neutralization therapy: an ex-vivo study. *Acad Emerg Med.* 1995;2:952–958.
132. Poison treatment in the home. American Academy of Pediatrics Committee on Injury, Violence, and Poison Prevention. *Pediatrics.* 2003; 112:1182–1185.
133. Merigian KS, Blaho KE. Single-dose oral activated charcoal in the treatment of the self-poisoned patient: a prospective, randomized, controlled trial. *Am J Ther.* 2002;9:301–308.

134. Scharman EJ, Cloonan HA, Durback-Morris LF. Home administration of charcoal: can mothers administer a therapeutic dose? *J Emerg Med.* 2001;21:357–361.
135. Donoso A, Linares M, Leon J, Rojas G, Valverde C, Ramirez M, Oberpaur B. Activated charcoal laryngitis in an intubated patient. *Pediatr Emerg Care.* 2003;19:420–421.
136. Dorrington CL, Johnson DW, Brant R. The frequency of complications associated with the use of multiple-dose activated charcoal. *Ann Emerg Med.* 2003;41:370–377.
137. Givens T, Holloway M, Wason S. Pulmonary aspiration of activated charcoal: a complication of its misuse in overdose management. *Pediatr Emerg Care.* 1992;8:137–140.
138. Kornberg AE, Dolgin J. Pediatric ingestions: charcoal alone versus ipecac and charcoal. *Ann Emerg Med.* 1991;20:648–651.
139. Pond SM, Lewis-Driver DJ, Williams GM, Green AC, Stevenson NW. Gastric emptying in acute overdose: a prospective randomised controlled trial. *Med J Aust.* 1995;163:345–349.
140. Kulig K, Bar-Or D, Cantrill SV, Rosen P, Rumack BH. Management of acutely poisoned patients without gastric emptying. *Ann Emerg Med.* 1985;14:562–567.
141. Albertson TE, Derlet RW, Foulke GE, Minguillon MC, Tharratt SR. Superiority of activated charcoal alone compared with ipecac and activated charcoal in the treatment of acute toxic ingestions. *Ann Emerg Med.* 1989;18:56–59.
142. Bond G. Home Syrup of ipecac use does not reduce emergency department use or improve outcome. *Pediatrics.* 2003;112:1061–1064.
143. Position paper: Ipecac syrup. *J Toxicol Clin Toxicol.* 2004;42:133–143.
144. Corby DG, Decker WJ, Moran MJ, Payne CE. Clinical comparison of pharmacologic emetics in children. *Pediatrics.* 1968;42:361–364.
145. Vasquez TE, Evans DG, Ashburn WL. Efficacy of syrup of ipecac-induced emesis for emptying gastric contents. *Clin Nucl Med.* 1988;13:638–639.
146. Saetta JP, Quinton DN. Residual gastric content after gastric lavage and ipecacuanha-induced emesis in self-poisoned patients: an endoscopic study. *J R Soc Med.* 1991;84:35–38.
147. Saetta JP, March S, Gaunt ME, Quinton DN. Gastric emptying procedures in the self-poisoned patient: are we forcing gastric content beyond the pylorus? *J R Soc Med.* 1991;84:274–276.
148. Czajka PA, Russell SL. Nonemetic effects of ipecac syrup. *Pediatrics.* 1985;75:1101–1104.

Editorial

Management of Conflict of Interest Issues in the Activities of the American Heart Association Emergency Cardiovascular Care Committee, 2000–2005

John E. Billi, MD; Brian Eigel, PhD; William H. Montgomery, MD; Vinay M. Nadkarni, MD; Mary Fran Hazinski, RN, MSN

In 2000 the American Heart Association (AHA), in conjunction with the International Liaison Committee on Resuscitation (ILCOR), sponsored the International Guidelines 2000 Conference on CPR and ECC. This conference led to the publication of the first international guidelines on CPR and ECC, *Guidelines 2000 for Cardiopulmonary Resuscitation and Emergency Cardiovascular Care: An International Consensus on Science.*[1] The conflict of interest (COI) policies governing the 2000 evidence discovery and consensus development process were consistent with the general COI policies in effect in the AHA at that time. Although these policies addressed disclosure and abstention from voting during subcommittee deliberations, they were, in retrospect, not sufficiently detailed to address the unique circumstances of a worldwide scientific review and consensus development process. In addition, they did not provide specific guidance for management of conflicts that arose among science reviewers, panelists, guidelines authors, and others involved in the complex guideline development process.

After publication of the *ECC Guidelines 2000,* the AHA was criticized for its management of potential conflicts among participants,[2] particularly those participants who received industry support for research or consultation. An intense debate took place in the literature, news sections of scientific journals, and Internet chatrooms. The AHA contended that the rigor of the scientific review and the multilayered peer-review process ensured that the guidelines were unbiased and that no individual or group could unduly influence guideline recommendations.

In preparation for the 2005 evidence evaluation process, the AHA Emergency Cardiovascular Care Committee began plans to create a new, more intensive, and more explicit approach to COI management and disclosure. The committee believed that public trust in the integrity of the scientific review process was so important that improvements were needed even if the existing safeguards had been effective. Therefore, in 2001 ECC leaders began broad discussions among the subcommittees about optimal management of conflicts of interest. These discussions continued at every meeting of the ECC Committee and its subcommittees from 2001 until the present.

In 2002 the ECC Committee invited Allan Detsky, an expert on the impact of commercial relationships on guideline development,[3] to discuss the risks of undisclosed and unmanaged conflicts. In addition, one of the authors of this editorial (J.B.) met with Sheldon Krimsky, author of *Science in the Private Interest,*[4,5] to review possible strategies to minimize potential commercial and intellectual conflicts. In addition to these discussions, about 100 AHA ECC committee and subcommittee volunteers responsible for setting policy and developing scientific consensus had multiple opportunities, in both formal and informal discussions, to consider optimal management of conflicts of interest and its effect on the guideline process. It was the consensus of this ECC leadership group that it was possible to design and implement a process to ensure that the AHA ECC review of science and development of guideline recommendations were truly and visibly free of commercial influence.

In 2002 the ECC Committee endorsed the Policy and Procedures for Disclosure and Management of Potential Conflict of Interest, which can be accessed on the AHA website: *http://www.c2005.org.* From that point forward all AHA ECC meetings were conducted in compliance with this policy and with routine AHA COI policies. Issues were brought to committee and task force chairs for resolution or sent to a higher level for decision.

In anticipation of the 2005 Consensus Conference, AHA volunteers worked with their international counterparts in ILCOR to develop a similar policy to govern all activities related to the 2005 evidence evaluation process. In 2004 ILCOR adopted a policy consistent with the AHA ECC policy, available at: *http://www.c2005.org.* All ILCOR meetings and activities since that time have complied with that policy, which governs all aspects of the evidence evaluation process, including selection of resuscitation topics for review, selection of worksheet authors to research the topics, presentation of findings in preliminary meetings and at the 2005 Consensus Conference, and drafting of consensus statements. ILCOR appointed two COI cochairs (J. Billi and D. Zideman) to oversee the process, adjudicate issues, and recommend solutions when problems arose.

The 2005 International Consensus Conference on Cardiopulmonary Resuscitation and Emergency Cardiovascular Care Science With Treatment Recommendations presented a special challenge to management and disclosure of conflicts of interest. How could an audience remain continuously aware of the industry relationships of a speaker in a way that

The opinions expressed in this article are not necessarily those of the editors or of the American Heart Association.

(*Circulation.* 2005;112:IV-204-IV-205.)

This special supplement to *Circulation* is freely available at http://www.circulationaha.org

DOI: 10.1161/CIRCULATIONAHA.105.170810

would allow listeners to keep those relationships in mind while weighing comments? ILCOR chose an approach to disclosure that, to our knowledge, has never been used before. For the duration of every speaker's comments, the speaker's COI disclosure slide was projected on a screen separate from the screen used to display presentation slides. This practice was followed for all scheduled speakers, panelists, and moderators as well as for anyone who asked questions or made comments from the floor. The disclosure slide listed research sponsored by industry, consultancies, paid speakers bureau roles and lectureships, gifts, investments, patents, and other relationships with the potential to influence the speaker. This novel disclosure method is described in detail in another editorial.[6] For the most part, participants responded favorably to the disclosure method, which was quick, unobtrusive, and uniform and offered the added benefit of reminding the audience of the speaker's name, especially important for speakers from the floor.

Although the COI management policies and practices used in 2005 by the AHA and ILCOR set a new standard for COI management and disclosure, the AHA and the rest of the scientific community should not yet be satisfied. Because substantial industry investment is often needed for scientific discovery and the invention of new technologies, those who commit to evidence review and development of guidelines must remain vigilant for new relationships that could pose a problem or the appearance of a conflict. The fact that most commercial relationships might not actually influence the scientists involved in the research or the review does not remove the potential for the public to be rightfully concerned about potential bias. The integrity of our current and future consensus statements and guidelines depends on the public trust. We must work to continue to earn it year after year.

References

1. American Heart Association in collaboration with International Liaison Committee on Resuscitation. Guidelines 2000 for Cardiopulmonary Resuscitation and Emergency Cardiovascular Care. *Circulation*. 2000; 102(suppl):I1-I384.
2. Kassirer J. *On the Take: How Medicine's Complicity with Big Business Can Endanger Your Health*. New York, NY: Oxford University Press; 2004.
3. Choudhry NK, Stelfox HT, Detsky AS. Relationships between authors of clinical practice guidelines and the pharmaceutical industry. *JAMA*. 2002; 287:612–617.
4. Krimsky S. *Science in the Private Interest: Has the Lure of Profits Corrupted Biomedical Research?* Lanham, Maryland: Rowman and Littlefield Publishers, Inc.; 2003.
5. Krimsky S, Rothenberg LS. Conflict of interest policies in science and medical journals: editorial practices and author disclosures. *Sci Eng Ethics*. 2001;7:205–218.
6. Billi JE, Zideman D, Eigel B, Nolan J, Montgomery W, Nadkarni V, from the International Liaison Committee on Resuscitation (ILCOR) and American Heart Association (AHA). 2005 American Heart Association Guidelines for Cardiopulmonary Resuscitation and Emergency Cardiovascular Care. Editorial: Conflict of interest management before, during and after the 2005 International Consensus Conference on Cardiopulmonary Resuscitation and Emergency Cardiovascular Care Science With Treatment Recommendations. *Circulation*. 2005;112:III-131–III-132.

Editorial

Major Changes in the 2005 AHA Guidelines for CPR and ECC

Reaching the Tipping Point for Change

Mary Fran Hazinski, RN, MSN; Vinay M. Nadkarni, MD; Robert W. Hickey, MD; Robert O'Connor, MD; Lance B. Becker, MD; Arno Zaritsky, MD

The emergency cardiovascular care (ECC) scientists involved in the 2005 evidence evaluation process and the revision of the *2005 AHA Guidelines for CPR and ECC* began and ended the process aware of the limitations of the resuscitation scientific evidence, optimistic about emerging data that documents the benefits of high-quality cardiopulmonary resuscitation (CPR), and determined to make recommendations that would increase survival from cardiac arrest and life-threatening emergencies. This editorial summarizes the factors that contributed to the tipping point, the point at which information and discussion either triggered support for major changes in the guidelines or reaffirmed existing recommendations.

The scientists critically reviewed the sequence and priorities of the steps of CPR to identify those factors with the greatest potential impact on survival. They then developed recommendations to support those interventions that should be performed frequently and well. There was unanimous support for increased emphasis on ensuring that rescuers deliver high-quality CPR: rescuers need to provide an adequate number and depth of compressions, allow complete chest recoil after each compression, and minimize interruptions in chest compressions.

The *2005 AHA Guidelines for CPR and ECC* are based on the most comprehensive review of resuscitation literature ever published.[1] The evidence evaluation process incorporated the input of 281 international resuscitation experts who evaluated research, topics, and hypotheses over a 36-month period before the 2005 Consensus Conference. The process included structured evidence evaluation, analysis, and documentation of the literature.[2] It also included rigorous disclosure and management of potential conflicts of interest, a process summarized in two editorials.[3,4]

The Challenge

Cardiopulmonary resuscitation and emergency cardiovascular care is a relatively new field. The epidemiologic data is incomplete, and high-level evidence is insufficient to support many recommendations. Although sudden cardiac arrest (SCA) is responsible for an estimated 250 000 deaths out of the hospital in the United States each year,[5] it is not yet a reportable cause of death to the National Center for Vital Statistics of the Centers for Disease Control and Prevention. This limits our ability to understand the true incidence of this leading cause of death and determine the impact of interventions.

Despite decades of efforts to promote CPR science and education, the survival rate for out-of-hospital cardiac arrest remains low worldwide, averaging 6% or less.[6–9] The low survival rate makes it difficult to perform clinical trials with sufficient power to demonstrate improved long-term outcomes (ie, neurologically intact survival to hospital discharge). As the experts evaluated current literature, they noted that clinical studies used a wide variety of short-term outcome end points, were underpowered or too small, were not randomized, or had other design factors that limited ability to evaluate the relative effects of many interventions. These difficulties have been compounded by the restrictions on research created by informed consent regulations in North America[10] and Europe.[11] Although researchers continue to try to identify therapies that may improve short-term outcomes, the goal of resuscitation research remains the identification of interventions that improve neurologically intact survival to hospital discharge following cardiac arrest.

Low rates of survival from out-of-hospital SCA are not inevitable. Increased survival rates were reported in a North American study of organized community lay rescuer CPR and automated external defibrillation (AED) programs.[12] In addition, survival rates from witnessed ventricular fibrillation (VF) SCA ranging from 49% to 74% have been reported in lay rescuer CPR and AED programs in airports[13] and casinos[14] and programs involving police officers.[15] These successful programs had several common elements, including the training of rescuers in a planned and practiced response, rapid recognition of SCA, prompt provision of bystander CPR, and defibrillation within 5 minutes of collapse.

A striking finding of the 2005 Consensus Conference was the contrast of data that showed the critical role of early, high-quality CPR in increasing rates of survival from cardiac arrest with data that showed that few victims of cardiac arrest receive CPR[16,17] and even fewer receive high-quality CPR.[18–20]

The Decisions: Factors Influencing the Major Changes in the *2005 AHA Guidelines for CPR and ECC*

Compression-Ventilation Ratio

No human data has identified the optimal compression-ventilation ratio for CPR for victims of all ages. The impetus

The opinions expressed in this article are not necessarily those of the editors or of the American Heart Association.

(*Circulation*. 2005;112:IV-206-IV-211.)

This special supplement to *Circulation* is freely available at http://www.circulationaha.org

DOI: 10.1161/CIRCULATIONAHA.105.170809

for a change in the recommended ratio was awareness that bystander CPR is performed infrequently and the rate of survival from SCA is low. Scientists agreed with the recommendation of the Utstein Conference on CPR Education to simplify CPR teaching.[21] Those recommendations are supported by evidence that participants often fail to master CPR skills during CPR courses[22] and that the quality of learned CPR skills rapidly declines after course completion.[23] The tipping point for the change in the compression-ventilation ratio came with evaluation and discussion of the cumulative evidence from recent clinical observations, theoretical calculations, and results of manikin and animal studies.

To be effective, CPR must restore adequate coronary and cerebral blood flow. Interruptions in chest compressions lower coronary perfusion pressure and decrease rates of survival from cardiac arrest.[24] In the first minutes of VF SCA, ventilation does not appear to be as important as chest compressions, but it does appear to contribute to survival from prolonged and asphyxial arrest.[25] Certainly the ventilation rate needed to maintain a normal ventilation-perfusion ratio during CPR is much smaller than normal because pulmonary blood flow is low.

In 2004 and 2005 several small case series in humans showed that during CPR healthcare providers delivered an inadequate number and depth of compressions, interrupted compressions frequently,[19,20] and provided excessive ventilation, particularly when victims were intubated.[18,20] Delivery of rescue breaths by lay rescuers was also likely to create long interruptions in chest compressions.[26,27] The combination of inadequate and interrupted chest compressions and excessive ventilation rates reduces cardiac output and coronary and cerebral blood flow[18,24] and diminishes the likelihood of a successful resuscitation attempt.

Once the experts agreed that a change in CPR recommendations was needed, the obvious challenge was how to translate that need into a specific recommendation that would be simple and appropriate for both asphyxial arrest and VF SCA and for attempted resuscitation of victims of all ages. Although continuous chest compressions alone could be appropriate in the first minutes of VF SCA, ventilations combined with minimally interrupted chest compressions would be more important for asphyxial arrest (including most pediatric arrests) and all forms of prolonged arrest. The experts also agreed that lay rescuers could not be expected to learn, select, and perform different sequences of CPR for victims with different causes of cardiac arrest.

Mathematical and animal models showed that matching of pulmonary blood flow and ventilation might be more appropriate at compression-ventilation ratios higher than 15:2.[28,29] There was concern, however, particularly among pediatric experts, that inadequate ventilation rates could reduce survival from pediatric and asphyxial (eg, drowning) arrest. To achieve optimal compression rates and reduce the frequency of interruptions in compressions, a universal compression-ventilation ratio of 30:2 for all *lone* rescuers of victims from infancy (excluding newborns) through adulthood is recommended by consensus, based on integration of the best human, animal, manikin, and theoretical data available. The 30:2 ratio is recommended to simplify training in 1-rescuer or 2-rescuer CPR for adults and all lay rescuer resuscitation. A compression-ventilation ratio of 15:2 is recommended for 2-rescuer CPR (a skill taught chiefly to healthcare providers and lifeguards) for infants and children (to the onset of puberty). This recommendation will result in the delivery of more rescue breaths per minute of CPR to victims with a high prevalence of asphyxial arrest.

Rescuers are encouraged to perform effective chest compressions (push hard, push fast), allow complete chest recoil after each compression, and minimize interruptions in chest compressions. Rescuers should take turns providing compressions during CPR because rescuers may tire after performing just a few minutes of compressions, and such fatigue can reduce the quality of compressions and chest recoil.

Compression First Versus Shock First for VF SCA

Recent data challenges the standard practice of providing defibrillation first to every victim with VF, particularly when more than 4 to 5 minutes has elapsed from collapse to rescuer intervention. In 2 studies of out-of-hospital VF arrest, when the interval between the call to the emergency medical services (EMS) system and delivery of the initial shock was 4 to 5 minutes or longer, a period of CPR before attempted defibrillation improved survival rates.[30,31] But one randomized study (LOE 2)[32] showed equivalent survival rates when either CPR or defibrillation was performed first for any EMS-call-to-shock interval.

The consensus was that there was insufficient data to recommend CPR before defibrillation for all victims of VF SCA. When participating in a public defibrillation program, lay rescuers should use the AED as soon as it is available. EMS rescuers may give about 5 cycles (about 2 minutes) of CPR before attempting defibrillation for treatment of out-of-hospital VF or pulseless ventricular tachycardia (VT) when the EMS response (call-to-arrival) interval is greater than 4 to 5 minutes or EMS responders did not witness the arrest. EMS medical directors may create system protocols based on the average response interval of their system. When multiple rescuers are present, one rescuer can perform CPR while the other readies the defibrillator, thereby providing both immediate CPR and early defibrillation.

The data was insufficient to determine (1) whether this recommendation should be applied to in-hospital cardiac arrest, (2) the ideal duration of CPR before attempted defibrillation, or (3) the duration of VF at which rescuers should switch from defibrillation first to CPR first.

1-Shock Versus 3-Shock Sequence for Attempted Defibrillation

The *ECC Guidelines 2000*[33] recommended the use of a so-called "stacked" sequence of up to 3 shocks, without interposed chest compressions, for the treatment of VF/pulseless VT. Although no studies in humans or animals specifically compared the 1-shock defibrillation strategy with the 3-stacked-shock sequence, other evidence created the tipping point for a change from a 3-shock sequence to 1 shock followed immediately by CPR.

The 3-shock recommendation was based on the low first-shock efficacy of monophasic damped sinusoidal waveforms and efforts to decrease transthoracic impedance with delivery of shocks in rapid succession. Modern biphasic defibrillators have a high first-shock efficacy (defined as termination of VF for at least 5 seconds after the shock), averaging more than 90%,[34,35] so that VF is likely to be eliminated with 1 shock. If 1 shock fails to eliminate VF, the VF may be of low amplitude and the incremental benefit of another shock is low. In such patients, immediate resumption of CPR, particularly effective chest compressions, is likely to confer a greater value than an immediate second shock.

After VF is terminated,[36–38] most victims demonstrate a nonperfusing rhythm (pulseless electrical activity or asystole) for several minutes; the appropriate treatment for such rhythms is immediate CPR. Yet in 2005 the rhythm analysis for a 3-shock sequence performed by commercially available AEDs resulted in delays of 29 to 37 seconds or more between delivery of the first shock and the beginning of the first post-shock compression.[38,39] This prolonged interruption in chest compressions cannot be justified for analysis of a rhythm that is unlikely to require a shock.

Experts recommend that rescuers resume CPR, beginning with chest compressions, *immediately after attempted defibrillation.* Rescuers should not interrupt chest compressions to check circulation (eg, evaluate rhythm or pulse) until after about 5 cycles or approximately 2 minutes of CPR. In specific settings (eg, in-hospital units with continuous monitoring in place), this sequence may be modified at the physician's discretion.

The recommendation for a 1-shock strategy creates a new challenge: to define the optimal energy for the initial shock. The consensus is that it is reasonable to use 150 J to 200 J for the initial shock with a biphasic truncated exponential waveform or 120 J with a rectilinear biphasic waveform. In recognition that many EMS systems may still be using monophasic defibrillators, the consensus recommendation for initial and subsequent monophasic waveform doses is 360 J. The goal of this recommendation is to simplify attempted defibrillation. For children, the consensus recommendation is an initial dose of 2 J/kg (monophasic or biphasic); for second and subsequent biphasic shocks, it is advisable to use the same or higher energy (2 to 4 J/kg). Manufacturers of defibrillators should ensure that each of their products clearly displays the range of energy levels at which each specific defibrillator waveform was shown to be effective at terminating VF. Healthcare providers should be aware of the range of energy levels of the specific device they are authorized to operate.

Vasopressors, Antiarrhythmics, and Sequence of Actions During Treatment of Cardiac Arrest

Despite the widespread use of epinephrine and several studies of vasopressin, no placebo-controlled study has shown that any medication or vasopressor given routinely at any stage during human cardiac arrest increases rate of survival to hospital discharge. Most out-of-hospital studies, however, are hampered by heterogeneous populations with prolonged arrest times, making it difficult to identify potentially successful therapies.

A meta-analysis of 5 randomized out-of-hospital trials showed no significant differences between vasopressin and epinephrine for return of spontaneous circulation, death within 24 hours, or death before hospital discharge.[40] A proposal to remove all recommendations for vasopressors was considered but not approved in the absence of a placebo versus vasopressor trial and the presence of laboratory evidence documenting the beneficial physiologic effects of vasopressors on hemodynamics and short-term survival.

There was no evidence that routine administration of any antiarrhythmic drug during human cardiac arrest increased rate of survival to hospital discharge. One antiarrhythmic, amiodarone, improved short-term outcome (ie, survival to hospital admission) but did not improve survival to hospital discharge when compared with placebo[41] and lidocaine.[42]

Given this lack of documented effect of drug therapy in improving long-term outcome from cardiac arrest, the sequence for CPR deemphasizes drug administration and reemphasizes basic life support. In the *ECC Guidelines 2000,*[43] pulse and rhythm checks were recommended after each shock. These recommendations contributed to prolonged interruptions in chest compressions. To minimize these interruptions in chest compressions, the *2005 AHA Guidelines for CPR and ECC* recommend that rescuers resume CPR beginning with chest compressions *immediately* after a shock, without an intervening rhythm (or pulse) check. Vasopressors or antiarrhythmics should be administered during CPR, as soon as possible after a rhythm check. The drug will be circulated by the CPR performed while the defibrillator charges or by the CPR that follows the shock. The most important part of the sequence is high-quality chest compressions with minimal interruptions. Providers should not interrupt compressions to check the rhythm after a shock is delivered until about 5 cycles or 2 minutes of CPR are provided. If an organized rhythm is present, the healthcare provider should check for a pulse.

Healthcare providers should practice coordination of CPR and shock delivery so that when a shock is indicated, it can be delivered as soon as possible after chest compressions are stopped and rescuers are "cleared" from contact with the victim. Studies have shown that a reduction in the interval between compression and shock delivery by as little as 15 seconds can increase the predicted shock success.[44,45] Defibrillator manufacturers are encouraged to develop AEDs that are capable of analyzing the heart rhythm during uninterrupted chest compressions.

Postresuscitation Care

Postresuscitation treatment is now receiving greater emphasis in emergency cardiovascular care, but there is little evidence to support specific therapies, and treatment is not standardized across healthcare communities.[46] After initial resuscitation, providers must be prepared to support myocardial and organ function. Support of blood pressure, control of temperature (particularly prevention or treatment of hyperthermia) and glucose concentration, and avoidance of routine hyperventilation are now recommended.

Therapeutic hypothermia has been shown to improve neurologic outcome among initially comatose survivors from out-of-hospital adult VF cardiac arrest.[47,48] Studies of newborns with asphyxia at birth suggest that brain cooling for selected patients may improve survival rates and neurologic outcomes.[49] But the role of this therapy after in-hospital cardiac arrest, across all age groups and arrest etiologies, requires further definition. Because of challenges in the practical application of therapeutic hypothermia, further research is needed to identify optimal methods of cooling and optimal timing, duration, and intensity of cooling that is likely to be effective.

Highlights of the *2005 AHA Guidelines for CPR and ECC* Recommendations

For further information about the evidence evaluated and treatment recommendations noted in this section, the reader is referred to relevant sections of this supplement. In many cases, as summarized below, there was insufficient evidence to create a tipping point toward a change in the guidelines; in others, accumulating data actually reaffirmed existing practices.

In pediatric resuscitation, emphasis is placed on provision of effective compressions and ventilations. A prospective randomized controlled trial confirmed that routine use of high-dose epinephrine was not beneficial and may actually increase rates of morbidity and mortality.[50]

In newborn resuscitation, a recent randomized controlled trial[51] showed no benefit for suctioning of the vigorous meconium-stained infant. This result reaffirmed the recommendations of the *ECC Guidelines 2000*.[52] There was inadequate data to indicate the superiority of room air to 100% oxygen for resuscitation. Evidence evaluation reaffirmed a focus on establishment of effective ventilation as the most important intervention in newborn resuscitation.

The Acute Coronary Syndromes Task Force confirmed the fundamental role of risk stratification involving the use of ECGs for classification and management of patients with acute coronary syndromes.[53] The task force reaffirmed the recommendation for out-of-hospital performance and prearrival transmission of either 12-lead ECGs or their interpretation to the receiving hospital to reduce time to reperfusion in acute myocardial infarction.[54] The recommendations for acute coronary syndromes have been simplified to focus on the first hours of therapy.

The Stroke Task Force reaffirmed the 2000 recommendation for use of tissue plasminogen activator (tPA) therapy for acute ischemic stroke[55] when administered by physicians in hospitals with stroke protocols that rigorously adhere to the eligibility criteria and therapeutic regimen of the National Institute of Neurological Disorders and Stroke (NINDS) protocol. Hospital commitment to stroke care can improve outcomes. A dedicated stroke unit with care provided by a multidisciplinary team experienced in managing stroke can improve survival rates, functional outcomes, and quality of life for patients with acute stroke.[56]

The First Aid Task Force evaluated the evidence supporting a number of first aid therapies, including the use of direct pressure versus tourniquets[57] for control of hemorrhage and treatment of ingestion and environmental emergencies. The recommendations of the task force form the basis of expanded guidelines for first aid.

Summary

This editorial summarizes several key changes in resuscitation skills and sequences recommended in the *2005 AHA Guidelines for CPR and ECC*. Simply put: rescuers should push hard, push fast, allow full chest recoil, minimize interruptions in compressions, and defibrillate promptly when appropriate. Many of these changes were not supported by level 1 evidence but were made by consensus, tipped by a combination of laboratory, clinical, and educational research and outcome data. Throughout the evidence evaluation document,[1] critical gaps in resuscitation knowledge were identified. Research in these issues has the potential to further improve CPR.

Further research is required in nearly all aspects of CPR and ECC. What is becoming clear is the need to focus on CPR performance and to integrate the performance of advanced cardiovascular life support skills into the continuous chest compression-ventilation sequence. There is no question that high-quality advanced cardiovascular life support depends on high-quality basic life support.

In the final analysis, the most important determinant of survival from sudden cardiac arrest is the presence of a rescuer who is trained, willing, able, and equipped to act in an emergency. Our greatest challenge and highest priority is the training of lay rescuers and healthcare providers in simple, high-quality CPR skills that can be easily taught, remembered, and implemented to save lives.

References

1. International Liaison Committee on Resuscitation. 2005 International Consensus on Cardiopulmonary Resuscitation and Emergency Cardiovascular Care Science with Treatment Recommendations. *Circulation*. 2005;112:III-1–III-136.
2. Zaritsky A, Morley P. 2005 American Heart Association Guidelines for Cardiopulmonary Resuscitation and Emergency Cardiovascular Care. Editorial: The evidence evaluation process for the 2005 International Consensus on Cardiopulmonary Resuscitation and Emergency Cardiovascular Care Science With Treatment Recommendations. *Circulation*. 2005;112:III-128–III-130.
3. Billi JE, Zideman D, Eigel B, Nolan J, Montgomery W, Nadkarni V, from the International Liaison Committee on Resuscitation (ILCOR) and American Heart Association (AHA). 2005 American Heart Association Guidelines for Cardiopulmonary Resuscitation and Emergency Cardiovascular Care. Editorial: Conflict of interest management before, during and after the 2005 International Consensus Conference on Cardiopulmonary Resuscitation and Emergency Cardiovascular Care Science With Treatment Recommendations. *Circulation*. 2005;112:III-131–III-132.
4. Billi JE, Eigel B, Montgomery WH, Nadkarni VM, Hazinski MF. Management of conflict of interest issues in the activities of the American Heart Association Emergency Cardiovascular Care Committee, 2000–2005. *Circulation*. 2005;112:IV-204–IV-205.
5. Zheng ZJ, Croft JB, Giles WH, Mensah GA. Sudden cardiac death in the United States, 1989 to 1998. *Circulation*. 2001;104:2158–2163.
6. Rea TD, Eisenberg MS, Sinibaldi G, White RD. Incidence of EMS-treated out-of-hospital cardiac arrest in the United States. *Resuscitation*. 2004;63:17–24.
7. Fredriksson M, Herlitz J, Nichol G. Variation in outcome in studies of out-of-hospital cardiac arrest: a review of studies conforming to the Utstein guidelines. *Am J Emerg Med*. 2003;21:276–281.
8. Nichol G, Stiell IG, Laupacis A, Pham B, De Maio VJ, Wells GA. A cumulative meta-analysis of the effectiveness of defibrillator-capable emergency medical services for victims of out-of-hospital cardiac arrest. *Ann Emerg Med*. 1999;34(pt 1):517–525.

9. Nichol G, Detsky AS, Stiell IG, O'Rourke K, Wells G, Laupacis A. Effectiveness of emergency medical services for victims of out-of-hospital cardiac arrest: a metaanalysis. *Ann Emerg Med.* 1996;27:700–710.
10. Hsieh M, Dailey MW, Callaway CW. Surrogate consent by family members for out-of-hospital cardiac arrest research. *Acad Emerg Med.* 2001;8:851–853.
11. Lemaire F, Bion J, Blanco J, Damas P, Druml C, Falke K, Kesecioglu J, Larsson A, Mancebo J, Matamis D, Pesenti A, Pimentel J, Ranieri M. The European Union Directive on Clinical Research: present status of implementation in EU member states' legislations with regard to the incompetent patient. *Intensive Care Med.* 2005;31:476–479.
12. The Public Access Defibrillation Trial Investigators. Public-access defibrillation and survival after out-of-hospital cardiac arrest. *N Engl J Med.* 2004;351:637–646.
13. Caffrey SL, Willoughby PJ, Pepe PE, Becker LB. Public use of automated external defibrillators. *N Engl J Med.* 2002;347:1242–1247.
14. Valenzuela TD, Roe DJ, Nichol G, Clark LL, Spaite DW, Hardman RG. Outcomes of rapid defibrillation by security officers after cardiac arrest in casinos. *N Engl J Med.* 2000;343:1206–1209.
15. White RD, Bunch TJ, Hankins DG. Evolution of a community-wide early defibrillation programme experience over 13 years using police/fire personnel and paramedics as responders. *Resuscitation.* 2005;65:279–283.
16. Herlitz J, Ekstrom L, Wennerblom B, Axelsson A, Bang A, Holmberg S. Effect of bystander initiated cardiopulmonary resuscitation on ventricular fibrillation and survival after witnessed cardiac arrest outside hospital. *Br Heart J.* 1994;72:408–412.
17. Stiell IG, Wells GA, Field B, Spaite DW, Nesbitt LP, De Maio VJ, Nichol G, Cousineau D, Blackburn J, Munkley D, Luinstra-Toohey L, Campeau T, Dagnone E, Lyver M. Advanced cardiac life support in out-of-hospital cardiac arrest. *N Engl J Med.* 2004;351:647–656.
18. Aufderheide TP, Sigurdsson G, Pirrallo RG, Yannopoulos D, McKnite S, von Briesen C, Sparks CW, Conrad CJ, Provo TA, Lurie KG. Hyperventilation-induced hypotension during cardiopulmonary resuscitation. *Circulation.* 2004;109:1960–1965.
19. Wik L, Kramer-Johansen J, Myklebust H, Sorebo H, Svensson L, Fellows B, Steen PA. Quality of cardiopulmonary resuscitation during out-of-hospital cardiac arrest. *JAMA.* 2005;293:299–304.
20. Abella BS, Alvarado JP, Myklebust H, Edelson DP, Barry A, O'Hearn N, Vanden Hoek TL, Becker LB. Quality of cardiopulmonary resuscitation during in-hospital cardiac arrest. *JAMA.* 2005;293:305–310.
21. Chamberlain DA, Hazinski MF. Education in resuscitation: an ILCOR symposium: Utstein Abbey: Stavanger, Norway: June 22–24, 2001. *Circulation.* 2003;108:2575–2594.
22. Brennan RT, Braslow A. Skill mastery in public CPR classes. *Am J Emerg Med.* 1998;16:653–657.
23. Kaye W, Mancini ME. Retention of cardiopulmonary resuscitation skills by physicians, registered nurses, and the general public. *Crit Care Med.* 1986;14:620–622.
24. Kern KB, Hilwig RW, Berg RA, Sanders AB, Ewy GA. Importance of continuous chest compressions during cardiopulmonary resuscitation: improved outcome during a simulated single lay-rescuer scenario. *Circulation.* 2002;105:645–649.
25. Berg RA. Role of mouth-to-mouth rescue breathing in bystander cardiopulmonary resuscitation for asphyxial cardiac arrest. *Crit Care Med.* 2000;28(suppl):N193–N195.
26. Assar D, Chamberlain D, Colquhoun M, Donnelly P, Handley AJ, Leaves S, Kern KB. Randomised controlled trials of staged teaching for basic life support, 1: skill acquisition at bronze stage. *Resuscitation.* 2000;45:7–15.
27. Heidenreich JW, Higdon TA, Kern KB, Sanders AB, Berg RA, Niebler R, Hendrickson J, Ewy GA. Single-rescuer cardiopulmonary resuscitation: 'two quick breaths'–an oxymoron. *Resuscitation.* 2004;62:283–289.
28. Babbs CF, Kern KB. Optimum compression to ventilation ratios in CPR under realistic, practical conditions: a physiological and mathematical analysis. *Resuscitation.* 2002;54:147–157.
29. Sanders AB, Kern KB, Berg RA, Hilwig RW, Heidenrich J, Ewy GA. Survival and neurologic outcome after cardiopulmonary resuscitation with four different chest compression-ventilation ratios. *Ann Emerg Med.* 2002;40:553–562.
30. Wik L, Hansen TB, Fylling F, Steen T, Vaagenes P, Auestad BH, Steen PA. Delaying defibrillation to give basic cardiopulmonary resuscitation to patients with out-of-hospital ventricular fibrillation: a randomized trial. *JAMA.* 2003;289:1389–1395.
31. Cobb LA, Fahrenbruch CE, Walsh TR, Copass MK, Olsufka M, Breskin M, Hallstrom AP. Influence of cardiopulmonary resuscitation prior to defibrillation in patients with out-of-hospital ventricular fibrillation. *JAMA.* 1999;281:1182–1188.
32. Jacobs IG, Finn JC, Oxer HF, Jelinek GA. CPR before defibrillation in out-of-hospital cardiac arrest: a randomized trial. *Emerg Med Australas.* 2005;17:39–45.
33. American Heart Association in collaboration with International Liaison Committee on Resuscitation. Guidelines 2000 for Cardiopulmonary Resuscitation and Emergency Cardiovascular Care: International Consensus on Science, Part 3: Adult Basic Life Support. *Circulation.* 2000; 102(suppl I):I22-I59.
34. White RD, Blackwell TH, Russell JK, Snyder DE, Jorgenson DB. Transthoracic impedance does not affect defibrillation, resuscitation or survival in patients with out-of-hospital cardiac arrest treated with a non-escalating biphasic waveform defibrillator. *Resuscitation.* 2005;64:63–69.
35. Morrison LJ, Dorian P, Long J, Vermeulen M, Schwartz B, Sawadsky B, Frank J, Cameron B, Burgess R, Shield J, Bagley P, Mausz V, Brewer JE, Lerman BB. Out-of-hospital cardiac arrest rectilinear biphasic to monophasic damped sine defibrillation waveforms with advanced life support intervention trial (ORBIT). *Resuscitation.* 2005;66:149–157.
36. Carpenter J, Rea TD, Murray JA, Kudenchuk PJ, Eisenberg MS. Defibrillation waveform and post-shock rhythm in out-of-hospital ventricular fibrillation cardiac arrest. *Resuscitation.* 2003;59:189–196.
37. White RD, Russell JK. Refibrillation, resuscitation and survival in out-of-hospital sudden cardiac arrest victims treated with biphasic automated external defibrillators. *Resuscitation.* 2002;55:17–23.
38. Rea TD, Shah S, Kudenchuk PJ, Copass MK, Cobb LA. Automated external defibrillators: to what extent does the algorithm delay CPR? *Ann Emerg Med.* 2005;46:132–141.
39. Yu T, Weil MH, Tang W, Sun S, Klouche K, Povoas H, Bisera J. Adverse outcomes of interrupted precordial compression during automated defibrillation. *Circulation.* 2002;106:368–372.
40. Aung K, Htay T. Vasopressin for cardiac arrest: a systematic review and meta-analysis. *Arch Intern Med.* 2005;165:17–24.
41. Kudenchuk PJ, Cobb LA, Copass MK, Cummins RO, Doherty AM, Fahrenbruch CE, Hallstrom AP, Murray WA, Olsufka M, Walsh T. Amiodarone for resuscitation after out-of-hospital cardiac arrest due to ventricular fibrillation. *N Engl J Med.* 1999;341:871–878.
42. Dorian P, Cass D, Schwartz B, Cooper R, Gelaznikas R, Barr A. Amiodarone as compared with lidocaine for shock-resistant ventricular fibrillation. *N Engl J Med.* 2002;346:884–890.
43. American Heart Association in collaboration with International Liaison Committee on Resuscitation. Guidelines 2000 for Cardiopulmonary Resuscitation and Emergency Cardiovascular Care: International Consensus on Science, Part 6: Advanced Cardiovascular Life Support: 7B: Understanding the Algorithm Approach to ACLS. *Circulation.* 2000; 102(suppl I):I140-I141.
44. Eftestol T, Sunde K, Steen PA. Effects of interrupting precordial compressions on the calculated probability of defibrillation success during out-of-hospital cardiac arrest. *Circulation.* 2002;105:2270–2273.
45. Steen S, Liao Q, Pierre L, Paskevicius A, Sjoberg T. The critical importance of minimal delay between chest compressions and subsequent defibrillation: a haemodynamic explanation. *Resuscitation.* 2003;58:249–258.
46. Langhelle A, Tyvold SS, Lexow K, Hapnes SA, Sunde K, Steen PA. In-hospital factors associated with improved outcome after out-of-hospital cardiac arrest. A comparison between four regions in Norway. *Resuscitation.* 2003;56:247–263.
47. Hypothermia After Cardiac Arrest Study Group. Mild therapeutic hypothermia to improve the neurologic outcome after cardiac arrest. *N Engl J Med.* 2002;346:549–556.
48. Bernard SA, Gray TW, Buist MD, Jones BM, Silvester W, Gutteridge G, Smith K. Treatment of comatose survivors of out-of-hospital cardiac arrest with induced hypothermia. *N Engl J Med.* 2002;346:557–563.
49. Gluckman PD, Wyatt JS, Azzopardi D, Ballard R, Edwards AD, Ferriero DM, Polin RA, Robertson CM, Thoresen M, Whitelaw A, Gunn AJ. Selective head cooling with mild systemic hypothermia after neonatal encephalopathy: multicentre randomised trial. *Lancet.* 2005;365:663–670.
50. Perondi MB, Reis AG, Paiva EF, Nadkarni VM, Berg RA. A comparison of high-dose and standard-dose epinephrine in children with cardiac arrest. *N Engl J Med.* 2004;350:1722–1730.
51. Vain NE, Szyld EG, Prudent LM, Wiswell TE, Aguilar AM, Vivas NI. Oropharyngeal and nasopharyngeal suctioning of meconium-stained

neonates before delivery of their shoulders: multicentre, randomised controlled trial. *Lancet*. 2004;364:597–602.

52. American Heart Association in collaboration with International Liaison Committee on Resuscitation. Guidelines 2000 for Cardiopulmonary Resuscitation and Emergency Cardiovascular Care: International Consensus on Science, Part 11: Neonatal Resuscitation. *Circulation*. 2000; 102(suppl I):I343-I357.
53. Ioannidis JP, Salem D, Chew PW, Lau J. Accuracy and clinical effect of out-of-hospital electrocardiography in the diagnosis of acute cardiac ischemia: a meta-analysis. *Ann Emerg Med*. 2001;37:461–470.
54. Wall T, Albright J, Livingston B, Isley L, Young D, Nanny M, Jacobowitz S, Maynard C, Mayer N, Pierce K, Rathbone C, Stuckey T, Savona M, Leibrandt P, Brodie B, Wagner G. Prehospital ECG transmission speeds reperfusion for patients with acute myocardial infarction. *N C Med J*. 2000;61:104–108.
55. Wardlaw JM, del Zoppo G, Yamaguchi T. Thrombolysis for acute ischaemic stroke. *Cochrane Database Syst Rev*. 2000;2:CD000213 [Record as supplied by publisher].
56. Organised inpatient (stroke unit) care for stroke. *Cochrane Database Syst Rev*. 2002:CD000197.
57. Pillgram-Larsen J, Mellesmo S. [Not a tourniquet, but compressive dressing. Experience from 68 traumatic amputations after injuries from mines]. *Tidsskr Nor Laegeforen*. 1992;112:2188–2190.

Additional Contributors

Tom P. Aufderheide, MD, *BLS*
Edward R. Stapleton, EMT-P, *BLS*
Andrea Gabrielli, MD, *BLS*
Thomas A. Barnes, EdD, RRT, *BLS*
Monica E. Kleinman, MD, *Pediatrics*
Ricardo A. Samson, MD, *Pediatrics*
Dianne L. Atkins, MD, *Pediatrics*
Susan Fuchs, MD, *Pediatrics*
Linda Quan, MD, *Pediatric Defibrillation*
Allan de Caen, MD, *Pediatrics*
Ashraf Coovadia, MD, *Pediatrics*
Charles L. Schleien, MD, *Pediatrics*
Venkataramani Ramesh, MD, *Pediatric Arrhythmias*
Elise van der Jaght, MD, MPH, *Pediatrics*
Vijay Srinivasan, MD, *Pediatrics*
Amelia Gorete Reis, PhD, *Pediatrics*
Melinda L. Fiedor, MD, Pediatrics
Paul Shore, MD, *Pediatrics*
Peter J. Kudenchuk, MD, *ACLS Arrhythmias*
Mark Link, MD, *ACLS Arrhythmias*
Henry R. Halperin, MD, *ACLS*
Hans-Richard Arntz, MD, PhD, *ACS*
Joseph P. Ornato, MD, *ACLS and ACS*
Michelle Welsford, MD, *ACS*
Warren Cantor, MD, *ACS*
Steven C. Brooks, MD, *ACS*
Carolyn Zelop, MD, *Special Resuscitation Situations*
John A. Morris, Jr, MD, *Special Resuscitation Situations*
Kathleen Jobe, MD, *Special Resuscitation Situations*
Jared Strote, MD, *Special Resuscitation Situations*
Leonard Frank, MD, *Special Resuscitation Situations*
Garry Lapidus, PA-C, MPH, *Pediatric Injury Prevention*
Karen Brock, MPH, *Pediatric Injury Prevention*
Curtis Snook, MD, *Special Resuscitation Situations*
Mary Ann Peberdy, MD, *ACLS Postresuscitation Care*
Robert Neumar, MD, *ACLS Postresuscitation Care*
David Gilmore, MD, *Special Resuscitation Situations*
Theodore Delbridge, MD, MPH, *ACLS*
Jeffrey L. Saver, MD, *Stroke*
Peter Viccellio, MD, *Stroke*
Les Wooldridge, RN, *Algorithms*
David Rodgers, MD, EdS, NREMT-P, *Education Chair-Elect*

ECC Committee, ECC Subcommittees, and ECC Task Forces

ECC Committee (July 2004–June 2005)

John E. Billi, MD, *Chair*
Robert W. Hickey, MD, *Chair (July 2005–Present)*
Vinay M. Nadkarni, MD
Robert E. O'Connor, MD, MPH, *Vice Chair (July 2005–Present)*
Max Harry Weil, MD, PhD
Graham Nichol, MD, MPH
Ahamed H. Idris, MD
Walt A. Stoy, PhD, EMT-P, CCEMTP
Stephen M. Schexnayder, MD
William E. McConnell, DO, MS
Mark Mattes, RRT, JD
Todd J. Crocco, MD
Theodore Delbridge, MD, MPH
Diana G. Fendya, RN, MSN R

ACLS Subcommittee (July 2004–June 2005)

Robert E. O'Connor, MD, MPH, *Chair*
Terry L. Vanden Hoek, MD, *Chair (July 2005–Present)*
Max Harry Weil, MD, PhD
Todd J. Crocco, MD
Henry R. Halperin, MD
Edward C. Jauch, MD, MS
Rashmi U. Kothari, MD
Steven D. Kronick, MD, MS
Charles W. Otto, MD, PhD
Norman A. Paradis, MD
Mary Ann Peberdy, MD
Edward Racht, MD

BLS Subcommittee (July 2004–June 2005)

Michael R. Sayre, MD, *Chair*
Graham Nichol, MD, MPH
Tom P. Aufderheide, MD
Lance B. Becker, MD
Diana Cave, RN, MSN
Andrea Gabrielli, MD
Keith Lurie, MD
Vincent N. Mosesso, MD
Tom Rea, MD
Wanchun Tang, MD
Roger D. White, MD

Subcommittee on Pediatric Resuscitation (July 2004–June 2005)

Stephen M. Schexnayder, MD, *Chair*
Arno Zaritsky, MD, *Chair (July 2005–Present)*
Robert W. Hickey, MD
Robert A. Berg, MD
Douglas S. Diekema, MD, MPH
Diana G. Fendya, RN, MSN (R)
George W. Hatch, Jr, EdD, LP, EMT-P
Jan Pankey, MD
Monica Kleinman, MD
Lester T. Proctor, MD
Ricardo A. Samson, MD
Marc D. Berg, MD, FAAP

Education Subcommittee (July 2004–June 2005)

Walt A. Stoy, PhD, EMT-P, CCEMTP, *Chair*
David Rodgers, EdS, NREMT-P
Shari Coleman, RN, MSN, CNS
Twink (Alice) Dalton, RN, MS
Cheryl Hamel, PhD
Richard Harper, MD, MS
Monna Johnson, PhD
Richard Judd, PhD, EMSI
Charles Mount, MEd, Capt, NC, USN (Ret)
Christopher Nollette, EdD, NREMT-P
Judy Ruple, PhD, RN, NREMT-P
Earl Shive, EdD
Mark Terry, EMT-P

Program Administration Subcommittee (July 2004–June 2005)

William E. McConnell, DO, MS, *Chair*
Mark Mattes, RRT, JD
Craig Day
Lynn Hunter-Wilson
RonDee Lockwood, RNC, CDE
John Mouw
Tinsla Trotter, RN
Elise W. van der Jagt, MD, MPH
Rosemary Adam, RN, EMT-P
Susan L. Engelbaugh, RN, MSN
Cathy Gagnon, RN, MSN
Dianne Molsberry, RNC, BSN, MA
Arlo F. Weltge, MD, MPH
Judy A. Young, RN, MSN, Lt Col, USAF, NC (Ret)

Stroke Task Force (July 2004–June 2005)

Michael R. Sayre, MD, *Cochair*
Todd J. Crocco, MD, *Cochair*
E. Brooke Lerner, PhD
Michael D. Hill, MD
Edward C. Jauch, MD
Andy Jagoda, MD
Terry L. Vanden Hoek, MD
Jeffrey L. Saver, MD
Brian A. Stettler, MD
Peter Viccellio, MD
William Barsan, MD
Sidney Starkman, MD

AHA-ARC First Aid Guidelines Writing Group (July 2004–June 2005)

William Hammill, MD, *Cochair*
David Markenson, MD, *Cochair*
Naomi Gauthier, MD
Adam J. Singer, MD
Christopher P. Holstege, MD
Donald J. Gordon, PhD, MD
Jonathan L. Epstein, MEMS, NREMT-P
Susan F. Wooley-Goekler, PhD

Neonatal Task Force (July 2004–June 2005)

John Kattwinkel, MD, *Chair*
Jeffrey M. Perlman, MB, ChB
David Boyle, MD
William A. Engle, MD
Marilyn B. Escobedo, MD
Jay P. Goldsmith, MD
Louis P. Halamek, MD
Jane E. McGowan, MD
Gary Weiner, MD
Thomas Wiswell, MD
Jeanette Zaichkin, RNC, MN
Nalini Singhal, MD
Wendy Marie Simon, MA, CAE

Acute Coronary Syndromes Task Force Writing Group

Laurie J. Morrison, MD, MSc, *Cochair*
P. Richard Verbeek, *Cochair*
Steven C. Brooks, MD
Warren Cantor, MD
Michelle Welsford, MD

Authors of Final Evidence Evaluation Worksheets, 2005 International Consensus on Cardiopulomonary Resuscitation and Emergency Cardiovascular Care With Treatment Recommendations Conference

Benjamin S. Abella, MD, MPhil
Riyad B. Abu-Laban, MD, MHSc
Imo P. Aisiku
Sherri-Lynne Almeida, DrPH
Hans-Richard Arntz, MD, PhD
Dianne L. Atkins, MD

Charles F. Babbs, MD, PhD
Gad Bar-Joseph
Thomas A. Barnes, EdD, RRT
Jason Bartsch
Michael Baubin, MSc
David G. Beiser, MD, MS
Robert A. Berg, MD
Ross Berringer
Adnan T. Bhutta
Dominique Biarent
Robert Bingham, MD
Richard Bissell, PhD
Bjug Borgundvaag, MD, PhD
Leo L. Bossaert, MD, PhD
Michael Bosse, MD
Bernd W. Böttiger, MD
David Boyle, MD
William Brady, MD
Richard Branson
Franklin H.G. Bridgewater, MD
Steven Brooks, MD
Fabrice Brunet, MD
Cartland Burns, MD
Steve Byrne
Rebecca Cain
Rick Caissie
Warren J. Cantor, MD
Pierre Carli, MD
Wally Carlo, MD
Renato Carrera, MD
Dan Cass
Antonio Celenza
Leon Chameides, MD
Ivy Cheng
Seshendra Chirumamilla
Gregory Christiansen, DO
Bill Clendenen, MBA
Sharon Coleman, RN, MSN, CNS
David C. Cone, MD
Arthur Cooper, MD, MS
Ashraf Coovadia, MD
Peter Cram, MD, MBA
Michelle Cretikos, MBBS, MPH
Todd J. Crocco, MD
Edward Crosby, MD
Ricky Davidson, MD
Mary Fry Davis, RN
Allan de Caen, MD
Edison Ferreira de Paiva, MD
Rien de Vos, MD
Charles D. Deakin, MD, MA
Jennifer Dennett
Andrew DePiero, MD
Douglas S. Diekema, MD, MPH
Burkhard Dirks, MD, PhD
Hans Domanovits, MD
Volker Dörges, MD
Trygve Eftestøl, DrIng
Christoph Eich, MD
Nabil El Sanadi, MD, MBA
William A. Engle, MD
Jonathan L. Epstein, MEMS, NREMT-P
Marilyn B. Escobedo, MD
Octavio A. Falcucci, MD
Peter Fenici, MD
Melinda L. Fiedor, MD
Judith Finn, PhD, RN
Matthias Fischer, MD
Richard T. Fiser, MD
Douglas Franzen
Ryan C. Fringer, MD
Andrea Gabrielli, MD
Naomi Gauthier, MD
Raul J. Gazmuri, MD, PhD
Hendrik W. Gervais, MD, PhD
Jay P. Goldsmith, MD
Monica Gope
Donald J. Gordon, PhD, MD
Munish Goyal, MD
Ruth Guinsburg
Kyle Gunnerson, MD
Francis Guyette
Werner Hacke, MD, PhD
Louis P. Halamek, MD
Henry R. Halperin, MD
Cheryl Hamel, PhD
William Hammill, MD
Anthony J. Handley, MD
George W. Hatch, Jr, EdD, LP, EMT-P
Jason S. Haukoos, MD, MS
Rita Ann Herrington
Robert W. Hickey, MD
Albert Hijdra, MD
Chris Hogan, MD
Christopher P. Holstege, MD
Dave Hostler, PhD, NREMT-P
Lei Huang
Ahamed H. Idris, MD
Kenneth V. Iserson, MD, MBA
Ian Jacobs, RN, PhD
Mike Jacobs, EMT-P
Andy Jagoda, MD
Edward C. Jauch, MD, MS
James A. Judge II, CEM, BPA, EMT-P
Richard E. Kerber, MD
Karl B. Kern, MD
Fulvio Kette, MD
Monica E. Kleinman, MD
Rudolph W. Koster, MD, PhD
Steven D. Kronick, MD, MS
Douglas F. Kupas, MD
David Lendrum, MD
E. Brooke Lerner, PhD
Swee Han Lim, MD
Charles M. Little, DO
Gayle Long, MD
Jesús López-Herce, MD
Jane Lukins, MD
Keith G. Lurie, MD
Russell D. MacDonald, MD
N. Clay Mann, PhD, MS
David Markenson, MD
Marcello Ricardo Paulista Markus, PhD
Jane E. McGowan, MD
Raina Merchant
Colin Morley, MD
Peter T. Morley, MD
Marilyn Morris
Vincent N. Mosesso, Jr, MD
Charles Mount, MEd, Capt, USN (Ret)
Rick Murray, EMT-P
Vinay M. Nadkarni, MD
Graham Nichol, MD
Susan Niermeyer, MD
Jerry Nolan, MD
Robert E. O'Connor, MD
Cathal O'Donnell
Deems Okamoto, MD
Andrzej Okreglicki, MD
Joseph P. Ornato, MD
Norman A. Paradis, MD
Michael Parr, MBBS, MRCP
Mary Ann Peberdy, MD
Debra G. Perina, MD
Gavin Perkins, MD
Jeffrey M. Perlman, MB, ChB
Lester T. Proctor, MD
Linda Quan, MD
Ana Paula Quilici
Bill Raynovich, EMSA
Tom Rea, MD
Amelia Gorete Reis, PhD
Sam Richmond, MD
Colin Robertson, MD
David Rodgers, EdS, NREMT-P
Antonio Rodriguez-Nuñez
Lynn Roppolo, MD
Ron Roth, MD
Miguel Ruano-Marco, MD
Sten Rubertsson, MD, PhD
Sebastian Russo, MD
Ricardo Samson, MD
Arthur B. Sanders, MD
Edward Sargeant
Jeffrey L. Saver, MD
Michael R. Sayre, MD
Anthony J. Scalzo, MD
Stephen M. Schexnayder, MD
Terri Schmidt, MD, MS
Ralph M. Shenefelt
Jonathan Sherbino, MD
Naoki Shimizu, MD, PhD
Paul M. Shore, MD
Michael Shuster, MD
Adam J. Singer, MD
Nalini Singhal, MD
Jasmeet Soar, MD
Michael Speer, MD
Carol Spizzirri
Vijay Srinivasan, MD
Edward R. Stapleton, EMT-P
Petter Andreas Steen, MD, PhD
Brian Steinhart
Ben J. Stenson, MD
Brian A. Stettler, MD
Ian G. Stiell, MD
Kjetil Sunde, MD, PhD
David Szpilman, MD
Edgardo Szyld, MD
Keiichi Tanaka, MD
Wanchun Tang, MD
Nicole Tenn-Lyn, MD
Andreas R. Thierbach, MD
Stephen H. Thomas, MD, MPH
James Tibballs, MD
Enrique Udaeta, MD
Elise W. van der Jagt, MD, MPH
Terry L. Vanden Hoek, MD
Sithembiso Velaphi, MB
Dharmapuri Vidyasagar
Wolfgang G. Voelckel, MD
Simone Wagner, MD
Tony Walker
Henry E. Wang, MD, MPH
Jeff Wassertheil, MD
Mike Watkinson, MD
Max Harry Weil, MD, PhD
Gary Weiner, MD
Michelle Welsford, MD
Arlo F. Weltge, MD, MPH
Volker Wenzel, MD
Lynn J. White, MS
Jane G. Wigginton, MD
Lars Widklund, MD
Benno Wolcke, MD
Susan F. Wooley, PhD
Myra H. Wyckoff, MD
Jonathan Wyllie, MD
Judy Young, RN, MSN, Lt Col, USAF (Ret)
Ting Yu, MD
Arno Zaritsky, MD
Uwe Zeymer, Priv. Doz. Dr. med.
David A. Zideman, MD
Thomas W. Zoch, MD

Conflict of Interest for Editors, Editorial Board, and Special Contributors and Reviewers

Writing Group	Member	Employment	Research Grant
Editors			
1	Hazinski, Mary Fran	Vanderbilt Children's Hospital	Served as uncompensated principal investigator for Medtronic Physio-Control, sponsored study of AEDs in children (1996–1999, published in 2003)
2	Chameides, Leon	Retired; Paid Editor/Writer 2005 AHA ECC Guidelines	None
3	Elling, Bob	Albany Medical Center	None
4	Hemphill, Robin	Vanderbilt University	None
Editorial Board			
1	Hickey, Robert W.	University of Pittsburgh	None
2	Billi, John E.	University of Michigan Medical School	None
3	Nadkarni, Vinay M.	University of Pennsylvania School of Medicine; Children's Anesthesiology Assoc, Division Critical Care	Research Grants: NIH/NICHD; Ross/Abbott; Sensormedics; Drager Medical
4	Montgomery, William H.	Straub Clinic and Hospital	None
5	O'Connor, Robert E.	Christiana Care Health Systems	None
6	Sayre, Michael R.	The Ohio State University	Research Grant: Zoll/Revivant
7	Vanden Hoek, Terry L.	University of Chicago	NIH, Grant support; DOD, Grant support; Alsius, Unrestricted grant, University of Chicago
8	Schexnayder, Stephen M.	University of Arkansas for Medical Sciences	Wyeth Laboratories, Madison, WI, recipient of grant support for salary (2%) for study of pantoprazole
9	Zaritsky, Arno	University of Florida College of Medicine	None
10	Jauch, Edward C.	University of Cincinnati College of Medicine	None
11	Morrison, Laurie	University of Toronto, Sunnybrook & Women's University, Academic Health Science Center	Grantee, Zoll Medical, Boston, MA; Grantee, Advantis; Grantee, Hoffman La Roche, Toronto, CA
12	Verbeek, Rick	The Ottawa Hospital, University of Toronto, and the Ottawa Health Research Institute	None
13	Perlman, Jeffrey M.	Weill-Cornell Medical Center, New York	None
14	Kattwinkel, John	University of Virginia	None
15	Hammill, William	University of Virginia	
			None
16	Markenson, David	Columbia University	None
17	Nichol, Graham	University of Washington	None
18	Field, John M.	Penn State University College of Medicine	None
19	Mattes, Mark	Clarian Health Partners, Inc	None
20	Shuster, Michael	Self-employed	None
21	Kloeck, Walter G. J.	Academy of Advanced Life Support	None
22	Stoy, Walt A.	Center for Emergency Medicine	None
23	Potts, Jerry	AHA Staff	None
24	Eigel, Brian	AHA Staff	None
Other			
1	Stoddard, F. G.	AHA Staff	None

Other Research Support	Speakers Bureau/Honoraria	Ownership Interest	Consultant/Advisory Board	Other
None	None	None	Senior Science Editor, American Heart Association; consultation fees for AHA ECC programs	None
None	None	None	None	None
None	None	High Quality Endeavors Ltd, co-owner	High Quality Endeavors Ltd, Senior Associate; AHA, paid consultant	None
None	None	None	AHA, paid ECC editor/writer	None
None	None	None	None	None
None	None	None	Editorial Board: *Resuscitation*	None
None	None	None	Unpaid education consultant: Laerdal, Medical Education Technologies, Inc	None
None	None	None	None	None
Research funding from AED manufacturers, Astra-Zeneca, McNeil, Pfizer; no salary support	None	None	President, National Association EMS Physicians; Chair, ACEP EMS Committee; Board, National Registry of EMTs	None
Travel reimbursement: Medtronic	None	None	Ohio Board of EMS, NHTSA Dept of Transportation	None
None	None	None	None	None
None	None	None	None	None
None	None	None	None	None
None	None	None	Consultant and grant recipient, Biosite, Inc, Consultant, Johnson & Johnson, Novo Nordisk, AstraZeneca, and Boeringer Ingelheim	None
None	None	None	None	None
None	None	None	None	None
None	None	None	None	None
None	None	None	None	None
Partner, IEC Inc, contract with Cardioconcepts to develop web-based BLS products for healthcare providers; Cardioconcepts has partnered with the AHA to develop this product line	None	None	None	None
None	None	None	None	None
Sponsor, Investigational Device Exemption; Wearable Cardioverter Defibrillator trial; RAFT Trial investigator (CIHR, Medtronic Inc); Sponsor, Wenabk Defibrillator IDF	None	None	None	None
None	None	None	None	None
None	None	None	Assistant Chief, Sugar Creek TWA Fire Department, New Palestine, IN	None
None	None	None	Chair, ECC Policy Advisory Committee, Heart & Stroke Foundation of Canada	None
None	None	None	Chairman, Resuscitation Council of Southern Africa	Distributor of AHA ECC Training Materials
None	None	President, Dr Walt Stoy and Associates; author, various publishers	None	None
None	None	None	None	None
None	None	700 shares Millennium Pharmaceuticals	None	None
None	None	None	None	None

Index